Research Methodologies in Human Diabetes
Part 1

Research Methodologies in Human Diabetes
Part 1

Editors: C. E. Mogensen, E. Standl

Walter de Gruyter
Berlin · New York 1994

Deutsche Bibliothek — Cataloging-in-Publication-Data

Research methodologies in human diabetes. — Berlin ; New York : de Gruyter.
Pt. 1. Ed.: C. E. Mogensen ; E. Standl. — 1994
ISBN 3-11-014248-1
NE: Mogensen, Carl E. [Hrsg.]

Medical science is constantly developing. Research and clinical experience expand our knowledge, especially with regard to treatment and medication.

For dosages and applications mentioned in this work, the reader may rely on the authors, editors and publisher having taken great pains to ensure that these indications reflect the standard of knowledge at the time this work was completed.

Nevertheless, all users are requested to check the package leaflet of the medication, in order to determine for themselves whether the recommentations given for the dosages or the likely contraindications differ from those given in this book. This is especially true for medication which is seldom used or has recently been put on the market and for medication whose application has been restricted by the German Ministry of Health.

Typesetting: Arthur Collignon GmbH, Berlin. — Printing: Gerike GmbH, Berlin. — Binding: Lüderitz & Bauer GmbH, Berlin. — Printed in Germany.

Editors

Prof. Dr. C. E. Mogensen
Medical Department M
Second University Clinic
of Internal Medicine
(Diabetes and Endocrinology)
Kommunehospitalet
DK-8000 Aarhus C
Denmark

Prof. Dr. E. Standl
Third Medical Department
City Hospital Schwabing
and Diabetes Research Unit
Kölner Platz 1
D-80804 München
Germany

List of first-mentioned contributors

H. Beck-Nielsen, M. D.
Diabetes Research Center
Department of Internal Medicine
and Endocrinology M
Odense University Hospital
DK-5000 Odense
Denmark

M. Bliss, M. D.
Department of History
University of Toronto
100 St. George Street
Toronto
Canada M5S 1A1

R. Bucala, Ph. D.
The Picower Institute
for Medical Research
350 Community Drive
Manhasset, New York 11030
USA

W. Creutzfeldt, M. D.
Gastroenterologie
und Endokrinologie
Medizinische Klinik und Poliklinik
Georg-August-Universität
Göttingen
Robert-Koch-Straße 40
D-37075 Göttingen
Germany

G. Dahlquist, M. D.
Department of Epidemiology
and Health Care Research
University of Umeå
S-901 85 Umeå
Sverige

Th. Danne, M. D.
Universitätsklinikum
Rudolf Virchow
Standort Charlottenburg/
Kinderklinik
Kaiserin-Auguste-Viktoria-Haus
Heubnerweg 6
D-14059 Berlin
Germany

G. Dowse, M. D.
International Diabetes Institute
260 Kooyong Road
Caulfield South, 3162
Australia

G. Eisenbarth, M. D. Ph. D
Barbara Davis Center
for Childhood Diabetes
University of Colorado
Health Sciences Center
4200 East 9th Avenue, Box B140
Denver, Colorado 80262
USA

A. Haddix, M. D.
Prevention Effectiveness Activity
Epidemiology Program Office
Centers for Disease Control
1600 Clifton Road, Mailstop F53
Atlanta, GA 30333
USA

S. M. Haffner, M. D.
Division of Clinical Epidemiology
Department of Medicine
University of Texas
Health Science Center
at San Antonio
7703 Floyd Curl Drive
San Antonio, Texas 78284-7873
USA

K. Hermansen, M. D.
Medical Department C
Diabetes and Endocrinology
Arhus amtssygehus
DK-8000 Arhus C
Denmark

S. L. Jones, M. D.
Guy's and St Thomas's
Medical and Dental School
Unit for Metabolic Medicine
Diabetes, Endocrinology,
Metabolism
London Bridge
GB-London SE1 9RT
England

R. Klein, M. D.
Department of Ophthalmology
University of Wisconsin-Madison
University Hospital & Clinics
600 Highland Avenue, F4/334
Madison, WI 53792
USA

A. Kofoed-Enevoldsen, M. D.
Steno Diabetes Center
Niels Steensens Vej 2
DK-2820 Gentofte
Denmark

E. M. Kohner, M. D.
Hammersmith Hospital
Du Cane Road
GB-London W12 OHS
England

H. Kolb, M. D.
Diabetes Forschungsinstitut
Auf'm Hennekamp 65
D-40225 Düsseldorf
Germany

R. R. Little, M. D.
University of Missouri
Department of Pathology
M 263 Helath Sciences Center
Columbia, MO 65212
USA

A. Maran, M. D.
Unit for Metabolic Medicine
4th floor Hunts House
Guy's Hospital
GB-London SE1 9RT
England

H. Molgaard, M. D.
Department of Cardiology
Skejby University Hospital
DK-8200 Arhus N
Denmark

I. Mühlhauser, M. D.
Medizinische Klinik
der Heinrich-Heine-Universität
Düsseldorf
Abteilung Stoffwechsel
und Ernährung
Moorenstr. 5
D-40225 Düsseldorf
Germany

H.-H. Parving, M. D.
Steno Diabetes Center
Niels Steensens Vej 2
DK-2820 Gentofte
Denmark

O. Pedersen, M. D.
Steno Diabetes Center
Niels Steensens Vej 2
DK-2820 Gentofte
Denmark

A. Rudenski, M. D.
Cambridge Health Authority
Department of
Clinical Biochemistry
Addenbrooke's Hospital
Hills Road
GB-Cambridge CB2 2QR
England

P. A. Rutherford, M. D.
Nephrology Research Laboratories
Podium Level 4
Freeman Hospital
High Heaton
GB-Newcastle-upon-Tyne
NE7 7DN
England

M.-R. Taskinen, M. D.
Third Department of Medicine
University of Helsinki
SF-00290 Helsinki
Finland

H. Tillil, M. D.
Department of Medicine
Ferdinand-Sauerbruch-Klinikum
Wuppertal
Arrenberger Str. 20
D-42117 Wuppertal
Germany

B. Willms, M. D.
Fachklinik für Diabetes
und Stoffwechsel
Kirchberg 21
D-37431 Bad Lauterberg/Harz
Germany

A.-G. Ziegler, M. D.
Third Med. Department
City Hospital Schwabing
and Diabetes Research Unit
Kölner Platz 1
D-80804 München
Germany

Preface

The number of research activities in the field of diabetes mellitus have exploded in recent years. This can come as no surprise in light of the complexity of the disorder – or better, family of disorders – with their multiple, yet distinct aetiopathogenic factors and many clinical manifestations and sequelae. The advent of new research technologies, e. g. derived from molecular biology, gene technology, applied biochemistry, computer methodology or refined ultrasound- and electrophysiology, has fostered a host of new theories and concepts on the development of various types of diabetes mellitus and related complications.

The previous three books of the *Diabetes Forum Series*, starting in 1989, have attempted to compile much of the progress made in modern diabetology. It is fascinating to observe the enormous spectrum of diabetes research and the intensive interaction with a diversity of other research areas such as immunology, epidemiology, endocrinology, cardiology, angiology, nephrology, neurology, opththamology, surgery, gynaecology, etc.; in this sense diabetology is truly an interdisciplinary subject. On the other hand, it has become impossible that a single researcher, or even research group, is able to maintain an overview of or provide all the research methodologies necessary for the investigation of human diabetes.

It is to this end that a book on "Research Methodologies in Human Diabetes" comes into play. It is geared to provide ready access to a wide array of investigative techniques in diabetology. In contrast to laboratory methods, mainly clinically oriented procedures quite often cannot be broken down into step-by-step instructions. Hence, for the various topics on research methodologies contained in this book, rather variable and individual organisations of each chapter have been chosen. We feel, however, that this is a strength of this book and has led to the best possible approach to each topic. In any case, the standard for investigative techniques within a given field of research has become quite apparent and also demarcates the present frontline of further research.

As editors, we feel highly privileged that top researchers in diabetology throughout the world have so willingly shared their particular expertise with the international community of diabetologists. As a result, a unique book has been made possible, representing the true state of the art of human diabetes research. In fact, during the preparation of this book it became obvious that the magnitude of material to be covered is so enormous that only two volumes could accommodate the present state of knowledge. Therefore a second volume will follow in 1994.

Above all, it should be remembered, but goes without saying, that research into human diabetes always deals with human beings and that the highest ethical standards have to be applied at all times. Therefore, the Declaration of Helsinki, which gives the ethical framework for any research in humans, concludes the first volume of "Research Methodologies in Human Diabetes".

We wish the diabetologists and the many friends throughout the world, a successful and meaningful use of these volumes on diabetes research methodologies.

Carl Erik Mogensen Eberhard Standl

Contents

Research methods and the discovery of insulin

M. Bliss

The "discovery" or isolation of insulin at the University of Toronto by a team of researchers in 1921 – 22 was a process that involved primitive research methods and the frequent misreading of results. Good luck was as important in determining the eventual outcome as good judgment. At the same time, however, the discovery was also made possible by the pooling of expertise in a well-funded collaborative project utilizing the most recent technological breakthroughs. Without the availability of newly-developed research tools and the pooling of research techniques as understood by advanced experts, the breakthrough could not have occurred in that place at that time.

The work of prior investigators

In 1889 Minkowski and von Mering in Germany observed the onset of severe diabetes mellitus in dogs following total pancreatectomy, and initiated the hypothesis of a relationship between the pancreas and diabetes [1]. It was necessarily a vague hypothesis because there was at that time little theoretical or practical understanding of endocrine activities.

Minkowski was the first of many researchers to attempt to restore the functions lost in diabetes by administering extracts of pancreas to experimental animals. All such methods failed for three reasons: (1) enzyme destruction of the active principle in oral administration; (2) toxic contaminants in extracts administered by injection; (3) inability to study the impact of injections because of imprecise measuring techniques.

The third point refers to the fact that it was not possible to do frequent serial measurements of blood sugar. Before 1910 Minkowski and other investigators had to rely primarily on measurements of glycosuria, which were extremely imprecise and time-consuming to make. Blood sugar estimates were even more difficult, requiring upwards of 20 cc. of blood and several hours' work. Until testing methods improved, observations of the impact of pancreastherapy on diabetes were fragmentary and subjective, albeit sometimes promising.

Offprint from
Research Methodologies in Human Diabetes – Part 1

These results, coinciding with the discovery and naming of several hormones, and the conceptual elaboration of the notion of the endocrine system, encouraged researchers to continue to search for an effective pancreatic extract. There was a rapid improvement in techniques to measure glycaemia between 1910 and 1920. Various researchers, including Scott [2], Kleiner [3], and Paulesco [4] now reported the ability to produce extracts of pancreas that reduced hyperglycaemia. All were still handicapped, baffled, or otherwise frustrated: Scott could not repeat his results; Kleiner and Paulesco reported fever and other toxic effects subsequent to injection. None was prepared to administer pancreas to a human diabetic. Scott gave up his work in frustration. Kleiner stopped when he took a job at a university which could not supply him with adequate numbers of research animals. Paulesco, working in war-torn Roumania, was handicapped by lack of financial resources, requiring him to use very primitive techniques. His blood sugar testing, for example, used the inadequate nineteenth century methods that had become obsolete in North America.

Banting's idea

The Toronto research originated in an idea that occurred to Frederick Banting, a physician and surgeon practising in the city of London, Ontario, Canada, in the night of October 30/31, 1920, while he was preparing to give a talk to medical students about the pancreas. He wrote it in his notebook as follows:

> Diabetus (sic!)
> Ligate pancreatic ducts of dog. Keep dogs alive till acini degenerate leaving Islets.
> Try to isolate the internal secretion of these to relieve glycosurea [5].

Banting took his interest to the Professor of Physiology at the University of Toronto, J. J. R. Macleod, and discussed with him the prospect of investigating the idea in the summer of 1921.

Banting's proposal was based on an assumption, not uncommon in the literature of the day, that efforts to isolate an internal secretion of the pancreas had failed in part because of the inability to prevent contamination and nullification by enzymes from the pancreas' external secretion. It was thought that ligation of the pancreatic ducts in the living animal would gradually destroy the trypsin-secreting acinar cells while preserving healthy islet cells which might be the seat of the internal secretion.

He did not specify it in his original note, but Banting also gleaned from the literature the thought that the most promising method of testing the activity of ligated, atrophied pancreas would be to graft or transplant portions of the organ into pancreatectomized animals. This surgically-trained young man was interested in what is today recognizable to us as a double surgical technique to achieve islet cell transplant [6].

Macleod agreed to allow Banting to begin work in his laboratory under his direction. Banting had little experience in research, and none at all working with the pancreas. He could not even spell "diabetes". Macleod explained to him the testing techniques that were available (note that Banting had expected to measure "glycosurea" rather than glycaemia). While sanctioning Banting's interesting in transplanting remnants of atrophied pancreas, Macleod also suggested the injection of aqueous extracts of the material. He gave Banting facilities, a supply of dogs, and the services of his two student summer assistants. One of the students, Charles Best, won a coin toss to see who would begin working with Banting in the summer of 1921. The other student later chose to let Best continue, a decision he regretted for the rest of his life.

Banting and Best's research

It cannot be too heavily emphasized that Banting had extremely limited research experience, and Best, a student, had none. Their experiments, which commenced on May 17, 1921 and carried on through the summer and into the autumn, were clumsily executed and subjectively and often erroneously interpreted. They had also been incorrectly conceived: a closer study of the literature would have shown that Banting's assumptions about the selective impact of duct-ligation on pancreatic degeneration, and on the menace of digestive ferments in pancreatic extracts, were wrong [7]. He was proposing to use a technique that would not work to address a problem that did not exist.

After the first month of preliminary experiments, Macleod left Banting and Best to carry on the work by themselves during an extremely hot summer. So many dogs died from infection and sloppy surgical procedures that Banting decided to postpone transplant experiments and move immediately to injections of extract of degenerated pancreas. These commenced on July 30.

Banting and Best's notebooks [8] indicate that the injections were administered intravenously. Their impact was to be measured by serial blood sugar readings made by Best, using the recently-developed Myers and Bailey modification of the Lewis and Benedict technique [9]. However the one-, two-, sometimes four-hour intervals used for the blood sugar readings almost certainly mean that Banting and Best were not accurately tracing the effects of their injections. The blood sugar data they reported was possibly – probably – meaningless.

They did not realize this. Their results, as recorded in their notebooks, were usually interpreted favourably. In their first publication [10] Banting and Best made a sweeping and untrue claim about their research in the period prior to November 14:

> In the course of our experiments we have administered over seventy-five doses of extract from degenerated pancreatic tissue to ten different diabetic animals. Since the extract has always produced a reduction of the percentage of sugar of the blood and of the sugar excreted in the urine, we feel justified in stating that this extract contains the internal secretion of the pancreas.

The notebooks actually contain data which, if meaning anything at all, suggest that the first 75 injections produced 42 favourable results, 22 unfavourable ones, and 11 inconclusive results. One August experiment clearly indicated that chilled whole pancreas was as potent as the ligated-atrophied pancreas. In both their notebooks and their first paper, Banting and Best interpreted this result exactly incorrectly.

Banting had made great material and emotional sacrifices to undertake his research. He was temperamentally inclined to believe passionately in the success of his efforts. He invariably interpreted his results positively, and he used these apparently favourable results to persuade Macleod to allow the work to continue and to suggest directions in which it might develop. Macleod dissuaded him from concentrating on his original interest in grafting. Longevity experiments were begun to see if the extract could maintain a diabetic animal indefinitely. Banting's interest in finding a source of "trypsin-free" pancreatic extract led him to experiments in the use of foetal calf pancreas and then to the realization by December that the whole endeavour to exclude the external secretion could be abandoned. An experiment at that time showed, as it had in August, that chilled fresh pancreas dissolved in alcohol was as effective as any of the extracts of ligated pancreas.

Admirers of the work of Paulesco and other prior researchers have noted correctly that the results of Banting and Best's animal research were not as impressive as those of Paulesco or Kleiner [11]. Banting and Best did not realize this because they were not inclined to spend time in the library learning about anyone else's research. When Best did attempt a quick study of the literature, he completely misread one of Paulesco's publications, which was in French, and reported the Roumanian's work negatively. Banting and Best did not appreciate the need to study the toxicity of their extracts, which was most commonly reflected in the development of high fever. Only once in all of their experiments did they record an animal's temperature. It was running a high fever immediately after injection of their extract.

Such extreme flaws and shortcomings in the research explain why the first public presentation of the work, at the December 1921 New Haven meeting of the American Physiological Society, was not enthusiastically received. It was not evident that Banting and Best had achieved results which justified their claim to have isolated the internal secretion of the pancreas. They had not gone beyond the accomplishment of other investigators, which was to produce extracts of pancreas that now and then reduced glycaemia. Neither the Canadians nor anyone else had as yet been able to prepare an extract of pancreas safe to test rigorously on human diabetics. The most interesting clinical tests of pancreatic extract remained those carried on by Georg Zuelzer in Berlin in 1908, and repeated by Forschbach in Minkowski's laboratory in 1909; they had been abruptly discontinued because of the extreme side effects they produced [12].

Collip's breakthrough

Having become convinced by Banting's enthusiastic presentation of his results that the extracts probably did contain the internal section, Macleod was willing to devote more resources to the isolation problem. Early in December he concurred with Banting's proposal to add a trained biochemist to the team. Banting had developed a friendship with J. B. Collip, a young biochemist from the University of Alberta who was visiting Toronto to work with Macleod on a different problem, but had several times expressed interest in the pancreas work. Banting apparently also realized that his assistant, Best, whose only training was an undergraduate program in physiology and biochemistry, was not sufficiently expert in extraction techniques. Macleod, too, possessed a confidence in Collip that he did not have in Banting or Best.

Collip was a well-trained, highly-skilled, innovative and energetic researcher. He plunged into the work, took daily advice from Macleod, and was soon expanding the findings dramatically. Collip introduced a new and quicker blood sugar test, the Shaffer-Hartmann method, and soon found that potent extract lowered the blood sugar of normal animals. Working with rabbits, he was able to carry out rapid testing of batches of the extract. Collip also produced the first results indicating that the team's extract (like Paulesco's) cleared ketone bodies from the urine of diabetic animals. More significantly, Collip conducted the experiments, suggested by both Banting and Macleod, which showed that potent extract enabled a diabetic liver to store glycogen. Here was increasing evidence that the extract was more than just a hypoglycemic agent [13].

Would it restore the metabolic functions impaired in diabetes in a human being? Banting, and all other investigators, had believed that the only conclusive test to prove the existence of an active principle in pancreatic extracts would be on humans. He and Best realized that their extract was too erratic and powerful in its effects (it sometimes caused anaphylactic shock, killing, for example, the first dog tested for longevity) for human trials. But when Macleod directed Collip to undertake the task of purification preparatory to clinical trials, Banting urged that he and Best ought to be allowed to make the first extract to be tested. There had been considerable friction among members of the team by that time, causing Banting, a narrow-minded, suspicious man, to believe that he was losing control of the work his idea had started.

By mid-December, 1921, the group was using a slightly acidic alcohol extract of chilled ox pancreas (no one agreed later on the origin of the suggestion to use alcohol). As Banting and Best's notebooks indicate, the extract still did not work consistently. On January 11, 1922 extract prepared by Banting and Best was given subcutaneously to a 14-year old diabetic patient, Leonard Thompson, in Toronto General Hospital. The injection caused only slight reductions in Thompson's glycosuria and hypoglycemia, no change in his ketonuria, and no change in his subjective presentation. A sterile abscess formed at the site of the injection. The clinicians concluded that this was a failed trial and discontinued administration of the extract [14]. One or two other patients may also have received Banting and Best's extract. Banting later wrote that "These results were not as encouraging as those obtained by Zuelzer in 1908" [15].

On January 23 tests on Thompson resumed, using extract that had been prepared by Collip. It was spectacularly effective in eliminating the symptoms of the boy's diabetes [14]. A letter that Collip wrote to the president of the University of Alberta on January 25 has recently come to light [16], and is published here for the first time:

> ... Last Thursday Jan. 19th I finally unearthed a method of isolating the internal secretion of the pancreas in a fairly pure and seemingly stable form suitable for human administration. It was tried out on one case in the clinic with such encouraging results that today $5000 has been placed at our disposal ... to rush the work. ...
>
> We some time ago succeeded in producing a potent extract which produced marvellous effects on dogs but which if injected into humans produced abscesses. While we were confident that we had established the potency of pancreatic extracts prepared in a definite manner an apparently insurmountable barrier

> lay before us. It was useless for human administration. The problem seemed almost hopeless so you can imagine my delight when about midnight one day last week I discovered a way to get the active principle free from all the "muck" with which it appeared to be inseparably bound.

Collip's method involved biochemical extraction techniques which by that time were becoming fairly commonplace. His problem had been to remove contaminants from the pancreatic solution while retaining the active principle. The group had discovered that the active principle was soluble in approximately 50 percent alcohol. Working long hours late into the night, with constant testing on his rabbits, Collip found he could precipitate out many of the contaminating proteins by increasing the concentration of alcohol in the solution. The group had gradually developed techniques of washing and filtration to remove fats and salts. Collip discovered that at approximately 95 percent concentration of alcohol, the active principle itself precipitated out of the solution [17].

By today's standards this precipitate was still grossly impure. In fact it was "clean" enough to act so effectively on a human diabetic that the scientific world, when presented with the reports of this and later trials, agreed that the Toronto team had finally succeeded in isolating the internal secretion of the pancreas [18].

Elaboration of the research

Because of the instant and dramatic therapeutic impact of insulin, an immediate effort was made to produce the extract in commercial quantities. This proved more difficult than anticipated for the Toronto group because of the limitations of its apparatus, because Collip's research methods tended to be intuitive and poorly-recorded, and because of intense continuing personal frictions which distracted everyone. The team eventually decided to pool its knowledge with an American ethical drug company, Eli Lilly and Company. Lilly played an important role in producing insulin for early clinical trials. In the late autumn of 1922 the Lilly chemists, simultaneously with a group from Washington University in St. Louis, discovered a technique of adjusting the iso-electric point in pancreatic solutions so as to facilitate the easy precipitation of much purer insulin. At that point the basic production problem was solved [6].

The impact of insulin on human diabetics was so obvious and measurable that it was never tested in anything like a double-blind clinical trial. No government standards existed that had to be met before insulin was sold commercially. Nonetheless, the discovery team, which patented its methods in the name of the University of Toronto, realized that significant testing was necessary to establish standards for human use. In North America, and to a degree in Denmark and the United Kingdom, two other early centres of production, insulin was at first distributed selectively to diabetes specialists for use in their most extreme cases. Only after the basic unit had been standardized and substantial clinical data had been accumulated (hypoglycemic reactions, which the group first observed in some of their rabbits, were of course a principal concern), was insulin released for general distribution. In other words, the discoverers realized that clinical research was a necessary complement to the laboratory/animal breakthrough. There was also, of course, an ongoing program at the University of Toronto, and many other centres, to explore the physiological and chemical activity of the magic hormone. Macleod directed much of this research. Banting, Best, and Collip left the field to search for other magic treatments.

Conclusions

Within a year or two of Toronto's research triumph, insulin was being produced by medical students as a laboratory exercise. In a moment of humility Collip once suggested that his role in the discovery of insulin was "only that which any well-trained biochemist could be expected to contribute" [19]. The truth in that remark lies in the fact that insulin had always been there in the pancreas waiting for someone to come along with the tools and techniques to get it out.

Like all of their predecessors, Banting and Best did not have the research skills to do the job. Their work was based on erroneous premises, was badly executed, and incorrectly interpreted. This was not widely realized at the time because of the tremendous excitement the discovery provoked, because of the urgent need to get on with the therapeutic application of insulin, and because both Banting and Best worked assiduously during their lifetimes to promulgate myths about their priority in the discovery [20]. As early as 1922, however, Banting and Best's fumbling papers were brilliantly dissected by an informed critic, Frangcon Roberts, who concluded that "the production of insulin originated in a wrongly conceived, wrongly conducted, and wrongly interpreted series of experiments" [21].

The limitations of Banting and Best's research methods were overcome when Banting's fierce enthusiasm convinced Macleod that there must be something in the extracts. Macleod commanded significant resources at the University of Toronto in the form of research animals, research money, and first-rate equipment. With his considerable knowledge of carbohydrate metabolism he was able to help redirect Banting and Best toward the problem of purifying the extract. He was also able to add a first-rate biochemist, familiar with the most advanced techniques of fractionation, to the team. Collip was on hand to be added to the team because he had been attracted by the reputation of Macleod and his laboratory at the University of Toronto. Banting became friends with Collip late in his life and would admit to friends that he and Best wouldn't have achieved a damned thing without Collip.

Until the work of the Toronto team, the problem of the pancreas had been tackled by isolated researchers, of limited expertise, often working alone and with inadequate resources. Even the Toronto research, by our standards was primitive, a product of the "horse-and-buggy" age. Given the right equipment and techniques – especially the methods for the micro-estimation of blood sugar – a few animals, and a trained biochemist, insulin was an "easy" discovery. It would soon have been made at some other centre, probably in the United States by researchers building on Paulesco's publications.

Fortunately for Canadian science, it happened that citizens' belief in the potential benefits of medical research had led to the equipment and staffing of the University of Toronto as a fully modern, well-funded research centre. A way had been prepared which made it possible for the strange sparks lit virtually accidentally by two determined amateurs to be developed by professional scientists into a beacon that still illuminates both the lives of people with diabetes and the history of medical research.

Note on sources

This account is based on the much more detailed history recounted in my book, *The Discovery of Insulin* (Chicago, University of Chicago Press, 1983). That narrative was constructed from a wealth of primary sources, including original research notebooks and correspondence, which have been preserved at the University of Toronto and other repositories. The references here are selective: for more detailed documentation of non-footnoted facts and interpretations consult *The Discovery of Insulin.*

References

[1] von Mering J, Minkowski O. Diabetes mellitus nach Pankreasextirpation. Archiv für Experimentelle Pathologie und Pharmakologie 1890; 26: 371–387.

[2] Scott EL. On the influence of intravenous injections of an extract of the pancreas on experimental pancreatic diabetes. Am J Phys 1912; 29: 306–310.

[3] Kleiner IS. The action of intravenous injections of pancreas emulsions in experimental diabetes. J Biol Chem 1919; 40: 153–170.

[4] Paulesco NC. Recherche sur le rôle du pancréas dans l'assimilation nutritive. Arch int de physiologie 1921; 17: 85–103.
[5] Banting FG. Notebook. Fisher Rare Book Library. University of Toronto.
[6] Bliss M. The discovery of insulin. University of Chicago Press. Chicago. 1983.
[7] Pratt JH. A reappraisal of researches leading to the discovery of insulin. J Hist Med 1954; 9: 281–289.
[8] Banting FG, Best CH. Notebooks. At the Fisher Rare Book Library. Univ. of Toronto.
[9] Myers VC, Bailey CB. The Lewis and Benedict Method for the estimation of blood sugar, With some observations obtained in disease. J Biol Chem 1916; 24: 147–161.
[10] Banting FB, Best CH. The internal secretion of the pancreas. J Lab Clin Med 1922: 7: 251–266.
[11] Murray I. Paulesco and the isolation of insulin. J Hist Med 1971; 26: 150–157; Pavel I. The priority of NC Paulesco in the discovery of insulin. Bucharest, 1976.
[12] Mellinghoff KH. Georg Ludwig Zuelzers Beitrag zur Insulinforschung. Düsseldorf 1971.
[13] Collip JB. History of the discovery of insulin. Northwest Med 1923; 22: 267–273.
[14] Banting FG, Best CH, Collip JB et al. Pancreatic extracts in the treatment of diabetes mellitus. Preliminary report. Can Med Ass J 1922: 141–146.
[15] Banting FG. The history of insulin. Edinburgh Med J 1929; Jan: 1–18.
[16] Collip JB. Letter to HM Tory, Jan. 25, 1922. Tory Papers, University of Alberta Archives. Drawn to my attention by Alison Li.
[17] Collip JB. The original method as used for the isolation of insulin in semipure form for the treatment of the first clinical case. J Biol Chem 1923; 55: xl–xli.
[18] Banting FG, Best CH, Collip JB et al. The effect produced on diabetes by extracts of pancreas. Trans Ass Am Physicians 1923; 1–11.
[19] Collip, JB. Frederick Grant Banting, discoverer of insulin. Scientific Monthly 1941; 52: 473–474.
[20] Bliss M, Banting FG. A Biography. Toronto: McClelland & Stewart, 1984; Bliss M. Rewriting Medical History: Charles Best and the Banting and Best Myth, [to read:] Hist Med 1993: 48: 253–274.
[21] Roberts F. Insulin. Letter. Brit Med J 1922; Dec 16: 1193–1194.

The discovery of the oral treatment of diabetes mellitus with sulphonylureas

W. Creutzfeldt

Introduction

When telling the story of the discovery of the sulphonylureas, one has to distinguish between the experimental research on the hypoglycaemic effect of sulphonamides which dates back to the year 1942, and the rather bold use of one of these substances in 1954 for the treatment of human diabetes mellitus by two clinicians who were not aware of any of the earlier experimental data [1]. After the publication of the clinically successful treatment of diabetes with sulphonylureas [1, 2], several authors claimed to have first tried using sulphonamides in diabetics [3–7]. However, these authors did not pursue the question of the potential usefulness of these substances for the therapy of diabetes mellitus and, therefore, cannot really be regarded as the initiators of the oral treatment of diabetes with sulphonamide-derivatives. One reason for the reluctance to make use of the hypoglycaemic side effect of the sulphonamides for therapy may have been the memory of the poor success of the guanidine derivatives (Synthalin A and B) as oral anti-diabetic drugs in the late twenties [8]. These substances had not been accepted by patients and physicians because of their anorectic effect and liver toxicity while insulin had proven to be not only life-saving, but also without side effects, except for hypoglycaemia. The only disadvantage of insulin was the inconvenience of daily subcutaneous injections.

Hypoglycaemia complicating sulphonamide treatment of patients with infectious diseases

On July 3, 1942, M. Janbon and co-workers [9] reported on serious side effects in patients with different infectious diseases (mainly typhoid fever) treated with a new sulphonamide, 2-[p-amino benzoylsulfamido]-5-isopropyl-thiodiazole ("IPTD"), synthesised by Vonkennel and Kimmig ("VK 57") [11] and produced by Rhone-Poulenc ("2254 RP").

Offprint from
Research Methodologies in Human Diabetes – Part 1

The clinical report by Janbon et al. [9] is worth reading. The authors describe in detail four patients, 15 to 46 years old (3 with typhoid fever, one with pneumonia) all of whom had classical neurological and psychiatric symptoms of hypoglycaemia after treatment for several days with high doses (8 – 12 g per day) of IPTD. They documented low blood glucose levels during the neuroglucopenic episodes and an immediate response to parenteral injection or infusion of glucose containing fluids. These case records are dated between March and April, 1942. After having proven reversible severe hypoglycaemic reactions as a side effect of the bacteriostatic treatment with IPTD, the authors suggested that the unexplained deaths in deep coma of two other young female patients with typhoid fever, which occurred during IPTD therapy in the autumn of 1941 were caused by undiagnosed hypoglycaemia. Altogether, they observed in 16 patients with typhoid fever, 8 cases, and in 12 patients with other infectious diseases, 1 case of severe hypoglycaemia. The high incidence in patients with typhoid fever was explained with the high doses used in these severely ill patients and their malnutrition. The authors stated that they had found a new serious side effect of chemotherapy with sulphonamides and proposed that the hypoglycaemic property of these otherwise non-toxic oral drugs should be pursued further. They conducted short-term studies with IPTD, tried to correlate the sulphonamide and glucose plasma levels and concluded that the hypoglycaemic effect was reproducible and specific for this sulphonamide [10]. Janbon also initiated Loubatières' extensive experimental work on the mechanism of the hypoglycaemia (see below) and conducted the first systematic studies on chemical structure and hypoglycaemic activity [12, 13], but did not report about a trial to treat patients with diabetes mellitus.

However, in 1971, in a long article about "The History of the Discovery of the Oral Anti-diabetic Drugs", Loubatières [14] mentioned that Janbon, in cooperation with Loubatières, had tried the IPTD-derivative, 2301 RP (P-Aminobenzen-sulfonamido-propylthiodiazole) in three patients with diabetes mellitus even before 1946 [14, p. 1193]: In a 30-year old female patient with pyoderma and hyperglycaemia, the elevated blood glucose level of 270 mg/dl fell within 4 days to 70 mg/dl. This patient had already been described in a short communication from Janbon et al. in 1943 as a hypoglycaemic complication [13]. Two female patients, aged 14 and 18 with acetonuria who had not yet been treated with insulin did not respond to 2301 RP. No further clinical trials with blood glucose lowering sulphonamides in diabetics were undertaken in Montpellier until 1955 despite a suggestion formulated by the physiologist A. Loubatières in his PhD thesis presented to the science faculty of the University of Montpellier and published in 1946 [14]. On page 77 of his thesis, he speculated about a form of diabetes due to a "paresis of the insulin secretory mechanisms" in which the use of hypoglycaemic sulphonamides would be indicated.

In December 1955, Loubatières reported the successful treatment of certain patients of diabetes mellitus with IPTD [3 – 5], finally confirming the extensive studies on the treatment of non-insulin-dependent diabetes with carbutamide which started in 1954 and were published in October 1955 [1, 2]. Despite 3 to 4 times higher doses of IPTD (2254 RP), this compound was less effective than carbutamide and only given for up to 4 weeks. Until 1955, the blood glucose lowering property of bacteriostatic sulphonamides had been regarded by the pharmaceutical industry as a serious side effect, limiting the use of these compounds as bacteriostatic agents and not as a quality for potential use as an anti-diabetic drug. This can clearly be seen from Kleinsorge's publications [6, 7].

In 1956, this author announced that since 1951 he had studied the hypoglycaemic side effect of two sulphonamides synthesised by the chemist E. Haak (who later left Dresden and worked for C.F. Boehringer, Mannheim) on behalf of Heyden, a pharmaceutical company in Dresden. The compounds were N1-sulfanilyl-N2-isopropylcarbamide (Loranil) and N1-sulfanilyl-N2-n-butylcarbamide (originally called Ca 1022 and, later, BZ 55 or carbutamide by Boehringer). Kleinsorge claims that hypoglycaemic complications following Loranil were well known to the company.

As a result, Kleinsorge was asked to investigate the same question with the bacteriostic carbutamide. He studied 94 patients and volunteers and observed 12 hypoglycaemic reactions. Thereafter, he advised that this compound should not be marketed. Kleinsorge also observed a blood glucose lowering effect in patients with diabetes. However, he refused treatment of diabetes mellitus with carbutamide because he was afraid of toxic effects during long-term treatment and the induction of bacterial resistance to sulphonamide [6].

Whether Kleinsorge's results and recommendations were known to E. Haak and the C.F. Boehringer Company in Mannheim is not documented and not known.

In the first publication on the oral treatment of diabetes with carbutamide, Franke and Fuchs claimed to have discovered hypoglycaemia as side effect of this compound when one of the authors (J. Fuchs) experienced symptoms of neuroglucopenia and a low blood glucose level while taking the drug for study purpose [1]. Thereafter, the authors decided to systematically treat patients with diabetes mellitus with carbutamide and reported on 50 patients in their first publication, of whom 80% responded and were treated up to

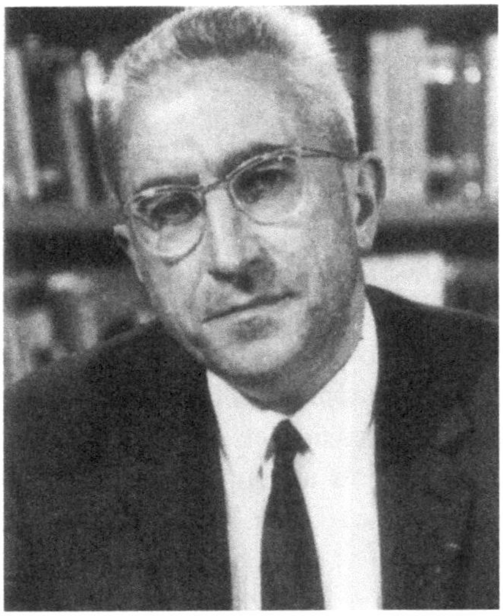

Fig. 1 Auguste Loubatières, Montpellier (1912–1977), the first investigator who systematically studied the mechanism of the hypoglycaemic side effect of a sulphonamide (1942–1946)

one year. M. Franke died before this publication. Therefore, in March 1955, the Boehringer Company asked F. Bertram, a leading German diabetologist, to continue with the study. The observations on 82 patients were published simultaneously [2] in the same issue of the "Deutsche Medizinische Wochenschrift" as Franke and Fuchs' work.

Studies on the mechanism of action of the blood glucose lowering sulphonamides

While it may be difficult to identify the person(s) who should be credited for the discovery of the oral treatment of diabetes with sulphonamide derivatives, there is no doubt that A. Loubatières (Fig. 1) in Montpellier was the first to experimentally study the mechanism by which IPTD caused the deleterious hypoglycaemic reactions in patients as observed by Janbon and co-workers in 1942 [9]. When Janbon informed him about his observations, Loubatières immediately started a series of experiments with dogs and rabbits. He described a reproducible decrease of the blood glucose level to 40 mg/dl after 0.2–0.4 g/kg IPTD orally or subcutaneously in dogs and reported severe irreversible hypoglycaemic reactions after treatment with 0.4 g/kg IPTD for several days which closely resembled the symptoms of glucopenia occurring after insulin overdose [16]. In the following years, research was hampered by the war and the German occupation of France. However, Loubatières pursued his research on IPTD and related compounds. Parts of the results were communicated in short papers [17–19] and, in 1946 published in extenso in his PhD thesis [15]. He found that IPTD intake of several days increased the glycogen content of the liver. IPTD was ineffective in pancreatectomised dogs and in those with diabetes due to injection of pituitary extracts. However, a definite effect on the blood sugar was proved in the 5/6 to 9/10th partially pancreatectomised animals. In alloxan diabetes of the rabbit of medium severity, IPTD suppressed glucosuria for the duration of medication. After withholding the drug, glucosuria recurred. In cross-circulation experiments (connecting the pancreatic vein of a donor dog with the jugular vein of a recipient dog), IPTD caused significant blood-sugar lowering in the recipient dog. Loubatières deduced from his experiments that IPTD stimulated insulin secretion from the islet B-cells.

Similar conclusions were reached by La Barre and Reuse after observing that IPTD depressed the blood-sugar level in cases of mild alloxan diabetes [20]. Research on the relationship of the chemical structure to the blood-sugar-lowering characteristic showed that the p-amino groups of the benzol ring are indispensable for the blood-sugar effect, while the aliphatic lateral chain of thiodiazole can be varied to a certain degree without loss of the hypoglycaemic effect [12, 18].

Retrospectively, it is of interest to note that the original (and correct) interpretation of hypoglycaemia by stimulation of insulin secretion through sulphonamides was abandoned even by Loubatières [3] during the years 1954 and 1955, i. e. at the time of the introduction of the sulphonylureas for the treatment of diabetes by German authors [1, 2]. This error was due to the supposition of damage and even complete destruction of the glucagon-producing α-cells of the pancreatic islets by IPTD in rabbits and rats [21–24], favouring the much debated "glucagon theory" of diabetes mellitus. However, significant α-cell damage could not be confirmed by other authors after treatment with either IPTD [25–27] or sulphonylureas [28–31]. Instead, increasing evidence supported Loubatières' original hypothesis [15], that hypoglycaemia following administration of certain sulphonamide derivatives is due to a direct interaction with endogenous insulin secretion. Thus, significant degranulation of the islet B-cells was a regular finding after acute or chronic application of tolbutamide, carbutamide or IPTD in different species [28, 29, 32–36]. Furthermore, after application of sulphonylureas, an enlargement of B-cell nuclei was documented by morphometry [33–36] and decreased pancreatic insulin concentration measured with bioassays in calves [34], dogs [37] and rats [38]. These indirect proofs of an interaction between the blood glucose-lowering sulphonamides and the B-cells were supported by the finding

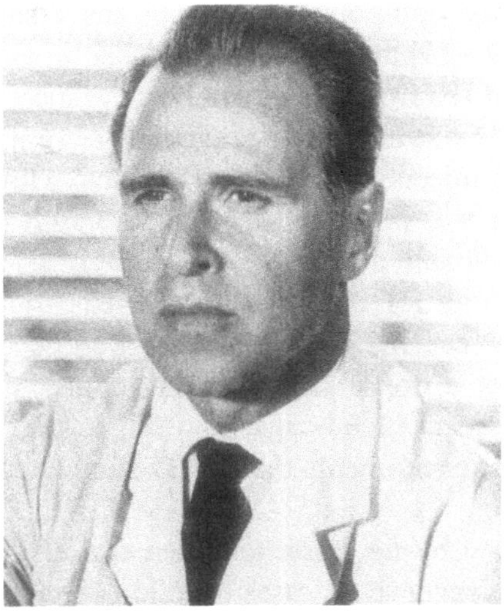

Fig. 2 Karl Joachim Fuchs, Berlin, the clinician who initiated in 1954 oral treatment of diabetes mellitus with the sulphonylurea carbutamide

of increased insulin levels in portal blood estimated with non-specific bioassay [39]. After the introduction of the radioimmunoassay for insulin by Berson and Yalow, stimulation of insulin secretion by hypoglycaemic sulphonamide derivatives was finally established by numerous authors.

Much later, the cell biology of this interaction was also explored. Specific receptors for sulphonylureas were demonstrated in B-cells [40, 41] and characterised as ATP-sensitive potassium channels which are inhibited by sulphonylureas [42].

Establishing oral treatment of diabetes with sulphonylureas

Despite the knowledge on the blood glucose-lowering property of sulphonamides since 1941, i. e. when Savagnone published an unheeded systematic study with three well known sulphonamides [43] and Janbon communicated severe hypoglycaemic reactions in patients with typhoid fever [9] which stimulated Loubatières to conduct his experimental studies, no serious attempts were made to use these compounds for the treatment of human diabetes mellitus. Kleinsorge [6] explained this by a reluctance to risk late toxicity during chronic use of a sulphonamide.

Fuchs (Fig. 2) had no scruples in this respect. When he noticed hypoglycaemic symptoms in himself and measured low blood glucose levels after taking carbutamide (BZ 55), he asked his boss, Franke, for approval for a systematic trial in diabetic patients with this compound.

Franke and Fuchs did not treat patients with diabetes mellitus with carbutamide because they knew about Janbon's observations [9, 10] or Loubatières' experimental work [15]. They did not ask the sophisticated question about the mechanism of action, but rather whether one could use the blood glucose-lowering property as remedy for diabetes, and they succeeded in 80% of the 50 patients treated [1]. This direct approach to the practical therapeutic question makes them the true discoverers of the oral treatment of diabetes with sulphonylureas. The Boehringer Company asked Bertram and co-workers to extend the observations in their specialised hospital for diabetics, and, in a very short time, established indications and contraindications for the sulphonylureas [2]. They showed that patients with insulin dependent diabetes mellitus did not respond, while most patients with non-insulin-dependent diabetes (at this time called "Gegenregulationsdiabetes") could be treated successfully. Even before the experiences of these authors were published, it had been shown that the hypoglycaemic activity was not related to the sulphanilyl group, but was also present in the related compound N-[4-methylbenzoylsulphonyl]-N1-butylcarbamide (D 860, tolbutamide) [44] which had no bacteriostatic properties. In a few months, a group of young investigators, in close co-operation, concluded a multicentre tolbutamide study with 781 patients [45, 46] which was published together with experimental investigations about tolbutamide (D 860) in one issue of the "Deutsche Medizinische Wochenschrift" [47, 48]. One year later (1957), the same investigators presented further clinical experiences and extensive experimental data on the clinical results and the mechanism of action of tolbutamide in another special issue of the same journal.

For many years, Tolbutamide became the most frequently used oral antidiabetic drug.

Summary

1. Severe hypoglycaemia as complication of treatment with certain sulphonamide derivatives was discovered by M. Janbon and co-workers in 1942. Janbon initiated clinical and experimental investigations about the mechanism of this serious side effect.
2. The first experimental investigations about the mechanism of action of the blood glucose-lowering sulphonamide IPTD were performed by A. Loubatières from 1942–1946. He provided evidence that the hypoglycaemic effect was dependent on the presence of functioning islet B-cells

and suggested to use the compound in patients, whose diabetes was due to "a paresis of the insulin secretory mechanisms". However, this plan was not realised.

3. Oral treatment of diabetes mellitus with a blood glucose-lowering sulphonamide (carbutamide, BZ 55) was discovered by H. Franke and J. Fuchs in 1954 after Fuchs had experienced hypoglycaemia as a serious side effect of this bacteriostatic sulphonamide.
4. Studies on the mechanism of action of the blood glucose-lowering sulphonamide derivatives since 1955 confirmed, with more sophisticated methods, Loubatières' thesis that the main effect of these compounds is a direct interaction with the pancreatic B-cells and, therefore, that they could only be successfully used in patients with non-insulin-dependent diabetes.

References

[1] Franke H, Fuchs J. Ein neues antidiabetisches Prinzip. Dtsch Med Wochenschr 1955; 40: 1449–1452.

[2] Bertram F, Bendfeldt E, Otto H. Über ein wirksames perorales Antidiabeticum (BZ 55). Dtsch Med Wochenschr 1955; 40: 1455–1460.

[3] Loubatières A. Les substances sulfamidèes dans le traitement du diabète sucré. La Presse Méd 1955; 63: 1728–1730.

[4] Loubatières A, Binet ML. Action curative du para-aminobenzène-sulfamido-isopropylthiodiazol dans le diabète sucré humain. C R Séanc Acad Sci (Paris) 1955; 241: 1422–1423.

[5] Loubatières A, Bouyard P, Fruteau de Laclos C. Etude expérimentale chez le diabétique humain du para-aminobenzène-sulfamido-isopropylthiodiazol. La Semaine des Hòpitaux de Paris (Annales de la Recherche Médicale 1956; 32: 1–6.

[6] Kleinsorge H. Bemerkung zu den Arbeiten über N1-sulfanilyl-N2-n-butylcarbamid als perorales Antidiabetikum. Dtsch Med Wschr 1956; 81: 750–751.

[7] Kleinsorge H. 1. Blutzuckersenkung durch Sulfonamidverbindungen. Z Ärztl Fortb 1956; 50: 407–411.

[8] Creutzfeldt W, Söling HD. Oral treatment of diabetes. Berlin, Göttingen, Heidelberg: Springer 1961.

[9] Janbon M, Chaptal J, Vedel A, et al. Accidents hypoglycémiques graves par un sulfamidothiodiazol (le VK 57 ou 2254 RP). Commun Soc Sci méd biol Montpellier 1942; 222–250; Montpellier Med 1942; 441.

[10] Janbon M, Lazerges P, Métropolitanski JH. Etude du métabolisme du sulfa-iso-propylthiodiazol (VK 57 ou 2254 RP) chez le sujet sain et en cours de traitement. Comportement de la glycémie. Commun Soc Sci méd biol Montpellier 1942, 212–221; Montpellier Med 1942; 489.

[11] Vonkennel J, Kimmig J. Versuche und Untersuchungen mit neuen Sulfonamiden. Klin Wschr 1941; 20: 2–8.

[12] Bovet D, Dubost P. Activitè hypoglycémiante des aminobenzenesulfamidoalkythiodiazols. C R Soc Sci Biol (Paris) 1944; 138: 764–765.

[13] Janbon M, Lazerges P, Metropolitanski JH et al. Action hypoglycémiante de certains composés sulfamides. Róle du radical propyl-thiodiazol. C R Soc Sci Biol Montpellier 1943; 132–133.

[14] Loubatières A. Zur Geschichte der Entdeckung der oralen Antidiabetica. In Handbuch des Diabetes mellitus. Pfeiffer EF, ed. Vol. II München: Lehmans Verlag, 1971; 1179–1207.

[15] Loubatières A. Physiologie et pharmacodynamie de certains dérivés sulfamidés hypoglycémiants. Contribution a l'étude des substances synthétiques a tropisme endocrinien. Thèses – A la faculté des sciences de l'université de Montpellier. Soutenues le 1er juin 1946 devant la Commission d'examen. Montpellier: Causse, Graille & Castelnau.
[16] Loubatières A, Godstein L, Metropolitanski J et al. Etude expérimentale chez le chien des accidents nerveux irréversibles consecutifs à l'hypoglycémie prolongée provoquée par le sulfa-isopropyl-thiodiazol. 43e Congrès des méd. alién. neurol. de France. Montpellier 1942; Paris Edit. Masson, 415.
[17] Loubatières A, Godstein L, Metropolitanski J et al. Analyse du mécanisme de l'action hypoglycémiante du P-Amino-benzène sulfamido thiodiazol (2254 R.P.) C R Soc Biol (Paris) 1944; 138: 766–767.
[18] Loubatières A, Godstein L, Metropolitanski J et al. Rélations entre la structure moléculaire et láctivité hypoglycémiante des amino-benzène-sulfamido-alkylthiodiazols. C R Soc Biol (Paris) 1944; 138: 830.
[19] Loubatières A, Godstein L, Metropolitanski J et al. Etude physiologique et pharmacodynamique de certains dévirés sulfamidés hypoglycémiants. Arch int Physiol 1946; 54: 174–177.
[20] La Barre J, Reuse J. A propos de láction hypoglycémiante de certains dérivés sulfamidés. Arch Néerland. Physiol 1947; 28: 475–480.
[21] von Holt C, Benedict I, Kühnau J. Chemische Ausschaltung der A-Zellen der Langerhansschen Inseln. Naturwissenschaften 1954; 41: 166.
[22] von Holt C, Benedict I, Kühnau J. Chemische Ausschaltung der A-Zellen der Langerhansschen Inseln. Nauyn-Schiedebergs Arch exp Path Pharmak 1955; 224: 66–77.
[23] von Holt C, Benedict I, Kühnau J. Über die Wirkung der chemischen Ausschaltung der A-Zellen der Langerhansschen Inseln auf den Alloxandiabetes. Naunyn-Schiedebergs Arch exp Path Pharmak 1955; 224: 78–94.
[24] von Holt C, Benedict I, Ferner H. Morphologie der A-Zellbildung und der Entinselung des Pankreas. Z Zellforsch 1955; 42: 305–330.
[25] Creutzfeldt W, Tecklenborg E. Synthalinhypoglykämie, A-Zellen und Glucagon. Klin Wschr 1955; 43–44.
[26] Creutzfeldt W, Tecklenborg E. Experimentelle Untersuchungen zur Funktion der A-Zellen der Pankreasinseln und zur Glucagonwirkung. Naunyn-Schmiedebergs Arch exp Path Pharmak 1955; 227: 23–61.
[27] Christophe J, Bellens R, Gepts W. Etude expérimentale d'un sulfamidé hypoglycémiant. II. Action du R.P. 2254 sur la glycémie, la tolérance glucidique et la sensibilité à l'insuline du rat normal et du rat diabétique. Annales d'Endocrinologie 1955; 16: 956–961.
[28] Christophe J, Bellens R, Gepts W. Etude expérimentale de l'action du BZ 55 sur le rat normal. II. Action sur la glycémie. Annales d'Endocrinologie 1956; 17: 291–298.
[29] Creutzfeldt W, Finter H. Blutzucker und histologische Veränderungen nach D 860 bei normalen Kaninchen. Dtsch med Wschr 1956; 892–896.
[30] Creutzfeldt W, Böttcher K. Die Wirkung des D 860 auf den Alloxandiabetes des Kaninchens. Dtsch med Wschr 1956; 896–899.
[31] Creutzfeldt W. Pankreasbefunde bei Diabetikern nach Behandlung mit D 860. Dtsch med Wschr 1956; 841–844.
[32] Bänder A, Häussler A, Scholz J. Ergänzende pharmakologische Untersuchungen über Rastinon. Dtsch med Wschr 1957; 36: 1557–1564.
[33] Creutzfeldt W, Detering L, Welte O. Das B-Zellensystem von normalen und hypophysektomierten Ratten sowie von Kaninchen unter D 860 und diabetogenen Hormonen. Dtsch med Wschr 1957; 36: 1564–1568.
[34] Pfeiffer EF, Steigerwald H, Sandritter W et al. Vergleichende Untersuchungen von Morphologie und Hormongehalt des Kälberpankreas nach Sulfonylharnstoffen (D 860). Dtsch med Wschr 1957; 36: 1568–1574.
[35] Kracht J, Rausch-Stroomann JG. Das Inselzellsystem unter N1-sulfanilyl-N2-n-butylcarbamid. Naturwissenschaften 1956; 43: 180.

[36] Kracht J, v. Holt C, v. Holt L. Morphologische Befunde zur Wirkungsweise oraler Antidiabetica. Endokrinologie 1957; 34: 129–146.
[37] Root MA. Effect of carbutamide on the insulin content of the dog pancreas. Diabetes 1957; 6: 12–16.
[38] Dulin WE, Johnston RL, Miller WL. Role of the pituitary in the response of rats to tolbutamide. Diabetes 1959; 8: 199–204.
[39] Pfeiffer EF, Pfeiffer M, Ditschuneit H et al. Clinical and experimental studies of insulin secretion following tolbutamide and metahexamide administration. Ann N Y Acad Sci 1959; 82: 479–495.
[40] Kaubisch N, Hammer R, Wollheim C et al. Specific receptors for sulfonylureas in brain and in a β-cell tumor of the rat. Biochem Pharmacol 1982; 6: 1171–1174.
[41] Geisen K, Hitzel V, Ökomonopoulos R et al. Inhibition of 3H-glibenclamide binding to sulfonylurea receptors by oral antidiabetics. Arzneim-Forsch/Drug Res 1985; 35: 707–712.
[42] Sturgess, NC, Cook DL, Ashford MLJ et al. The sulphonylurea receptor may be an ATP-sensitive potassium channel. Lancet 1985; II: 474–475.
[43] Savagnone L. Sulfamidi e ricambio idrocarbonato influenza della somministrazione di sulfamidi sul tasso glicemico in condizioni normali e patologiche. La Settimana Medica 1941; 19: 1005–1012.
[44] Ehrhart G. Über neue peroral wirksame blutzuckersenkende Substanzen. Naturwissenschaften 1956; 43: 93.
[45] Mohnike G, Stötter G. Klinische Ergebnisse mit D 860. Dtsch med Wschr 1956; 81: 826–835.
[46] Creutzfeldt W, Ehrhart H, Marx R et al. The treatment of diabetes with D 860. German Medical Monthly 1956; 8: 1–18.
[47] Bänder A, Creutzfeldt W, Dorfmüller T et al. Über die orale Behandlung des Diabetes mellitus mit N-[4-Methyl-benzolsulfonyl]-N'-butyl-harnstoff(D 860). Dtsch med Wschr 1956; 21: 823–846.
[48] Creutzfeldt W. D860: a new oral antidiabetic drug. German Medical Monthly 1956; 8: 1–11.

Epidemiological research methodologies for the study of the aetiology of IDDM

G. Dahlquist

Epidemiology is a scientific theory and method aimed at studying disease occurrence in a defined population and relating the occurrence rate to certain characteristics of the individual. The ultimate aims are to define the risk determinants for the disease, to indicate disease causation and to find effective prevention strategies. Historically, this method was developed and used mainly for epidemic diseases. The best known successful study was John Snow's, who indicated an effective preventive strategy for cholera as early as in 1884 by identifying water from a specific source in London as a risk factor, long before the knowledge of the cholera vibrion. During the past decades, the scientific theories of epidemiology as well as the biostatistical techniques have rapidly developed parallel with the development of computer technology. Epidemiological techniques have also been successfully used for the study of the aetiology of non-communicable and chronic diseases. The epidemiological approaches have been rewarding, especially in diseases which are supposed to have a multiplex aetiology, i. e. caused by a combination of genetic and non-genetic factors . Perhaps, the best examples of successful epidemiological research in such diseases are lung cancer and cardiovascular diseases. Evidence of a similar complexity of the aetiology of insulin-dependent diabetes mellitus (IDDM) is accumulating. Not only the genetic prerequisites for disease susceptibility seem to be multiplex and permissive rather than decisive, but they also seem to interact in a complex manner with different non-genetic exposures.

The previously reported concordance rate of IDDM in monozygotic twins of 50% [1] has recently been shown to be even lower [2] when using an unbiased selection of twin pairs as the study base. These findings point to the huge importance of non-genetic risk factors for the aetiology of IDDM. The findings of marker genes for IDDM in the HLA-region of chromosome 6 strongly suggested an auto-immune pathogenesis of IDDM, and, as a result of extensive experimental and clinical research, several elegant hypotheses on the immune pathogenic mechanism of β-cell destruction have been suggested [3 – 5]. To fully understand the cause of IDDM, it is necessary to identify

Offprint from
Research Methodologies in Human Diabetes – Part 1

risk factors that may initiate the auto-immune process in the genetically susceptible individuals. An increased workload as well as increased levels of interleukin 1 [5] have been shown to accelerate the β-cell destructive process. Risk factors which act as promoters such as these may also be important to identify for preventive purposes, since only a fraction of individuals who develop auto-immunity against β-cells, as reflected by the presence of islets cell antibodies, will develop the clinically overt disease [2].

For identification of risk determinants which may be causally related to the disease occurrence and also to assess the relative importance of the risk factors on the incidence rate of IDDM, epidemiological, i. e. population-based research strategies, are necessary.

The tools

The basic tool for epidemiological research is a reliable case registry. Since the most interesting measure for etiological studies is the *disease occurrence* rate, both the diagnosis and the time at onset of the disease must be well defined. For insulin-dependent diabetes, the diagnostic criteria have been based on: age at onset, degree of metabolic disturbance, i. e. ketoacidosis at onset, as well as of insulin dependence. C-peptide measurements have been of little value as a clinical diagnostic tool, since many type 1 diabetics, at least in the clinical remission phase, may secrete considerable amounts of C-peptide. Low age at onset has proven to be the best criterion for discrimination between IDDM and non-IDDM at onset. Consequently, most IDDM registries used for a etiological studies have covered age groups 0–14 years of age. In these age groups, probably less than 1% of insulin-treated individuals are not classically insulin-dependent or type 1 diabetics. The time of diagnosis or rather the time of the first insulin injection has often been the pragmatic definition of disease occurrence. In growing individuals, the time-lag between clinical diagnosis and clinical onset, i. e. a clinically important relative insulin deficiency, will not be very long but may vary in different age groups.

In family studies, in which first degree relatives, including twins and siblings, have been followed up for the study of the natural history of IDDM, it has been shown that the markers of auto-immunity, i. e. islet cell antibodies, can occur many years before the clinical onset of the disease. Thus, the induction time may be long and varied and this is important when interpreting studies based on registries measuring date of clinical diagnosis.

The study base for a case registry is defined as the individuals living ineg a specified area (nation, county etc.) during a specific observation time. Within this study base, all individuals developing the disease should be covered by the register which may not include any other cases. If, for example, a certain hospital is used as the source of registration, it has to be clearly ascertained that only cases recruited from the specified study base are registered and also that patients from the specified study base who have been diagnosed in private practice or in another hospital must be included. For validation of population-based case registries, the double source method, or "capture-recapture" method, has often been used in IDDM research [7].

In practice, incidence data could be collected either by a continuous registration of diagnosed cases [8] or by regular repeated surveys [9]. A continuous registration has advantages, since it provides a possibility to continuously follow incidence rates over time and to rapidly collect incident cases for incident case-control studies. It is important, then, to perform regular validation procedures to assure a stable quality of the register. Repeated surveys are often more expensive and there is a risk that each survey will not be performed by identical methods. During the past few years, population-based registers for childhood IDDM have been set up in many parts in Europe [10] and all over the world [11] thanks to the activities of the EURODIAB collaborative study and the DIAMOND/WHO-project. These registers provide an excellent basis, not only for etiologic studies of the disease, but also for the study of the natural history of IDDM and its complications.

Epidemiological strategies for etiological research

Ecological studies

This kind of study compares the incidence rates of a disease in different populations to mean exposure rates of, for example, mean milk or coffee consumption. The obvious bias that may occur in this kind of comparison is that an association between variables on an aggregated level may not mean that the same association exists on an individual level. Still, some interesting ecological studies have been performed in IDDM research, e. g. the Icelandic study showing a higher incidence of IDDM in males born in October which was nine months after a period of traditionally high intake of nitrosamin rich food [12] or the study showing a correlation between the mean incidence of child IDDM and the mean consumption of cow's milk [13].

Descriptive epidemiological studies

For a etiological research the dynamic measure of disease, i. e. the incidence rate, is the most effective, since it measures the number of new cases occurring in a specified population during a specified time in contrast to the prevalence which only yields a measure of the total number of cases in a population at one time point. The study of patterns of disease occurrence measured as incidence rates, e. g. by age, by sex, by time or by geographical location, yields basic knowledge essential for the formulation of causation theories.

When comparing age standardised data from the population-based and validated IDDM registries in different populations, huge differences in incidence rates have been indicated with the highest rates appearing in Scandinavia (Finland, Sweden and Norway) and the lowest rates in Japan [11]. Such differences may be explained by both genetic or life style related exposures varying in different populations. Even if strong correlations have been shown between the presence of some of the genetic markers for IDDM [14] and incidence rates, clear outliers from such correlations are described [15, 16]. Furthermore, a five to six fold variability in incidence rate have been described between genetically very similar populations such as the Finnish and the Estonian [17], thus indicating other than genetic effects.

The world-wide geographical variability to some extent also is correlated to latitude which has been interpreted as an effect of relatively colder climates in the northern part of the world [11]. Colder environment as a risk factor, perhaps precipitating the disease occurrence in IDDM, is also indicated by the seasonal variability described in most epidemiological studies from all over the world showing the lowest incidence rates during the warmer period of the year (for review see 18). This is also in accordance with experimental studies in both animals and man showing an increased insulin need in the winter time.

Very specific pattern of disease occurrence has also been repeatedly shown by age in IDDM [18]. Thus, there is a low incidence rate among children below 5 years of age. Thereafter, a steady increase is noted with a maximum incidence rate occurring at puberty for both boys and girls. After puberty, the incidence decreases to a rather stable level between the ages of 20 to 34 [19]. The puberty peak has been interpreted as a result of the high pubertal growth rate since growth hormone increases the peripheral insulin resistance and may, thus, precipitate the disease occurrence [20].

Descriptive studies have also revealed interesting sex differences in IDDM incidence. Before puberty, incidence rates are very similar with a slight male predominance. In contrast, in the age group 20 to 34, the disease occurrence is almost twice as common among males compared to women [19]. During the past decade is has become evident that the incidence of IDDM is increasing in many countries [21]. This increase is much too rapid to be explained by an increase in the genetic pool of the disease, e. g. due to the successful outcome of pregnancy in diabetic mothers, since the genetic markers thus far found for the disease seem to be common in the general population, varying from 20 to 60% [22]. Therefore, the increasing trend probably depends on an increased exposure to one or several non-genetic risk factors which must be identified.

Analytical studies

Basically, in analytical epidemiological studies, the incidence rates of the disease under study are compared between exposed and non-exposed individuals. This comparison can be performed either by measuring exposure rates in a total *cohort* and, after follow-up, identify who will become cases or, as in the *case-control* study, by identification of the cases and comparing their exposure levels to that of relevant controls. In case-control studies, the exposures may either have been measured before or after the identification of cases. The basic difference between the two strategies is, that in the cohort design exposure data are collected for all individuals, whereas in the case control study design, exposure information is collected for the cases and, in addition, a representative sample only of the non-cases. Traditionally, cohort studies have been regarded as superior to the case-control design in a etiological studies, but this view has changed a lot during the past decade [23], since there are pros and cons to both strategies when validity aspects are balanced against effectiveness. For the study of a low prevalent disease like IDDM, case-control studies may, in reality, be the only choice. In Sweden, a country with a comparably high incidence rate of IDDM, 350–400 incident cases could be collected during one year and compared to data from representative controls with a rather high statistical power for a lot of interesting exposures. To collect a similar number of cases and, thus, achieve a similar precision in a cohort study, it would be necessary to follow around 100 000 children from birth and up to 15 years of age and continuously collect data on exposures from the whole cohort. Obviously, such a study would not only be rather ineffective and expensive, but would also encounter problems of validity because of the probable high dropout rate among the families being followed.

The main problem in case control designs is the possibility of a disease-dependent bias which largely depends on how exposure data are collected and also on the type of variable under study. If data on exposures operating before the onset of diabetes are collected from, for example, hospitals or health care centre records or registries, then the sensitivity and specificity of such data may be similar among cases and controls, whereas some data collected from questionnaires or interviews might be biased if, e. g. the diseased respondent might have an idea that the exposure may be a risk factor and, therefore, tend to recall such information differently than controls. Therefore, obviously the interpretation of such data must be carefully considered and double checking questions should be added to questionnaire or interview protocols.

When planning a case-control study, preferably based on a case registry, the most important considerations will be the size of the study and the choice of controls. The size of a study is, of course, dependent on economical realities as well as on power considerations. In case control studies, it can be shown

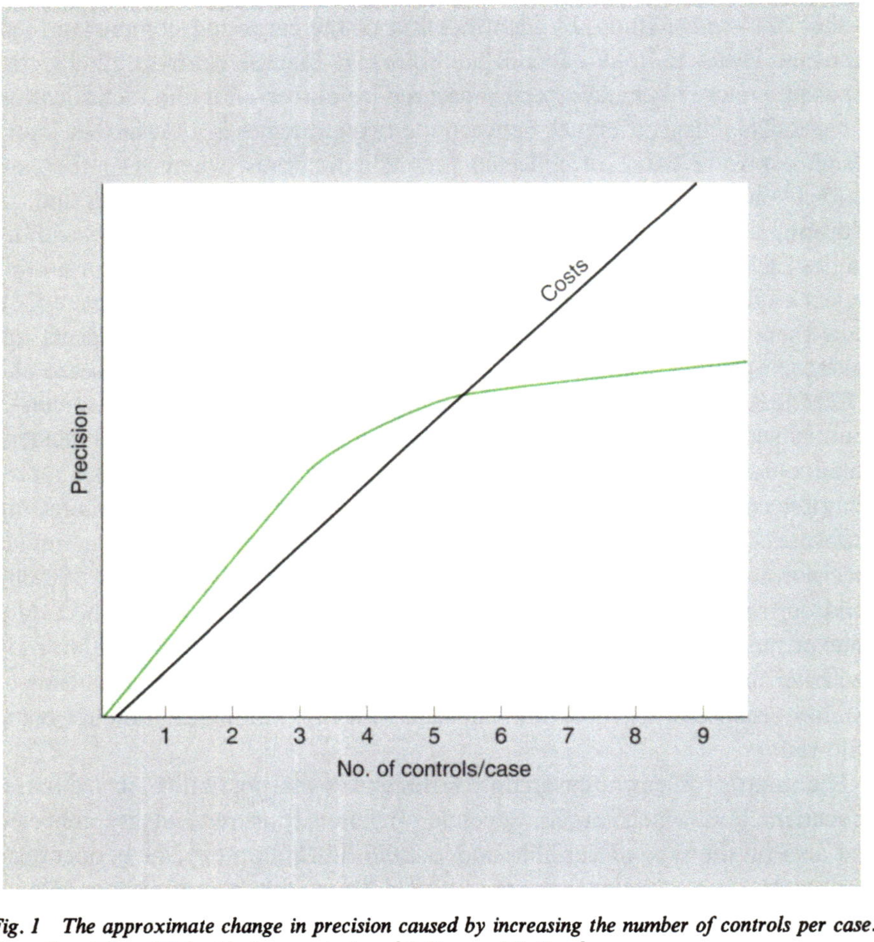

Fig. 1 The approximate change in precision caused by increasing the number of controls per case. Reproduced from [25] with the permission of S Karger AB, Basel

that the gain in precision will change with the number of controls per case [24] as shown in Fig. 1. Obviously, it is rarely motivated to increase the number of controls per case more than three or four. The power of the study is a measure of the potential of the study to detect a real difference (e. g. 1 minus the probability of a type 2 error). The power depends on the number of case-control sets, the level of statistical significance (for type 1 errors) chosen, the risk increase or relative risk judged to be of interest, but also on the frequency of exposed controls (Fig 2). Such considerations are naturally important to consider in the planning of a study but also in the case of "negative" result. (See [26] for further power discussions).

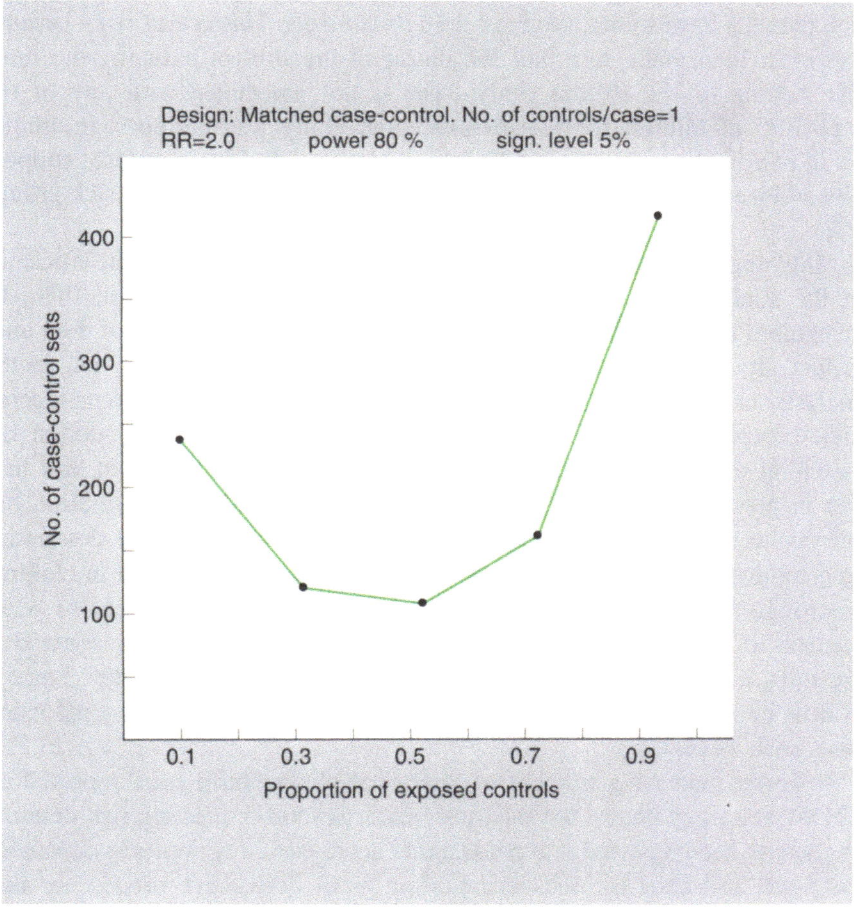

Fig. 2 The relationship between the required number of case-control sets and the proportion of exposed controls in a matched case-control study. Reproduced from [25] with the permission of S Karger AB, Basel

The basic concept of a proper control in an epidemiological study is that they should mirror the exposure of the study base (study population x observation time) from which the cases are recruited. For practical reasons, siblings and schoolmates or neighbours have often been used as controls. Such selection of controls may lead to overmatching since lifestyle habits or viral infections, which may be interesting risk factors for IDDM, may be shared by the cases and their schoolmates or neighbours, and, thus, not appear as a risk factor. In a recent discussion on a case control study of IDDM, it was claimed that such strategy may exaggerate risk estimates of socio-psychological variables as well [7]. Since it has been claimed that sick persons have a characteristic way of answering questions or interviews, other sick patients have sometimes been used as controls. This is also risky because one must then make sure that the illness of the control patient (who must also belong to the correct study base) is not associated with any of the exposures of interest for the disease under study. Furthermore, in studies using two control groups, one healthy and one sick, little empirical support was adduced for different patterns of reply between healthy and sick groups [28].

Matching controls to the cases has often been used to increase the efficiency of the study and to control some of the confounding. It must, then, be recognised that confounding could be controlled in the analyses of data and, in fact, matching does not guarantee control for confounding, but, in the analysis, must be taken into account anyway. It must also be remembered that, except for the risk of overmatching, in a matched study design the matching should be preferably kept in all the analyses. This might lead to a loss in precision, since not all pairs or triplets from which information has been collected might be useful because of non-responding. Since descriptive epidemiological studies have shown that the incidence of IDDM in children is strongly age and sex dependent, it might, however, be efficient to select controls at random within age and sex strata. Controls could be selected at the start, at the end or, continuously, during the study. This latter choice is of little importance for a low-prevalent chronic disease with a long induction time, such as diabetes.

A slowly increasing number of analytical studies have been reported on IDDM aetiology during the past few years. Several interesting risk determinants have been reported that could either act as initiating events by damaging the β-cell and start the self-perpetuating β-cell destructive process, or that may simply act to promote this pathogenic process. The following risk determinants have be identified which may act as initiators of the autoimmune process: Foetal rubella infections [29], maternal-child blood group incompatibility [30], early exposure of cow's milk proteins [31 – 37], later exposure of nitrosamines and other proteins [38]. Frequent intake of carbohydrate and protein-rich food [38] may promote or accelerate the autoimmune process by increasing the workload on the β-cells. This type of promoting effect is also indicated by risk determinants which may act through an increase of the peripheral insulin demand, such as frequent infections [39], a high growth rate [40] and stressful life events [41]. Different risk profiles have been shown to emerge in different age groups [42] and a possibility of synergism between nitrosamines and infections is also indicated [42] and a multiplex causation model has been proposed [43].

Intervention studies

To further test the cause effect relationship between an identified risk determinant and the disease, the proposed risk determinant may be modified in the population and the incidence rate can be followed. The strategies have many basic similarities with pharmaceutical clinical trials, but when applied to the general population, huge difficulties occur. Again, the characteristics of IDDM as a low-prevalent disease with a long induction time, will render such studies extremely time consuming and costly, but they will be necessary. Thus far, no intervention studies have been started to study the incidence rate of IDDM after modification of any of the suggested risk factors. It may be more effective to study the effect of intervention in high risk groups, such as HLA-identical and/or islet cell antibody-positive first degree relatives of IDDM patients.

Intervention studies, trying to arrest an already on-going β-cell destructive process by immunomodulating agents, such as cyklosporine and other immune suppressants and free radical scavengers such as nicotinamide, have been reported. For the planning and, also importantly, for the interpretation of such studies, an epidemiological perspective is also important since (1) the predictive value of a marker used to select individuals at risk will differ tremendously between high risk and low risk populations due to the dependence of the predictive value on the prevalence of the disease [44], and (2) the effect of the treatment may not be similar among high risk individuals belonging to the two different populations. These considerations are especially important in the case of IDDM where only about 10% of the cases are derived from high risk groups, i. e. families with an IDDM proband.

Analysis of data

The analysis of data basically depends on the a priori hypothesis of causation, but also on the study design. In essence, the same biostatistical methods could be used whether the study is a cohort or a case-control design. The measure of effect in cohort studies is often that of a relative risk whereas in a case-control study the odds ratio is to be used. But since IDDM is a low-prevalent disease, the odds ratio will be similar to the relative risk (Table 1).

Table 1 Some definitions

Risk (P)	The probability that an event will occur. This probability may be measured as a cumulative incidence rate.
Odds $\frac{P}{1\text{-}P}$	The probability that an event occurs relative to the probability that it does not.
Relative risk $\frac{Pe}{Pu}$	The ratio between the risk among exposed (e) and that among unexposed (u) individuals.
Odds ratio $\frac{Pe}{1\text{-}Pe} : \frac{Pu}{1\text{-}Pu}$	The ratio between the odds among exposed and that among the unexposed individuals.
Risk difference (Pe-Pu)	The absolute difference in risk between an exposed and an unexposed group of individuals.
Etiologic fraction (in population)	The proportion by which the incidence rate in the population will be reduced if an exposure is eliminated.

As already stated, the concept of cause of diabetes is that different non-genetic risk factors alone or in concert will initiate or promote the disease occurrence in genetically susceptible individuals. Some of these risk factors may be necessary, but not sufficient, and others may be contributing risk factors. For both economical and scientific reasons, several exposures are, therefore, often studied in the same, for example, case control study. To identify which risk factors will independently affect the risk for disease occurrence, and to identify possible interactions, such as synergism between risk factors, either stratification techniques or multivariate modelling techniques must be used. The most comprehensive method is the use of stratifications to standardise for possible confounders and the use of the Mantel-Haenszel methods to calculate combined or weighted risk estimates [45]. The most comprehensive way of evaluating the effect estimates is to calculate the confidence limits which tells within which limits the true risk value is to be found with a chosen probability of, e. g. 95%. Many modern biostaticians and epidemiologists consider the commonly used P-values, i. e. an arbitrarily chosen point of the probability function, as more important for decision making in clinical situations than for the presentation of scientific results where confidence limits or even the complete probability function would be more useful to consider [23].

The obvious advantage of analysis of multifactorial problems by stratifications is that the researcher maintains close contact with the original data set and will not miss, for example, non-linear trends, inconsistencies or even errors in the data set. On the other hand, the now rapidly developing multivariate strategies are necessary when working with many possible risk determinants in a limited number of case-control sets, for example. In this study design, the logistic regression analysis has become popular [26]. Several handy epidemiological computer software programs have been developed in the past years for multivariate analysis. When using these, it is of the utmost importance to start with a comprehensive biological hypothesis and sufficient knowledge of the multivariate modelling process. The researcher will immediately lose contact with the original data set which is squeezed into exponential log functions which deliver smoothed estimates of risk factors and predictive models. The odds ratios may also become very "shaky". The obvious advantage of multivariate analyses is that one preserves precision while controlling for many variables and thus the data will be efficiently used.

Since several exposures are often examined in the same study in epidemiological studies, it has often been claimed that significance has occurred by chance due to the so-called mass significance problem. It is certainly true that when doing multiple analyses, 5% of those will, by chance, reach the 5% significance level. A traditional statistical approach to this problem has been to correct for this by increasing the p-values by some factor that depends on the number of comparisons made. However, the problem of mass significance is highly dependent on the a priori hypothesis to be tested. If, as in sequential analyses, for example, the same hypothesis is repeatedly tested using the same or partly the same data set, then the significance level must be corrected. If, in epidemiological studies, different a priori hypotheses are tested, for example, that different exposures may, probably by different mechanisms, affect the risk for the disease occurrence, each analysis should be regarded as separate from the other and correction of the p-value is not relevant [23]. The problem with increasing the significance level is that when trying to avoid a type 1 error, one simultaneously increases the risk of a type 2 error. It is, then, important to consider which error might have the more serious consequences. To avoid wasting important new knowledge, perhaps one should completely avoid regarding a risk estimate as "significant" depending on a chosen p-value, but rather, as previously discussed, use confidence limits as the method of presentation of the risk estimate and its precision. The risk estimate could, then, be judged as to scientific, biological or clinical significance by the reader.

The inference of epidemiological studies

Clearly, the inference of epidemiological studies as well as that of other studies are dependent on the study design, the precision as well as the possibilities of systematic errors in either the selection of cases and controls or of the estimates of exposures. The possibility that non-responders might differ from responders in either disease status or as to some important exposure may also be considered. It is important that the study base is clearly specified and to remember that results from one specified type of study base can rarely be generalised to another.

Misclassification errors are common in epidemiological research, since especially exposure data are very often indirectly collected through registries, records or questionnaires. For some exposures collected after the onset of diabetes, certainly the possibility of disease-dependent information bias must be carefully considered. It is, however, important to remember that unless a misclassification of exposure is dependent on disease status, a low sensitivity and/or specificity of the exposure data will only lead to that the odds ratio or the relative risk will tend to approach 1.0 [44]. This dilution effect is, however, often balanced by the possibility of studying much larger groups of individuals using a more inexpensive, but less precise method to measure exposures. Experimental and clinical researchers who often study small groups of animals or patients are eager to find as precise methods as possible for the measure of effect. In epidemiological studies, it is often more cost-effective to use less precise instruments that could be applied to larger groups of individuals. Similar reasoning is applicable to diagnostic tests, i. e. the classification of the outcome variable. Unless it could be expected that the classification procedure is associated with an exposure under study, then the misclassification of cases and controls will be similar among exposed and unexposed individuals and such misclassification will never lead to an overestimation of the effect of an exposure. In the study of type 1 diabetes, misclassification of disease is rare if the population under study is younger than 15 years old, for example, when type 2 diabetes is rare.

For the interpretation of the results, it is important to have a model of causation based on a biologically reliable hypothesis. In fact, analytical epidemiological studies can only define risk determinants, i. e. exposures, that increase the probability of occurrence of disease or risk markers which are attributes associated with an increased probability of a specified outcome, such as disease occurrence. Neither risk determinants nor risk markers are necessarily causally related to the disease. If, in a population-based intervention study, the probability of disease occurrence could be modified by modifying a risk determinant or a risk marker, causality is more probable and one may then speak of a risk factor [46]. It is also important to note that some risk factors may operate in certain age groups only, and some may be dependent on the simultaneous occurrence of other risk factors. A confounder is a risk factor that is associated to an exposure under study which has been found to be associated with an increase in the disease risk. It is, then, of course important to examine whether the association is independent of that of the confounder. If the confounder is known, it could be taken into account both in the study design and in the analysis of data. Unknown or unmeasured confounders may always exist and, therefore, one must always be careful to interpret epidemiological studies as to causation.

On the other hand, as pointed out in the beginning of this chapter, the epidemiological observational studies will provide necessary input of knowledge concerning exposures which may be causally related to disease occurrence, and without this perspective, the full aetiology of, e. g. lung cancer and cardiovascular disease and probably IDDM, will not be disclosed. The pathogenesis of disease occurrence and the mechanism of operation of a risk factor at the organ-, cellular- and DNA-levels certainly must be explored using experimental techniques, but based on the knowledge derived from observational, epidemiological studies. For prevention strategies, however, epidemiological studies may sometimes be sufficient, if strong evidence exists of an association between a risk factor and a disease, even though the exact mechanism of action is not yet explored. This is especially relevant if it could be shown that the etiologic fraction (Table 1) of a specific exposure is large, meaning that a large proportion of incident cases could be reduced if the exposure could be eliminated as is the case of smoking and lung cancer, for example.

Conclusions

Epidemiological theory and methodology have developed rapidly during the past decade and are important for the study of the aetiology of diseases with a multiplex mode of causation such as IDDM. Epidemiological study techniques have been increasingly applied in the study of the aetiology of IDDM. Several risk determinants have been identified which could initiate or promote the auto-immune β-cell destruction and others have been suggested which may precipitate the clinical onset by increasing the peripheral insulin need. These risk determinants must be further explored in epidemiological, analytical and intervention studies. Experimental studies are further needed to explain the mechanism of action of these possible risk factors.

References

[1] Tattersall RB, Pyke DA. Diabetes in identical twins. Lancet 1992; II: 1120–1125.
[2] Kapio J, Toumilehto J, Koskenvuo M et al. Concordance for type 1 (insulin-dependent) and type 2 (non-insulin-dependent) diabetes mellitus in a population-based cohort of twins in Finland. Diabetologia 1992; 35: 1060–1062.
[3] Eisenbarth GS. Type 1 diabetes mellitus: a chronic autoimmmune disease. New Engl J Med 1986; 314: 1360–1368.
[4] Bottazzo GF, Pujol-Borrell R, Gale EAM. Autoimmunity and type 1 diabetes. Bringing the story up to date. In Alberti KGMM. Krall LP, eds. The Diabetes Annual/3. Amsterdam: Elsevier Science Publ, 1987: 15–38.
[5] Mandrup-Poulsen T. On the pathogenesis of insulin-dependent diabetes mellitus. Dan Med Bull 1988; 35: 438–460.
[6] Landin-Olsson M, Karlsson A, Dahlquist G et al. Islet cell and other organ-specific autoantibodies in all children developing diabetes during one year and matched controls. Diabetologia 1989; 32: 387–395.
[7] Bishop YMN, Fienberg SE, Holland PW. Estimating the size of a closed population. In: Discrete multivariate analysis, 5th edn. Cambridge, Mass: MIT, 1978; 229–256.
[8] Dahlquist G, Gustavsson KH, Holmgren G et al. The Incidence of Diabetes Mellitus in Swedish Children 0–14 Years of Age. Acta Paediatr Scand 1982; 71: 7–14.
[9] Wagener DK, Sacks JM, LaPorte RE et al. The Pittsburgh Study of Insulin-dependent Diabetes Mellitus. Risk for Diabetes Among Relatives of IDDM. Diabetes 1982; 31: 136–144.
[10] Green A. Gale EAM, Pattersson CC for the EURODIAB ACE Study Group. Incidence of childhood onset insulin-dependent diabetes mellitus: The EURODIAB ACE study. Lancet 1992; 339: 905–909.
[11] Diabetes epidemiology research international group. Geographic patterns of insulin-dependent diabetes mellitus. Diabetes 1988; 37: 1113–1119.
[12] Helgason T, Ewen SW, Ross IS et al. Diabetes produced in mice by smoked/cured mutton. Lancet 1982; II: 1017–1022.
[13] Scott FW. Cow milk and insulin-dependent diabetes mellitus: is there a relationship. Am J Clin Nutr 1990; 51: 489–491.
[14] Dorman JS, LaPorte RE, Stone RA et al. Worldwide differences in the incidence of type 1 diabetes are associated with amino-acid variation at position 57 of the HLA-DQß chain. Proc Natl Acad Sci USA 1990; 87: 7370–7374.
[15] Baisch JM, Weeks T, Giles R et al. Analysis of HLA-DQ genotypes and susceptibility in insulin-dependent diabetes mellitus. N Engl J Med 1990; 322: 1836–1841.
[16] Reijonen H, Ilonen J, Knip M et al. HLADQB1 alleles and absence of Asp57 as susceptibility factors of IDDM in Finland. Diabetes 1991; 40: 1640–1644.
[17] Tuomilehto J, Podar T, Brigis G et al. Comparison of the incidence of insulin-dependent diabetes mellitus in childhood among five Baltic populations during 1983-88. Int J Epidemiol 1992; 21: 518–527.
[18] Dahlquist G. Epidemiological studies of childhood insulin-dependent diabetes. Rewiev article. Acta Paediatr Scand 1991; 80: 583–589.

[19] Nyström L, Dahlquist G, Östman J et al. Developing diabetes before 35 years of age – risk assessment based on a 5-year nationwide surveillance system. Int J Epidemiol 1992; 21: 352–558.
[20] Dahlquist G, Blom L, Holmgren G et al. The epidemiology of diabetes in Swedish children 0–14 years – a six-year prospective study. Diabetologia 1985; 28: 802–808.
[21] Diabetes Epidemiology Research Group. Secular Trends in Incidence of Childhood IDDM in 10 Countries. Diabetes 1990; 39: 858–864.
[22] Deschamps J, Bevessi JP, Khalil J et al. The role of genetic predisposition to type 1 (insulin-dependent) diabetes mellitus. Ann Med 1991; 23: 427–435.
[23] Rothman KJ. Modern epidemiology. Boston, Toronto: Little Brown and Company, 1986.
[24] Morgenstern H, Winn DAM. A method for determining the sampling ratio in epidemiologic studies. Statistics Med 1983; 2: 387–396.
[25] Dahlquist G. The Swedish childhood diabetes study: Methodological aspects. In Levy-Marchal C, Czernikow P (eds). Epidemiology and Etiology of Insulin-dependent diabetes in the young. Pediatr. Adolesc Endocrinol Vol 21. Basel: Karger, 1992; 11–21.
[26] Breslow NE, Day NE. Statistical methods in cancer research. Vol II. International Agency for Research on Cancer. Oxford: Oxford Univ Press, 1989.
[27] Siemiatycki J. Second Thoughts. Friendly control bias. Clin Epidemiol 1989; 42: 687–688.
[28] Norell S, Ahlbom A. Hospital versus population referents in two case-referent studies. Scand J Work Environ Health 1987; 13: 62–66.
[29] Menser MA, Forrest JM, Bransby RD. Rubella infection and diabetes mellitus. Lancet 1978; 1: 57–60.
[30] Dahlquist G, Källén B. Maternal-child blood group incompatibility and other perinatal events increase the risk for early onset type 1 (insilin-dependent) diabetes mellitus. Diabetologia 1992; 35: 671–675.
[31] Borch-Johnsen K, Mandrup-Poulsen T, Lachan-Christiansen B et al. Relation between breast-feeding and incidence rates of insulin-dependent diabetes mellitus. Lancet 1984; II: 1083–1086.
[32] Blom L, Dahlquist G, Nyström L et al. The Swedish childhood diabetes study – Social and perinatal determinants for diabetes in childhood. Diabetologia 1989; 32: 7–13.
[33] Virtanen SM, Räsänen L, Aro A et al. Infant feeding in Finnish children <7 year of age with newly diagnosed IDDM. Diabetes Care 1991; 14: 415–417.
[34] Glatthaar Ch, Whittall DE, Welborn TA et al. Diabetes in Western Australian children: descriptive epidemiology, Med. J. Austr 1988; 148: 117–123.
[35] Siemiatycki J, Colle E, Campbell S et al. Case-control study of IDDM. Diabetes Care 1989; 12: 209–216.
[36] Mayer EJ, Hamman RF, Gay EC et al. Reduced risk of IDDM among breast-fed children. Diabetes 1988; 37: 1625–1632.
[37] Kostraba JN, Dorman J, LaPorte R et al. Early infant diet and risk of IDDM in blacks and whites. Diabetes Care 1988; 15: 626–631.
[38] Dahlquist G, Blom L, Persson LÅ et al. Dietary factors and the risk of developing diabetes in childhood. Br Med J 1990; 300: 1302–1306.
[39] Blom L, Dahlquist G, Sandström A et al. The Swedish childhood diabetes study – infectious disease and vaccinations as risk determinants for diabetes in childhood. Diabetologia 1991; 34: 176–181.
[40] Blom L, Persson LÅ, Dahlquist G. A high linear growth and risk for diabetes. Diabetologia 1992; 35: 528–533.
[41] Hägglöf B, Blom L, Dahlquist G et al. The Swedish childhood diabetes study: indications of severe psychological stress as a risk factor for Type 1 (insulin-dependent) diabetes in childhood. Diabetologia 1991; 34: 589–593.
[42] Dahlquist G, Blom L, Lönnberg G. The Swedish childhood diabetes study – a multivariate analysis of risk determinants for diabetes in different age groups. Diabetologia 1991; 34: 757–762.

[43] Dahlquist G. Etiological aspects of insulin-dependent diabetes – an epidemiological perspective. Hypothesis. Autoimmunity. In press.
[44] Ahlbom A, Norell S. Introduction to modern epidemiology. Chestnut Hill MA: Epidemiology resources inc. 1984.
[45] Armitage P, Berry G. Statistical methods in medical research, 2nd ed. Oxford: Blackwell Scientific Publications, 1988.
[46] Last J. A dictionary of epidemiology. New York: Oxford Univ Press, 1988.

Epidemiological research methodologies for NIDDM

G. Dowse, P. Zimmet

Introduction

Epidemiological studies of NIDDM are being increasingly performed in both developed and developing countries. These studies take various forms, from examination of routinely available morbidity and mortality data, to complex longitudinal investigations of aetiology and pathogenesis in defined populations.

Interest in the epidemiology of NIDDM was first aroused in the 1960s after the distinction between IDDM and NIDDM became clear, and expanded throughout the 1970s as it was realized that there was considerable variation in the frequency of NIDDM between populations [1, 2]. However, comparison of results from these early studies was hampered by inconsistency in the diagnostic criteria for diabetes, including the size and nature of glucose loads, and the blood glucose cut-off points which were used. Recognition of these and other problems led ultimately to the development of the now internationally accepted criteria for classification and diagnosis of diabetes [3–5], and to recommendations for the reporting of epidemiological studies [2, 6, 7].

Although the US National Diabetes Data Group (NDDG) [3] and the World Health Organization (WHO) [4, 5] criteria for diabetes are essentially the same, they differ in their definition of impaired glucose tolerance (IGT). Popular usage over the past decade, even in the US, has decided in favour of the simpler WHO criteria [8–10]. The general acceptance of these criteria has corresponded with a considerable increase in the number of epidemiological studies of NIDDM, associated with concern over the increasing frequency of the disease, particularly in populations which have experienced rapid modernization of lifestyle in recent decades [9, 10].

This review will focus on some important practical aspects of the organization and conduct of field surveys of NIDDM which use reliable but relatively simple methods for assessment of risk factors and complications. Other means of epidemiological study of NIDDM will be considered briefly.

Offprint from
Research Methodologies in Human Diabetes – Part 1

Study Types

Routine Data

In general, it is always worthwhile examining routine sources of data which might yield information appropriate to a particular research question. Most countries collect at least some information on cause of death and hospitalisation. Although this may be incomplete in developing countries, and unsuitable for international comparisons, it may still be reasonable to compare rates within the population, over time, by region, and by age, for instance, in order to identify coarse patterns.

Routine data may also yield information on complications such as diabetic coma, ketoacidosis, sepsis and gangrene, amputations and renal failure. The availability of such data will vary depending on the degree of development of the country and its medical record systems. However, even in countries with little routine data collection, for example, individual hospitals may maintain a register of operations performed, which can be used to trace the records of subjects who have had amputations. Hospital notes can then be checked to identify amputees with diabetes.

Similarly, particularly in small countries, it may be possible to get albeit limited information on trends in the frequency of diabetic retinopathy and renal failure by examining records at government or private clinics where laser and dialysis services are available.

Registers

In some situations, it may be feasible to establish local or national registers of cases of diabetes, which distinguish NIDDM and IDDM. These might be created primarily for epidemiological monitoring and research, or alternatively, be used for purposes of patient follow-up. With increasing sophistication, such registers might be computerised, and contain information such as age at diagnosis, treatment, and presence of complications.

Registers for monitoring of and research into the genetic and environmental causes of IDDM have been established in many countries in recent years, usually on a local or regional basis, and procedures for planning and organizing such registers have been well described [11]. These methods could be modified to allow registration of NIDDM in situations where this is feasible and desirable.

Special studies and surveys

It is axiomatic that given the current definition of NIDDM, a relatively high proportion of total cases are asymptomatic, possibly for some years prior to recognition of the disease. In both developed [12, 13] and under-developed countries [9, 14], population surveys have shown that as many as 50% or more of all cases may be unknown. Moreover, these asymptomatic individuals have often already developed at least the preclinical stages of both microvascular and macrovascular complications associated with diabetes [15, 16].

Therefore, for both public health information and academic research purposes, population-based surveys are required to detect asymptomatic or undetected (there may be a difference between the two) cases of NIDDM and to define the total prevalence and incidence of the disease and its complications. For aetiologic enquiry, cross-sectional, longitudinal and case-control study variants may all be used for epidemiological investigation of NIDDM. Studies of prevention, whether of disease itself in subjects with IGT, or of complications in subjects who already have NIDDM, should follow classical design theory for randomized controlled clinical trials, as detailed elsewhere [17].

In practice, the case-control format has been little used in epidemiological studies of NIDDM, probably because surveys need to be performed to define glucose tolerance anyway, so analyses are then performed within the entire data set. Additionally, because NIDDM is a relatively common disease, with prevalence in adults ranging from around 3% to levels as high as 30% or more in some populations, the "rare disease" statistical assumptions underlying the use of the odds ratio as an estimate of relative risk are not satisfied. Nevertheless, case-control studies, particularly "nested" designs within larger studies offer advantages in terms of cost for exploration of particular hypotheses linking risk factors with NIDDM and its complications. For example, the association with NIDDM of a newly-discovered genetic marker could be investigated by testing sera/DNA (fresh or stored) from cases and appropriately selected controls from within a larger study population. Similarly, the relationship of specific dietary components or foods with disease could be studied by performing diet questionnaires on cases newly-detected during a cross-sectional population survey (but not yet aware of their disease status) and a group of controls with normal glucose tolerance matched on basic characteristics such as age and sex.

Study design

Sampling strategies for surveys

The particular sampling strategy used and the size of sample required for a study of NIDDM prevalence and/or incidence will vary depending on the objectives, available resources, and logistic details including geography and transport systems in the survey area. The ideal of a simple random sample, whereby all individuals in a defined population have an equal chance of being chosen is rarely possible. Some possible strategies are outlined below.

Selected community samples: Most commonly, NIDDM surveys are performed on all individuals within a required age-range living in pre-selected communities. These are usually chosen because of convenience and/or because they are judged to be "typical" of the background population, given the a priori objectives of the investigators. For example, geographically defined villages/towns may be chosen because they are thought to typify rural or urban dwellers, or a particular ethnic group in a country or region [9, 12, 18–20]. This design has often been used in studies examining the effect of modernization of lifestyle in developing countries.

Random cluster sampling: This design retains the logistic advantages of working in whole areas, but is an attempt to draw a sample which is more likely to be representative of the target population. In essence, geographically defined clusters of population are given an equal chance of being selected, and the larger the number of clusters the more representative the sample. If the population within clusters varies then selection should be with "probability proportional to size" [21]. Use of clusters previously defined for administrative or electoral reasons is preferred. For example, a two-stage random cluster sampling scheme was employed in a national study of NIDDM prevalence in the Indian Ocean island nation of Mauritius [14].

Random sampling of individuals: Where a complete sampling frame, such as electoral rolls or national identity registration is available, randomization of individuals is possible. However, completion of survey procedures in individuals whose places of residence are separated by potentially large distances is logistically much more complex than inviting all adults living in a defined area to a central survey site. For example, a recent estimate of diabetes prevalence in Australia was derived from a national population sample selected from electoral rolls, but compromises based on logistic concerns meant that the sample was limited to residents of large cities, and an oral glucose tolerance test could not be performed [22]. In this instance, it is arguable that more useful data for the prevalence of NIDDM in Australia may actually be found in the study of adults living in Busselton, a small rural town [12]. A more complete national study of diabetes prevalence was performed in the USA, whereby a complex stratified sampling scheme was applied to the total population, and glucose tolerance was assessed at multiple locations across the country according to a standardized protocol [13]. However, the resources required to undertake such studies are rarely available.

Non-response: Experience suggests that response rates in surveys involving individual randomization tend to be considerably lower than those where all subjects in a defined population cluster are eligible. A community survey, particularly in a developing country, can become an important social event, and individuals are much more likely to attend if their neighbours and relatives are also invited. It is worth considering whether a response rate of 60% in a national or regional study involving individual randomization, may be more or less representative of the target population than a study involving a number of randomly or deliberately chosen clusters where the overall response rate is 85%.

In the first instance, bias may be introduced because of selective attendance of "worried well", sick individuals or a particular socio-economic group. In the second scenario, particularly where estimates are based on small sample size and few clusters, there will always be doubts as to how well a sample may represent a particular target population, whether it be a country, ethnic group or stage of development. Unfortunately, some form of compromise is usually necessary. Most importantly, investigators must be aware of potential biases in whichever approach they use, and consider the likely effect when analysing data.

Demographic characteristics of non-responders (such as age, sex and ethnic group), which should be available from either a pre-existing sampling frame or a household census performed prior to the survey, can be compared with those of responders. Where possible, all or at least a sub-sample of non-responders should be contacted following a survey and asked a simple questionnaire to identify reasons for non-attendance and to assess the frequency of self-reported end-points of interest, such as diabetes, hypertension or ischaemic heart disease. Comparison of the latter with prevalence in the responder group can help in the detection of response bias.

Additional sampling stages: Stratification, with over- and/or under-sampling of a particular sub-group (such as an age-group or ethnic group) and randomization (usually "systematic", whereby, for example, every nth individual enumerated in every kth household along a street might be chosen) can be added as additional stages to either community samples selected purposively, or to randomly-selected cluster samples [21].

Sample size

Statistical advice should be sought in the early phases of planning an epidemiological study, both with respect to the method of sampling and the sample size required to meet the main study objectives. Determination of sample size will be based on various parameters including estimates of the major study end-points (e. g. difference in prevalence between two sub-groups), the level of statistical significance (usually $p < 0.05$) accepted as indicating a real difference, and the power or likelihood of the study to demonstrate such a difference if it really exists. More detailed consideration of sampling and statistical aspects, including calculation of sample size, can be found elsewhere [21, 23].

Study variants

Cross-sectional epidemiological studies of NIDDM have taken advantage of several design variants which have helped to define the importance of both genetic and environmental factors in determining disease occurrence [2]. Some major forms are outlined below.

Rural-urban comparisons: Here the prevalence of NIDDM and risk factor levels are compared in populations of similar genetic background but different lifestyles. Such studies in Pacific island countries have shown much higher NIDDM prevalence in urban areas where diet and physical activity patterns are more modernized relative to the more traditional pattern observed in rural areas [9, 18, 19].

Migrant studies: Similarly, the importance of lifestyle in modulating risk of NIDDM has been demonstrated by studies which have shown increased prevalence of NIDDM in migrants relative to their peers remaining in the place of origin [24–26]. Less directly, the results of unconnected studies of groups of similar ethnicity living in different environments can be compared [27]. For example, migrant Chinese living in Singapore [28], Taiwan [29] and

Mauritius [14] have moderate to high prevalence of NIDDM, in contrast to the low prevalence found in separate studies performed in mainland China [30].

Comparison of different ethnic cohabitants: Studies comparing disease prevalence and risk factor levels in different ethnic groups living similar lifestyles in the same country have helped to illustrate the importance of genetic factors related to ethnicity. For example, NIDDM prevalence is higher in people of Asian Indian origin than in their cohabitants in many countries [19, 27, 28, 31], and urbanized Australian Aborigines have been shown to have much higher NIDDM prevalence than European-origin Australians [32]. The pronounced difference in prevalence and incidence of NIDDM observed in epidemiological studies of American Pima Indians and other Americans [33] has spawned a series of clinical and genetic studies directed toward identifying the basis of the Pima's susceptibility [34, 35].

Studies of genetic admixture: Studies in Nauruans [36], Mexican-Americans [37] and Australian Aborigines [38] have shown that the prevalence of NIDDM decreases as the proportion of European admixture increases, highlighting the relatively greater susceptibility of the "native" genotype in these groups.

Field survey methodology

Specific techniques which are commonly used in epidemiological field surveys of NIDDM have been well described previously [7, 23, 39, 40], as have practical suggestions for the structure and conduct of field surveys [40]. Therefore, this section will highlight only certain critical aspects of preparation for, and performance of, field survey work, based on the authors' experience. These methods have been used successfully over many years in rural and urban areas of developing countries of the Pacific Ocean region [9, 15, 19] as well as in newly-industrialized Mauritius [14, 40], and developed Singapore [41].

Preparation of survey manual

An early stage in planning for a field survey must be the preparation of a detailed study protocol/survey manual [40]. This should include information such as that listed in Table 1.

Table 1 Information which should be included in a survey manual and protocol for an epidemiological study of NIDDM

1. The main objectives of the study.
2. A timetable from commencement to completion.
3. A list of personnel and their duties.
4. Details of sample selection, including any special census performed to enumerate the sample.
5. Clear step-by-step instructions for each procedure (registration, venesection, glucose load, height and weight measurement, etc.).
6. A flow-chart of the sequence in which procedures should be undertaken and a pictorial representation of the preferred lay-out of the survey site.
7. A chart detailing precisely how all blood, urine or other biological samples should be processed, including information on centrifugation, number and size of aliquots, storage temperature, location of storage, and ultimate purpose and destination for each aliquot.
8. Details of quality assurance for each procedure.
9. A statement regarding ethical clearance for the survey.
10. An outline of arrangements for entry and editing of data, and the likely format of main statistical analyses.
11. A policy on preparation of publications (particularly for large studies involving multiple investigators).

Survey manuals provide crucial information not only during field-work, but are also invaluable documents in later years as aids to memory for the preparation of manuscripts, and for the planning of longitudinal phases of a study, even if these were not part of the original design. A clear and detailed survey manual is absolutely crucial in situations where there are multiple investigators and/or field staff, and when staff and senior investigators may change over the duration of a longitudinal study.

Training of staff

Rigorous training of staff is required as part of attempts to ensure the validity of data collected. For most routine procedures this can usually be undertaken in the week before commencement of the survey, so that methods remain fresh in the memory. Measurement techniques and questionnaire administration can be refined by practise on groups of volunteers and amongst the staff themselves. Individual staff who do not perform satisfactorily in training for a particular procedure should be replaced.

The amount of training required will depend on the nature of the task. Even for a procedure as relatively simple as measuring height and weight, an hour or more of instruction and practice will be required, covering details which include: checking calibration and zeroing of the machine; allowable clothing and stance of participants; rounding of measurements and recording on the survey form; accuracy and repeatability of measurements; and method of packing the machine for transportation between survey sites. For blood pressure measurement, however, proper training is more complex, and may take two or more days, using video and/or audio-tapes, and cross-checks using a double-headed stethoscope against a certified "gold-standard" observer [23].

Variation between obervers can be minimized by limiting the number of staff performing each survey task as far as is practicable. Additionally, where there may be more than one observer for a measurement task, it is important that there is not a systematic difference in the manner in which groups of participants present to the observers. For example, if different observers record blood pressure in each of two survey locations, and one location is subsequently shown to have higher mean blood pressure than the other, then it will be unclear whether the difference is real or may be due to systematic measurement differences between the observers, even when both underwent careful, standardized training. It is therefore important to ensure that observers perform the same tasks throughout the duration of a survey or clinical study.

Census of survey population

Unless a pre-existing sampling frame such as an up-to-date electoral roll is used, it will usually be necessary to perform a census immediately prior to the conduct of a survey. This defines the denominator prior to any additional sampling stages, and allows for assessment of response and representativeness of the final survey population. In a community or cluster survey the census will generally be on a house-to-house basis. In rural villages, and even in urban areas of under-developed countries where there may be no street and house number information, it will be necessary to allocate numbers to dwellings and to draw a map showing these houses in relation to each other and landmarks such as rivers, roads and school-buildings. These methods have been applied commonly in surveys of NIDDM in island nations of the Pacific region [9, 18, 19].

The name, age/birth-date, sex, and employer of all "usual residents" of each household who fall within the required age-range are enumerated [40]. At the time of the census verbal and, when appropriate, written information should be given to each household concerning the reasons for the survey and what it might entail for each individual.

Promotion, invitations and consent

Prominent members of the community such as local politicians, and village and church leaders should be approached for support in promoting the survey. Where feasible, newspaper advertisements, posters in survey areas, and radio and television announcements are also helpful. A few days prior to their appointment, individual households should be given an invitation letter listing the names of those eligible for the survey, and detailing instructions for fasting. Explanatory letters for employers can also be included at this time. If subjects are illiterate, invitations must be given verbally.

Where ethical clearance for a particular study requires written consent, it is usually most convenient to ask subjects to sign a consent form at the time they register for the survey. In non-literate societies, it may be reasonable to assume that attendance is sufficient indication of consent but, if necessary, thumb-prints can be taken.

Survey site and number of staff

The site chosen for survey activities will depend on factors such as: proximity and accessibility to the invited population; available facilities, including electricity, toilets and running water; and adequate space in relation to the range of procedures to be undertaken and the number of subjects to be invited at any one time. For large surveys, schools (during holidays) are especially suitable as procedures can be undertaken sequentially in different rooms, but community halls, health centres or even outdoor areas can be used, depending on circumstances.

Similarly, the number of staff required will vary depending on the scope of a particular survey. As previously described, the critical factors which determine staff numbers include the number of subjects invited per day, the time taken for each procedure, and the number of procedures [40]. As subjects are fasting, one should aim for the last subject to have completed all procedures, including the 2-hour blood collection, by midday. If few staff are available, then either fewer procedures should be undertaken, or fewer subjects should be invited each day.

Practical structures for surveys of NIDDM and cardiovascular disease have been described whereby 120–150 subjects could be comfortably surveyed, and plasma glucose measured and other specimens aliquotted and stored, by around midday, using 15–20 well trained staff [14, 40]. The range of procedures included in a study performed recently in Mauritius, and which

Table 2 Model flow-sheet for a large scale NIDDM field survey, requiring 15 – 20 team members and allowing 120 – 150 subjects to undertake 'core' procedures

Procedure	Number of staff
Core activities	
1. Registration	2 – 3
2. Venesection (fasting and 2-hour)	3
3. Glucose load	1
4. Height and weight	1
5. Waist and hip girth	1
6. Lean body mass[a]	1
7. General questionnaire[b]	1
8. Activity questionnaire[a]	1
9. Blood pressure	2
10. Electrocardiogram[a]	2
[11. Laboratory	2 – 4]
Complications screening[a] (all diabetic subjects and sample of IGT and normals: performed on day following core procedures)	
1. Early morning urine	–
2. Visual acuity and mydriasis	1
3. Vibration threshold	1
4. Retinal photography	1

[a] non-essential procedures, depending on population and resources
[b] general questionnaire: demographic details, socio-economic status, personal and family medical history, cigarette and alcohol consumption, simple index of physical activity

followed this model (but with two complete teams working independently in different survey locations), are listed in Table 2.

As another example, 5 – 6 team members could process 60 – 100 subjects per morning in the situation where only two-hour blood was collected, ECGs and special complications screening were not undertaken, and staff performed more than one procedure [40, 42].

Survey procedures

Descriptions of methodology for specific survey procedures such as those listed in Table 2 have been published previously [7, 23, 39, 40]. Only brief comments and less obvious practical suggestions concerning some of these procedures are outlined below.

Registration: It is usually advisable to allocate each responding subject a unique sequential survey number at this point, by recording their name and household number from the census book against the next number in the "daily register". This number is subsequently used on blood collection and serum aliquot tubes, electrocardiogram tracings, and so on. Attendance should also be ticked off in the census book and the newly allocated survey number should be cross-referenced there. These details are important for ensuring correct identification of responders, for issuing of re-invitations to non-responders, and ultimately for calculating response rates and characteristics of non-responders. Subjects should be given their survey forms at the registration station, and carry these with them as they move from station to station [40].

Venesection: In field survey conditions, particularly where blood is to be collected into two or more tubes containing different preservatives, the use of vacuum tube and multi-sample needle systems is preferred. In a standard survey of NIDDM prevalence and risk factors, it is usually sufficient to use a small (e. g. 2 ml draw) fluoridated tube for glucose estimation, and a larger (e. g. 10 ml for fasting, 5 ml for 2-hour) plain tube from which multiple aliquots of sera can be taken for lipids and routine automated biochemistry, insulin, and other variables of interest. Tubes collected at different times during the OGTT should be marked simply (e. g. "F" for fasting and "T" for two hour samples, alongside the subject's unique survey number).

Glucose load: For field studies where large numbers of subjects are being tested, and particularly in less developed countries, it is most convenient and least expensive to prepare large containers of the appropriate concentration of glucose solution on the evening prior to each day's testing. Dextrose monohydrate is easier to work with than anhydrous glucose. In urban and developed settings it may be possible to have this job performed in a hospital laboratory, but in remote areas, as long as there is a reliable water source available, pre-weighed bags of dextrose monohydrate powder can be used to make up solution in enclosed containers of known volume. Required equipment for the glucose load station includes a battery-operated digital clock; a jug; a measuring cylinder; a book to record survey number, time, and name; and sufficient disposable or washable cups of at least 250 ml volume [40].

As previously pointed out [2, 40], glucose loads containing either 75 g of anhydrous glucose or equivalent (the official recommendation of WHO [5]), or 75 g of dextrose monohydrate (equivalent to 68 g of the anhydrous form), have been commonly used in epidemiological studies. New studies should probably attempt to follow the WHO recommendations.

Blood pressure: As discussed elsewhere [23], and earlier in this review, strict attention should be paid to the training of blood pressure observers. Depending of preference, either random zero or standard sphygmomanometers can be used, but it is important to ensure an adequate cuff and bladder size. Routinely available cuffs are often too short, and it is preferable to use a longer cuff with a bladder which completely encircles the arm [23, 40].

Measurement of glucose: In general, the use of dry chemistry test strips and reflectance meters to measure glucose in epidemiological studies is not advised [43]. If there is no alternative, then there must be meticulous attention to training of observers and ongoing quality assurance checks throughout the survey [40, 43, 44]. Even so, at least in tropical climatic conditions, doubts remain as to the reliability of dry chemistry systems, and their use should be discouraged pending further evaluation [43, 45].

The preferred method is to measure the glucose, most usually in plasma, using reliable laboratory analysers. Where adequate laboratory-based equipment is available close to the survey site, such as in developed countries and in urban settings in some under-developed countries, separated plasma may be transported to that facility on the same day for glucose estimation using a variety of continuous auto-analysers and dedicated single sample analysers [43].

In remote locations, it may be necessary to freeze plasma samples for later measurement. However, experience has shown that glucose can be measured accurately and reliably in the field, even in relatively rugged and inaccessible parts of some Pacific island countries, using portable semi-automated machines which can be powered by generator if required [9, 19, 40]. The authors prefer this method as it allows results to be given to subjects within a day, ensures that results are not lost due to spoilage of specimens in storage or during transport, and allows subjects with abnormal results to be called back immediately for additional procedures such as complications screening with urine collection and retinal photography.

Whichever of the above options is preferred, it is still recommended that specimens for glucose estimation should be collected into fluoridated tubes on all occasions, and centrifuged immediately, in order to avoid the known deterioration in glucose concentration which follows collection (for the first 1 – 2 hours this occurs *irrespective* of the use of preservative) [43, 46]. Glucose can then be measured in separated fresh, cooled or frozen plasma, depending on the different strategies outlined above. Even if the intention is to centrifuge specimens immediately, keep them cool at 0 – 4 °C, or to measure glucose immediately in whole blood, any of which might obviate the use of preservatives, equipment failure or an unforeseen back-log of samples is always possible, and preservatives will guard against loss of glucose, at least after the first 1 – 2 hours following collection [43, 46].

Regular calibration of equipment, and internal and external quality assurance involving routine measurement of duplicate samples and use of low-normal-high control solutions are vital to ensure the accuracy and precision of glucose measurements in population research.

Genetic studies: Studies of the association between NIDDM and specific genes or gene markers are made difficult because of the possibility that controls may actually have the diabetic genotype, but have not yet expressed it. In cross-sectional studies it is possible to diminish this risk somewhat by choosing controls from elderly subjects shown to be normal on the glucose tolerance test, irrespective of the age of the cases. A method of integrating collection of blood samples for genetic studies into the fasting test, and avoiding additional venesection has been described previously [40].

Assessing complications

Cross-sectional versus longitudinal studies: Under field survey conditions it is usually necessary to make some compromises in technique to allow practical but standardized assessment of complications. Nevertheless, cross-sectional population surveys are valuable in defining the true spectrum of complications in the diabetic sub-population, as they detect undiagnosed complications in both previously known and newly-diagnosed diabetic subjects. However, the information from cross-sectional studies is biased against the more severe end of the spectrum, due to selective non-attendance in surveys by persons with severe complications, due to both disability and higher mortality rates relative to those with no or less severe complications.

Therefore, if resources permit, more complete information on the frequency of and risk factors for complications is provided by longitudinal studies where standardized tests such as urinary microalbumin and retinal photography can be repeated at regular intervals. Additionally, some form of surveillance should be instituted to detect important end-points. The nature of any surveillance system will depend on a number of factors, including the size and stability of the study cohort, the degree of sophistication and accessibility of the health record system, and the resources available to the investigators.

In countries where record linkage is possible via unique identity numbers it may be relatively straight-forward to track major end-points by computer, but in most cases effective surveillance will rely on regular (e. g. annual) personal contact with the subject. At this time changes to address, and events such as death, myocardial infarction, stroke and amputations can be recorded, along with details including the dates and place of hospitalisation or death, and the attending doctor's name. If the subject is dead, not available, or untraceable, then as much information as possible should be collected from relatives, neighbours, village chiefs, postal workers, or whichever local sources are most appropriate. Providing that proper consent for viewing of records has been collected at the beginning of the study, sources such as death certificates and medical records can then be traced for the purpose of validating diagnoses.

Macrovascular disease: Prevalent coronary heart disease is most commonly assessed by classification of electrocardiograms according to the Minnesota Code [23, 39, 40, 47]. In populations where they have been validated, questionnaires for assessing the frequency of angina and myocardial infarction may be used, with or without recording of the electrocardiogram [23]. There is usually little point in performing assessment of CHD in subjects younger than 35 years of age.

Past history of stroke can usually be adequately assessed by simple questions concerning the duration of typical signs and symptoms, and in many cases can be verified by residual disability. Similarly, any past history of amputation can be readily verified during a cross-sectional survey, although the usefulness of such data can be questioned. Methods of measuring peripheral blood flow are addressed elsewhere in this volume, but in general these techniques are not readily adaptable to epidemiological studies.

Microvascular disease: These assessments are performed infrequently in population surveys, probably related to the time-consuming nature of some of the tests, the extra resources required, and the relatively low yield of diabetics in many studies. However, at least from the public health view-point, some information on the frequency of these complications in the diabetic subpopulation is likely to be of interest in highlighting the magnitude of the problem in both known and newly-detected cases. This applies particularly in less developed countries where clinical care and compliance with treatment is often unsatisfactory, tertiary treatment facilities such as laser photocoagulation and renal dialysis are limited or non-existent, and clinical data on the frequency of complications are unavailable.

A successful strategy for integrating special complications screening tests into surveys has been to perform these only on subjects with diabetes, and if necessary on sub-samples of IGT and normal subjects [40]. As results of glucose tolerance tests will often not be available until after subjects have left the survey site, even when glucose is measured on-site, this means that selected subjects not previously known to be diabetic must be invited back on another day.

At the time subjects are issued with an invitation to return for further assessment such as retinal photography and/or ophthalmological examination, and tests of peripheral nerve function, it may be convenient to issue them with instructions and a jar for collection of urine, which can be returned at the time of their second attendance [40]. Although 24-hour or other timed collections are optimal as they permit calculation of the albumin excretion rate, early morning or casual specimens are more practical, and microalbumin concentration or microalbumin/creatinine ratio in such a specimen generally provides adequate information for epidemiological studies [15].

Retinopathy is best assessed by trained ophthalmologists, either during the survey using a standardized reporting form [7, 48], and/or by later reading of a standard series of retinal photographs [49, 50]. The latter have the particular advantages that results can be verified by an independent observer, and they are available for later comparison in longitudinal studies. Whichever system is used, it is important that the observers are masked as to the glucose tolerance status of the subject.

In large field surveys, it may not be practicable to take the full series of photographs recommended by Klein and associates [49, 50]. A workable alternative used recently by the authors in surveys in Western Samoa and Mauritius has been to take 45° stereo photographs in one eye only, in three fields (centred on disc, macula, and nasal to disc), and to grade the photographs according to Airlie House criteria [51]. Using this system, around 50 subjects could be photographed in one day by a single photographer, with an assistant to measure visual acuity and apply mydriatic drops.

While subjects waited for photography, a third observer measured vibration perception thresholds, as an index of peripheral sensory neuropathy, using a commercially available electronic instrument [52]. Simpler means of assessing vibration thresholds using a calibrated tuning fork are also available [53]. More complex methods of investigating diabetic neuropathy are discussed elsewhere in this volume, although these are not readily adapted to the field survey setting.

Conclusions

Epidemiological studies have contributed much to present knowledge of the aetiology, natural history and pathogenesis of NIDDM and its complications. Complementing basic, clinical, and genetic studies, an epidemiological approach will continue to contribute substantially to progress in understanding of this complex disease.

Particularly in epidemiological field surveys, it may be necessary to make some compromises in measurement methods, relative to those that might be applied in clinical laboratories. Nevertheless, it is essential to ensure that the methodology is sufficiently accurate and precise to produce meaningful results. This requires that techniques should be validated against standard methods, that there must be rigorous training of observers, and that quality assurance procedures should be applied at all stages.

References

[1] West KM. Epidemiology of diabetes and its vascular lesions. New York: Elsevier, 1978.
[2] Dowse GK, Zimmet PZ. The prevalence and incidence of non-insulin-dependent diabetes mellitus. In: Alberti KGMM, Mazze R, eds. Frontiers of diabetes research: current trends in non-insulin-dependent diabetes mellitus. Amsterdam: Elsevier, 1989; 37–59.
[3] National Diabetes Data Group. Classification and diagnosis of diabetes mellitus and other categories of glucose intolerance. Diabetes 1979; 28: 1039–1057.
[4] World Health Organization Expert Committee on Diabetes Mellitus. Second report. Technical Report Series 646. Geneva: WHO, 1980.
[5] World Health Organization Study Group. Diabetes Mellitus. Technical Report Series 727. Geneva: WHO, 1985.
[6] West KM. Standardization of definition, classification, and reporting in diabetes-related epidemiologic studies. Diabetes Care 1979; 2: 65–76.
[7] Bennett PH. Recommendations on the standardization of methods and reporting of tests for diabetes and its microvascular complications in epidemiologic studies. Diabetes Care 1979; 2: 98–104.
[8] Harris MI, Hadden WC, Knowler WC et al. International criteria for the diagnosis of diabetes and impaired glucose tolerance. Diabetes Care 1985; 8: 562–567.
[9] Zimmet P, Dowse G, Finch C et al. The epidemiology and natural history of NIDDM – lessons from the South Pacific. Diabetes/Metabolism Reviews 1990; 6: 91–124.
[10] King H, Rewers M, WHO Ad Hoc Diabetes Reporting Group. Global estimates for prevalence of diabetes mellitus and impaired glucose tolerance in adults. Diabetes Care 1993; 16: 157–177.
[11] WHO DIAMOND Project Group. The WHO multinational project for childhood diabetes – DIAMOND: Diabetes Mondiale. Diabetes Care 1990; 13: 1062–1068.
[12] Glatthaar C, Welborn TA, Stenhouse NS et al. Diabetes and impaired glucose tolerance: a prevalence estimate based on the Busselton 1981 survey. Med J Aust 1985; 143: 436–440.
[13] Harris MI, Hadden WC, Knowler WC et al. Prevalence of diabetes and impaired glucose tolerance and plasma glucose levels in US population aged 20–74 yr. Diabetes 1987; 36: 523–534.

[14] Dowse GK, Gareeboo H, Zimmet PZ et al. High prevalence of NIDDM and impaired glucose tolerance in Indian, Creole and Chinese Mauritians. Diabetes 1990; 39: 390–396.
[15] Collins VR, Dowse GK, Finch CF et al. Prevalence and risk factors for micro- and macro-albuminuria in diabetic subjects and entire population of Nauru. Diabetes 1989; 38: 1602–1610.
[16] Tuomilehto J, Li N, Dowse G et al. The prevalence of coronary heart disease in the multi-ethnic and high diabetes prevalence population of Mauritius. J Internal Med 1993; 233: 187–194.
[17] Bulpitt CJ. Randomised controlled clinical trials. The Hague: Martinus Nijhoff, 1983.
[18] Zimmet P, Faaiuso S, Ainuu J et al. The prevalence of diabetes in the rural and urban Polynesian population of Western Samoa. Diabetes 1981; 30: 45–51.
[19] Zimmet P, Taylor R, Ram P et al. Prevalence of diabetes and impaired glucose tolerance in the biracial (Melanesian and Indian) population of Fiji: a rural-urban comparison. Am J Epidemiol 1983; 118: 673–688.
[20] McLarty D, Swai ABM, Kitange HM et al. Prevalence of diabetes and impaired glucose tolerance in rural Tanzania. Lancet 1989; 1: 871–875.
[21] Armitage P, Berry G. Statistical methods in medical research. 2nd ed. Oxford: Blackwell Scientific Publications, 1987.
[22] Welborn TA, Glatthaar C, Whittall D et al. An estimate of diabetes prevalence from a national population sample: a male excess. Med J Aust 1989; 150: 78–81.
[23] Rose GA, Blackburn H, Gillum RF et al. Cardiovascular survey methods. 2nd ed. WHO Monograph Series No. 56. Geneva: WHO, 1982.
[24] Ostbye T, Welby TJ, Prior IAM et al. Type 2 (non-insulin-dependent) diabetes mellitus, migration and westernization. The Tokelau Island migrant study. Diabetologia 1989; 32: 585–590.
[25] Taylor R, Bennett P, Uili R et al. Diabetes in Wallis Polynesians: a comparison of residents of Wallis Island and first generation migrants to Noumea, New Caledonia. Diabetes Res Clin Practice 1985; 1: 169–178.
[26] Kawate R, Yamakido M, Nishimoto Y et al. Diabetes mellitus and its vascular complications in Japanese migrants on the island of Hawaii. Diabetes Care 1979; 2: 161–170.
[27] Taylor R, Zimmet P. Migrant studies in diabetes epidemiology. In: Mann JI, Pyorala K, Teuscher A, eds. Diabetes in epidemiological perspective. Edinburgh: Churchill Livingstone, 1983: 58–77.
[28] Thai C, Yeo PPB, Lun KC et al. Changing prevalence of diabetes mellitus in Singapore over a ten year period. In: Vannasaeng S, Nitianant W, Chandraprasert S, eds. Epidemiology of diabetes mellitus: proceedings of the International Symposium on Epidemiology of Diabetes Mellitus. Bangkok: Crystal House Press, 1987; 63–67.
[29] Tai TY, Yang CL, Chang CJ et al. Epidemiology of diabetes mellitus among adults in Taiwan, ROC. In: Vannasaeng S, Nitianant W, Chandraprasert S, eds. Epidemiology of diabetes mellitus: proceedings of the International Symposium on Epidemiology of Diabetes Mellitus. Bangkok: Crystal House Press, 1987; 42–48.
[30] Pan X-R, Hu Y-H, Li G-W et al. Impaired glucose tolerance and its relationship to ECG-indicated coronary heart disease and risk factors among Chinese. Da Qing IGT and diabetes study. Diabetes Care 1993; 16: 150–156.
[31] Omar MAK, Seedat MA, Dyer RB et al. The prevalence of diabetes mellitus in a large group of South African Indians. S Afr Med J 1985; 67: 924–926.
[32] Guest C, O'Dea K, Hopper JL et al. The prevalence of glucose intolerance in Aborigines and Europids of south-eastern Australia. Diabetes Res Clin Practice 1992; 15: 227–235.
[33] Knowler WC, Bennett PH, Hamman RF et al. Diabetes incidence and prevalence in Pima Indians: a 19-fold greater incidence than in Rochester, Minnesota. Am J Epidemiol 1978; 108: 497–505.
[34] Bogardus C, Lillioja S, Nyomba BL et al. Distribution of in vivo insulin action in Pima Indians as mixture of three normal distributions. Diabetes 1989; 38: 1723–1732.

[35] Saad MF, Lillioja S, Nyomba BL et al. Racial differences in the relation between blood pressure and insulin resistance. N Engl J Med 1991; 324: 733–739.
[36] Serjeantson SW, Owerbach D, Zimmet P et al. Genetics of diabetes in Nauru: effects of foreign admixture, HLA antigens and the insulin-gene-linked polymorphism. Diabetologia 1983; 25: 13–17.
[37] Gardner LI, Stern MP, Haffner SM et al. Prevalence of diabetes in Mexican Americans: relationship to percent of gene pool derived from native American sources. Diabetes 1984; 33: 86–92.
[38] Williams DRR, Moffitt PS, Fisher JS et al. Diabetes and glucose tolerance in New South Wales coastal Aborigines: possible effects of non-Aboriginal genetic admixture. Diabetologia 1978; 30: 72–77.
[39] Rose G, Keen H, Jarrett J. Epidemiologic methods in diabetic macrovascular disease. Diabetes Care 1979; 2: 91–97.
[40] Dowse GK, Zimmet PZ. A model protocol for a diabetes and other noncommunicable disease field survey. World Health Stat Q 1992; 45: 360–372.
[41] Research and Evaluation Department. National health survey, 1992. Highlights of main survey findings. Singapore: Ministry of Health, 1993.
[42] King H, Finch C, Collins A et al. Glucose tolerance in Papua New Guinea: ethnic differences associated with environmental and behavioural factors and the possible emergence of glucose intolerance in a highland community. Med J Aust 1989; 151: 204–210.
[43] Burrin JM, Alberti KGMM. What is blood glucose: can it be measured? Diabetic Med 1990; 7: 199–206.
[44] Campbell EM, Redman S, Dunkley PR et al. The use of portable blood glucose monitors by trained lay operators. Med J Aust 1992; 157: 446–448.
[45] Ducorps M, Papoz L, Cuisinier-Raynal JC et al. Reliability of glucose measurement by glucose test strips in tropical conditions. Diabetes Res Clin Practice 1992; 17: 51–54.
[46] Chan AYW, Swaminathan R, Cockram CS. Effectiveness of sodium fluoride as a preservative of glucose in blood. Clin Chem 1989; 35: 315–317.
[47] Nan L, Tuomilehto J, Dowse G et al. Electrocardiographic abnormalities and associated factors in Chinese living in Beijing and in Mauritius. Br Med J 1992; 304: 1596–1601.
[48] King H, Balkau B, Zimmet P et al. Diabetic retinopathy in Nauruans. Am J Epidemiol 1983; 117: 659–667.
[49] Diabetic Retinopathy Study Research Group. A modification of the Airlie House classification of diabetic retinopathy. Diabetic retinopathy study report No. 7. Invest Ophthalmol Vis Sci 1981; 21: 210–226.
[50] Klein R, Klein BEK, Moss SE et al. The Wisconsin epidemiologic study of diabetic retinopathy. II. Prevalence and risk of diabetic retinopathy when age at diagnosis is less than 30 years. Arch Ophthalmol 1984; 102: 520–526.
[51] Plehwe WE, Dowse, GK, Zimmet et al. A high prevalence of diabetic retinopathy in Western Samoa (Abstract). Proceedings, Australian Diabetes Society, 1992.
[52] Wiles PG, Pearce SM, Rice PJS et al. Vibration perception threshold: influence of age, height, sex, and smoking, and calculation of centile values. Diabetic Med 1991; 8: 157–161.
[53] Thivolet C, Farkh JE, Potlot A et al. Measuring vibration sensations with graduated tuning fork. Simple and reliable means to detect diabetic patients at risk of neuropathic foot ulceration. Diabetes Care 1990; 13: 1077–1080.

Methodological concerns in diagnosing the prediabetic state

S. M. Haffner

Introduction

Interest in the possible diagnosis of the prediabetic state has increased in recent years. The precise identification of the prediabetic state may aid in studies of aetiology such as the relative importance of insulin secretion versus insulin resistance in the pathogenesis of non-insulin-dependent diabetes. While both of these defects occur in the established subjects with non-insulin-dependent diabetes mellitus (NIDDM) [1], which one is primary is still hotly debated [2, 3]. Identification of the precise metabolic lesion in the prediabetic state may help to screen potential candidate genes for NIDDM.

Identification of the prediabetic state may also help in patient counseling. Subjects at particularly high risk of diabetes may need special interventions to prevent diabetes. This may be especially important since some data suggest that the risk of cardiovascular disease, the major cause of death in NIDDM, is as great in newly discovered diabetic subjects as in subjects with longer duration of diabetes [4–6]. Thus intervention before the onset of the diabetic state may be important in the prevention of the excess risk of coronary heart disease in NIDDM. The National Institute of Health will start a 5-year multicenter trial in 3,000 subjects with impaired glucose tolerance to prevent diabetes in 1994.

The optimal approach to understand the prediabetic state would be to study subjects longitudinally. However, in most populations the annual rate of conversion to NIDDM is low and so many subjects must be followed for several years to obtain enough converters for statistical analysis. Some types of metabolic studies (such as glucose potentiation) [7] are expensive and thus not suitable for the large numbers of subjects required for a longitudinal study. Thus a number of alternative approaches to gain information on the prediabetic state have been used. I will review risk factors for diabetes identified through a number of methods, including:

Offprint from
Research Methodologies in Human Diabetes — Part 1

1. Longitudinal studies.
2. Non-diabetic subjects with a parental history of diabetes.
3. Non-diabetic subjects in high risk populations for NIDDM.
4. Insulin Resistance Syndrome.
5. Impaired glucose tolerance.
6. Upper-body adiposity.
7. Multivariate predicting equations.

Longitudinal studies

Several studies have examined risk factors for NIDDM prospectively. Impaired glucose tolerance has been related to the incidence of NIDDM [8–13]. In addition, elevated insulin concentration has been a strong predictor of the incidence of NIDDM [10–14]. The latter studies suggest that insulin resistance may be a risk factor for the development of NIDDM, since in non-diabetic subjects, insulin concentrations and insulin resistance are very highly correlated ($r = -.6$ to $-.7$) [15, 16]. Insulin resistance as measured by the euglycaemic clamp has been associated with increased risk of NIDDM in Pima Indians [17]. Similarly, insulin resistance as measured by the intravenous glucose tolerance has been associated with increased risk of NIDDM in Caucasian children of two diabetic parents [18]. In the same population, low non-insulin mediated glucose disposal also predicted the incidence of NIDDM [19]. In a study of Japanese men, increased C-peptide but not insulin concentrations predicted the incidence of NIDDM [20].

Overall adiposity has also been associated with an increased risk of diabetes in Pima Indians [10], Nauruans [11], Caucasians [13, 14], Mexican Americans [12], Swedish men [21] and Swedish women [22]. In several of the studies, the effect of obesity was not statistically independent of insulin and glucose concentrations [10–12] suggesting that the effect of obesity was to make individuals more insulin resistant. In addition, an unfavorable body fat distribution ("apple shaped adiposity") has been shown to predict NIDDM in Finnish men and women [13] and Swedish men [21] and women [22]. Increased subscapular-to-triceps skinfold ratio also predicts NIDDM in Mexican Americans [12]. Increased visceral fat as measured by computerized axial tomography predicts NIDDM in Japanese American men [20].

Relatively fewer studies have examined the role of physical activity. Physical activity has also been associated with a decreased risk of NIDDM [23, 24]. The effect of physical activity was independent of baseline adiposity.

A number of other metabolic abnormalities have been associated with an increased risk of developing NIDDM. Decreased levels of sex hormone binding globulin (an indirect measure of androgenicity [25]) have been associated with increased conversion to NIDDM in women [26, 27] but not in men. Nestler has recently proposed that sex hormone binding globulin may be a marker for insulin resistance [28].

Prediabetic subjects have increased blood pressure and triglyceride and decreased high density lipoprotein cholesterol concentration prior to the onset of diabetes [29, 30], suggesting increased risk of cardiovascular disease even prior to the onset of clinical elevations in blood sugar. Traditionally, the major risk factors for microvascular complications (retinopathy and nephropathy) were thought to be mainly dependent on hyperglycaemia and to some extent on hypertension [4, 6]. Recently, increased albumin excretion, traditionally associated with microvascular complications, has been shown to predict the onset of NIDDM thus suggesting that it may also form part of the prediabetic state. Thus, the traditional distinctions between risk factors for microvascular and macrovascular complications may be less clear than previously thought [31]. As the above material suggests, risk factors for the development of NIDDM are similar in high risk populations for NIDDM [9–12, 20] and lower risk Caucasian populations [13, 14].

Parental history of diabetes

In a number of populations, it has been reported that the prevalence of NIDDM in the offspring of two NIDDM parents may reach 60–70% [18, 32, 33]. Thus, comparing non-diabetic subjects with a very strong family history of diabetes to non-diabetic subjects without a family history of diabetes represents an indirect approach to the study of precursors of diabetes. Since the numbers of subjects can be small, this approach offers the possibility of using very sophisticated metabolic ward studies. Also, cases (subjects with a family history of diabetes) and controls (subjects without a family history of diabetes) can be matched on important confounding variables such as obesity and body fat distribution.

In a population-based study, insulin concentrations have been shown to be higher in non-diabetic subjects with a parental history of diabetes than in non-diabetic subjects without such a history [34]. Similarly, normoglycaemic subjects with two diabetic parents have decreased non-oxidative glucose disposal but relatively normal glucose oxidation and hepatic glucose production [35, 36] relative to normoglycaemic subjects without a family history of diabetes. This suggests that a defect in non-oxidative glucose disposal may represent a very early lesion in the etiology of NIDDM. Insulin resistance has been shown to be strongly familial in Pima Indians [37]. However, one study found an increase in hepatic glucose production in non-diabetic subjects with a family history of diabetes [38]. O'Rahilly et al [39] has suggested that the earliest lesion in individuals who are first degree relations of NIDDM patients is a loss of pulsatile insulin secretion. Because insulin is biologically more effective when delivered in pulses [40], this defect might have important pathogenic consequences.

Non-diabetic subjects in high risk populations for NIDDM

One inexpensive way to examine possible risk factors for the development of NIDDM is to examine non-diabetic subjects in high and low risk populations for NIDDM. Presumably, the non-diabetic subjects in the high risk population for NIDDM will contain a larger number of genetically susceptible individuals than in the low risk population. This type of study is ecological in nature and is limited because it deals with characteristics of populations rather characteristics of individuals. Thus, only weak inferences can be made from this type of study. A number of studies have shown that non-diabetic subjects in high risk populations such as Pima Indians [41], Mexican Americans [42] and Nauruans [43] are hyperinsulinaemic compared to low risk Caucasian populations. Recently, high insulin and C-peptide were shown in Hispanics [44]. Increased insulin resistance has been shown in Pima Indians by the euglycaemic clamp [45, 46] and in Mexican Americans by the intravenous glucose test compared to NHWs matched for obesity [47]. In addition, increased first phase insulin secretion and decreased hepatic clearance of insulin was observed in Mexican Americans using the frequently sampled intravenous glucose test with C-peptide kinetics [48]. All of the ecological studies of insulin concentrations and insulin resistance have shown high risk populations to have insulin resistance rather than impaired insulin secretion. The high risk populations were all obese and frequently had an unfavorable body fat distribution [41 – 44]. However, in these studies, statistical control for differences in obesity or matching for obesity was done.

The Insulin Resistance Syndrome ("Syndrome X")

Reaven suggested in his 1988 Banting Lecture that insulin resistance may underlie a cluster of related diseases including impaired glucose tolerance, coronary heart disease, hypertension and dyslipidaemia (especially increased triglyceride and decreased high density lipoprotein cholesterol) [49]. A number of cross-sectional studies have suggested an association of hyperinsulinaemia and insulin resistance with cardiovascular disease and risk factors studies

Table 1 Prevalence of clusters of impaired glucose tolerance (IGT), hypertriglyceridemia (hyper TG), low HDL-cholesterol (low HDL), and hypertension (HT), risk of developing non-insulin-dependent diabetes mellitus in various clusters of these risk factors, and plasma insulin level in various risk factor clusters: Kuopio, eastern Finland, 1986 – 1991

	Prevalence			2-hour plasma insulin
	% (cases)	OR*	95% CI	(pmol/l)
No risk factors	30.2 (269)	1.00	–	232 ± 11
Clusters of two risk factors				
Low HDL and HT	10.3 (92)	7.40	3.07 – 17.8	835 ± 68
HyperTG and HT	8.1 (72)	9.32	3.80 – 22.8	974 ± 89
HyperTG and low HDL	6.1 (54)	10.3	4.04 – 26.5	975 ± 108
IGT and HT	15.7 (140)	11.7	5.28 – 26.0	903 ± 52
IGT and low HDL	5.4 (48)	17.9	7.14 – 44.9	1152 ± 111
IGT and hyperTG	4.6 (41)	28.2	11.1 – 71.7	1200 ± 127
Clusters of three risk factors				
HyperTG and low HDL and HT	3.7 (33)	12.2	4.32 – 34.6	1077 ± 151
IGT and low HDL and HT	3.4 (30)	28.5	10.4 – 78.0	1202 ± 155
IGT and hyperTG and HT	3.5 (31)	30.6	11.3 – 82.8	1210 ± 153
IGT and hyperTG and low HDL	2.5 (22)	39.1	12.1 – 117	1394 ± 209
Cluster of four risk factors				
IGT and hyperTG and low HDL and HT	1.6 (14)	58.7	16.0 – 215	1520 ± 289

* OR, odds ratio compares odds of developing NIDDM for subjects with a stated risk factor cluster to odds for subjects with no risk factors.
CI, confidence interval.
Reproduced with the permission of Diabetologia (reference [13]).

[50 – 57], although the association of insulin resistance with hypertension remains controversial [58 – 61]. Only two studies had considered the Insulin Resistance Syndrome [IRS] in a prospective fashion. Mykkänen et al. [13] considered four possible components of the IRS (hypertension, impaired glucose tolerance, low HDL cholesterol and high triglyceride) as predictors of the incidence of NIDDM in elderly Finnish subjects (Table 1). There was a stepwise increase in the risk of developing NIDDM with increasing numbers of IRS-related metabolic disorders at baseline. Subjects with all four disorders related to the IRS had a 58.7 fold increased risk of NIDDM compared to subjects with no IRS-related disorders at baseline (Table 1). The increase in IRS-related disorders was paralleled by higher insulin concentrations at baseline. In another prospective study [62] increased insulin concentrations were observed at baseline in subjects who subsequently developed several disorders related to the IRS as opposed to those who developed only one IRS related disorder. Thus, the existence of multiple metabolic disorders related to the IRS is associated with a very high probability of developing NIDDM.

Recent interest has focused on the possible role of proinsulin in the Insulin Resistance Syndrome. Many of the studies describing the association of insulin resistance and/or hyperinsulinaemia with cardiovascular risk factors have been limited by the fact that insulin was measured with an assay that cross reacts with proinsulin. Temple et al. [63] have suggested that proinsulin comprises the majority of circulating immunoreactive insulin in subjects with NIDDM. Several studies have suggested that proinsulin is disproportionately elevated in subjects with NIDDM [64, 65]. Furthermore, proinsulin is more strongly associated with cardiovascular risk factors in diabetic subjects than is insulin [66]. In non-diabetic subjects, both proinsulin and insulin (measured by a specific RIA which does not cross react with proinsulin) are both associated with metabolic disorders linked to the Insulin Resistance Syndrome [67] suggesting that contamination of conventional insulin assays with proinsulin does not explain the previously reported associations between insulin concentrations and cardiovascular risk factors. In non-diabetic subjects, an increased fasting proinsulin/insulin ratio was observed in subjects with multiple metabolic disorders [68] suggesting a selective increase in proinsulin relative to insulin in the Insulin Resistance Syndrome.

Impaired glucose tolerance

Impaired glucose tolerance is one of the most consistent predictors of the development of NIDDM [8–13]. In middle-aged Caucasian populations, the rate of conversion to diabetes is about 15% during a 5–10 year interval [9, 14, 69]. In high risk populations such as Pima Indians [10] and Nauruans [9], the rate of conversion to NIDDM is about 25% over 5 years. However, even in lower risk populations the rate of conversion to NIDDM from IGT is very high in elderly subjects (23% in 3.5 years in a study from Finland [13]). In the Finnish study [13], more than two thirds of subjects who become diabetic had impaired glucose tolerance at baseline, whereas the subjects with impaired glucose tolerance comprised only 20% of all subjects at baseline.

Subjects with impaired glucose tolerance also have increased cardiovascular risk factors including dyslipidaemia (especially elevated triglyceride and decreased HDL cholesterol levels) and increased blood pressure [70, 71]. These subjects also have increased overall adiposity [9–11] and an unfavorable body fat distribution [72]. Although subjects with impaired glucose tolerance have relatively normal LDL cholesterol levels, they have altered LDL composition (increased small dense LDL [71]) which may also increase their risk of atherosclerosis [73, 74].

Visceral fat

Upper body adiposity has been associated with increased glucose and insulin concentrations in both metabolic ward studies [75, 76] and population-based studies [77, 78]. Increased waist-to-hip ratio has also been associated with insulin resistance in a number of studies [75, 79, 80]. In the two studies which utilized indirect calorimetry together with the hyperinsulinaemic euglycaemic clamp, upper body adiposity was associated with non-oxidative glucose disposal rather than glucose oxidation in women [79] and men [80]. As mentioned previously, this is the pattern of insulin resistance observed in non-diabetic relatives of NIDDM subjects [35, 36] thus further suggesting that unfavorable body fat distribution is an important part of the prediabetic state. An unfavorable body fat distribution has also been associated with an increased incidence of NIDDM in Swedish women [22] and men [21], Japanese men [20], Mexican Americans [12] and elderly Finnish subjects [13]. An unfavorable body fat distribution is also associated with lipoprotein abnormalities [16, 77, 78, 81] and hypertension [78].

Recent interest has focused on visceral fat as possibly being more metabolically active than subcutaneous abdominal fat [82, 83]. In some studies, visceral adiposity was much more strongly associated with insulin concentrations [20] or insulin resistance [84, 85] than was subcutaneous fat. A number of mechanisms specific to visceral fat may be important in increasing risk of diabetes. An enlarged portal fat tissue depot results in high concentrations of portal vein free fatty acids [86]. High concentrations of portal free fatty acids can cause an increased hepatic secretion of very low density lipoproteins [87]. Furthermore, exposure of the liver to high portal concentrations of free fatty acids will also increase hepatic production of glucose by stimulating gluconeogenesis [88, 89]. In isolated hepatocytes, free fatty acids inhibit insulin binding, degradation, and function [90]. Decreased hepatic clearance of insulin is associated with increased abdominal adiposity in premenopausal women [91]. The latter observation suggests another reason why subjects with abdominal adiposity might have increased insulin concentrations in addition to increased insulin secretion compensatory to increased insulin resistance.

Upper body adiposity is also associated with a variety of changes in sex hormones. In premenopausal women, abdominal adiposity is associated with decreased sex hormone binding globulin and increased free testosterone [92,

93]. In contrast, increased upper body adiposity is associated with *decreased* testosterone concentrations in men [76, 80]. The latter observation may help explain why low levels of sex hormone binding globulin predict the incidence of NIDDM in women [26, 27] but not in men [27].

Multivariate predicting equations

Although impaired glucose tolerance has classically been the most important risk factor for the development of NIDDM [8–13], it has a number of limitations. The oral glucose tolerance test is known to have considerable intraindividual variability [94–97]. Administration of oral glucose is burdensome to patients in terms of expense, time, and sometimes unpleasant side effects. In addition, impaired glucose tolerance most likely represents a heterogeneous disorder [98]. Subjects who display impaired glucose tolerance on a given occasion may represent not only subjects with persistently impaired

Table 2 Multivariate predicting equations for the 8-year incidence of NIDDM based on the San Antonio Heart Study

Equations for the various predicting models are as follows:

1. Optimal model, overall population (n = 1272):
$$\text{Ln}(P/1\text{-}P) = -16.8547 + (0.0909 \times FPG) + (0.0237 \times 2\text{-}hPG) + (0.0966 \times BMI) + (-0.0397 \times HDL) + (0.0318 \times PPr)$$
2. Reduced model*, overall population (n = 1453):
$$\text{Ln}(P/1\text{-}P) = -15.6863 + (0.1120 \times FPG) + (0.1008 \times BMI) + (-0.0477 \times HDL) + (0.0433 \times PPr) + (-0.8659 \times sex)$$
3. Reduced model, men (n = 612):
$$\text{Ln}(P/1\text{-}P) = -12.9642 + (0.0936 \times FPG) + (0.0614 \times PPr) + (-0.0443 \times HDL) + (0.8707 \times HT)$$
4. Reduced model, women (n = 841):
$$\text{Ln}(P/1\text{-}P) = -19.6987 + (0.1295 \times FPG) + (0.1029 \times BMI) + (-0.0519 \times HDL) + (0.0382 \times SBP) + (-1.1159 \times HT)$$
5. Reduced model, Mexican American (n = 825):
$$\text{Ln}(P/1\text{-}P) = -19.1121 + (0.1107 \times FPG) + (0.0983 \times BMI) + (-0.9800 \times sex) + (0.6915 \times LnTG)$$
6. Reduced model, non-Hispanic white (n = 628):
$$\text{Ln}(P/1\text{-}P) = -22.6261 + (0.1170 \times FPG) + (0.0691 \times SBP) + (-0.0605 \times HDL) + (0.0982 \times BMI)$$

Where 2-hPG = 2-h plasma glucose (mg/dl): Ln = natural log; sex: 1 = male, 0 = female; HT = hypertension (1 = present, 2 = absent); FPG (mg/dl); BMI (kg/m^2); HDL (mg/dl); SBP (mmHg); pulse pressures (PPr) (mmHg).

* "Reduced" models excluded non-clinical variables, specifically, insulin, skinfolds, and post glucose load values.

Reproduced with the permission of Diabetes (reference [99]).

glucose tolerance, but also subjects who may actually have diabetes but have lower glucose levels on the day of the examination as well as subjects whose glucose tolerance is normal, but happens to fall in the upper range of the normal plasma glucose distribution [98]. Thus, many subjects with impaired glucose tolerance category may represent individuals who will ultimately regress to the mean of either the diabetic or the normoglycaemic distribution. If this is true, one might expect that subjects with impaired glucose tolerance would be more likely to progress to NIDDM if they came from a high risk population for NIDDM than if they came from a low risk population.

To avoid some of the problems in using impaired glucose tolerance, Stern et al have developed multivariate predicting equations based on 1485 subjects in the eight-year follow-up of the San Antonio Heart Study [99]. For all multivariate models, the stepwise process selected a mixture of anthropometric, glycaemic, lipid and haemodynamic variables (Table 2). The top 15% of the risk continuum for each model was defined as high risk to compare the performance of the models with the performance of impaired glucose tolerance (15% prevalence) as a predictor of diabetes. The relative risk of being high

Table 3 Test parameters for overall and sex- and ethnic-specific IGT and reduced models for the development of type 2 diabetes. San Antonio Heart Study (8-year follow-up)

	Overall population	Men	Women	Mexican American	Non-Hispanic white
IGT models					
n	1419	604	815	796	623
Sensitivity (%)	59.2	62.1	57.4	60.4	56.5
Specificity (%)	87.3	88.3	86.6	86.1	88.8
Percentage correctly classified	85.8	87.1	84.9	84.4	87.6
Predictive value of a positive test (%)	20.9	21.2	20.8	23.7	16.3
Predictive value of a negative test (%)	97.4	97.9	97.1	96.8	98.2
RR	8.04	10.0	7.11	7.46	8.82
Reduced models					
n	1453	612	841	825	628
Sensitivity (%)	69.6	67.7	81.3	72.7	83.3
Specificity (%)	88.1	88.0	88.0	87.0	89.9
Percentage correctly classified	87.1	86.9	87.6	86.1	89.6
Predictive value of a positive test (%)	25.2	23.1	29.1	28.6	24.7
Predictive value of a negative test (%)	98.1	98.1	98.7	97.8	99.3
RR	13.26	12.16	22.38	13.00	35.29

* n for IGT models slightly smaller than for corresponding reduced models, as a result of missing values for 2-h plasma glucose concentrations.
Reproduced with the permission of Diabetes (reference [99]).

risk ranged from 12.2 to 35.3 whereas the relative risk of having impaired glucose tolerance ranged from 7.1 to 10.0 (Table 3). The sensitivity of the multiple logistic regression models ranged from 68% to 82% compared with 57% to 62% for impaired glucose tolerance and the positive predictive values of the multivariate models ranged from 23 to 29% compared to 16–24% for IGT. The results indicate that multivariate predictive models perform at least as well, if not better than, impaired glucose tolerance in predicting NIDDM, but need not require an oral glucose load. These predicting equations need to be tested in other populations.

Conclusions

We have shown that using a variety of approaches to define the prediabetic state there is remarkable similarity between the risk factors identified by each approach. In almost all cases, increased glucose and insulin concentrations or insulin resistance, obesity and an abnormal body fat distribution are identified as strong risk factors for NIDDM. A selective decrease in non-oxidative glucose disposal has been identified both from studies of non-diabetic relatives of NIDDM subjects and studies of patients with increased visceral fat. It has been more difficult to identify abnormalities in insulin secretion in prediabetic subjects but this may be because some of secretory defects (loss of glucose potentiation, loss of insulin pulsatility, etc.) require more sophisticated assessment techniques than other potential risk factors.

The choice of methods to identify the prediabetic state may therefore depend on the goal of a particular study. Longitudinal studies, of course, would be preferred because only in this case is the investigator certain that the subject is actually prediabetic. However, the period of follow-up is likely to be prolonged and large numbers of subjects are required since in most studies the rate of conversion to NIDDM is low. Thus, longitudinal studies are not likely to be appropriate for expensive metabolic ward techniques. For metabolic ward studies, comparing non-diabetic subjects with a strong family history of diabetes to non-diabetic subjects without a family history of diabetes would be desirable. For clinical purposes, in preventing the development of NIDDM in high risk subjects, selecting subjects by IGT status, multivariate models and the occurrence of two or more Insulin Resistance Syndrome related metabolic disorders are particularly attractive. As discussed in the previous section, impaired glucose tolerance has a number of limitations including poor reproducibility, administration of a glucose load and lower sensitivity than multivariate predicting models. However, further tests of the performance of multivariate models are needed. Lastly, the selection of subjects with an unfavorable body fat distribution (such as high waist-to-hip ratio) as an initial screen is useful since it does not require blood sampling. This measurement could be combined with questions about parental history of diabetes. After the initial screening, subjects with upper body adiposity could be referred for fasting blood measurements of lipids and lipoproteins, glucose and insulin concentrations to further define their risk for developing diabetes.

A second issue is that prediabetic subjects, by most of the definitions we have considered in this report, have been shown to have increased risk factors for cardiovascular disease, including dyslipidaemia and elevated blood pressure and in some cases, increased cardiovascular disease itself. This suggests that interventions armed at reducing the risk of NIDDM should also include measures to reduce the risk of cardiovascular disease.

References

[1] DeFronzo RA. Lilly Lecture 1987: the triumvirate: β-cell, muscle, liver: a collusion responsible for NIDDM. Diabetes 1988; 37: 667–687.

[2] Cerasi E, Efendic S, Luft R. Dose-response relation between plasma insulin and blood glucose levels in prediabetic subjects. Lancet 1973; 1: 794–797.

[3] Reaven GM, Bernstein R, Davis B et al. Nonketotic diabetes mellitus: insulin deficiency or insulin resistance? Am J Med 1976; 60: 80–88.

[4] West KM; Ahoja MMS, Bennett PH et al. The role of circulating glucose and triglyceride concentrations and their interactions with other "risk factors" as determinants of arterial disease in nine diabetic population samples from the WHO Multinational Study. Diabetes Care 1983; 6: 361–369.

[5] Fuller JH, Shipley MJ, Rose G et al. Coronary heart disease risk and impaired glucose tolerance: the Whitehall Study. Lancet 1980; 1: 1373–1376.

[6] Haffner SM, Stern MP, Rewers M. Diabetes and atherosclerosis: epidemiologic considerations in diabetes and atherosclerosis: molecular basis and clinical aspects. New York: Elsevier, 1993; 229–254.

[7] Porte D. β-cells in type 2 diabetes mellitus. Banting Lecture 1990. Diabetes 1991; 40: 166–180.

[8] Jarrett RJ, Keen H, Fuller JH et al. Worsening of diabetes in men with impaired glucose tolerance ("borderline diabetes"). Diabetolgoia 1979; 16: 25–30.

[9] King H, Zimmet P, Roper LR et al. The natural history of impaired glucose tolerance in the Micronesian population of Naurau: A six-year follow-up study. Diabetologia 1984; 26: 39–43.

[10] Saad MF, Knowler WC, Pettitt DJ et al. The natural history of impaired glucose tolerance in the Pima Indians. N Engl J Med 1986; 319: 1500–1506.

[11] Sicree RA, Zimmet PZ, King HVM et al. Plasma insulin response among Nauruans. Prediction of deterioration in glucose tolerance over 6 years. Diabetes 1987; 36: 179–186.

[12] Haffner SM, Stern MP, Mitchell BD et al. Incidence of type 2 diabetes in Mexican Americans predicted by fasting insulin and glucose levels, obesity, and body fat distribution. Diabetes 1990; 39: 283–288.

[13] Mykkänen L, Kuusisto J, Pyörälä K et al. Cardiovascular disease risk factors as predictors of type 2 (non-insulin-dependent) diabets mellitus in elderly subjects. Diabetologia 1993; 36: 553–559.

[14] Charles MA, Fontbonne A, Thibault N et al. Risk factors for NIDDM in white population. Paris Prospective Study. Diabetes 1991; 40: 796–799.
[15] Hollenbeck CB, Chen N, Chen YDI et al. Relationship between the plasma insulin response to oral glucose and insulin stimulated glucose utilization in normal subjects. Diabetes 1984; 33: 460–463.
[16] Mykkänen L, Haffner SM, Rönnemaa T et al. Is there a sex difference in the association of plasma insulin level and insulin sensitivity with serum lipids and lipoproteins? Metabolism, in press.
[17] Bogardus C, Lillioja S, Foley J et al. Insulin resistance predicts the incidence of non-insulin dependent diabetes mellitus in Pima Indians (Abstract). Diabetes 1987; 36 (Suppl. 1): 47A.
[18] Warram JH, Martin BC, Krolewski AS et al. Slow glucose-removal rate and hyperinsulinemia precede the development of type 2 diabetes in offspring with diabetic parents. Ann Intern Med 1990; 113: 909–915.
[19] Martin BC, Warram JH, Krolewski AS et al. Role of glucose and insulin resistance in development of type 2 diabetes mellitus: results of a 25-year follow-up study. Lancet 1992; 340: 925–929.
[20] Bergstrom RW, Newell-Morris LL, Leonetti DL et al. Association of elevated fasting C-peptide level and increased intra-abdominal fat distribution with development of NIDDM in Japanese-American men. Diabetes 1990; 39: 104–111.
[21] Ohlson LO, Larrson B, Svardsudd K et al. The influence of body fat distribution on the incidence of diabetes mellitus. 13.5 years of follow-up of the participants in the study born in 1913. Diabetes 1985; 34: 1055–1058.
[22] Lundgren H, Bengtsson C, Blohme G et al. Adiposity and adipose tissue distribution in relation to the incidence of diabetes in women: results from a prospective population study in Gothenburg, Sweden. Int J Obesity 1989; 13: 413–423.
[23] Manson JE, Nathan DM, Krolewski AS et al. A prospective study of exercise and incidence of diabetes among U. S. male physicians. JAMA 1991; 268: 63–67.
[24] Manson JE, Rimm EB, Stampfer MJ et al. Physical activity and incidence of non-insulin dependent diabetes in women. Lancet 1991; 338: 774–778.
[25] Anderson DC. Sex hormone binding globulin. (Clin Oxf) 1974; 3: 69–96.
[26] Lindstedt G, Lundberg PA, Lapidus et al. Low sex hormone binding globulin as independent risk factor for development of NIDDM. 12-year follow-up of population study in Gothenburg, Sweden. Diabetes 1991; 40: 123–128.
[27] Haffner SM, Valdez RA, Morales PA et al. Decreased sex hormone binding globulin predicts the incidence of non-insulin-dependent diabetes mellitus. J Clin Endocrin Metab 1993; 77: 56–60.
[28] Nestler JE. Sex hormone binding globulin: a marker for hyperinsulinemia and/or insulin resistance (Editorial). J Clin Endocrinol Metab 1993; 76: 273–274.
[29] Haffner SM, Stern MP, Hazuda HP et al. Cardiovascular risk factors in confirmed prediabetic individuals. Does the clock for coronary heart disease start ticking before the onset of clinical diabetes? JAMA 1990; 263: 2893–2898.
[30] McPhillips JB, Barrett-Connor E, Wingard DL. Cardiovascular disease risk factors prior to othe diagnosis of impaired glucose tolerance and non-insulin-dependent diabets mellitus in a community of older adults. Am J Epidemiol 1990; 131: 443–453.
[31] Mykkänen L, Haffner SM, Kuusisto J et al. Microalbuminuria predicts the development of non-insulin-dependent diabetes mellitus. Submitted.
[32] Viswanathan M, Mohan M, Snehalatha C et al. High prevalence to type 2 (non-insulin-dependent) diabetes among the offspring of conjugal type 2 diabetic parents. Diabetologia 1985; 28: 907–910.
[33] Kahn CB, Soeldner JS, Gleason RE et al. Clinical and chemical diabetes in offspring of diabetic couples. N Engl J Med 1969; 281: 343–347.
[34] Haffner SM, Stern MP, Hazuda HP et al. Increased insulin concentrations in non-diabetic offspring of diabetic parents. N Engl J Med 1988; 319: 1297–1301.

[35] Gulli G, Ferrannini E, Stern MP et al. The metabolic profile of NIDDM is fully established in glucose-tolerant offspring of two Mexican-American NIDDM parents. Diabetes 1992; 41: 1575–1586.
[36] Eriksson J, Fransilla-Kallunki A, Ekstrand A et al. Early metabolic defects in persons at increased risk for non-insulin dependent diabetes mellitus. N Eng J Med 1989; 321: 337–343.
[37] Bogardus C, Lillioja S, Nyomba BL et al. Distribution of in vivo insulin action in Pima Indians as mixture of three normal distributions. Diabetes 1989; 38: 1423–1432.
[38] Osei K. Increased basal glucose production and utilization in non-diabetic first degree relatives of patients with NIDDM. Diabetes 1990; 39: 597–601.
[39] O'Rahilly S, Turner RC, Mathews DR. Impaired pulsatile secretion of insulin in relatives of patients with non-insulin dependent diabetes. N Engl J Med 1988; 318: 1225–1230.
[40] Paolisso G, Sgamboto S, Passariello N et al. Greater efficacy of pulsatile insulin in type 1 diabetes critically depends on plasma glucose levels. Diabetes 1987; 36: 566–570.
[41] Aronoff SL, Bennett PH, Gorden P et al. Unexplained hyperinsulinemia in normal and "prediabetic" Pima Indians compared with normal Caucasians: an example of racial differences in insulin secretion. Diabetes 1977; 26: 827–840.
[42] Haffner SM, Stern MP, Hazuda PH et al. Hyperinsulinemia in a population at high risk for non-insulin dependent diabetes mellitus. N Engl J Med 1986; 315: 220–224.
[43] Balkau B, King H, Zimmet P et al. Factors associated with the development of diabetes in the Micronesian population of Nauru. Am J Epidemiol 1985; 122: 594–605.
[44] Boyko EJ, Keane EM, Marshall JA et al. Higher insulin and C-peptide concentrations in Hispanic population at high risk for NIDDM. San Luis Valley Study. Diabetes 1991; 40: 509–515.
[45] Naguelesparan M, Savage PJ, Knowler WC et al. Increased in vivo insulin resistance in non-diabetic Pima Indians compared with Caucasians. Diabetes 1982; 31: 952–956.
[46] Elahi D, Nagulesparan M, Herschopf RJ et al. Feedback of insulin secretion by insulin: relation to hyperinsulinemia of obesity. N Engl J Med 1982; 306: 1196–1202.
[47] Haffner SM, Stern MP, Dunn JF et al. Diminished insulin sensitivity, and increased insulin response in non-obese, non-diabetic Mexican Americans. Metabolism 1990; 39: 842–847.
[48] Haffner SM, Stern MP, Watanabe R et al. Relationship of insulin clearance and insulin secretion to insulin sensitivity in Mexican Americans. Eur J Clin Invest 1992; 22: 147–153.
[49] Reaven GM. Banting Lecture 1988. Role of insulin resistance in human disease. Diabetes 1988; 37: 1595–1607.
[50] Modan M, Halkin H, Almos S et al. Hyperinsulinemia: a link between hypertension, obesity and glucose intolerance. J Clin Invest 1985; 75: 807–817.
[51] Zavaroni I, Bonora E, Pagliara M et al. Risk factors for coronary artery disease in healthy persons with hyperinsulinemia and normal glucose tolerance. N Engl J Med 1989; 320: 702–706.
[52] Orchard TJ, Becker DJ, Bates M et al. Plasma insulin and lipoprotein concentrations: an atherogenic association? Am J Epidemiol 1983; 118: 326–337.
[53] Haffner SM, Fong D, Hazuda HP et al. Hyperinsulinemia, upper body adiposity and cardiovascular risk in non-diabetics. Metabolism 1988; 37: 338–345.
[54] DeFronzo RA, Ferrannini E. Insulin resistance: a multifaceted syndrome responsible for NIDDM, obesity, hypertension, dyslipidemia and atherosclerotic cardiovascular disease. Diabetes Care 1991; 14: 173–194.
[55] Ferrannini E, Buzziogli G, Bonadonna R et al. Insulin resistance in essential hypertension. N Engl J Med 1987; 317: 350–357.
[56] Garg A, Helderman JH, Huffler et al. Relationship between lipoprotein levels and in vivo insulin action in normal young white men. Metabolism 1988; 37: 982–987.
[57] Abbott WGH, Lillioja S, Young AA et al. Relationships between plasma lipoprotein concentrations and insulin action in a obese hyperinsulinemic population. Diabetes 1987; 36: 897–904.

[58] Mbanya JCN, Thomas TH, Wilkinson R et al. Hypertension and hyperinsulinemia: a relation in diabetes but not in essential hypertension. Lancet 1988; 1: 733–734.
[59] Saad MF, Lillioja S, Nyomba BL et al. Racial differences in the relation between blood pressure and insulin resistance. N Engl J Med 1991; 324: 733–739.
[60] Haffner SM, Ferrannini E, Hazuda HP et al. Clustering of cardiovascular risk factors in confirmed prehypertensive individuals. Hypertension 1992; 20: 38–45.
[61] Haffner SM. Insulin and blood pressure: fact or fantasy? (Editorial). J Clin Endocrinol Metab 1993; 76: 541–543.
[62] Haffner SM, Valdez RA, Hazuda HP et al. Prospective analysis of the Insulin Resistance Syndrome. Diabetes 1992; 41: 715–722.
[63] Temple RC, Carrington CA, Luzio SD et al. Insulin deficiency in non-insulin-dependent diabetes. Lancet 1989; 1: 293–295.
[64] Temple RC, Clark P, Schneider A et al. Radioimmunoassay may overestimate insulin in non-insulin-dependent diabetics. Clin Endocrinol 1990; 32: 689–693.
[65] Ward WK, La Cova EC, Paquette TL et al. Disproportionate elevation of immunoreactive proinsulin in type 2 (non-insulin dependent) diabetes mellitus and in experimental insulin resistance. Diabetologia 1987; 30: 698–702.
[66] Nagi DK, Hendra TJ, Tyle AJ et al. The relationships of concentrations of insulin intact proinsulin and 32–33 split proinsulin with cardiovascular risk factors in type 2 (non-insulin dependent) diabetic subjects. Diabetologia 1990; 32: 532–537.
[67] Haffner SM, Mykkänen L, Stern MP et al. Relationship of proinsulin and insulin to cardiovascular risk factors in non-diabetic subjects. Diabetes 1993; 42: 1297–1302.
[68] Haffner SM, Stern MP, Bowsher R. Increased proinsulin levels are association with the insulin resistance syndrome. Submitted.
[69] Keen H, Jarrett RJ, McCarthney P. The year follow-up of the Bedford survey (1962–1972) glucose tolerance and diabetes. Diabetologia 1982; 22: 72–78.
[70] Mykkänen L, Laakso M, Pentillä I et al. Asymptomatic hyperglycemia and cardiovascular risk factors in the elderly. Atherosclerosis 1991; 88: 153–161.
[71] Barakat HA, Carpenter JW, McLendon VD et al. Influence of obesity, impaired glucose, and NIDDM on LDL structure and composition. Possible link between hyperinsulinemia and atherosclerosis. Diabetes 1990; 39: 1527–1533.
[72] Mykkänen L, Laakso M, Uusitupa M et al. Prevalence of diabetes and impaired glucose tolerance in elderly subjects and their association with obesity and family history of diabetes. Diabetes Care 1990; 13: 1099–1105.
[73] Austin MA, Breslow JL, Hennekens CHD et al. Low density lipoprotein subclass patterns and risk of myocardial infarction. JAMA 1988; 260: 1917–1921.
[74] Campos H, Genest JJ, Blijlevens E et al. Low density lipoprotein particle size and coronary artery disease. Arteriosclerosis 1992; 12: 187–195.
[75] Evans DJ, Hoffman RG, Kalkhoff RK et al. Relationship of body fat topography to insulin sensitivity and metabolic profiles in premenopausal women. Metabolism 1984; 33: 68–75.
[76] Seidell JC, Björntorp P, Sjöstrom L et al. Visceral fat accumulation in men is positively associated with insulin, glucose and C-peptide levels, but negatively with testosterone levels. Metabolism 1990; 39: 897–901.
[77] Krotkiewski M, Björntorp P, Sjöstrom L et al. Impact of obesity on metabolism in men and women: importance of regional adipose tissue distribution. J Clin Invest 1983; 72: 1150–1162.
[78] Haffner SM, Fong D, Hazuda HP et al. Hyperinsulinemia, upper body adiposity, and cardiovascular risk factors in a non-diabetic population. Metabolism 1988; 37: 338–346.
[79] Bonora E, Del Prato S, Bonadonna RC et al. Total body fat content and fat topography are associated differently with in vivo glucose metabolism in non-obese and obese non-diabetic women. Diabetes 1992; 41: 1151–1159.
[80] Haffner SM, Karhapää P, Mykkänen L et al. Insulin resistance, body fat distribution and sex hormones in men. Diabetes, in press.

[81] Coon PJ, Bleacker ER, Drinkwater DT et al. Effects of body fat composition and exercise capacity on glucose tolerance, insulin, and lipoprotein lipids in healthy older men: A cross-sectional and longitudinal intervention study. Metabolism 1989; 38: 1201 – 1209.
[82] Kissebah AH, Peiris AN, Evans DJ. Mechanisms associating body fat distribution to glucose intolerance and diabetes mellitus: window with a view: health implications of regional obesity. Eds. Björntorp P, Smith U, Lönnroth P. Acta Medica Scandinavia 1988; 723: 79 – 80.
[83] Björntorp P. Abdominal obesity and risk. Clin Exp Hypertension. Theory and Practice 1990; 12: 783 – 794.
[84] Fujioka S, Matsuzawa Y, Tokanaga K et al. Contribution of intra-abdominal fat accumulation to the impairment of glucose and lipid metabolism in human obesity. Metabolism 1987; 36: 54 – 59.
[85] Björntorp P. Abdominal obesity and the development of non-insulin-dependent diabetes mellitus. Diabetes/Metabolism Reviews 1988; 4: 615 – 622.
[86] Strömblad G, Björntorp P. Reduced hepatic clearance in rats with dietary-induced obesity. Metabolism 1986; 35: 323 – 328.
[87] Carlson LA, Boberg J, Högstedt B. Some physiological and clinical implications of lipid mobilization from adipose tissue. In: Eds. Renold AE and Cahill GF, Jr. Handbook of physiolgoy. Section V; Washington: Williams and Wilkins, 1985; 625 – 644.
[88] Williamson JR, Kreisberg RA, Felts PW. Mechanisms for the stimulation of gluconeogenesis by fatty acids in the profused rat liver. Proc Natl Acad Sci, USA 1966; 56: 247 – 254.
[89] Blumenthal SA. Stimulation of gluconeogenesis by palimitic acid in rat hepatocytes: evidence that these effects can be associated from provision of reducing equivalents. Metab Clin Exp 1983; 32: 971 – 981.
[90] Björntorp P. "Portal" adipose tissue as a generator of risk factors for cardiovascular disease and diabetes. (Editorial). Arteriosclerosis 1990; 10: 493 – 496.
[91] Peiris AN, Meuller RA, Smith GA et al. Splanchnic insulin metabolism in obesity: influence of body fat distribution. J Clin Invest 1986; 78: 1648 – 1657.
[92] Evans DJ, Hoffman RG, Kalkhoff RK et al. Relationship of androgenic activity to body fat topography, fat cell morphology and metabolic abnormalities in premenopausal women. J Clin Endocrinol Metab 1983; 57: 304 – 310.
[93] Haffner SM, Katz MS, Stern MP et al. The relationship of sex hormones to hyperinsulinemia and hyperglycemia. Metabolism 1988; 37: 683 – 688.
[94] Toeller M, Knussman R. Reproducibility of oral glucose tolerance tests with three different loads. Diabetologia 1973; 9: 102 – 107.
[95] Riccardi G, Vaccaro O, Rivellese A et al. Reproducibility of the newly diagnostic criteria for impaired glucose tolerance. Am J Epidemiol 1985; 121: 422 – 429.
[96] Yudkin JS, Alberti KGMM, McLarty DG et al. Impaired glucose tolerance. Is it a risk factor for diabetes or a diagnostic ragbag? Br Med J 1990; 301: 397 – 402.
[97] Feskens EJM, Bowles CH, Kromhout D. Intra- and interindividual variability of glucose tolerance in an elderly population. J Clin Epidemiol 1991; 44: 947 – 953.
[98] Stern MP, Rosenthal MP, Haffner SM. A new concept of impaired glucose tolerance: relation to cardiovascular risk. Arteriosclerosis 1985; 5: 311 – 314.
[99] Stern MP, Morales PA, Valdez RA et al. Predicting diabetes. Moving beyond improved glucose tolerance. Diabetes 1993; 42: 700 – 714.

Genetic patterns of IDDM related to environmental factors

A.-G. Ziegler, E. Standl

Accumulating evidence suggests that type 1 (insulin-dependent) diabetes is an autoimmune disease which predominantly occurs in genetically susceptible individuals [1 – 3]. Approximately 5 percent of first degree relatives of patients with type 1 diabetes will develop the disease and approximately 30 – 50% of identical twins are concordant for the disease. The great majority of individuals who develop type 1 diabetes has alleles within the major histocompatibility region of the sixth chromosome associated with the disorder. In addition, world-wide regional differences in the incidence of type 1 diabetes and the high rate of discordance between monozygotic twins suggest an important role for environmental factors.

HLA-molecules

Type 1 diabetes (IDDM) occurs predominantly in individuals who express the serologically defined HLA class II molecules DR4 and DR3 on their immune cells [4, 5]. HLA DR2, however, is negatively associated with the disease. Studies at the gene level have elucidated that DR alleles are associated with specific DQ alleles and that susceptibility or resistance to develop type 1 diabetes are even more closely determined by particular DQ genes. For example, only individuals carrying the haplotype DR4-DQB1*0302, and not those being DR4-DQB1*0301, are at increased risk for IDDM. Thus, the DR4 association is apparently caused by linkage disequilibrium to DQB1*0302.

Both the HLA DQ and the HLA DR molecules are heterodimers made up of an alpha chain and a beta chain and both subunits are intrinsic membrane proteins. Most of the variability is found in the outer domains of these class II molecules, and the regions of polymorphism are probably linked to disease susceptibility [6]. Using allele-specific oligonucleotides, several investigators have reported that the absence of an aspartic acid at position 57 (Asp-57) of the DQ beta chain provides an excellent marker for IDDM [7, 8]. According to a model of HLA class II molecule structure, position 57 of DQB1 is

Offprint from
Research Methodologies in Human Diabetes – Part 1

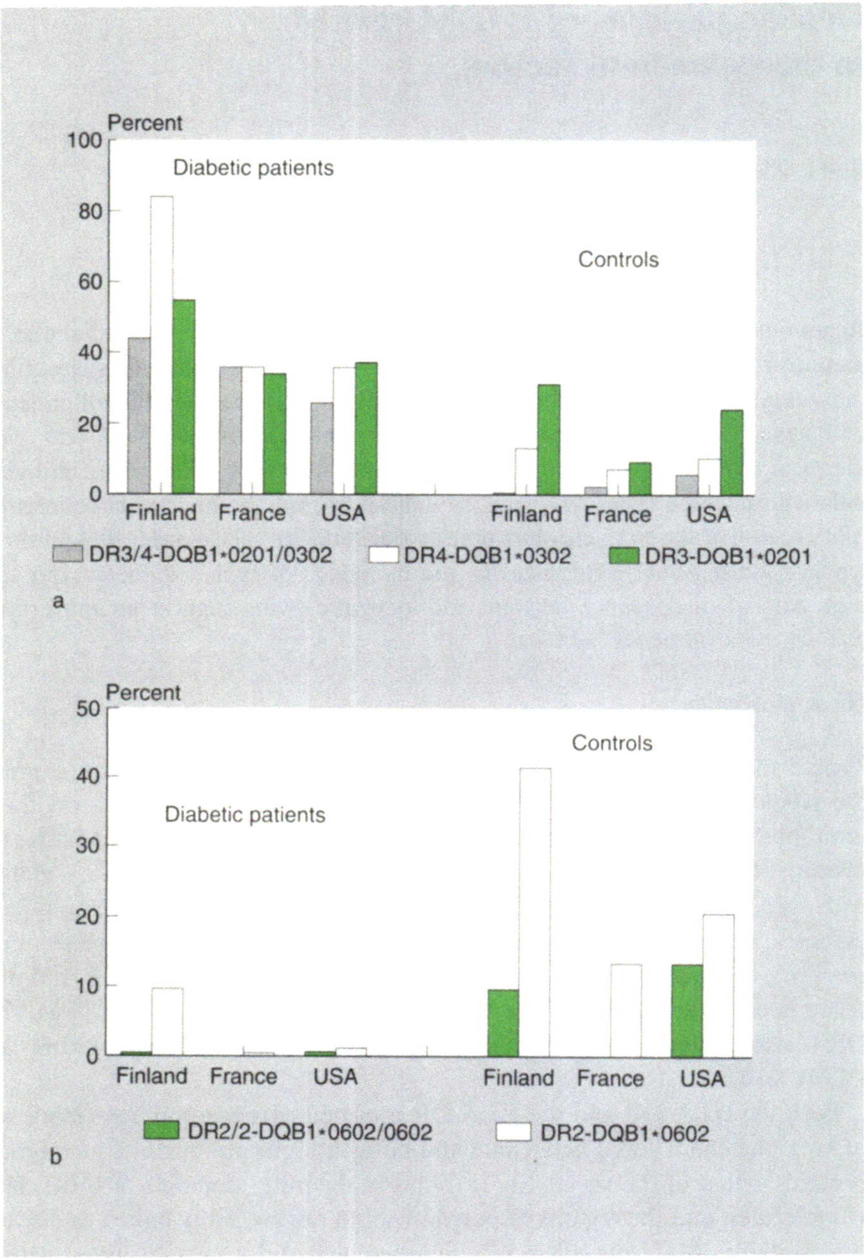

*Fig. 1 Genotype- and haplotype-frequency of DR4-DQB1*0302 and DR3-DQB1*0201 (a) and DR2-DQB1*0602 (b) in type 1 diabetic patients and healthy controls of Finland, France, and USA (modified from [12, 14, 15])*

located in an important position of the molecule which possibly affects the antigen binding and T-cell recognition, so that the charge of this amino acid may contribute to the autoimmune process leading to the destruction of insulin producing beta cells.

However, several exceptions to the Asp-57 hypothesis have been reported. For example, in Japanese patients, the major susceptibility haplotypes are DR4-DQB1*0401 and DR9-DQB1*0303, both of which carry Asp at DQB1-57 [9]. In addition, certain haplotypes encoding Asp-negative chains such as for example the DR7-DQw2 haplotype (Asp-) are not increased in Caucasians, whereas they are positively associated with the diseases in Black populations [10]. This latter distinction is thought to be due to the DQ alpha locus difference, DQA1*0201 in Caucasians and DQA1*0301 in Black populations [11]. The contributions of DQalpha in Caucasians was also reported by Khalil et al., who proposed that cis or trans encoded DQ molecules consisting of a DQ alpha chain having arginine (Arg) at position 52 and a non-Asp DQ beta chain were most strongly associated with type 1 diabetes susceptibility, and that susceptibility correlated quantitatively with the expression of such cis or trans encoded DQ molecules [12]. In contrast, DQ molecules being DQ alpha non-Arg and DQ beta Asp were supposed to confer protection. Other studies indicated also a significant contribution of particular DRB1 genes encoding given variants of DR4. Among the DR4-DQB1*0302 haplotype, only the DRB1*0401 (Dw4) and DRB1*0402 (Dw10) subtypes are positively associated with IDDM [13].

In summary, it is concluded that a single amino acid residue alone might be insufficient to determine susceptibility or resistance to IDDM in different ethnic groups. The accurate assessment of susceptibility to type 1 diabetes requires rather the complete characterization of the HLA DR-DQ haplotype, including alpha and beta chain typing.

Fig. 1a, b illustrates the frequency of diabetic risk alleles and protective alleles in different populations such as Finland, France, and USA [12, 14, 15]. The results clearly demonstrate that in all three Caucasian countries type 1 diabetes susceptibility was most strongly associated with the genotype DR3-DQB1*0201/DR4-DQB1*0302 (type 1 diabetic patients: Finland 44%, France 36%, USA 26% versus healthy individuals: Finland 0%, France 2%, USA 5%; Fig. 1a). The relative risk (RR) of an individual carrying this genotype to develop overt type 1 diabetes, however, was different between the three populations and highest in Finland with 91 in comparison to France (RR = 32) and USA (RR = 6, Fig. 2a). Unlike many previous investigators, these studies did not find that HLA DR3-DQB1*0201 was associated with IDDM except when it was paired with DR4-DQB1*0302. The degree of protection provided by the HLA DR2-DQB1*0602 haplotype in both the heterozygous and the homozygous states was remarkable in all three populations. Fig. 1b illustrates the frequency of DR2-DQB1*0602 in type 1 diabetic individuals and healthy controls. It is evident that healthy individuals carry this haplotype more frequently than diabetic patients. The relative risk for individuals expressing this haplotype is significantly decreased (RR < 0.1 for all countries in both heterozygous and homozygous states, Fig. 2b). This implies, that the DR-DQ associated resistance is often dominant over the DR-DQ associated susceptibility.

As part of the 11th International Histocompability Workshop (1991), 981 unrelated Black, Caucasian or Japenese type 1 diabetes patients were genomically typed for HLA class II alleles, and the results compared with those obtained by typing 2228 healthy control subjects [16]. DQA1*0301 together with DQB1*0302 (associated with DR4), and DQA1*0501 together with DQb1*0201 (associated with DR3) were found associated with type 1 diabetes in all three ethnic groups. Among Blacks, a significant association was also found with DQA1*0301 together with DQB1*0201 (often together with genes encoding DR7), whereas in Japanese patients susceptibility was also associated with DQA1*0301 together with DQB1*303, and DQA1*0301 together with DQB1*0401. The Caucasian genotype most often involved was again DR3-DQB1*0201/DR4-DQB1*0302. Resistance against development of type 1 diabetes in all three ethnic groups was found with DQA1*0102 together with DQB1*0602 (associated with DR2). The DQ-associated resistance again was partly, but not completely dominant over the DQ-associated susceptibility.

One explanation for the increased frequency of certain haplotypes in patients with type 1 diabetes is that the antigen-binding pocket or the region of T-cell interaction of a particular DQ molecule may have higher affinity for a relevant antigen in diabetes or be more conductive to interaction with the T-cell receptor of the responding T-cell. The finding that certain DQ molecules may determine IDDM susceptibility may lead to new concepts for preventing the development of IDDM in susceptible individuals, the use of blocking peptide analogues, for example. At a practical level, it is now possible – utilizing polymerase chain reaction technology – to amplify specific regions of class II alleles and to rapidly type individuals. In the general population it is conceivable that individuals be identified carrying the high risk genotype DR3/4 DQB1*0201/0302 at birth. If clinical prevention of IDDM becomes a reality, genetic screening, coupled with autoantibody screening, may extend prediction of type 1 diabetes to the general population.

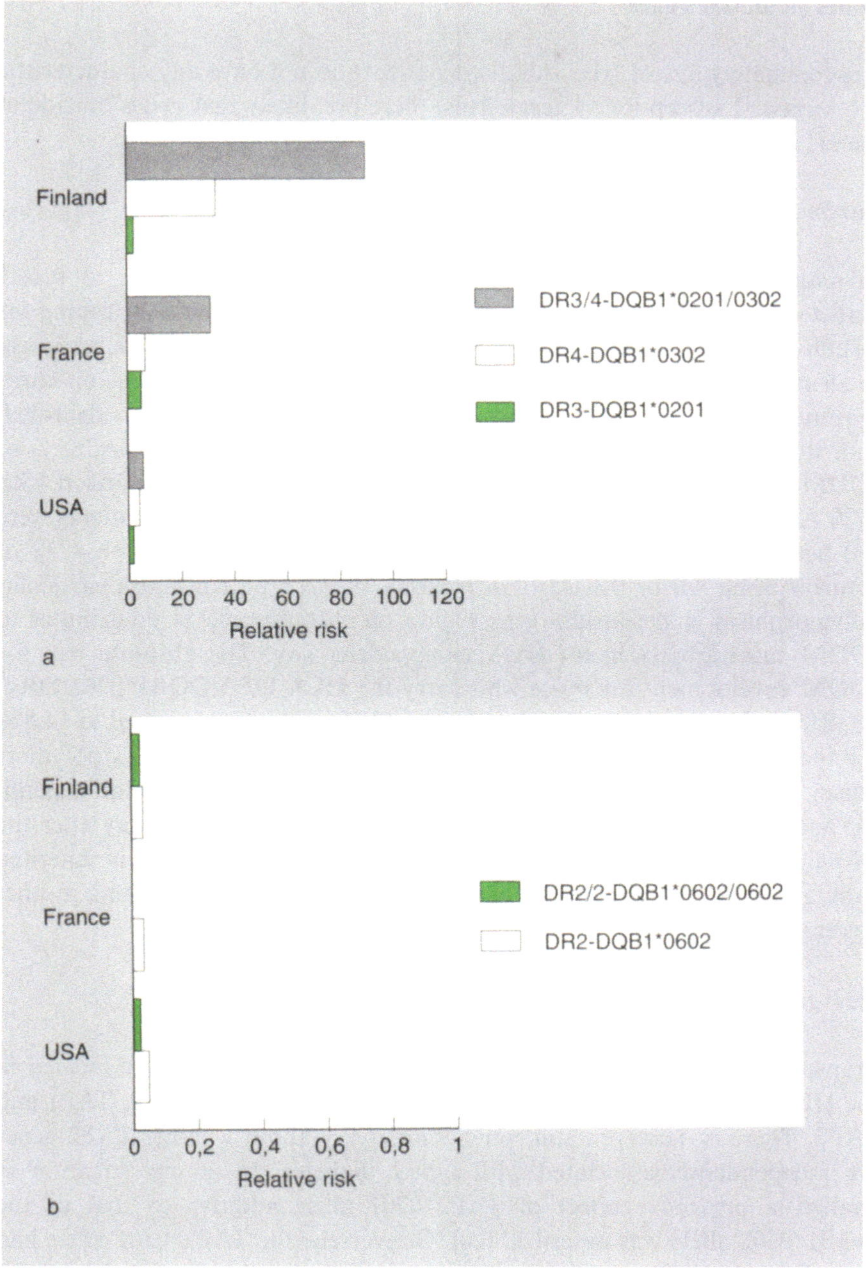

*Fig. 2 Relative risk to develop type 1 diabetes according to genotype- and haplotype-frequency of DR4-DQB1*0302 and DR3-DR3-DQB1*0201 (a) and DR2-DQB1*0602 (b) in Finland, France, and USA (modified from [12, 14, 15])*

Other potential genes

Approximately 3% of type 1 diabetic patients do not have any characteristic HLA class II susceptibility genes. It is, therefore, likely that genes outside of the HLA complex also contribute to diabetes susceptibility.

Insulin gene

In man, the only region outside of the MHC currently linked to type 1 diabetes lies within the insulin gene close to the IGF-II-gene [17]. Typing for insulin gene polymorphism shows a consistent association with diabetes risk in all populations studied to date [17–19]. The insulin gene locus on chromosome 11 is polymorphic and two INS alleles (A and B) have been identified. In a study of 124 IDDM patients and 38 controls in Denver, USA, 85% of IDDM patients were identified to be AA homozygous in comparison with 52% AA homozygosity in controls. In contrast, 15% of IDDM patients were AB heterozygous, none were BB homozygous in comparison with 48% of controls being AB or BB. Also, in Norway, it was reported that a particular polymorphism in the insulin gene region on chromosome 11 contributes to IDDM susceptibility in an HLA independent way. The absolute risk for IDDM development for those who carry the HLA DR3-DQB1*0201/DR4-DQB1*0302 genotype was reported to be 13.5%, while it increased to 14.8% for those also being homozygous for the IDDM associated INS polymorphism. The strength of this association may, however, be population-dependent and a study from France suggests that genetic imprinting may alter the effect of these alleles. In particular, if the uncommon B allele is inherited from a father, it may protect from diabetes, while inheritance from a mother has no influence.

TAP genes

Transporter genes (TAP) associated with antigen processing, are located in the HLA class II region. Two TAP genes were recently identified, TAP1 and TAP2. There is, however, still some controversy about whether TAP2 genes are independently associated with type 1 diabetes. In an investigation in France, a protective effect of TAP2*0201 allele additive to that of the DQB1*0602 allele was described [20]. Conversely, the TAP2*0101 allele had a predisposing effect in the homozygous state and reinforced the DR3/4 susceptibility. In contrast, a studied performed in Norway and Finland [21] found a strong linkage disequilibrium with DR and DQ genes. When they compared HLA DR and DQ identical patients and controls, an association of TAP genes was no longer detectable. They conclude that the association is secondary to a primary association between IDDM and DQ molecules.

"Type 2 diabetes" gene

A popular hypothesis is that separate major genes are responsible for type 1 and type 2 diabetes susceptibility. Type 1 diabetes is considered to be autoimmune by nature and is clearly associated with specific HLA antigens. Type 2 diabetes is thought neither to be autoimmune nor has it shown a consistent association or linkage with genes in the HLA region. On the other hand, several studies have documented the increased type 1 diabetes risk to siblings of a type 1 diabetic proband when a parent has type 2 diabetes [22]. This increase in risk was similar in magnitude to that seen for siblings of a type 1 diabetes proband when a parent had type 1 diabetes. In addition, we were able to demonstrate a striking frequency of type 2 diabetes among second degree relatives of type 1 diabetic probands (Table 1, [23]). Of 192 type 1 diabetic probands, 47% had second degree relatives with type 2 diabetes compared to only 19% of 72 non-diabetic controls ($p = 0.0003$). The highest incidence of type 2 diabetes was found in grandmothers on father's side ($p < 0.05$). With multiple loci required for both type 1 diabetes and type 2 diabetes, the possibility exists that a single locus may contribute to the susceptibility to both diseases. A genetic relationship between susceptibility

Table 1 Frequency of type 1 and type 2 diabetes in first and second degree relatives of type 1 diabetic probands

	Controls n = 72	Type 1 diabetic patients n = 192	p
Type 1			
First degree relatives	*	9%	
Second degree relatives	*	7%	
1st or 2nd degree relatives	*	16%	
Type 2			
First degree relatives	10%	5%	n. s.
Second degree relatives	19%[3]	47%[4]	0.0003
1st or 2nd degree relatives	28%[6]	49%[7]	0.001

* per definitionem excluded

to both diseases may allow for exploration of some of the observed clinical heterogeneity and expression of both type 1 and type 2 diabetes.

Environmental factors and unknown genes

The discordance for type 1 diabetes between identical twins has been cited as evidence that environmental factors acting on a genetically-predisposed individual may initiate autoimmune beta cell destruction. Major geographic variations in the occurrence of type 1 diabetes have been recognized with a polar to equator gradient for the risk of diabetes [24]. It has been reported that the risk for type 1 diabetes appears to correlate with the average yearly temperature of the environment, the distance from the equator, and the frequency of HLA risk alleles (such as Asp-57-negative DQ molecules) in the population at risk [25]. One exception to the north to south gradient – the population of Sardinia – has been described. This population was discovered to have a higher frequency of Asp-57-negative DQ alleles (similarly to Norway and Finland with the highest rates of IDDM) among non-diabetic control subjects than do populations with low rates of IDDM. An understanding of the geographic differences will, therefore, be important to the identification of factors related to the etiology of IDDM.

Diet

Exclusive breast feeding for the first 3–4 months of life was found to protect from later development of diabetes in Finnish children [26]. In addition, diabetes does not occur in diabetes-prone BB rats nor in NOD mice (both animal models for autoimmune diabetes) reared on a diet free of cow's milk for the first two to three months of life [27]. With respect to cow's milk as a potential trigger of the immune response in type 1 diabetes, it is of interest, that Karjalainen et al. observed elevated antibodies to bovine serum albumin antibodies in 100% of newly diagnosed diabetic children compared to only 2.5% of control children by a particle concentration fluoroimmunoassay [28]. Similarly, anti-BSA antibodies were significantly higher in diabetes-prone BB rats than in control animals. The anti-BSA-antibodies found in patients with type 1 diabetes as well as in BB rats were mostly of the IgG isotype; most interestingly, they were shown to crossreact with a pancreatic beta-cell surface 69 kd protein that is inducible by interferon gamma. It is proposed by the authors that a BSA-induced, p69-crossreactive immune response could be the link between milk protein and beta-cell specific immunity in patients with type 1 diabetes. Subsequently, a small peptide of BSA containing 17-amino

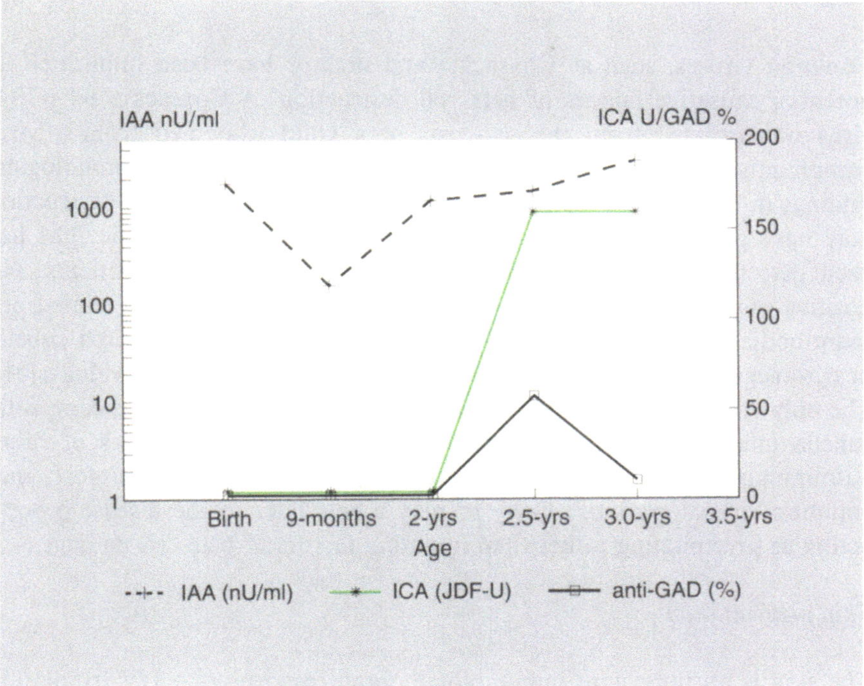

Fig. 3 Appearance of islet cell autoimmunity in an offspring of a type 1 diabetic mother. Insulin autoantibodies (nU/ml) are present from birth, ICA (JDF-U) and GAD-antibodies (%) appear at 2.5 years of age (modified from [29])

acids was identified ("ABBOS"). It was shown that, most of the diabetes-associated antibodies in diabetic children are directed against this epitope and that, immunization with synthetic ABBOS induced the formation of antibodies capable of reacting with p69. In this context, it may be of interest that we discovered islet cell autoimmunity within the first months of life in offspring of type 1 diabetic mothers. To date, of 70 neonates followed up to the age of 2 years, 4% were found to have positive insulin autoantibodies (IAA) before age 2 (Fig. 3) and all IAA-positive offspring later developed positive ICA and anti-GAD-antibodies [29]. These data would suggest that an antigen-driven immune response against insulin secreting beta cells is initiated very early in life. It is not unlikely that a dietary manipulation early in life such as exclusive breast feeding or the prevention of exposure to cow's milk, therefore, might influence the initiation of autoimmune beta cell destruction.

Virus

Common viruses, such as Coxsackie and mumps have been implicated as potential causative factors of beta cell destruction. A Coxsackie B4 (CB4) virus was isolated from the pancreas of a child who died from a viral encephalitis and diabetic ketoacidosis [30]. Later reports of the pathological findings in the child's pancreas, however, indicated that beta cell destruction may have preceded the virus infection. Coxsackie-B-virus specific IgM has been detected frequently in newly diagnosed type 1 diabetic patients. No positive association, however, between the presence of islet cell-related autoantibodies and Coxsackie B, recent mumps, postnatally acquired rubella or cytomegalovirus infection has been found in non-diabetic individuals [31]. The only virus clearly associated with type 1 diabetes of humans is congenital rubella infection, which also increases the incidence of a series of other autoimmune disorders (e. g. thyroiditis) [32]. It is suggested, therefore, that common viruses are more likely to play a role later in the disease process acting as precipitating rather than initiating factors of beta cell damage.

Skin pigmentation

The skin is an important immunologic organ responsive to UV irradiation and environmental agents. We therefore studied skin pigmentation and reactivity to UV light in association with susceptibility to type 1 diabetes in Germany. We found that significantly more type 1 diabetic patients showed increased reactivity to UV light, fair skin type and blue eye color compared to age matched controls [33]. The relative risk for susceptibility to type 1 diabetes in subjects with low pigment eye color was 3.1, in subjects with fair skin type 3.4, and in subjects with increased UV sensitivity 5.8. The highest risk for the development of diabetes was seen in subjects who had low pigment eye color and/or increased UV sensitivity (17.4). The significance of these findings remains unknown, but one might hypothesize that a low pigment skin type may predispose for the development of type 1 diabetes in genetically-predisposed individuals.

Immune related hormones

In view of the immune mediated nature of IDDM and its association with low pigment skin type we have begun to investigate pigment related hormones such as 1,25-dihydroxyvitamin D3, 25-hydroxyvitamin D3, alpha-MSH, and ACTH in newly diagnosed type 1 diabetic patients. Evidence has been accumulated in recent years that these hormones, in addition to their effect on skin pigmentation, have a large spectrum of immunoregulatory properties, and the discovery of receptors for 1,25-dihydroxyvitamin D3 in cells in the immune system has raised the possibility that 1,25-dihydroxyvitamin D3 is a potent agent in the modulation of the immune response [34, 35]. A marked decrease of 1,25-$(OH)_2D_3$-levels was found at onset of IDDM compared to normal controls [36]. Grouping patients according to season (winter or summer) of diabetes onset and blood sampling, it was demonstrated that the decrease of 1,25-$(OH)_2D_3$ was primarily present during summer season and due to a loss of the seasonal rhythm of this hormone observed in healthy controls (Figure 4). No difference, however, was found in mean and median

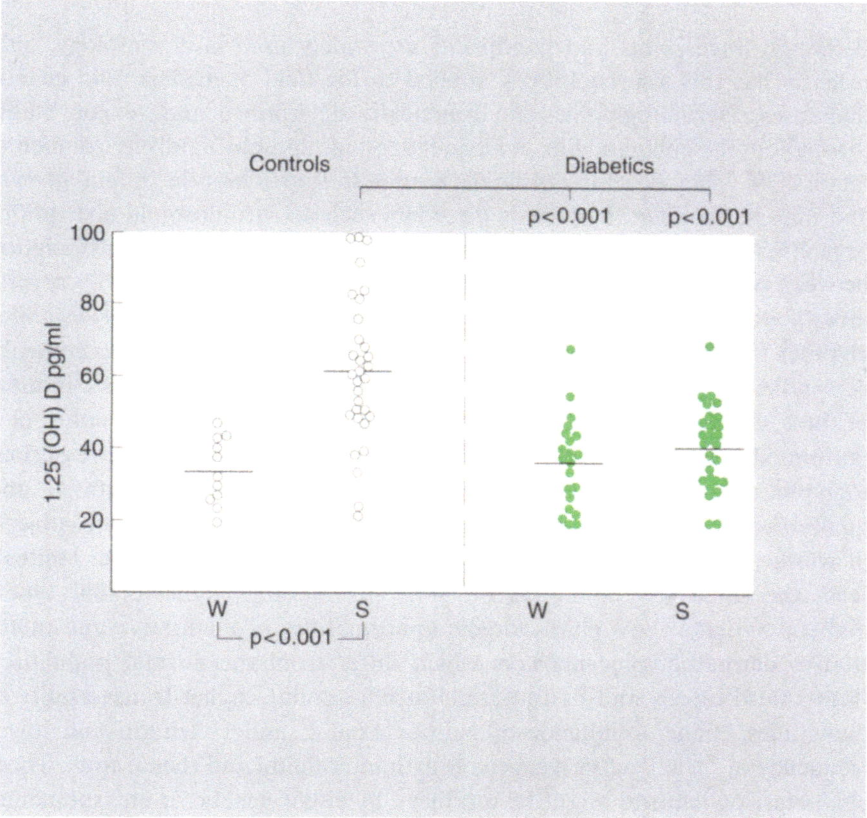

Fig. 4 Serum concentrations of 1,25-dihydroxyvitamin D_3 in nondiabetic controls (left panel) and new onset type 1 diabetic patients (right panel) according to time of blood drawing and diabetes onset, respectively (W = winter = November until April, S = summer = May until October). Mean values of 1,25-$(OH)_2D_3$ are indicated by horizontal lines [36]

values of alpha-MSH and ACTH between IDDM patients and controls. These data suggest a possible involvement of skin pigmentation related hormones such as 1,25-$(OH)_2D_3$ in the pathogenesis of type 1 diabetes. Investigations of 1,25-$(OH)_2D_3$ as immunosuppressive substance in combination with Cyclosporin A (CsA) have recently shown, that 1,25-$(OH)_2D_3$ enhances the immunosuppressive effects of CsA on lymphocytes of patients with rheumatoid arthritis in vitro [37]. Furthermore, it was reported that 1,25 $(OH)_2$ vitamin D_3 was able to prevent insulitits in the animal model of NOD mice [38]. In view of human type 1 diabetes, it remains to be seen whether higher serum concentrations of 1,25$(OH)_2D_3$ may mitigate its natural course.

Dermatoglyphics

Although fingerprints and handprints are widely used in criminology, only recently has this approach been applied to the field of medical and genetic diagnoses. Dermatoglyphics are genetically determined and remain stable throughout the postnatal life, independent of age and postnatal environmental factors [39]. They develop during the second to fourth months of fetal growth and may be modified by genetic disorders such as chromosomal aberrations or environmental factors during fetal life. In more recent years, an association between dermatoglyphics and diabetes mellitus has been studied by several investigators [41 – 43]. Although distinct characteristic patterns of dermatoglyphics have been described for diabetic patients in comparison to controls, contradictory results have been published from different laboratories. In most of these studies, no separate analysis was performed for patients with type 1 (autoimmune-) diabetes and type 2 diabetes. In order to investigate dermatoglyphics in type 1 diabetic patients, we have analyzed quantitative and qualitative characteristics of fingers and palms in 196 type 1 diabetic subjects of southern Germany and compared with the data of 199 normal controls from the same geographic region [44]. Our findings indicate that type 1 diabetic patients show characteristic abnormalities of qualitative and quantitative dermatoglyphic markers which differ from the normal population (lower third finger- and first interdigital ridge count, higher transversality of main lines, higher frequency of palmar axial t′ and t″ triradii and lower frequency of "true" patterns in the fourth interdigital and thenar area. These characteristic features might be produced by either genetic or environmental factors acting early in pregnancy in the aetiology of the disease. It is known that congenital rubella infection, which is associated with the subsequent development of type 1 diabetes, is associated with abnormal dermatoglyphic findings. In addition, genetic illnesses such as Down's syndrome, Turner's syndrome, Klinefelter's syndrome and others can be detected by characteristic patterns of dermatoglyphics. The origination of dermatoglyphics during the 2nd to 4th months of fetal growth is influenced by three factors: the thickness of the epidermis, the width of epidermal padding and the fluid content of epidermal vesicles. Tissue pressure and fluid content are suggested to be susceptible to environmental factors during pregnancy and fluctuations of such parameters might subsequently be responsible for abnormalities of dermatoglyphics in certain diseases such as type 1 diabetes. In our study, by multivariate analysis of quantitative and qualitative variables, a predictive value of 78.6% and 77.3%, respectively, for male, and 81.4% and 82.2%, respectively, for female type 1 diabetics was found. Therefore, dermatoglyphics seem to be an interesting tool for genetic studies and studies related to the prediction of type 1 diabetes.

Conclusions

As a basis, every study on genetic patterns of IDDM related to environmental factors or pinpointing the genetic versus the environmental impact in IDDM, has to take HLA DR antigens into account and probably HLA DQ antigens, too. In addition, the assessment of HLA DRB1 subtypes, insulin gene polymorphism or transporter gene subtypes may be useful. Although we are still short of an unequivocally established factor, the environmental influence appears to be a significant possibility which modulates the preexisting genetic predisposition in the pathogenesis of IDDM. The high discordance rate for IDDM of monocygotic twins is believed to be the most convincing argument for the importance of non-genetic factors. In this regard, major interest presently concentrates on the role of breast feeding, early nutrition with cow's milk, social factors, or additional infectious disease. Independently of or in conjunction with these environmental factors, the distance from the equator, the average annual temperature, ultraviolet light exposure, vitamin D metabolism might affect the genetic predisposition. Also intrauterine effects cannot be ruled out, perhaps in conjunction with the maternal predisposition for NIDDM or with gestational diabetes. As in the animal models of IDDM, i. e. in the BB rat and the NOD mouse, where two independent genes apparently determine the occurrence of IDDM, this possibility of a second genetic predisposition which may be more generally effective and again be modulated by environmental factors, also exists for the human situation. This may apply to the findings in relation to the skin type, skin pigmentation, ultraviolet light reactivity, and dermatoglyphics. Whatever the hypothesis, studies on the environmental impact depend critically on the selection of clearly defined IDDM patients, clearly defined ethnical groups, perfectly matched control groups and – last, but not least – clearly defined environmental factors. Only if these precautions are provided, can it be hoped that more light can be shed into the complex pathogenesis of IDDM originating both from genetic and environmental factors.

References

[1] Ziegler AG, Eisenbarth GS. Immunology of Diabetes. In: Alberti KGMM, Krall LP, eds. The Diabetes Annual/5. Amsterdam: Elsevier Science Publishers, 1990; 22–50.

[2] Ziegler AG, Ziegler R, Vardi P et al. Life table analysis of progression to diabetes of anti-insulin-autoantibody positive relatives of Type 1 diabetics. Diabetes 1989; 38: 1320–1325.

[3] Ziegler AG, Herskowitz R, Jackson RA et al. Predicting Type 1 diabetes. Diabetes Care 1990; 13: 762–775.

[4] Thorsby E, Ronningen KS. Particular HLA-DQ molecules play a dominant role in determining susceptibility or resistance to type 1 diabetes mellitus. Diabetologia 1993; 36: 371–377.

[5] Nepom GT. A unified hypothesis for the complex genetics of HLA associations with IDDM. Diabetes 1990; 39: 1153–1157.

[6] Brown JH, Jardetzky T, Sarper MA et al. A hypothetical model of the foreign antigen binding site of class II histocompatibility molecules. Nature 1989; 338: 587–589.

[7] Todd JA, Bell JI, McDevitt HO. HLA-DQ beta gene contributes to susceptibility and resistance to insulin dependent diabetes mellitus. Nature 1987; 329: 599–604.

[8] Vallet-Colom I, Levy-Marchal C, Zarrouk D et al. HLA-DQB1 codon 57 and genetic susceptibility to type 1 (insulin-dependent) diabetes mellitus in french children. Diabetologia 1990; 33: 174–176.

[9] Awata T, Kuzuya T, Matsuda A et al. Genetic analysis of HLA class II alleles and susceptibility to type 1 diabetes mellitus in japanese subjects. Diabetologia 1992; 35: 419–424.

[10] Mijovic CH, Jenkins D, Jacobs KH et al. HLA-DQA1 and -DQB1 alleles associated with genetic susceptibility to IDDM in a black population. Diabetes 1991; 40: 748–753.

[11] Todd JA, Fukui Y, Kitagawa T et al. The A3 allele of the HLA-DQA1 locus is associated with susceptibility to type 1 diabetes in Japanese. Proc natl Acad Sci USA 1990; 87: 1094–1098.

[12] Khalil I, Auriol L, Gobet M et al. A combination of HLA-DQb Asp 57 negative and HLA DQa Arg 52 confers susceptibility to IDDM. J Clin Invest 1990; 85: 1315–1319.

[13] Sheehy MJ, Scharf SJ, Rowe RJ et al. A diabetes-susceptible HLA haplotype is best defined by a combination of HLA DR and -DQ alleles. J Clin Invest 1989; 83: 830–835.

[14] Reijonen H, Ilonen J, Knip M et al. HLA-DQB1 alleles and absence of Asp 57 as susceptibility factors of IDDM in Finland. Diabetes 1991; 40: 1640–1644.

[15] Baisch JM, Weeks T, Giles R et al. Analyses of HLA-DQ genotypes and susceptibility in insulin-dependent diabetes mellitus. N Engl J Med 1990; 322: 1836–1841.

[16] Ronningen KS, Spurklamd A, Tait BD et al. HLA class II associations in insulin-dependent diabetes mellitus among Blacks, Caucasoids and Japanese. In: HLA 1991. Oxford: Oxford University press.

[17] Bell GI, Horita S, Koram JH. A polymorphic locus near the human insulin gene is associated with insulin dependent Diabetes. Diabetes 1983; 33: 176–183.

[18] Pugliese A, Bain SC, Todd JA et al. INS polymorphism in chromosome 11 in type 1 diabetes. J Autoimmunity 1993: 15 (suppl) A.

[19] Ronningen KS, Unlien DE, Thorsby E. Genetic markers in IDDM patients. J Autoimmunity 1993: 15 (suppl) A.

[20] Boitard C, Assan R, Bach JF. Protection from insulin dependent diabetes mellitus is linked to a peptide transporter gene. J Autoimmunity 1993: 15 (suppl) A.
[21] Ronningen KS, Unlien DE, Ploski R et al. Allelic variants of the human putative peptide transporter TAP2 and susceptibility to type 1 diabetes. Diabetes 1993 (a); in press.
[22] Rich SS, Panter SS, Goetz FC et al. Shared genetic susceptibility of type 1 and type 2 diabetes mellitus: contributions of HLA and haptoglobin. Diabetologia 1991; 34: 350–355.
[23] Ziegler AG, Baumgartl HJ, Mühlbauer K et al. Familienuntersuchung bei Typ-I-Diabetes. Hinweise für eine gemeinsame genetische Komponente von Typ-I- und Typ-II-Diabetes. Diabetes und Stoffwechsel 1992; 1: 14–17.
[24] Diabetes Epidemiology Research International Group. Geographic patterns of childhood insulin-dependent Diabetes mellitus. Diabetes 1988; 37: 1113–1119.
[25] Dorman JS, Laporte RE, Stone RA et al. Worldwide differences in the incidence of type 1 diabetes are associated with amino acid variation at position 57 of the HLA-DQ beta chain. Proc Natl Acad Sci USA 1990; 87: 7370–7374.
[26] Virtanen SM, Räsänen L, Aro A et al. Infant feeding in finnish children < 7 yr of age with newly diagnosed IDDM. Diabetes Care 1991; 14: 415–417.
[27] Elliott RB, Martin JM. Dietary protein: a trigger of insulin-dependent diabetes in the BB rat? Diabetologia 1981; 20: 87–93.
[28] Karjalainen J, Martin JM, Knip M et al. A bovine albumin peptide as a possible trigger of insulin-dependent diabetes mellitus. N Engl J Med 1992; 327: 302–307.
[29] Ziegler AG, Hillebrand B, Rabl W et al. On the appearance of islet cell associated autoimmunity in offspring of diabetic mothers: a prospective study from birth. Diabetologia 1993; 36: 402–408.
[30] Yoon JW, Austin M, Onodera T et al. Virus-induced diabetes mellitus: isolation of a virus from the pancreas of a child with diabetic ketoacidosis. N Engl J Med 1979; 300: 1173–1179.
[31] Scherbaum WA, Hampl W, Muir P et al. No association between islet cell antibodies and coxsackie B, mumps, rubella and cytomegalovirus antibodies in non-diabetic individuals. Diabetologia 1991; 34: 835–838.
[32] Ginsberg-Fellner F, Witt ME, Yagihashi S et al. Congenital rubella syndrome as a model for type 1 diabetes mellitus: increased prevalence of islet cell surface antibodies. Diabetologia 1984; 27: 87–89.
[33] Ziegler AG, Baumgartl HJ, Ede G et al. Low pigment skin type and predisposition for development of type 1 diabetes? Diabetes Care 1990; 13: 529–531.
[34] Ranson M, Posen S, Mason RS. Human melanocytes as a target tissue for hormones: in vitro studies with 1 alpha-25 dihydroxyvitamin D3, alpha-melanocyte stimulating hormone, and beta-estradiol. Soc Invest Dermatol: 1989; 593–598.
[35] Manolagas SC, Hustmyer FG, Yu XP. 1,25-dihydroxyvitamin D3 and the immune system. Soc Exp Biol Med: 1989; 238–245.
[36] Baumgartl HJ, Standl E, Schmidt-Gayk H et al. Changes of Vitamin D_3 serum concentrations at the onset of immune-mediated type 1 (insulin-dependent) diabets mellitus. Diabetes Research 1992; 16: 145–148.
[37] Gepner P, Amor B, Fournier C. 1,25-dihydroxyvitamin D3 potentiates the in vitro inhibitory effects of cyclosporin A on T cells from rheumatoid arthritis patients. Arth Reum 1989; 32: 31–36.
[38] Mathieu C, Laureys J, Waer M et al. 1,25 $(OH)_2$ Vitamin D prevents insulitis in NOD mice. Diabetologia 1992; 35: 217A.
[39] Rodewald A, Zankl H. Hautleistenfibel. Stuttgart: Gustav Fischer Verlag, 1981; 21.
[40] Verbov JL. Dermatoglyphics in early-onset diabetes mellitus. Heredity 1973; 23: 535–539.
[41] Chakravartti MR. Association between diabetes mellitus and dermatoglyphics. In: Hirsch W. Hautleisten und Krankheiten. Berlin: Grosse-Verlag, 1969; 157–161.

[42] Eswaraiah G, Bali RS. Palmar flexion creases and dermatoglyphics among diabetic patients. Am J Phys Anthrop 1977; 47: 11 – 13.
[43] Iqbal MA, Sahay BK, Ahuja YR. Finger and palmar ridge counts in diabetes mellitus. Acta Anthropogenetica 1978; 2: 35 – 38.
[44] Ziegler AG, Mathies R, Ziegelmayer G et al. Dermatoglyphics in type 1 diabetes. Diabetic Medicine 1993; 10: 720 – 724.

Immune mechanisms of beta cell destruction in the prediabetic phase of IDDM patients: research methodologies identifying susceptible individuals

G. S. Eisenbarth

Abstract

During the past decade it has become clear that type 1 diabetes develops gradually in the great majority of individuals [1]. The slowness of diabetes development allows the detection of immunologic abnormalities prior to diabetes onset. Though the natural history of the appearance of autoantibodies is still incomplete (in particular for children less than age 5), the discovery, sequencing and utilization of a series of autoantigens (e. g. insulin, GAD, ICA69, GM2-1) is rapidly improving the identification of at risk relatives. Conversion to autoantibody positivity usually occurs in infancy. The levels of all biochemically defined autoantigens are remarkably constant over time, are regulated at different levels for different prediabetics, and such levels are in part determined by alleles within the major histocompatibility complex. In that different prediabetic individuals independently express different autoantibodies, we are developing combinatorial predictive algorithms (e. g. expression of ≥2 autoantibodies). A general rule is that almost all prediabetics express more than one autoantibody and that the expression of a single autoantibody is rarely associated (e. g. restricted ICA which represents a subtype of "GAD" ICA) with progression to diabetes. In addition to determination of autoantibodies we utilize metabolic testing to aid in defining when diabetes will develop. The identification of high risk individuals can greatly increases the efficiency of trials for the prevention of type 1 diabetes.

Introduction

The identification of individuals at increased risk for type 1 diabetes could be based upon determination of (1) genetic risk, (2) exposure to environmental

Offprint from
Research Methodologies in Human Diabetes – Part 1

triggers of the disease, (3) detection of autoantibodies, (4) detection of autoreactive T cells, (5) detection of tissue damage (e.g. release of islet components upon lysis of cells), (6) metabolic abnormalities and (7) a combination of abnormalities. Because of their identification, specificity, sensitivity, and ease of determination, factors 1, 3, and 6 are the current mainstays of identifying at risk individuals, and will be reviewed in this chapter.

Genetic risk

Individuals who develop type 1 diabetes share alleles within the major histocompatibility complex associated with diabetes susceptibility [2]. In Caucasians the highest risk haplotypes are associated with DR3 and DR4, and in particular with specific DQbeta alleles, DR3, DQA1*0501, DQB1*0201 and DR4, DQA1*0301, DQB*0302. More than 90% of patients developing type 1 diabetes express either DR3 and DR4 and approximately 40% of patients with type 1 diabetes express both of these high risk haplotypes (in contrast to 2% of the general population). In addition, selective alleles appear to provide in a dominant fashion protection from type 1 diabetes. The DR2 associated haplotype with DQA1*0102, DQB1*0602 [3] almost completely protects from type 1 diabetes in many ethnic groups including Caucasians and Japanese populations. Individuals with insulin-dependent diabetes and DQB1*0602 should be evaluated for unusual genetic syndromes such as Wolfram's syndrome (DIDMOAD, diabetes insipidus, diabetes mellitus, optic atrophy and nerve deafness [4]) or the polyendocrine type I autoimmune syndrome [5] with mucocutaneous candidiasis, hypoparathyroidism, and Addison's disease. Additional protective haplotypes are being defined in other ethnic groups such as American hispanics. Actual determination of DQbeta alleles is superior to simply determining whether there is an aspartic acid at position 57 of the BQbeta chain [6], as there is relatively little correlation between diabetes risk and aspartic acid at position 57 in contrast to typing for complete alleles (e.g. DQB1*0602, DQB1*0301, and DQB1*0402 all contain Asp 57; while *0602 is protective, *0301 neutral, and *0402 diabetogenic [2, 3]).

It is almost certain that alleles outside of the major histocompatibility complex also contribute to diabetes susceptibility. To date, only alleles associated with insulin gene/IGF2 gene polymorphisms [7[are firmly associated with diabetes risk. The inheritance of such alleles appear to be complex, with the potential for maternal imprinting. In that the diabetes associated allele is very common in the general population, at present typing for such alleles does not aid in the prediction of type 1 diabetes. It is likely that other genes will be discovered to contribute to diabetes susceptibility, similar to animal models of the disorder [8, 9]. Approximately 70% of identical twins expressing DR3/4 are concordant for type 1 diabetes. This gives an approximate upper limit for genetic penetrance of the disorder [10].

Both HLA alleles and insulin gene alleles are currently typed following amplification of DNA with the polymerase chain reaction (PCR) [11]. For example, typing for HLA DQalpha alleles can be performed within hours with a reverse dot blot "kit" which does not utilize radioactivity. It is likely that a similar kit for DQbeta alleles will soon be available. It is currently possible to screen large populations for DR3/4 heterozygosity utilizing oligonucleotide probes following PCR amplification. Such individuals from the general Caucasian population would have a genetic risk of type 1 diabetes similar to offspring of a patient with type 1 diabetes (approximately 1/16). More than 85% of patients developing type 1 diabetes do not have a first degree relative with the disease. The ability to initially genetically identify a high risk group which comprises approximately 40% of patients with type 1 diabetes will likely find utility in identifying members of the general population for preventive trials.

First degree relatives of patients with type 1 diabetes (1/20 risk of diabetes with one diabetic relative, increasing to almost a 1/3 risk with two diabetic first degree relatives (e. g. two parents, parent and sibling)) and patients with the polyendocrine syndrome type II [12] are at increased genetic risk. In the polyendocrine syndrome type II, with associated autoimmune disorders including Addison's disease, type 1 diabetes, myasthenia gravis, pernicious anaemia, Graves' disease, vitiligo, alopecia totalis, there is an inherited tendency to break tolerance to multiple tissues. In general, the rarer the autoimmune disease (e. g. Addison's versus Graves' disease), the more likely that an individual will develop type 1 diabetes. Caution in predicting diabetes in ICA positive individuals with polyendocrine autoimmunity is required. A significant proportion of such patients express a subset of cytoplasmic islet cell antibodies ("restricted", "selective", "GAD-ICA") which are not predictive of diabetes [13, 14].

Autoantibodies

Table 1 lists a series of molecularly characterized autoantigens. It is likely that biochemical assays for specific autoantibodies will rapidly replace testing for cytoplasmic islet cell antibodies.

Table 1 Molecularly characterized autoantigens

Insulin
Glutamic acid decarboxylase (GAD65 and GAD67)
ICA 69 (milk albumin related)
Carboxypeptidase H
Gangliosides GT3, GM2-1

ICA

Cytoplasmic islet cell antibodies (ICA) reflect a series of different autoantibodies and many biochemically detectable autoantibodies (insulin, most GAD autoantibodies) do not give rise to islet staining in standard tests for ICA. Of even more concern it has been difficult to standardize ICA testing, and there is large variation between laboratories. A portion of this variation has been ameliorated with international utilization of titers of ICA expressed in JDF units [15], and with proficiency test kits provided by the Immunology of Diabetes workshop Committee, through Gainesville. Nevertheless, the ICA test which predominantly utilizes frozen sections of human pancreas is markedly dependent upon the human pancreas utilized and a laboratories performance can vary over time as new pancreatic substrate is obtained. Despite the above caveats, the detection of high titers of ICA (> 20 JDF units) is associated with more than a 50% risk of future type 1 diabetes after five years of follow up amongst first degree relatives of patients with type 1 diabetes [1, 16, 17]. Applying Bayes' theorem, it is likely that the positive predictive value of the same titers of ICA applied to the general population would be less than 10%.

In the past, ICA was spoken of in the singular. It is now clear that there is heterogeneity in what is termed ICA, and importantly, a subset of high titer ICA is not associated with appreciable risk of future type 1 diabetes [14]. This form of ICA which we termed "restricted" and which Bottazzo and coworkers have termed "selective" [13] has been found in both first degree relatives and in polyendocrine patients. Restricted ICA was initially identified because it failed to stain mouse islets while reacting with human and rat islets (Fig. 1). Correlates of restricted ICA include absorption by affinity purified glutamic acid decarboxylase [18], association with extremely high levels of anti-GAD autoantibodies as detected with a radioassay, ability to Western blot GAD, and ability to stain GABA-ergic neurons. Relatives expressing restricted ICA have antibodies which to date are not distinguishable from the antibodies of patients with Stiff Man Syndrome. It appears that the ability

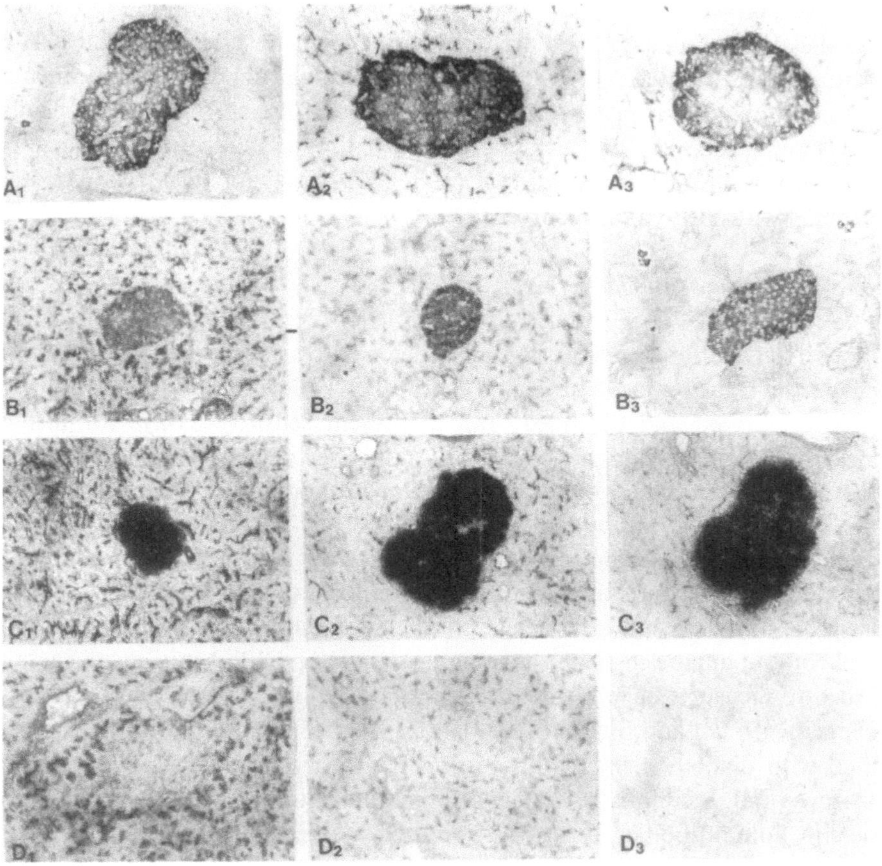

Fig. 1 Immunoperoxidase staining of rat (A_1-A_3, and C_1-C_3) and mouse (B_1-B_3 and D_1-D_3) pancreas with sera. Restricted ICA is beta cell specific (for rat) and reacts strongly with rat pancreas (C_1-C_3) but is non-reactive with mouse pancreas (D_1-D_3) while non-restricted ICA reacts equally well with mouse and rat pancreas (A_1-A_3 and B_1-B_3). Panels 1, 2, 3, sera diluted 1 : 5, 1 : 25 and 1 : 125. From Diabetes 1992; 41: 347–353

to simply absorb high dilutions of ICA positive sera with GAD does not suffice to identify restricted ICA, as studies which have utilized only this criteria have failed to distinguish antibody subsets with prognostic significance [19]. Of eight relatives we have studied whose ICA is absorbed with GAD, six have extremely high titer anti-GAD autoantibodies, and of these six, none has progressed to overt diabetes, none express other autoantibodies (insulin, ICA69), and all have maintained normal first phase insulin secretion with more than 5 years of follow up. In contrast, of two relatives whose sera could be absorbed with GAD, but who do not have high titer anti-GAD autoantibodies by radioassay, one developed type 1 diabetes and expressed ICA69 autoantibodies and the other has both ICA69 autoantibodies and anti-insulin autoantibodies. It is noteworthy that restricted ICA and high levels of anti-GAD autoantibodies, and lack of progression to type 1 diabetes are associated with the protective HLA allele DQB1*0602 both amongst relatives and patients with Stiff Man Syndrome [20].

Anti-insulin autoantibodies

Insulin autoantibodies were originally detected by Palmer and coworkers in new onset patients prior to insulin therapy [21]. This initial observation has been confirmed and extended, and at present sensitive assays for insulin autoantibodies provide one of the best assays for detection of individuals at risk for type 1 diabetes. In addition, insulin autoantibodies are unique in that the levels of such antibodies appear to inversely correlate with the age at which type 1 diabetes develops [22]. We currently determine insulin autoantibodies with a competitive fluid phase radioassay which utilizes relatively large volumes of sera (150 ul of sera $\times$ 4 for duplicate measurement with and without unlabeled insulin). Attempts to develop ELISA anti-insulin assays failed to measure diabetes predictive antibodies, probably related to the low capacity (10^{-12}) and high affinity (10^{10}) of the insulin autoantibodies associated with diabetes risk. In this respect the antibodies which follow insulin therapy and therefore subcutaneous immunization appear to differ from insulin autoantibodies. Insulin autoantibodies recognize a limited conformational epitope of the insulin molecule critically dependent upon A13 leucine and involving both the A and B chains. Of note, removal of the B chain terminal eight amino acids which abolishes bioactivity does not alter binding to autoantibodies. In addition, proinsulin is as immunoreactive as insulin.

Insulin autoantibodies are present in approximately 70% of the relatives we have followed to overt diabetes. There is some evidence that such antibodies are the first antibodies to appear in many individuals and we frequently detect insulin autoantibodies preceding ICA in young children (Fig. 2). For children under the age of 5, almost all who express insulin autoantibodies subsequently develop ICA. The levels of insulin autoantibodies do not appear to be directly correlated with age, but rather with the age at which type 1 diabetes develops [22]. Thus, cytoplasmic islet cell antibody positive children under the age of 5, who lack detectable insulin autoantibodies, remain insulin autoantibody negative and to date have not developed diabetes with follow up. In contrast to young children, adults often express insulin autoantibodies for years as their only immunologic abnormality. Risk of diabetes, though present, appears to be low in such IAA+/ICA− relatives.

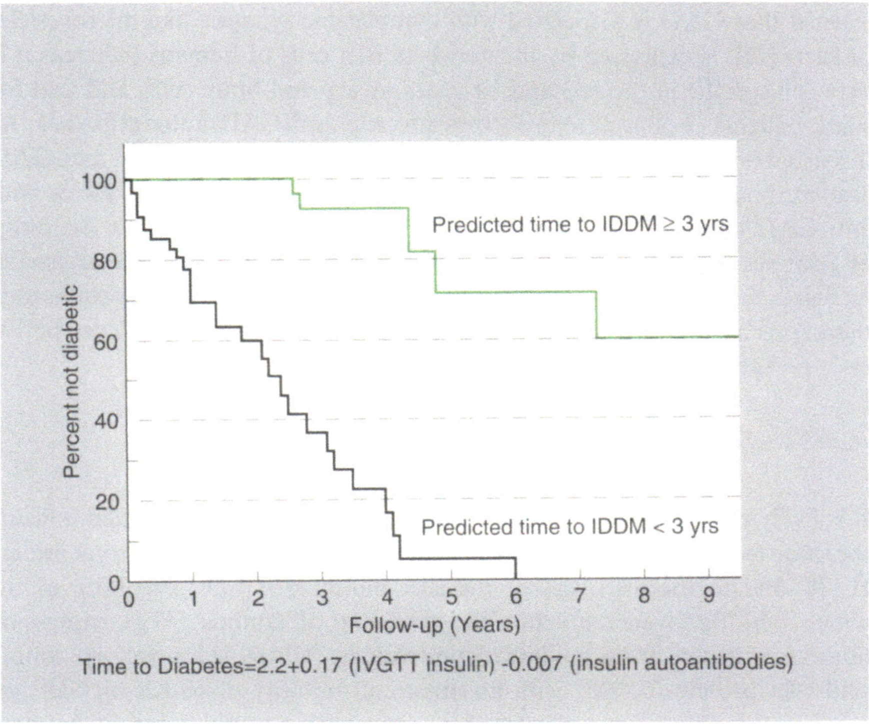

Fig. 2 Illustrated are levels of insulin autoantibodies and cytoplasmic islet cell antibodies for two offspring of a patient with type 1 diabetes. For both children, insulin autoantibodies preceded ICA. Insulin autoantibodies < 39 mU are normal while both siblings developed levels in the hundreds (sibling 1) to thousands (sibling 2)

Anti-GAD autoantibodies

Studies of anti-GAD autoantibodies illustrate the rapidity of progress with the biochemical identification of putative autoantigens. Antibodies to a 64 Kd protein of islets were first described in 1982 [23]. The difficulty of the assay for such antibodies greatly hindered their study and led to considerable confusion as to their importance, with claims that the target antigen was beta cell specific, present on the surface of beta cells, and the first antigen to which antibodies are formed [24]. It now appears that none of the above were correct. In 1990 DeCamilli, Baekkeskov and coworkers, following studies of Stiff Man Syndrome [25], discovered that glutamic acid decarboxylase was the antigen of the 64 Kd reactivity [25]. With its biochemical characterization and the availability of monoclonal anti-GAD antibodies it has rapidly been learned that GAD is associated with cytoplasmic synaptic like microvesicles of islets [26], is expressed by the non-beta islet cells of humans (whereas it is beta cell specific in the rat) and by testes, ovary and brain cells, and that for some patients insulin autoantibodies precede anti-GAD autoantibodies. As discussed under ICA, a subset of relatives with the highest levels of anti-GAD autoantibodies rarely progress to overt diabetes [14], but for relatives with anti-GAD autoantibodies exceeding the normal range, but below the range of relatives with restricted ICA, the presence of anti-GAD autoantibodies increases the risk of type 1 diabetes [27]. In contrast to insulin autoantibodies, there does not seem to be a correlation between levels of anti-GAD antibodies and the age at which type 1 diabetes develops.

ICA69 autoantibodies

It is likely that an enlarging family of autoantigens will be identified utilizing the same technique applied to the detection of antibodies to carboxypeptidase H [28] and to the discovery of the islet molecule ICA69 [29]. Both of the above were discovered utilizing the screening of lambda GT11 expression libraries with sera from prediabetic individuals. ICA69 is a novel 483 amino acid islet protein (55 Kd) with an apparent mobility of 69 Kd on SDS gel chromatography. Using a Western blot assay with recombinant protein, more than 40% of prediabetic individuals produce antibodies to ICA69. It is very likely that the large majority of prediabetics will be found to produce autoantibodies to ICA69 when a radioassay for such antibodies is developed. In the rat, ICA69 is beta cell specific, but it is not currently known whether it is also beta cell specific for human islets (note that GAD is beta cell specific for the rat but not man). A search of GenBank revealed no molecules homologous to ICA69, though it does share two short sequences with bovine albumin. ICA69 appears to be identical to the milk albumin related protein sought by Dosch and coworkers [30].

Anti-37 Kd autoantibodies

At present, autoantibodies capable of precipitating a 38 Kd islet protein and reactivity of T cell lines from diabetics with a 37 Kd islet molecule have generated considerable interest [31, 32]. It is becoming clear that these molecules are not derivatives of GAD, despite initial assays which involved immunoprecipitation of labeled and trypsin digested 64 Kd antigen preparations [31]. It is likely that antibodies to these molecules will aid in the prediction of the risk of type 1 diabetes, but comparisons between their predictive potential comparing (a) patients with restricted ICA and anti-GAD (64 Kd) autoantibodies (a single autoantibody), and (b) patients expressing ICA and anti-37 Kd autoantibodies (two different autoantibodies) are likely to exaggerate the positive predictive value of antibodies to this molecule alone [31].

Anti-ganglioside autoantibodies

Beginning with studies of monoclonal antibody A2B5 [33], it has become apparent that islets share with neurons a series of complex glycolipids [34, 35]. Early studies indicated that glycolipid extracts of human pancreas could be utilized to block ICA staining [36, 37]. On thin layer chromatography, blocking activity migrated between gangliosides GM2 and GM1 and at the TLC front. The ganglioside between GM2 and GM1 has been biochemically characterized by Dotta and coworkers, and of note it is an unusual ganglioside similar to LM1 gangliosides which are the targets of anti-neuronal autoimmunity, and which have a terminal sialic acid residue [38]. The recent identification of the GM2-1 molecule will hopefully facilitate the production of the molecule for autoantibody assays.

Other autoantibodies

A series of other islet autoantigens are in various stages of characterization both biochemically and in terms of their ability to aid in the prediction of type 1 diabetes. One difficulty presented by the finding of such a large group of autoantibodies relates to distinguishing which antigens are central to the pathogenic process and which are secondary. It is likely that the order in which antibodies first appear will aid in such discrimination, but definition of this order will almost certainly require the prospective evaluation of children less than age 5. In addition, one can hypothesize that crucial autoantigens will be absent from pseudoatrophic islets (islets from long term patients with type 1 diabetes which contain only non-beta cells). To date, insulin and proinsulin are the only beta cell specific antigen identified.

Combinatorial prediction of type 1 diabetes

Though the existence of a series of autoantigens will complicate the search for "pathogenic" autoantigens, such a family of biochemically defined autoantigens should greatly facilitate the prediction of type 1 diabetes. Our initial studies of autoantibodies to insulin, GAD and ICA69 indicate that autoantibodies appear to each molecule independently in prediabetics. Thus it is possible to identify relatives expressing two out of the three antibodies, and thereby greatly increase specificity without impacting on sensitivity of detecting at risk relatives [39].

Metabolic testing

The presence of autoantibodies identifies relatives with an increased risk of type 1 diabetes, but for the most part does not aid in estimating when overt diabetes will develop (a potential exception is the presence of high levels of insulin autoantibodies associated with a more rapid progression to diabetes) [16]. Metabolic abnormalities preceding diabetes can be subdivided by when they occur prior to overt diabetes.

We have now followed more than 40 ICA positive individuals who have had intravenous glucose tolerance testing prior to overt diabetes. Loss of first phase insulin secretion usually but not always precedes all other metabolic abnormalities. Thus at a time when oral glucose tolerance testing is normal, K rate on intravenous glucose tolerance testing is normal, fasting glucose is below 90 mg%, HbA1 is normal, first phase insulin response is frequently below the first percentile of normal individuals [40–45]. A standardized protocol for intravenous glucose tolerance testing has been developed. Profound abnormalities of first phase insulin secretion can precede diabetes (as diagnosed with oral glucose tolerance testing) by more than three years. Closer to the development of overt diabetes, ICA positive relatives frequently evidence sporadic elevations of fasting glucose, and a fasting glucose greater than 108/dl has in our studies been associated with a positive predictive value for overt diabetes of close to 100% within 1.5 years [43]. The fasting glucose usually does not begin to rise until 1.5 years prior to overt diabetes.

Problems with intravenous glucose tolerance testing include an approximate 30% coefficient of variation [46], occasional observation of a "first" test effect in children under age 7, age related changes in intravenous glucose tolerance testing [47], abnormalities of first phase secretion in essentially all forms of diabetes, and the existence of a subset of relatives who rapidly lose first phase insulin secretion only shortly prior to overt diabetes. The only method to date to dramatically reduce the coefficient of variation of "testing" is repetition of the test. Repeating the test twice reduces the coefficient of variation from 30% to 21%, and with three repetitive tests to 18%. We utilize such repetitive testing to evaluate ICA positive relatives who might be eligible for entry into trials for the prevention of type 1 diabetes. In addition, a problem in the testing of young children appears to be the frequent occurrence of a markedly abnormal first test, followed by "normal" subsequent testing. After puberty there is little change in first phase secretion, and a major portion of lower values for pre-pubertal children appears to be this first test effect. Variation of first phase secretion is so large in normal populations [42] that we have not found correction by age to be of use in developing predictive models.

Fig. 3 illustrates the utilization of a linear predictive model to subdivide relatives into "short" (less than three years) and long (> 3 years) time to overt diabetes [48, 49]. The model, years to DM = 2.2 ± 0.17 (IVGTT

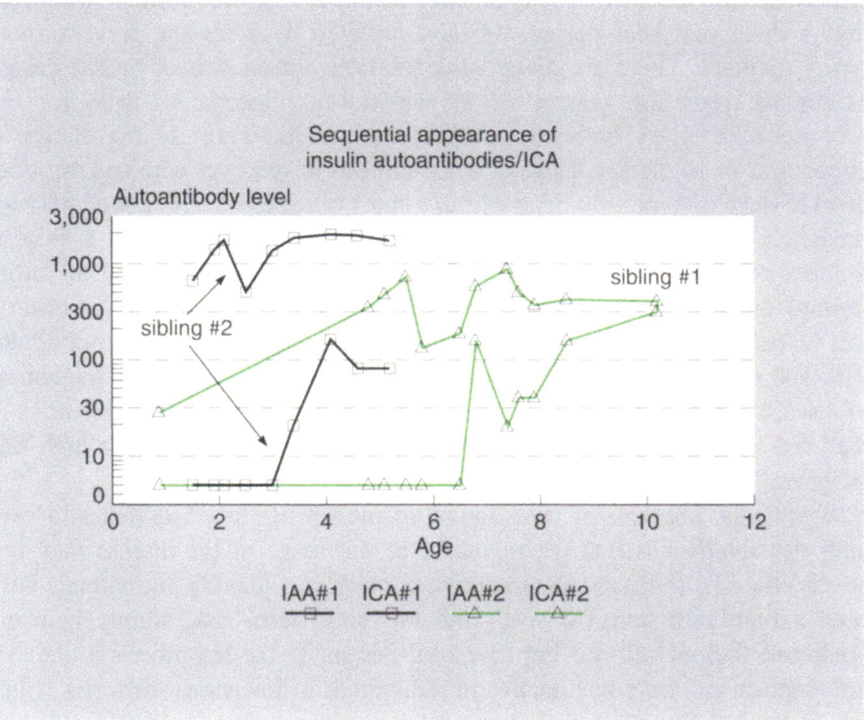

Fig. 3 Life table analysis of progression to overt diabetes in ICA+ relatives subdivided by "dual" parameter predicted time (> or < 3 years)

insulin) − 0.007 (Insulin autoantibodies) gives a life table very similar to that generated when ICA+ relatives only subdivided on the basis of first phase insulin secretion. Though the two life tables appear similar, the major advantage of the model is the initial identification of almost 1/2 of the ICA positive relatives at high risk rather than 1/3. Thus the model allows earlier entry of ICA positive relatives into preventive trials. As more experience has been gained with such a linear regression model we find significant inter-individual heterogeneity [50]. Time to diabetes can accurately be predicted for approximately 3/4 of ICA positive relatives followed to diabetes, while for 1/4, at all time points there is a significant overestimation of time to diabetes. Factors distinguishing between these two groups of relatives need to be developed to improve the sensitivity of diabetes prediction.

Trials for the prevention of type 1 diabetes

With the ability to identify relatives at very high risk for the development of type 1 diabetes and at the same time identify relatives with a much lower risk over a three year time period, we have initiated trials for the prevention of type 1 diabetes. There are many considerations which impact on the design of clinical trials and sample size considerations. Specific to trials for the prevention of type 1 diabetes, considerations of the stage of the disease is important. In particular, trials of interventions in relatives who can be identified to develop type 1 diabetes within a short time period with a high positive predictive value can enter few individuals (e.g. 20) and screen a limited number of first degree relatives (1/150 relatives are at high risk at initial testing). In contrast, trials which utilize only ICA positivity as an entry criteria can be calculated to require the screening of as many as 45,000 individuals with 900 relatives randomized if an intervention fails to influence the course of disease in very high risk relatives. Even if an intervention were effective in high risk individuals, screening and entry could be reduced for the high risk subgroup by specific identification.

A potential negative of trials aimed at preventing type 1 diabetes in very high risk relatives is that interventions at this stage of the disease may not be effective. In that current predictive models can identify individuals with both a high short-term (3 year) and low short-term risk, simply ignoring predictive factors will not improve trial design. If the hypothesis is that an intervention will only be effective in individuals at low short-term risk, trials would need to focus on individuals who would not develop diabetes in the next two to three years and use as their outcome those developing diabetes three to more years after the beginning of an intervention.

Consideration of trial design for the prevention of type 1 diabetes is certainly no longer simply an academic consideration. Trials have begun in the United States and Europe. At the Barbara Davis Center and the Joslin Diabetes Center we have treated 7 individuals at high risk for type 1 diabetes with nicotinamide and 6/7 are now diabetic. In contrast, both institutions are now collaborating in a trial of high dose intravenous insulin (5 days per 9 months) followed by low dose subcutaneous insulin. Preliminary data (7/7 diabetic amongst non-treated versus 1/5 versus treated) suggests that such a regimen may delay or prevent diabetes [51] and a randomized, IV placebo controlled multicenter trial of such therapy has begun.

The future

It is very likely that therapies to delay or prevent type 1 diabetes will shortly become available. It is hoped that effective therapies will utilize antigen specific interventions such as oral insulin for "oral tolerance" [52] or parenteral insulin for "beta cell rest" [51] rather than general immunosuppressives. If any of the current trials are successful, laboratory based assays will need to be converted to biochemical "kit" like assays for application to large populations. If one estimates that there are 2,000,000 first degree relatives of patients with type 1 diabetes in the United States, 13,000 would be eligible as high risk individuals. Amongst the whole U. S. population it is likely that there are more than 100,000 individuals at high risk for type 1 diabetes. In that the prior probability of diabetes is 3/1,000 in the general population versus 50/1,000 amongst first degree relatives, prediction in the general population will require combinatorial strategies to obtain acceptable positive predictive values. Screening initially for DR3/4 heterozygous individuals in the general population with PCR based methods followed by autoantibody testing is currently feasible. The screening for autoantibodies will almost certainly utilize a family of defined autoantigens (replacing ICA testing). There is much yet to be learned concerning the natural history and pathogenesis of type 1 diabetes, but I am hopeful that even without a fundamental increase in our knowledge, diabetes for a subset of individuals will become preventable.

References

[1] Thai A-C, Eisenbarth GS. Natural history of IDDM. Diabetes/Metabolism Reviews 1993; in press.
[2] Nepom GT, Erlich H. MHC class-II molecules and autoimmunity. Ann Rev Immunol 1991; 9: 493–525.

[3] Erlich HA, Griffith RL, Bugawan TL et al. Implication of specific DQB1 alleles in genetic susceptibility and resistance by identification of IDDM siblings with novel HLA-BQB1 allele and unusual DR2 and DR1 haplotypes. Diabetes 1991; 40: 478–481.
[4] Karasik A, O'Hara C, Srikanta S et al. Genetically programmed selective islet beta-cell loss in diabetic subjects with Wolfram's syndrome. Diabetes Care 1989; 12: 135–138.
[5] Ahonen P, Myllarniemi S, Sipila I et al. Clinical variation of autoimmune polyendocrinopathy-candidiasis – ectodermal dystrophy (apeced) in a series of 68 patients. New Eng J of Med 1990; 322: 1830–1836.
[6] Morel PA, Dorman JS, Todd JA et al. Aspartic acid at position 57 of the HLA-DQ beta chain protects against type 1 diabetes: a family study. Proc Natl Acad Asi USA 1988; 85: 8111–8115.
[7] Julier C, Hyer RN, Davies J et al. Insulin-IGF2 region encodes a gene implicated in HLA-DR4-dependent diabetes susceptibility. Nature 1991; 354: 155–159.
[8] Todd JA, Aitman TJ, Cornall RJ et al. Genetic analysis of autoimmune type 1 diabetes mellitus in mice. Nature 1991; 351: 542–547.
[9] Jacob HJ, Pettersson A, Wilson et al. Genetic dissection of autoimmune type 1 diabetes in the BB rat. Nature Genetics 1992; 2: 56–60.
[10] Johnston C, Pyke DA, Cudworth AG et al. HLA-DR typing in identical twins with insulin dependent diabetes, difference between concordant and discordant pairs. BR J 1983; 286: 253–255.
[11] Bugawan L, Erlich HA. Rapid typing of HLA-DQB1 DNA polymorphism using nonradioactive oligonucleotide probes and amplified DNA. Immunogenetics 1991; 33: 163–170.
[12] Eisenbarth GS, Jackson RA. The immunoendocrinopathy syndromes. In: Wilson JD, Foster DW, eds. Williams Textbook of Endocrinology. 8th ed. Philadelphia: W. B. Saunders Company, 1992: 1555–1566.
[13] Genovese S, Bonifacio E, McNally JM et al. Distinct cytoplasmic islet cell antibodies with different risks for type 1 (insulin-dependent) diabetes mellitus. Diabetologia 1992; 35: 385–388.
[14] Gianani R, Pugliese A, Bonner-Weir S et al. Prognostically significant heterogeneity of cytoplasmic islet cell antibodies in relatives of patients with type 1 diabetes. Diabetes 1992; 41: 347–353.
[15] Greenbaum CJ, Palmer JP, Nagataki S et al. Improved specificity of ICA assays in the Fourth International Immunology of Diabetes Exhange Workshop. Diabetes 1992; 41: 1570–1574.
[16] Ziegler AG, Ziegler R, Vardi et al. Life table analysis of progression to diabetes of anti-insulin autoantibody-positive relatives of individuals with type 1 diabetes. Diabetes 1989; 38: 1320–1325.
[17] Bonifacio E, Bingley PJ, Shattock M et al. Quantitative islet cell antibody measurement assists in the prediction of insulin-dependent diabetes. Lancet 1990; 335: 147–149.
[18] Gianani R, Jackson R, Eisenbarth GS. Evidence that the autoantigen of restricted ICA is GAD. Diabetes Research and Clinical Practice 1991; 14 (suppl. 1): S13 (abstract).
[19] Atkinson MA, Kaufman DL, Newman D et al. Islet cell cytoplasmic autoantibody reactivity to glutamate decarboxylase in insulin-dependent diabetes. J Clin Invest 1993; 91: 350–356.
[20] Pugliese A, Gianani R, Solimena M et al. Association of HLA-DQB1*0201 and DQB1*06 Alleles with Stiff-Man Syndrome. Diabetes 1993; in press (abstract).
[21] Kuglin B, Kolb H, Greenbaum C et al. The fourth international workshop on the standardisation of insulin autoantibody measurement. Diabetologia 1990; 33: 638–639.
[22] Vardi P, Ziegler AG, Matthews JH et al. Concentration of insulin autoantibodies at onset of type 1 diabetes: inverse log-linear correlation with age. Diabetes Care 1988; 11: 736–739.
[23] Baekkeskov S, Nielsen JH, Marner B et al. Autoantibodies in newly diagnosed diabetic children immunoprecipitate specific human islet cell proteins. Nature 1982; 298: 167–169.
[24] Baekkeskov S, Landin M, Kristensen JK et al. Antibodies to a 64,000 M, human islet antigen precede the clinical onset of insulin dependent diabetes. J Clin Investigation 1987; 79: 926–934.

[25] Solimena M, Folli F, Aparisi R et al. Autoantibodies to GABA-ergic neurons and pancreatic beta cells in Stiff-Man Syndrome. New England Journal of Medicine 1990; 322: 1555–1560.
[26] Reetz A, Solimena M, Matteoli M et al. GABA and pancreatic beta-cells: colocalization of glutamic acid decarboxylase (GAD) and GABA with synaptic-like microvesicles suggests their role in GABA storage and secretion. EMBO Journal 1991; 10: 1275–1284.
[27] Rowley MJ, Mackay IR, Chen Q et al. Antibodies to glutamic acid decarboxylase discriminate major types of diabetes mellitus. Diabetes 1992; 41: 548–551.
[28] Castano L, Russo E, Zhou L et al. Identification and cloning of a granule autoantigen (carboxypeptidase H) associated with type 1 diabetes. J Clin Endo Metab 1991; 73: 1197–1201.
[29] Pietropaolo M, Castano L, Babu S et al. Islet cell autoantigen 69 kDa (ICA69): molecular cloning and characterization of a novel diabetes associated autoantigen. J Clin Invest 1993; (in press).
[30] Karjalainen J, Martin JM, Knip M et al. A bovine albumin peptide as a possible trigger of insulin-dependent diabetes mellitus. The New England Journal of Medicine 1992; 327: 302–307.
[31] Christie MR, Richard YM, Tun RYM et al. Antibodies to GAD and tryptic fragments of islet 64K antigen as distinct markers for development of IDDM: Studies with identical twins. Diabetes 1992; 41: 782–787.
[32] Roep BO, Kallan AA, Hazenbos WLW et al. T-cell reactivity to 38kD insulin-secretory-granule protein in patients with recent-onset type 1 diabetes. Lancet 1991; 337: 1439–1441.
[33] Eisenbarth GS, Shimizu K, Bowring MA et al. Expression of receptors for tetanus toxin and monoclonal antibody A2B5 by pancreatic islet cells. Proc Natl Acad Sci (USA) 1982; 79: 5066–5070.
[34] Gillard BK, Thomas JW, Nell LJ et al. Antibodies against ganglioside GT3 in the sera of patients with type 1 diabetes mellitus. Journal Immunol Methods 1989; 142: 3862–3832.
[35] Alejandro R, Shienvold FL, Hajek SAV et al. A ganglioside antigen on the rat pancreatic B cell surface identified by monoclonal antibody R2D6. J Clin Invest 1984; 74: 25–38.
[36] Dotta F, Colman PG, Nayak RC et al. Ganglioside expression in human pancreatic islets. Diabetes 1989; 38: 1478–1483.
[37] Colman PG, Nayak RC, Campbell IL et al. Binding of cytoplasmic islet cell antibodies is blocked by human pancreatic glycolipid extracts. Diabetes 1988; 37: 645–652.
[38] Dotta F, Previti M, Tiberti C et al. Identification of the GM2-1 islet gnaglioside: Similarities with a major neuronal autoantigen. Diabetes 1992; 41: 365A.
[39] Eisenbarth GS. Combinatorial autoantibody screening for prediction of type 1 diabetes. Clinical Research 1993; in press: (abstract).
[40] Srikanta S, Ganda OP, Eisenbarth GS et al. Islet cell antibodies and beta cell function in monozygotic triplets and twins initially discordant for type 1 diabetes mellitus. New England Journal of Medicine 1983; 308: 322–325.
[41] Ganda OP, Srikanta S, Brink WJ et al. Differential sensitivity to beta cell secretagogues in "early" type 1 diabetes mellitus. Diabetes 1984; 33: 516–521.
[42] Srikanta S, Ganda OP, Soeldner JS et al. First degree relatives of patients with type 1 diabetes mellitus: islet cell antibodies and abnormal insulin secretion. New England Journal of Medicine 1985; 313: 461–464.
[43] Bleich D, Jackson RA, Soeldner JS et al. Analysis of metabolic progression to type 1 diabetes in islet cell antibody positive relatives of patients with type 1 diabetes. Diabetes Care 1990; 13: 111–118.
[44] Vardi P, Crisa L, Jackson RA et al. Predictive value of intravenous glucose tolerance test insulin secretion less than or greater than the first percentile in islet cell antibody positive relatives of type 1 (insulin-dependent) diabetic patients. Diabetologia 1991; 34: 93–102.
[45] Tarn AC, Smith CP, Spencer KM et al. Type 1 (insulin-dependent) diabetes mellitus: a disease of slow clinical onset? British Medical Journal 1987; 294: 342–345.

[46] Smith CP, Tarn AC, Thomas JM et al. Between and within variation of the first phase insulin response to intravenous glucose. Diabetologia 1988; 31: 123–125.
[47] Smith CP, Thomas JM, Tarn AC et al. Basal and stimulated insulin levels rise with advancing puberty. Clinical Endocrinology 1988; 28: 7–14.
[48] Vardi P, Dib S, Herskowitz RD et al. Multiparameter prediction of months to overt diabetes in ICA positive first degree relatives. Diabetes 1988: 37 (Suppl): 21A (abstract).
[49] Ziegler AG, Ziegler R, Jackson RA et al. Testing the linear destruction hypothesis in type 1 diabetes: The Joslin Study. In: Adreani D, Kolb H, Pozzilli P, eds. Immunotherapy of type 1 diabetes. John Wiley and Sons Ltd, 1989: 155–167.
[50] Verge CF, Eisenbarth GS, Chase HP. Interindividual variation in accuracy of a dual parameter predictive model. Diabetes 1993; abstract.
[51] Keller RJ, Jackson RA, Eisenbarth GS. Preservation of beta cell function in islet cell antibody (ICA) positive first degree relatives treated with insulin. Diabetes 1992; 41 (Suppl 1): 50A.
[52] Zhang JZ, Davidson L, Eisenbarth GS et al. Suppression of diabetes in nonobese diabetic mice by oral administration of porcine insulin. Proc Natl Acad Sci (USA) 1991; 88: 10252–10256.

Interventions attempting at preventing or ameliorating the development of type 1 diabetes

H. Kolb

Who should read this chapter?

Most clinicians and researchers looking through this book probably do not intend to embark on intervention trials in (pre)type 1 diabetes. Hence, this chapter is meant for the diabetologist who seeks an update on results of immunotherapy studies and information about ongoing trials. In addition, a critique is provided of past and current attempts of intervention.

Lessons from the past — intervention trials at onset of IDDM

Attempts to ameliorate the natural course of type 1 diabetes by immune intervention have been reported since 1978 [1]. The decision in favour of such trials is based on two reasons. For one, insulin substitution therapy to date has not prevented the occurrence of late complications and early death, although considerable progress has been achieved [2]. Secondly, evidence is accumulating that immune reactions contribute to beta cell loss in type 1 diabetes [3]. Thus, immune intervention might prevent, halt or significantly delay progression of the disease.

Immunosuppression

In recent onset type 1 diabetes, immunosuppression has been tried following protocols known to be effective in other auto-immune diseases or in graft recipients. A summary of immunosuppression trials is given in Table 1. The large majority of these studies have to be refuted because of questionable scientific value. That is, most of these studies lack a randomised control group and/or recruited only small numbers of patients so that only enormous therapeutic effects could have been detectable. Most of these studies have been described in earlier reviews [1, 4] and, therefore, will not be discussed again.

Offprint from
Research Methodologies in Human Diabetes — Part 1

Table 1 List of published trials with immunosuppression protocols in recent onset type 1 diabetes

Azathioprine	Gamma irradiation of pancreas
Azathioprine + Prednis(ol)one	Monoclonal anti T-cell antibodies
Azathioprine + Prednis(ol)one et al.	Plasmapheresis
Azathioprine + Thymic Extract	Prednis(ol)one
Cyclosporin A	Prednis(ol)one + ATGAM

Relevant information was gained from two placebo-controlled trials with cyclosporin A [5, 6] and from a randomised, but not placebo-controlled trial of azathioprine plus glucocorticoids [7]. In fact, the outcome of the two cyclosporin-A-trials is considered a landmark, since it was shown for the first time that treatment with an immunosuppressive drug has beneficial effect on the course of the disease, in terms of reduced mean insulin requirements [5] and of preserved beta cell function (glucagon-stimulated C-peptide secretion) [6].

Results of the cyclosporin-A-trials can be summarised as follows:

- Continuous treatment with cyclosporin A (12 h trough level in whole blood 300 – 600 ng/ml, polyclonal antibody RIA) enhances the remission rate (approx. doubled after 1 year) and prolongs the remission phase. For effect, cyclosporin A must be introduced within weeks after diagnosis of IDDM.
- Continuous treatment with cyclosporin A increases and preserves beta cell function during the first year. However, even during insulin-independent remission with normal metabolic control (HbA1 levels within normal range), beta cell function is subnormal with loss of the first phase insulin response to intravenous glucose.
- Discontinuation of immunosuppressive treatment is followed by deterioration of metabolic control within 4 – 10 weeks and remission of abnormal blood and biochemical parameters within 3 – 6 months.
- Cyclosporin A effects on the course of diabetes are not long-lasting. Within 6 months after discontinuation, insulin requirements and beta cell function drop to the level of the control group [8].
- Even continuous administration of cyclosporin A was not able to prevent loss of remission after, at the longest, 2 – 3 years.

Conclusion: The immunosuppressive intervention after onset of IDDM has shown only transient efficacy. In view of the substantial risk of side-effects, the use of immunosuppressants must, thus, remain limited to well planned clinical trials. In addition, such trials should be supported only if the protocol differs significantly and convincingly from the prior studies. Because of the known long-term risks of immunosuppressive therapy, follow up of patients beyond drug discontinuation seems advisable. For further discussion, see below, "Ongoing trials".

Immunomodulation

A list of published immunointervention trials at onset of IDDM using so-called immunomodulatory approaches is given in Table 2. The common use of the term immunomodulation excludes immunosuppression but summarises types of intervention which aim at restoring a normal immunoregulatory balance. Thus, it is assumed that the immune attack against beta islet cells in type 1 diabetes is a consequence of immune dysregulation.

Table 2 List of published trials with immunomodulatory treatment protocols in recent onset type 1 diabetes

Ciamexone	Theophylline
Gammaglobulin	Thymopentin (TP5)
Indomethacin	$\text{Thymopoetin}_{32-36}$ +/− Glutathione
Inosine Pranobex	Thymostimulin (TP1)
Interferon	Transfusion
Levamisole	

Nearly all such intervention trials published to date lack a proper randomised control group or included only small numbers of patients, so that effects of the magnitude observed in the cyclosporin A trials would have gone unnoticed. Most of these studies have been described in earlier reviews [1, 4, 9] and, therefore, will not be discussed again.

Relevant information was gained from the placebo-controlled studies of interferon (no effect, but only 2 weeks of treatment) [10] and ciamexone (borderline significant effect, study discontinued because of uncertainty about the risk of adverse effects regarding liver function, observed in a randomised study in rheumatoid arthritis).

Conclusion: The published experience with immunomodulatory treatment protocols after onset of IDDM is not encouraging, but not unexpected. Past experience in other chronic inflammatory diseases has shown that these approaches offer only limited beneficial outcome. Thus, only large trials could have proven such effects. For further discussion, see below, "Ongoing trials".

Beta cell protection

Pancreatic islet cells have been found to be highly susceptible to the toxic effects of oxygen radicals [11, 12], nitric oxide [13] and interleukin 1 [14], the latter acting through the induction of NO synthesis and release of nitric oxide [15]. Thus, antioxidants or compounds supporting the beta cell defences are regarded as potential therapeutics in type 1 diabetes.

Nicotinamide is the only compound for which data from completed and published trials at onset of IDDM are available. This water-soluble vitamin was found previously to improve beta cell survival in various animal models and in tissue culture, including alloxan, streptozocin, oxygen radical and nitric oxide toxicity, partial pancreatectomy, and beta cell proliferation in vitro [13, 16–20]. Nicotinamide was able to prevent diabetes development in NOD mice when given from early in life and in high doses (500 mg/kg body weight/day) [21]. However, treatment with nicotinamide failed to prevent diabetes in the BB rat model [9, 22]. Four modes of protective action are presently discussed for nicotinamide (Fig. 1). Mechanism 1 foresees the action as an oxygen radical scavenger. However, nicotinamide is a weak radical scavenger, even potent oxygen radical scavengers do not match nicotinamide in diabetes prevention in animals nor do oxygen radical scavengers protect islet cells from nitric oxide toxicity [9, 13]. Mechanism 2 expects nicotinamide to act as precursor of NAD, thus stabilising NAD-levels in islet cells under immune attack. In vitro, this possibility has been ruled out since structurally related compounds without NAD precursor activity also protect islet cells [13]. Mechanism 3 describes nicotinamide as an inhibitor of poly-ADP-ribosylation. Poly-ADP-ribosylation occurs early during the repair of DNA damage which is expected to occur in islet cells under immune attack. Consumption of ADP-ribose leads to the depletion of NAD, subsequent loss of ATP and plasma membrane lysis [23]. Mechanism 4 is based on the finding that nicotinamide also inhibits mono(ADP-ribose)transferases, albeit to a lesser degree [24]. Mono-ADP-ribosylation of proteins often regulates protein function; any interference with this activity will affect cell function. The concentration of nicotinamide needed for 50% inhibition of mono(ADP-ribose)transferases is in the millimolar range. Such high levels will not be reached in vivo, unless there is active accumulation of nicotinamide in islets.

It is estimated that more than 400 recently diagnosed IDDM patients have been treated with nicotinamide to date. A detailed account of the individual trials has recently been published [4]. In summary, most trials applied doses between 10 and 50 mg/kg body weight/d. They were randomised, often placebo-controlled and included children, adolescents and adults [25–31].

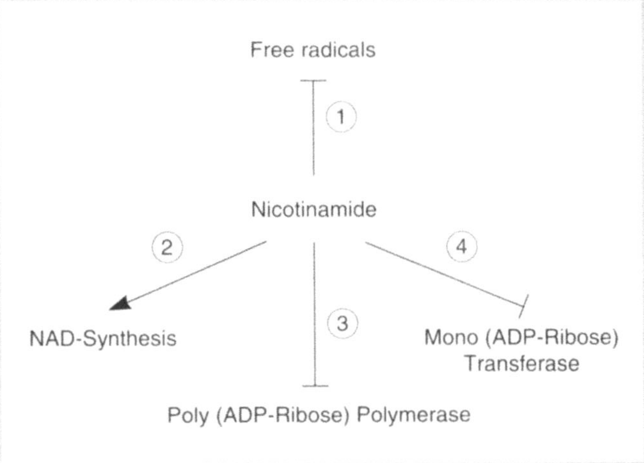

Fig. 1 Possible modes of action of nicotinamide. (1) Scavenging of free radicals. (2) Action as precursor of NAD. (3) Inhibition of poly(ADP-ribose)polymerase. (4) Inhibition of mono(ADP-ribose)transferases. The actual mechanism responsible for diabetes prevention in animals and possibly in humans is not yet identified

There was consensus among the reports, except for one small trial [25], that daily administration of nicotinamide had no substantial impact on the course of metabolic control, as determined by HbA1 measurements, the length of remission periods and beta cell function. Adverse effects of nicotinamide treatment were not noted. A more detailed analysis of possible side-effects is underway (Pozzilli et al., to be published). The concern about possible adverse effects of high dose nicotinamide therapy focuses on the risk of accumulation or facilitation of DNA alterations as known for inhibitors of poly(ADP-ribose)polymerase. Although this is at present a theoretical risk, long term follow up of nicotinamide receiving patients seems advisable.

Conclusion: The approach of beta cell protection by administration of high dose nicotinamide after onset of IDDM was, apparently, unsuccessful. To the knowledge of this author none of the diabetes centres involved in these trials has decided to use nicotinamide as an adjunct to insulin in newly diagnosed IDDM patients. This also holds for centres which reported limited beneficial effects of nicotinamide. For further discussion, see below, "Ongoing trials".

Lessons from the past – prevention of IDDM

The published experience of IDDM prevention studies in individuals at high risk is very limited. Thus, a rigid test of the hypothesis that preventive therapy can delay or inhibit the clinical manifestation of IDDM has not been undertaken.

One limitation of pilot trials with one or few individuals is that the prediction of insulin dependency to occur in the next few years is hardly possibly with 100% certainty. This statement does not disregard opposite claims from individual diabetes centres. However, full reliability of a diabetes prediction procedure requires reproducibility in other diabetes centres and regions, which is severely hampered by the lack of fully standardised ICA assays (differences in the tissue substrate) and differences in IAA assays and beta cell function tests. The other limitation is that lifestyle and environmental factors appear to have a significant impact on diabetes risk [32]. This is more than a theoretical concern since the knowledge about impending insulin dependency has a psychological impact and thus may affect diet and lifestyle of probands within a diabetes prevention trial. Daily intake of a drug and repeated hospital visits for follow up testing are appropriate to reinforce this "study effect".

Azathioprine: A single case has been reported where an adolescent with immunological and metabolic signs of imminent IDDM received azathioprine because of concomitant rheumatoid arthritis. Metabolic status improved and she remained normoglycaemic for over 5 years now [33].

Cyclosporin A: Two individuals at risk of IDDM received cyclosporin A and showed improvement of the first phase insulin response to intravenous glucose [34, 35].

Nicotinamide: Three individuals with high titer ICA and near absent first phase insulin response to intravenous glucose received nicotinamide (43 mg/

kg/d) but nevertheless progressed to overt IDDM within 0.5 to 1.7 years [36]. The other published trial comprises a combination of cases treated in Auckland, New Zealand and Denver, USA and historical controls (only Denver). The children and adolescents had high titer ICA and a low first phase insulin response to i.v. glucose (< 67 μUnits/ml, 1 + 3 min). At the time of publication (mean duration of treatment 17 months), all controls had developed diabetes but only 1 of 14 individuals receiving nicotinamide. Subsequently, further individuals in the nicotinamide group developed diabetes [4], including 3 of 4 patients from Denver [37]. For further discussion, see "Ongoing trials".
Conclusion: The published results of diabetes prevention trials are insufficient to value the feasibility of this approach. Larger studies presently underway promise better insight for the near future (see below).

Ongoing trials

Current approaches of intervention at IDDM onset

Ongoing and planned trials of intervention shortly after diagnosis of IDDM focus on selective immunosuppressive approaches. In one series of studies, improving the efficacy of (low dose) cyclosporin-A-therapy is being tried by initial additive immunotherapy aimed at stimulated lymphocytes only. For example, patients receive monoclonal antibody to the IL-2 receptor, a marker of activated T-cells, or a toxic conjugate of IL-2 with diphtheria toxin [38, 39] during the first 1 – 2 weeks of immunotherapy.

Another approach is to inactivate stimulated peripheral lymphocytes (which are supposed to comprise islet-specific T-cells) by photophoresis followed by reinfusion (T-cell vaccination). For this purpose, blood cells are incubated with 8-methoxypsoralen and irradiated with UVA light [40]. A further approach is to specifically hit CD5 positive T- and B-lymphocytes by a conjugate of a CD5-specific monoclonal antibody and the A chain of ricin. CD5 positive B-cells comprise the majority of auto-antibody-producing lymphocytes. Because of the risk of anaphylactic reactions, the treatment period was limited to 1 week. It is hoped that long term effects on the immunoregulatory balance will be reached [41].

Novel, rather broadly-acting immunosuppressive agents are presently being tested in pilot trials or are considered for study. These drugs include FK506, rapamycin, cyclosporin G and pentoxifylline, among others.

"Milder" approaches with immunomodulatory or beta cell protective compounds have also been announced to the registry of the International Diabetes Immunotherapy Group (IDIG). These include nicotinamide, nicotinamide +

deflazocort, ascorbic acid + β-carotene + nicotinamide + selenium + vitamin E, glipizide.

Comment: For many of these studies, a convincing new rationale is not obvious, given the fact that continuous cyclosporin-A-treatment in general did not maintain, but only prolonged clinical remission. Many of these drugs are not appropriate for long term administration in young diabetic patients. Short term treatment protocols, on the other hand, should offer the promise of long term effects. Appropriate studies of this aspect in IDDM animal models are almost entirely lacking.

Current approaches of diabetes prevention

The planned and ongoing trials of diabetes prevention are receiving considerable attention, outside the diabetological community, also. It is hoped that early intervention has a better chance of success because a larger beta cell mass is still available, because the disease process may be less aggressive and because mere slowing down of the disease process may extend considerably the time until insulin dependency.

Ketotifen: This histamine/serotonin antagonist is presently being tried in a placebo-controlled trial in high titer ICA positive individuals with low first phase insulin response to i.v. glucose. The approach was based on the observation of vascular leakage in inflamed islets of animal modes, such as the BB rat [42] and on the positive outcome of treatment with an serotonin antagonist in the low dose streptozocin model [43]. A 3-month treatment period did not prevent the deterioration of beta cell function and, thus, makes a beneficial effect of anti-allergic therapy in late pre-diabetes improbable (Böhmer et al., manuscript in preparation).

Nicotinamide: The IDIG registry indicates several ongoing trials with high dose nicotinamide (20 – 50 mg/kg/d) in ICA positive first degree relatives of IDDM patients and in school children. Interim data for the largest trial in the general population have been reported by Dr. R.B. Elliott on the occasion of the Immunology of Diabetes Workshop, April 1993 in Orlando, Florida, USA. In the Greater Auckland Area (N.Z.), 400 schools were randomised into two groups. The treatment arm comprised 33,600, 5 – 7 year-old children. In 20,200 children, ICA tests could be done and the 150 children with ICA titers of $\geq$ 20 JDF unit were started on nicotinamide. After approx. 2.5 years, diabetes had occurred at a rate of 1.1 per 10,000 children per year in the treatment arm (including the total of 33,600 children). The control group of 48,300 children had a diabetes rate of 2.0 per 10,000 children per year after approx. 4.5 years of follow up. Since no placebo was applied, it remains open if the difference observed is due to a "study effect" as discussed above. A study effect will become improbable if the different diabetes incidence in the two groups persists in the following years.

An international placebo-controlled trial of nicotinamide (ENDIT) in ICA positive (≥ 20 JDF units) relatives of IDDM patients is about to start in autumn 1993. Presently 20 national study groups have expressed their desire to participate. Co-ordinator of ENDIT is Dr. E. Gale, London, UK. The German nicotinamide trial (DENIS) is restricted to children with high risk, i. e. ICA positive (≥ 20 JDF units) siblings ≤ 12 years of age of IDDM patients. This study began in early 1993. Contact person of the DENIS trial is Dr. E. Lampeter, Düsseldorf, Germany.

The meager results with nicotinamide in recent onset IDDM and in pre-diabetic subjects with deficient first phase insulin response (see above) have led to the assumption that this approach is effective only in early pre-diabetes. This view is supported by the encouraging interim results of Dr. Elliott's study in school children. However, the available data were not regarded as solid enough to exclude probands with deficient beta cell function from the ENDIT and DENIS trials.

Insulin: Prophylactic insulin therapy has been shown to partially suppress insulitis and diabetes in animal models [44, 45]. The several possible modes of action of insulin are depicted in Fig. 2. The hormone may directly modulate immune cell function, it may act as antigen and alter the immune reactivity towards beta cells because of the repeated immunisations ("immune deviation") or it may be acting via its suppressive action on beta cell function (beta cell rest hypothesis). The latter effect would lead to a lesser auto-antigen expression on beta cells with subsequent less auto-immune reactivity and a potentially better resistance of resting cells towards the immune attack. Prophylactic insulin treatment in pre-diabetic individuals was started by Dr. G. Eisenbarth, Denver, USA, followed by other collaborating centres. The interim status of these studies is described in the chapter by Dr. Eisenbarth. The difference in progression to diabetes between the insulin treatment group and a non-randomised control group is strongly encouraging [46]. A randomised placebo-controlled multicentre trial of such therapy has begun.

It is probable that the remission phase seen after the start of insulin therapy in acute IDDM is the direct consequence of insulin administration. This effect of insulin apparently also involves partial recovery and better survival of beta

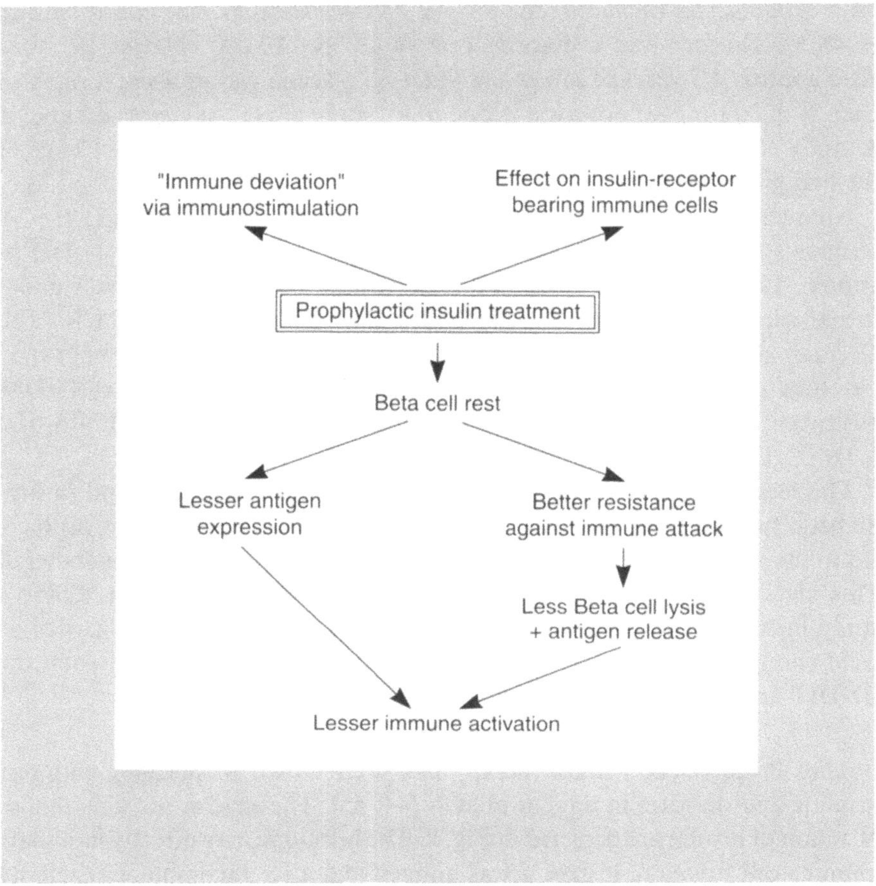

Fig. 2. Possible modes of action of prophylactic insulin treatment in pre type 1 diabetes. The 4 mechanisms indicated are based on findings of animal models and in vitro studies. The actual mechanism responsible for diabetes prevention in animals and possibly in humans is not yet identified

cells. Most interestingly, remission induction was not accelerated by cyclosporin A immunosuppression [5]. Thus, at least transient recovery of beta cell function is to be expected from prophylactic insulin therapy.

Breast feeding and cow's milk free diet: Earlier studies have shown that complex proteins represent "diabetogenic" factors in the diet of spontaneously diabetic BB rats and NOD mice [47] and that prolonged breast feeding is correlated with slightly lower diabetes risk [32]. Furthermore, the presence of antibodies in IDDM to peptide epitopes common to bovine serum albumin and a beta cell surface antigen has led to the hypothesis that cow's milk proteins may represent a dietary trigger of IDDM [48]. A study has been initiated by Dr. H.-M. Dosch, Toronto, Canada and Dr. H. Akerblom, Helsinki, Finland, to determine the effect of prolonged breast feeding and subsequent cow's milk-free formula in children with first degree relatives with type 1 diabetes.

Further studies: The observation that auto-antigens given orally may reinforce tolerance or suppression of auto-immunity because of interaction with the gut-associated immune system [49] has led to plans for trials with oral insulin or with other orally administered islet antigens. Oral insulin induced partial suppression of diabetes and insulitis in NOD mice [50], while it failed in the low dose streptozocin model [51]. In the latter model, partial diabetes prevention was reached by oral administration of an extract of streptozocin treated islets [51]. T-cell vaccination with peripheral blood lymphocytes exposed to phototherapy (see above) is being tried in a pilot trial [40]. A number of other modes of intervention is being considered for pre type 1 diabetes, including thymopentin and low-dose cyclosporin A, but a formal trial has not been announced to the IDIG registry.

Comment: The growing awareness of the fact that it is possible to diagnose a high risk of later insulin dependency in seemingly healthy subjects with reasonable certainty is presently stimulating an increasing number of prevention trials. Although it may be tempting to try any promising new protocol or drug very soon in (pre)type 1 diabetes, the risks associated with such intervention should be carefully weighed. In most cases, the chances of a new therapy can be assessed if tested first in animal models of type 1 diabetes. This step should not be omitted. Secondly, for new drugs, sufficient knowledge about adverse effects should be available. Other, more severe, chronic inflammatory diseases offer a better risk-benefit ratio for first testing of new modes of immune intervention than does pre type 1 diabetes.

References

[1] Andreani D, Kolb H, Pozzilli P. Immunotherapy of diabetes. Chichester: John Wiley & Sons, 1989.

[2] Diabetes Epidemiology Research International Mortality Study Group. Major cross-country differences in risk of dying for people with IDDM. Diabetes Care 1988; 37: 1591–1594.

[3] Boitard C. The differentiation of the immune system towards anti-islet autoimmunity. Clinical prospects. Diabetologia 1992; 35: 1101–1112.

[4] Skyler JS, Marks JB. Immune intervention in type I diabetes mellitus. Diabetes Reviews 1993; 1: 15–42.

[5] Canadian European Diabetes Study Group . Cyclosporin-induced remission of IDDM after early intervention. Association of 1 yr of cyclosporin treatment with enhanced insulin secretion. Diabetes 1988; 37: 1574–1582.
[6] Feutren G, Papoz L, Assan R et al. Cyclosporin increases the rate and length of remissions in insulin-dependent diabetes of recent onset: results of a multicentre double-blind trial. Lancet 1986; 2: 119–124.
[7] Silverstein J, Maclaren NK, Riley WJ, et al. Immunosuppression with azathioprine and prednisone in recent onset insulin-dependent diabetes mellitus. N Engl J Med 1988; 319: 599–604.
[8] Martin S, Schernthaner G, Nerup J et al. Follow-up of cyclosporin A in Type 1 (insulin-dependent) diabetes mellitus: lack of long term effects. Diabetologia 1991; 34: 429–434.
[9] Kolb H, Schmidt M, Kiesel U. Immunomodulatory drugs in type 1 diabetes. In: Eisenbarth GS, ed. Immunotherapy of type 1 diabetes and selected autoimmune diseases. Boca Raton: CRC Press, 1989: 111–122.
[10] Koivisto VA, Aro A, Cantell K et al. Remissions in newly diagnosed type I (insulin-dependent) diabetes mellitus: influence of interferon as an adjunct to insulin therapy. Diabetologia 1984; 27: 193–197.
[11] Malaisse WJ, Malaisse-Lagae F, Sener A et al. Determinates of the selective toxicity of alloxan to the pancreatic B cell. Proc Natl Acad Sci U S A 1982; 79: 927–933.
[12] Sumoski W, Baquerio H, Rabinovitch A. Oxygen free radical scavengers protect rat islet cells from damage by cytokines. Diabetologia 1989; 32: 792–796.
[13] Kallmann B, Burkart V, Kröncke K-D et al. Toxicity of chemically generated nitric oxide towards pancreatic islet cells can be prevented by nicotinamide. Life Sci 1992; 51: 671–678.
[14] Mandrup-Poulson T, Bendtzen K, Nerup J et al. Affinity-purified human interleukin 1 is cytotoxic to isolated islets of Langerhans. Diabetologia 1986; 29: 63–67.
[15] Bergmann L, Kröncke K-D, Suschek D et al. Cytotoxic action of IL-1ß against islets is mediated via nitric oxide formation and is inhibited by N^G-monomethyl-L-arginine. FEBS Lett 1992; 103–106.
[16] Lazarow A. Protection against alloxan diabetes. Anat Rec 1947; 97: 353.
[17] Schein PS, Cooney DA, Vernon ML. The use of nicotinamide to modify the toxicity of streptozotocin diabetes without loss of antitumor activity. Cancer Res 1967; 27: 2324–2332.
[18] Burkart V, Koike T, Brenner H-H et al. Oxygen radicals generated by the enzyme xanthine oxidase lyse pancreatic islet cells in vitro. Diabetologia 1992; 35: 1028–1034.
[19] Sugiyama K, Yonemura Y, Okamoto H. Effects of poly(ADP-ribose)synthetase inhibitor on B-cells of a canine pancreas after massive pancreatectomy. Int J Pancreatol 1991; 8: 85–95.
[20] Sandler S, Andersson A. Long-term effects of exposure of pancreatic islets to nicotinamide in vitro on DNA synthesis, metabolism and B-cell function. Diabetologia 1986; 29: 199–206.
[21] Yamada K, Nonaka K, Hanafusa T et al. Preventive and therapeutic aspects of large dose nicotinamide injections on diabetes associated with insulitis: an observation in non-obese diabetic (NOD) mice. Diabetes 1982; 31: 749–753.
[22] Hermitte L, Viallettes B, Atlef N et al. High dose nicotinamide fails to prevent diabetes in BB rats. Autoimmunity 1989; 5: 79–86.
[23] Okamoto H. Regulation of proinsulin synthesis in pancreatic islets and a new aspect to insulin-dependent diabetes. Mol Cell Biochem 1981; 37: 43–61.
[24] Banasik M, Komura H, Shimoyama M et al. Specific inhibitors of poly(ADP-ribose)synthetase and mono(ADP-ribosyl)transferase. J Biol Chem 1992; 267: 1569–1575.
[25] Vague P, Viallettes B, Lassman-Vague V et al. Nicotinamide may extend remission phase in insulin-dependent diabetes. Lancet 1987; 1: 619–620.
[26] Pozzilli P, Visalli N, Ghirlanda G et al. Nicotinamide increases C-peptide secretion in patients with recent onset type I diabetes. Diab Med 1989; 6: 568–572.
[27] Vague P, Picq R, Bernal M et al. Effect of nicotinamide on the residual insulin secretion of type I (insulin-dependent) diabetes patients. Diabetologia 1989; 32: 316–321.

[28] Mendola G, Casamitgana R, Gomis R. Effects of nicotinamide therapy upon B-cell function in newly diagnosed type I (insulin-dependent) diabetic patients. Diabetologia 1989; 32: 160–162.
[29] Chase HP, Butler-Simon N, Garg S et al. A trial of nicotinamide in newly diagnosed patients with type I (insulin-dependent) diabetes mellitus. Diabetologia 1990; 33: 444–446.
[30] Lewis MC, Canafx DM, Sprafka JM et al. Double-blind randomized trial of nicotinamide on early diabetes. Diabetes Care 1992; 15: 121–123.
[31] Viallettes B, Picq R, Du Rostu M et al. A preliminary multicentre study of the treatment of recently diagnosed type I diabetes by combination nicotinamide-cyclosporin therapy. Diab Med 1990; 7: 731–735.
[32] Blom L, Dahlquist G, Nyström L et al. The Swedish childhood diabetes study – social and perinatal determinants for diabetes in childhood. Diabetologia 1989; 32: 7–13.
[33] Riley WJ, Maclaren NK, Spillar R. Reversal of deteriorating glucose tolerance with azathioprine in prediabetes. Trans Proc 1986; 18: 819–822.
[34] Levy-Marchal C, Czernichow P, Quiniou MC et al. Cyclosporin administration reversed abnormalities in a prediabetic child (Abstract). Diabetes 1984; 33 (Suppl. 1): 183A.
[35] Assan R, Feutren G, Bougneres PH et al. Treatment of a glucose intolerant pre-type I diabetic twin with ciclosporin (Abstract). Diabetes Res Clin Prac 1991; 14 (Suppl. 1): S51.
[36] Dumont-Herskowitz R, Jacksonl RA, Soeldner JS et al. Pilot trial to prevent type I diabetes: progression to overt IDDM despite oral nicotinamide. J Autoimmunity 1989; 2: 733–737.
[37] Eisenbarth GS. Immune mechanisms of beta cell destruction in the pre-diabetic phase of IDDM patients: Research methodologies identifying susceptible individuals (see this volume).
[38] Pacheco-Silva A, Bastos MG, Muggia RA et al. Interleukin 2 receptor targeted fusion toxin (DAB486-IL-2) treatment blocks diabetogenic autoimmunity in non-obese diabetic mice. Eur J Immunol 1992; 22: 697–702.
[39] Boitard C, Timsit J, Assan R et al. Treatment of type I diabetes mellitus with DAB486-IL-2, a toxin conjugate which targets activated T-lymphocytes (Abstract). Diabetologia 1992; 35 (Suppl. 1): A218.
[40] Harrison LC, Honeyman M, Steele C et al. Photophoresis trial in IDDM: an interim report. Proc Aust Diabetes Soc 1992; 91.
[41] Skyler JS, Byers V, Einhorn D et al. Effects of an anti-CD5 immunoconjugate (H65-RTA) on pancreatic islet beta cell function in type I diabetes mellitus (Abstract). Diabetes Res Clin Prac 1991; 14 (Suppl. 1): S54.
[42] De Paepe ME, Corriveau M, Tannous WN t al. Increased vascular permeability in pancreas of diabetic rats: detection with high resolution protein A-gold cytochemistry. Diabetologia 1992; 35: 1118–1124.
[43] Martin S, Kolb-Bachofen V, Kiesel U et al. Pathogenesis of low dose streptozotocin induced diabetes: Requirement for alpha 1 – adrenoreceptor activation and vaso-active amine release. Diabetologia 1989; 32: 140–142.
[44] Gotfredsen GF, Buschard K, Frandsen EK. Reduction of diabetes incidence of BB Wistar rats by early prophylactic insulin treatment of diabetes-prone animals. Diabetologia 1985; 28: 933–935.
[45] Atkinson MA, Maclaren NK, Luchetta R. Insulitis and insulin-dependent diabetes in NOD mice reduced by prophylactic insulin therapy. Diabetes 1990; 39: 933–937.
[46] Keller RJ, Eisenbarth GS, Jackson RA. Insulin prophylaxis in individuals at high risk of type I diabetes. Lancet 1993; 341: 927–928.
[47] Scott FW, Elliott RB, Kolb H. Diet and autoimmunity: Prospects of prevention of Type I diabetes. Diabetes Nutr Metab 1989; 2: 61–74.
[48] Karjalainen J, Martin JM, Knip M et al. A bovine albumin peptide as possible trigger of insulin-dependent diabetes mellitus. N Engl J Med 1992; 327: 302–307.
[49] Thompson HSG, Staines NA. Could specific oral tolerance be a therapy for autoimmune disease? Immunology Today 1990; 11: 396.

[50] Zhong ZJ, Davidson L, Eisenbarth GS et al. Suppression of diabetes in nonobese diabetic mice by oral administration of porcine insulin. Proc Natl Acad Sci USA 1991; 88: 10252–10256.
[51] Kolb H, Zielasek J, Berschick P et al. Oral prevention of type 1 diabetes. Autoimmunity 1991; 11: 133.

Assays for measuring proinsulin, insulin, and related peptides

A. S. Rudenski, N. J. Crowther and C. N. Hales

Introduction

The method of choice for the assay of a biologically active polypeptide might at first sight seem to be a bioassay. Bioactivity is, however, often the net response to a number of different biologically active molecules with similar or antagonistic effects. A more profound understanding is therefore provided by the specific determination of the chemical amount of each of these molecules.

It is becoming increasingly recognised that some polypeptide hormones are subject to chemical heterogeneity, so there may be difficulties in accurately quantifying them [1]. Fortunately, at least to date, there is no evidence that the active insulin molecule is subject to chemical modifications.

The other major problems of bioassay in general are that they are cumbersome, imprecise, and insensitive. Trethewey has written an account of the development and problems of bioassays for insulin over a 30 year period [2].

The only methods available at present which have adequate sensitivity and specificity to detect polypeptides in the picomolar range are those employing antibodies. Methods based on the use of receptor binding, whilst theoretically advantageous, have rarely proved to have adequate sensitivity.

Immunoassays for human insulin have been commercially available since the 1960's. At present, research workers in diabetes are confronted with a large variety of methods with different labels and varying degrees of automation. Possibly as a consequence, there exists in the literature a disconcertingly wide range of reported concentrations for the amount of insulin in human plasma after an overnight fast and following an oral glucose tolerance test, even when apparently comparable groups of subjects have been studied. Apart from the inherent problem of artefacts due to individual methods, there are two major difficulties in measuring insulin, which will be the main topics with which this chapter will be concerned. The first is sensitivity. Many assays have sensitivity characteristics which result in their being barely able to detect insulin in the low-normal concentration range as observed after an

Offprint from
Research Methodologies in Human Diabetes – Part 1

overnight fast in non-obese subjects. The consequence is a lack of precision and specificity when the assay has a relatively large signal-to-noise ratio. The second problem is that of specificity, in the presence of the cross-reacting precursor molecules proinsulin and partially processed proinsulin.

Structure of insulin and related peptides

Essential to an understanding of the problems of assay of insulin and related peptides is a knowledge of how these peptides are related to each other in structure. Steiner and Oyer discovered proinsulin, the precursor of insulin in 1967 [3], and since then it has been shown that proinsulin is converted to insulin and C-peptide via a series of intermediate compounds, which have similar structures. Fig. 1 illustrates in diagrammatic form how proinsulin is converted to insulin via the action of three peptidase enzymes. Endopeptidase type 1 acts specifically at the Arg^{32}-Arg^{33} site, whereas the type II endopeptidase acts specifically at the Lys^{64}-Arg^{65} site [4]. After cleavage at the AC and BC junctions, each resultant split product undergoes further processing by carboxypeptidase H, losing a pair of basic amino acids to form des-64,65 proinsulin, and des-32,32 proinsulin. These products are then acted upon by the type I and type II endopeptidases respectively and by carboxypeptidase H to yield insulin and C-peptide. It is not clear whether there is a preferred processing route. Although there is evidence that the type II endopeptidase is active first, before the type I endopeptidase, in the Golgi apparatus [4], in-vitro studies indicate that while the type I enzyme acts equally on proinsulin or des-64,65 proinsulin, the type II enzyme has a marked preference for des-31,32 proinsulin over intact proinsulin as a substrate [5]. It has been observed that there is a preponderance of des-32,33 split proinsulin over des-64,65 split proinsulin in the pancreas [6] and circulation [7].

Clearly, there is much common structure among the different proinsulin-derived peptides. The insulin moiety of intact proinsulin and its partially processed derivatives is known to be very similar in structure to that of the mature insulin molecule [8], whilst the C-peptide has a much less well defined structure. Although much is known of the crystal structure of insulin [9], less is known about the exact conformation taken up by insulin in physiological solution. From X-ray analysis of insulin crystals, two distinct insulin conformations have been identified [10]. These have been termed the R and T conformations and are depicted in Fig. 2. Determination of the conformation taken up by insulin in solution has been attempted using NMR technology, but this technique requires the use of non-physiological conditions [11] or engineered insulins [12], to prevent insulin from self-associating at the high

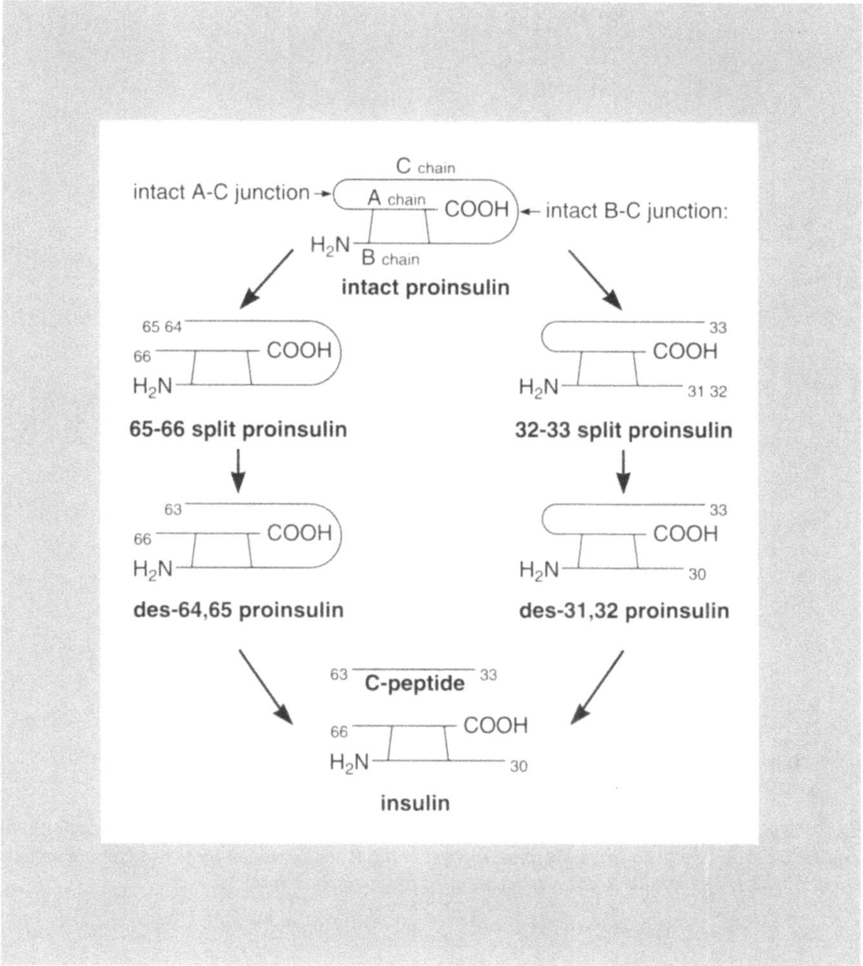

Fig. 1 Diagram of processing of proinsulin via split products to insulin and C-peptide. The numbers refer to the sequence of the amino acids when in the parent molecule, proinsulin

concentrations necessary for these type of studies. The active form of insulin is thought to be the monomer [13], and theoretical considerations point to the T conformation as being the major species in solution [10, 14], but this has yet to be proven conclusively. In terms of measuring insulin in solution, the assumptions of all assays to date, is that they measure all insulin present, irrespective of conformation or degree of association. The latter assumption is likely in view of the fact that dimerisation has been reported to occur at concentrations of insulin well above those occurring physiologically [13].

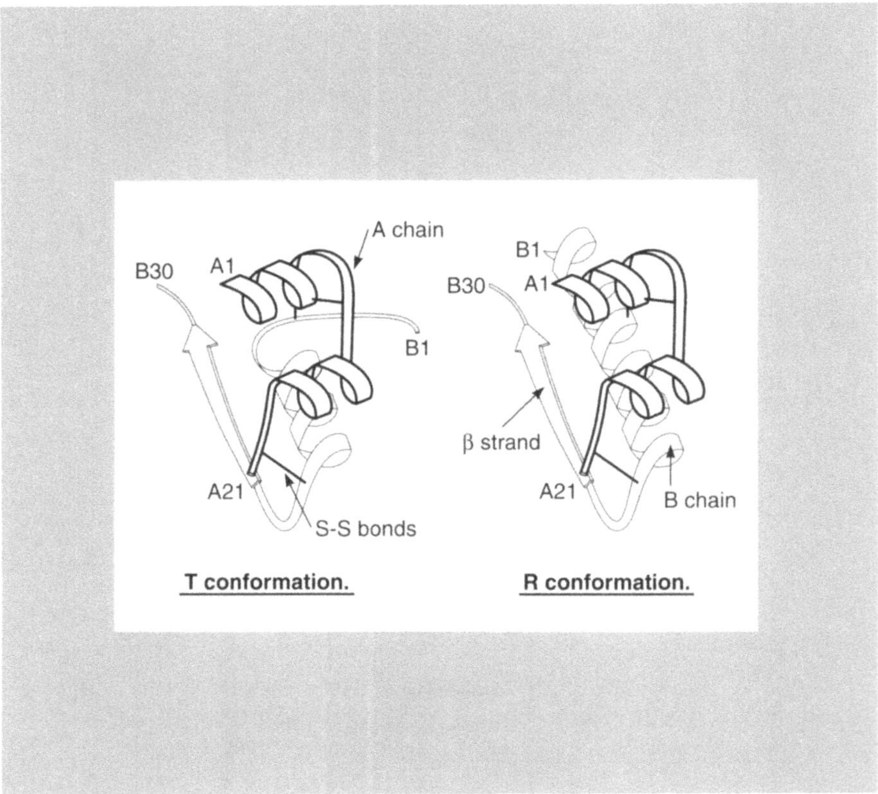

Fig. 2 Diagrammatic representation of the R and T conformations of insulin. In the T conformation residues B1 to B9 are in an extended format whilst in the R conformation these residues are arranged into a α helix. (The insulin A chain is represented by the thicker line)

Immunoassay techniques

Preparation and modification of antibodies

The insulin molecule is immunogenic to a varying degree, depending upon the species of insulin and the species of the immunised animal. In the optimal conditions, it is capable of generating antibodies that will bind it with high affinity. The best source of such antibodies against human, porcine or bovine insulin, all of which have very similar amino acid sequences is the guinea pig, probably because the sequence of its insulin is very different from that of other mammalian species [15]. Many commercially available insulin assay kits include guinea pig derived antisera. Methods for producing human insulin in large quantities from bacteria [16] and yeast [17] have permitted the large scale production of anti-insulin antibodies.

The preparation of antibodies was transformed by the development of monoclonal methodology [18]. These procedures facilitated the production of antibodies whose binding to a specific protein could be limited to a particular epitope. Cohen, for example, was able to raise an antibody specifically against the intact B-C junction of proinsulin, which was used to measure intact proinsulin and 65-66 split proinsulin [19]. Those interested in the methodology of antibody production are referred to a detailed review of the subject by Burrin and Newman [20].

Further advances in methods of monoclonal antibody production and modification may be expected from the use of the techniques of molecular biology [21]. To an ever increasing extent, the antibody production repertoire of the immune system is being reproduced in vitro, by the use of the polymerase chain reaction to amplify the cDNA coding for the hypervariable regions of immunoglobulin molecules [22]. These methods involve less animal work, and should be less time-consuming than present production methods.

Radioimmunoassay

The first highly sensitive immunoassay was described in 1959 by Yalow and Berson [23], and this was for the assay of insulin. The method used a polyclonal antiserum to insulin derived from human subjects with diabetes mellitus who had been treated with bovine and porcine insulins. In this assay protocol, insulin in the sample competed for binding sites with ^{131}I-labelled insulin. Free, labelled insulin was separated from antibody-bound, labelled insulin by chromatoelectrophoresis. The hormone concentration was inversely related to the quantity of bound label. This basic assay principle has changed little, although many technical improvements have been made: purer, specific insulin antibodies are now easily available; ^{125}iodine is usually used to label the competing ligand; and other methods of separating bound from free label, such as precipitating antibody with anti-immunoglobulin [24, 25], salt precipitation [26], coated charcoal [27] and polyethylene glycol [28], have been developed.

Single antibody techniques are still used for the measurement of C-peptide. Since the C-peptide sequence is present in intact and split proinsulin products, such assays are theoretically capable of cross-reacting with such products. In practice, however, this does not present a problem, because the concentrations of C-peptide are so much greater than those of proinsulin, or of its split products (Table 1).

Table 1 Concentrations of insulin and proinsulin related peptides in human serum

	Basal concentration (pM)	Stimulated concentration (pM)
Insulin	27	101
Proinsulin	2.1	4.7
32-33 split proinsulin	3.0	6.4
65-66 split proinsulin*	< 1.0	3.8 †
C-peptide	499	1410

Mean fasting concentrations in 12 non-diabetic subjects from Clark et al. 1992, and (*) in 8 subjects from Sobey et al. 1989. The stimulated values are the concentrations achieved at the end of a 60 minute 5 mg/kg ideal body weight glucose infusion, or (†) the maximal concentration achieved after a 75 g oral glucose stimulus.

Immunoradiometric assays

In radioimmunoassay, labelled antigen competes with the analyte of interest for a limited quantity of antibody binding sites. In these assays, known also as competitive assays, the amount of label bound varies in inverse relation to the analyte concentration. In 1968, Miles and Hales suggested the use of an immunoradiometric assay, where the antibody is labelled, and in excess [29]. The amount of label bound should then be in direct proportion to the concentration of the analyte to be measured. The first such assay was described for growth hormone in 1971 [30].

The development of the production of monoclonal antibodies has significantly contributed to the development of two-site immunoassays. In two-site assays, one antibody (sometimes termed the 'capture antibody') is bound to or adsorbed onto a solid phase, whilst the other is labelled and involved in the signalling process. Capture antibodies may be conveniently bound non-covalently to fixed surfaces such as plastic microtitre well plates, or test tubes, when simple decanting/aspiration will separate bound from free molecules. Another convenient method is to attach antibody to particles, such as magnetic particles [31], where a magnet is used to effect the separation, or to attach the antibody to a large molecule such as cellulose [32] which can be separated by centrifugation.

The use of two antibodies in an assay has expected advantages over the use of a single antibody in the measurement of molecules in the presence of different, but closely related substances. A cross-reacting substance would have to share two, as opposed to one, specific epitopes. This advantage has been exploited in the measurement of insulin and related molecules. Sobey et al. [7] described the use of a panel of monoclonal antibodies against the different epitopes. The specificity of the antibodies meant that in paired combinations, they could be used in immunoradiometric assays for insulin, proinsulin, and 65-66 split proinsulin. The antibodies available did not, however, allow a specific combination for the detection of 32-33 split proinsulin, whose concentration could be calculated as the difference between two different paired-antibody assay formats. Similar assays using an amplified immunoenzymometric format have been described subsequently [33].

Sensitivity

The degree of sensitivity required of an assay is clearly dependent upon the expected concentrations of peptides to be measured and ideally should be well in excess of that necessary for measurement of values at the lower end of the normal range. Basal and stimulated concentrations of insulin and related peptides in human serum are shown in Table 1. Because of its longer half-life, C-peptide, secreted equimolarly with insulin [34], is present in plasma in molar concentrations an order of magnitude greater than insulin concentrations [35]. Proinsulin, and 32-33 split proinsulin are present in concentrations lower than those of insulin [35], whilst 65-66 split proinsulin has a still lower concentration [7]. The detection limit attainable is dependent on many factors, including the affinity of the antibodies used, and the specific activity of the labels used. Ekins has reviewed the topic recently [36]. The sensitivity of an assay increases with increasing affinity of the antibody, and with increasing precision of the zero standard. This precision increases as the specific activity of the label does. Ekins used a mathematical model to demonstrate that in a competitive assay, little gain in sensitivity is obtained by using a label with a specific activity greater than that of ^{125}iodine, if the affinity of the antibody is less than 10^{10}. In a non-competitive assay, minimisation of non-specific binding is crucial. If it is kept below 0.01%, then a sensitivity 10,000 times greater than that attainable in a competitive assay can be achieved. In this case, however, the label used must have a specific activity greater than that of ^{125}iodine. Numerous labels are available, and those which have a particularly high specific activity are the fluorescent labels, such as europium chelates, enhanced luminescence systems, and enzyme amplification systems, where detection limits for proinsulin as low as 0.1 pmol/l have been reported [37]. As well as allowing greater sensitivity, non-isotopic labels do not have the hazards of radioactivity, and generally have a longer shelf life.

Specificity and cross-reactivity

In the early days, considerable ingenuity was required to develop ways of measuring proinsulin, because antibodies against insulin would cross-react with proinsulin and vice-versa. Gel chromatography was used to separate a higher molecular weight fraction, which was then tested by straightforward insulin radioimmunoassay [38]. The differences in insulin immunoreactivity before and after treatment with a protease, specific for insulin, was used by Kitabchi [39]. It was then demonstrated that this method gave high results because the enzyme only partially degraded insulin [40]. Heding precipitated insulin and proinsulin with insulin antibody, and then measured proinsulin in the precipitate with an antibody against C-peptide [41]. Ward carried out the converse procedure, by extracting proinsulin with C-peptide antibody, and then testing for insulin immunoreactivity [42].

The possibility that the partially processed intermediates of proinsulin conversion to insulin might be present in human plasma was raised by Gray et al. [43]. These workers found that a two-site assay developed for the measurement of intact proinsulin and based upon an antiserum to human insulin and one to human C-peptide detected intact proinsulin poorly, if at all. However, partial tryptic digestion of the then newly produced bioengineered human proinsulin greatly increased its immunoreactivity. It was found that the assay cross-reacted well with either of the partially split products of proinsulin. Since the assay detected proinsulin-like material in human plasma, it was concluded that at least some of this material must be the split products rather than intact proinsulin. Subsequently, with the advent of assays capable of measuring specifically all of these variants, this was confirmed. It was found that the major split product was the 32-33 form, and that the 65-66 split product could not be detected [7]. Studies of non-insulin-dependent diabetics revealed elevated concentrations of both intact and 32-33 split proinsulin [44, 45]. Sufficient of these materials are present to result in erroneously high 'insulin' concentrations being observed if these were measured by a non-specific radioimmunoassay method. Specificity of an assay may not be the most important requirement. The low levels of cross-reacting 65-66 split proinsulin, which cross reacts in the specific insulin assay described by Sobey [7], do not significantly interfere with this insulin assay. There may be situations, such as screening for an insulinoma, where an assay which detects both proinsulin and insulin is desired. In cases where proinsulin-related peptides need to be measured specifically, a two-site immunoassay format has advantages over other protocols. The modification of antibodies (attachment to solid phase or label) required by such a format does, however, have some potential drawbacks. Attachment of antibodies to a solid phase can alter binding properties, such as the affinity constant [46], which will have implications with regard to the sensitivity of an assay. Also, the binding of one antibody to an antigen may induce conformational changes within the antigen, affecting its interaction with the second antibody in an assay. An example of this was reported by Sobey et al. [7], who found that in the presence of the monoclonal antibody A6, the monoclonal antibody 14B was able to bind proinsulin, whereas it showed no affinity for proinsulin when A6 was not present. Temple et al. [47] reviewed the characteristics, including sensitivity and cross-reactivities, of several insulin and proinsulin assays.

A further potential problem of specificity of insulin and proinsulin assays relates to the steps involving removal of the basic amino acids exposed in the new C-terminal sequences of the endo-protease cleaved split proinsulins. The amount of the carboxypeptidase enzyme responsible for removing these basic amino acids greatly exceeds the amounts of the two endopeptidases described above. Thus either or both des-32 or des-31,32 and des-65 or des-64,65 split products may exist in plasma. The assays described by Sobey at al. [7] were not capable of discriminating between the various possibilities or indeed the possibility that there might be some incompletely processed insulin which retained one or two basic amino acids at the C-terminus of the B-chain.

Assay interference

A common problem of assays measuring analyte levels in serum is that of matrix effects. Human serum contains a number of solutes that may cause assay interference [48]. Large errors in immunoassays can be caused by heterophilic antibodies, which are capable of binding to the immunoglobulins used in the assay [49]. Thus, Alpha et al. reported spurious proinsulin values, which were shown to be the result of endogenous serum antibodies [33]. The problem was alleviated by preincubating plasma samples with goat antisera directed against human immunoglobulins. Alternatively, the sample to be assayed can be incubated with serum from the species from which the assay antibodies were derived, so that any heterophilic antibodies can become saturated by non-specific immunoglobulin. In general, matrix effects are best dealt with by choice of antibodies and reagents that produce low non-specific binding and by careful assay validation [48].

Chromatography

HPLC is the primary chromatographic method for analysis of insulin and proinsulin and its products, with variations such as high-performance capillary electrophoresis proving less satisfactory [50]. The choice of columns, buffers, and detectors is large, and very often dependent upon the apparatus already available, and manufacturers usually offer helpful advice to those wishing to set up a system. Even then, the setting up of any chromatographic system requires a large amount of time, involving much trial and error, since overall performance depends upon the inter-relation of components, such as buffer and stationary phase [51]. On its own, a system can be set up to quantitate proinsulin and related peptides in fluids such as commercially produced insulin solutions, where concentration and purity are likely to be high. Analysis of human samples, however, poses further demands on a system: the ability to detect low concentrations against a background of numerous other peptides and proteins. To meet this demand, the specificity and sensitivity of the detection system is provided by immunological techniques. The chromatographic phase of the analysis is able to separate related peptides, such as split proinsulins from their des-diamino-derivatives, and these are then detected in their separate fractions by immunoassay. When a system is up and running, analysis of large numbers of samples is slow by comparison with most immunoassay techniques. For further information, the reader is advised to consult descriptions of working systems [52].

In a recent study comparing the immunoradiometric assay of 32-33 split proinsulin with an HPLC-based assay of des-31,32 split proinsulin in human plasma, good agreement was found between the two methods [53]. This confirms that the main split form of proinsulin in plasma lacks the C-terminal basic amino acids and indicates that this is the main material measured by the immunoradiometric assay of '32-33' split proinsulin.

Standards

A study reported in 1969 of insulin measurements in different laboratories showed great disparity [54]. In 1982, Shishiba et al. reported that the large difference in results between different kits for insulin assay was due primarily to differences in concentrations of standards [55]. The question of standardisation of assays is not unique to insulin, and has been addressed by analytical chemists. An international reference preparation for insulin is now available. Nevertheless, matrix differences between standards and patient samples are likely to be accentuated to different degrees in different assay formats, resulting in different degrees of bias. This can be minimised by diluting standards and samples in similar buffers, another advantage of having assays of high sensitivity.

In 1984, Kruse et al. reported that early pancreatic-derived proinsulin standards were wrong, and had resulted in a positive bias in proinsulin assays [56]. The advent of biosynthetic human proinsulin [57] not only provided a source of material for immunisation, to raise new antibodies, but also a source of pure material suitable for use as standards in assays.

Quality control

Special care should be taken to minimise damage to blood samples prior to insulin analysis, since haemolysis is known to reduce the insulin concentration [58]. Whilst the effects of temperature and timing of specimen separation and storage have been studied for insulin [59], little is known about the effects on the different proinsulin-derived molecules, and whether any effects observed would differ in different assays. Therefore, the normal procedure is for blood specimens to be collected into tubes containing heparin anticoagulant, and for plasma to be separated promptly by centrifugation, and frozen rapidly for storage at a temperature of -20 °C or lower. As with standards, particular care also needs to be taken in the preparation of internal and external quality assurance materials.

The subject of quality assurance is covered in great depth in most textbooks of clinical (bio)chemistry. This will include the use of internal controls, and rejection of assays on the basis of criteria such as those proposed by Westgard [60]. External quality control schemes are available in the UK for insulin, but not for the less frequently analysed proinsulin-derived peptides. Such schemes can provide useful information about the performance of an assay. One should be aware, however, that when many of the participants in such a scheme are using a method which is inaccurate, or subject to interference, comparison of one assay's performance with the consensus mean may lead to false conclusions. This will be more of a problem when no definitive or reference methods have been established.

Conclusions

The importance of measuring insulin accurately and specifically, when possible disorders of insulin secretion and action are being investigated, has been discussed. Researchers interested in possible disorders of insulin biosynthesis and proinsulin processing will also wish to take advantage of the now available specific assays for intact proinsulin and its split products. Some of the problems and advances in the development of assays have been mentioned, since known and potential limitations of an assay need to be borne in mind by those using available assays, as well as by those wishing to develop their own assays.

References

[1] Jeffcoate SL. Analytical and clinical significance of peptide hormone heterogeneity with particular reference to growth hormone and luteinizing hormone in serum. Clin Endocrinol 1993; 38: 113–121.
[2] Trethewey J. Bio-assays for the analysis of insulin. J Pharmaceutical & Biomedical Analysis 1989; 7: 189–197.
[3] Steiner DF, Oyer PE. The biosynthesis of insulin and a probable precursor of insulin by a human islet cell adenoma. Proc Natl Acad Sci USA 1967; 67: 473–480.
[4] Davidson HW, Rhodes CJ, Hutton JC. Intraorganelle Ca^{2+} and pH control proinsulin cleavage in the pancreatic B-cell via two distinct site-specific endopeptidases. Nature 1988; 333: 93–96.
[5] Rhodes CJ, Lincoln B, Shoelson SE. Preferential cleavage of des-31,32-proinsulin over intact proinsulin by the insulin secretory granule type II endopeptidase. J Biol Chem 1992; 267: 22719–22727.
[6] Given BD, Cohen RM, Shoelson SE et al. Biochemical and clinical implications of proinsulin conversion intermediates. J Clin Invest 1985; 76: 1398–1405.
[7] Sobey WJ, Beer SF, Carrington CA et al. Sensitive and specific two-site immunoradiometric assays for human insulin, proinsulin, 65-66 split proinsulin and 32-33 split proinsulins. Biochem J 1989; 260: 535–541.
[8] Frank BH, Pekar AH, Veros AJ. Physical studies on proinsulin – comparison of titration behaviour of tyrosine residues in insulin and proinsulin. Biochemistry 1972; 11: 4926–4931.
[9] Blundell TL, Cutfield JF, Cutfield SM et al. Atomic positions in rhombohedral 2-zinc insulin crystals. Nature 1971: 231: 506–511.
[10] Bentley G, Dodson E, Dodson G et al. Structure of insulin in 4-zinc insulin. Nature 1976; 261: 166–168.
[11] Kline AD, Justice RM. Complete sequence-specific ^1H NMR assignments for human insulin. Biochemistry 1990; 29: 2906–2913.
[12] Weiss MA, Nguyen T, Khait I et al. Two-dimensional NMR and photo-CIDNP studies of the insulin monomer: assignment of aromatic resonances with application to protein folding, structure and dynamics. Biochemistry 1989; 28: 9855–9873.
[13] Pekar AH, Frank BH. Conformation of proinsulin: a comparison of insulin and proinsulin self-association at neural pH. Biochemistry 1972; 11: 4013–4016.
[14] Kruger P, Strabburger W, Wollmer A et al. The simulated dynamics of the insulin monomer and their relationship to the molecules structure. Eur Biophys J 1987; 14: 449–459.
[15] Blundell T, Dodson G, Hodgkin D et al. Insulin: the structure in the crystal and its reflection in chemistry and biology. Advan Protein Chem 1972; 26: 279–402.
[16] Goeddel DV, Kleid DG, Bolivar F et al. Expression in Escherichia coli of chemically synthesized genes for human insulin. Proc Natl Acad Sci USA 1979; 76: 106–110.
[17] Thim I, Hansen MT, Norris K et al. Secretion and processing of insulin precursors in yeast. Proc Natl Acad Sci USA 1986; 83: 6766–6770.
[18] Köhler G, Milstein C. Continuous cultures of fused cells secreting antibody of predefined specificity. Nature 1975; 256: 495–497.
[19] Cohen RH, Nakabayashi T, Blix PM et al. A radioimmunoassay for circulating human proinsulin. Diabetes 1985; 34: 84–91.
[20] Burrin J, Newman DJ. Production and assessment of antibodies. In: Price CP, Newman DJ, eds. Principles and Practice of Immunoassay. Macmillan Publishers UK, 1991; 19–52.
[21] Winter G, Milstein C. Man-made antibodies. Nature 1991; 349: 293–299.

[22] Huse WD, Sastry L, Iverson SA et al. Generation of a large combinatorial library of the immunoglobulin repertoire in phage lambda. Science 1989; 246: 1275–1281.
[23] Yalow RS, Berson SA. Assay of plasma insulin in human subjects by immunological methods. Nature 1959; 184: 1648–1649.
[24] Hales CN, Randle PJ. Immunoassay of insulin with insulin-antibody precipitate. Biochem J 1963; 88: 137–146.
[25] Morgan CR, Lazarow A. Immunoassay of insulin: two antibody system. Plasma insulin levels of normal, subdiabetic and diabetic rats. Diabetes 1963; 12: 115–126.
[26] Grodsky GM, Forsham PH. An immunochemical assay of total extractable insulin in man. J Clin Invest 1960; 39: 1070–1079.
[27] Herbert V, Lau KS, Gottlieb CW et al. Coated charcoal immunoassay of insulin. J Clin Endocrinol 1965; 25: 1375–1384.
[28] Desbuquois B, Aurbach GD. Use of polyethylene glycol to separate free and antibody-bound peptide hormones in radioimmunoassays. J Clin Endocrinol 1971; 33: 732–738.
[29] Miles LEM, Hales CN. Labelled antibodies and immunological assay systems. Nature 1968; 219: 186–189.
[30] Addison GM, Hales CN. Two site assay of human growth hormone. Horm Metab Res 1971; 3: 59–60.
[31] Sturgess ML, Weeks I, Mpoko CN et al. Chemiluminescent labeled-antibody assay for thyroxin in serum with magnetic separation of the solid-phase. Clin Chem 1986; 32: 532–535.
[32] Hales CN, Woodhead JS. Labelled antibodies and their use in the immunoradiometric assay. Methods Enzymol 1980; 70: 334–355.
[33] Alpha B, Cox L, Crowther N et al. Sensitive amplified immunoenzymometric assays (IEMA) for human insulin and intact proinsulin. European J Clinical Chemistry & Clinical Biochemistry 1992; 30: 27–32.
[34] Kemmler W, Peterson JD, Steiner DF. Studies on the conversion of proinsulin to insulin. J Biol Chem 1971; 246: 6786–6791.
[35] Clark PM, Levy JC, Cox L et al. Immunoradiometric assay of insulin, intact proinsulin and 32-33 split proinsulin and radioimmunoassay of insulin in diet-treated type 2 (non-insulin-dependent) diabetic subjects. Diabetologia 1992; 35: 469–474.
[36] Ekins R. Immunoassay design and optimisation. In: Price CP, Newman DJ, eds. Principles and Practice of Immunoassay. Macmillan Publishers UK, 1991; 96–153.
[37] Dhahir FJ, Cook DB, Self CH. Amplified enzyme-linked immunoassay of human proinsulin in serum (detection limit: 0.1 pmol/L). Clin Chem 1992; 38: 227–232.
[38] Roth J, Gorden P, Pastan I. "Big insulin": a new component of plasma insulin detected by immunoassay. Proc Soc Natl Acad Sci USA 1968; 61: 138–145.
[39] Kitabchi AC, Duckworth WC, Brush JS et al. Direct measurement of proinsulin in human plasma by the use of an insulin-degrading enzyme. J Clin Invest 1971; 50: 1792–1799.
[40] Cresto JC, Lavine RL, Fink G et al. Plasma proinsulin. Comparison of insulin specific protease and gel filtration assays. Diabetes 1974; 86: 631–637.
[41] Heding L. Specific and direct radioimmunoassay for human proinsulin in serum. Diabetologia 1977: 13: 467–474.
[42] Ward WK, Paquette TL, Frank BH et al. A sensitive radioimmunoassay for human proinsulin, with sequential use of antisera to C-peptide and insulin. Clin Chem 1986; 32: 726–733.
[43] Gray IP, Siddle K, Docherty K et al. Proinsulin in human serum; problems in measurement and interpretation. Clin Endocrinol 1984; 21: 43–47.
[44] Temple RC, Carrington CA, Luzio SD et al. Insulin deficiency in non-insulin-dependent diabetes. Lancet 1989; I: 293–295.
[45] Temple RC, Clark PMS, Nagi DK et al. Radioimmunoassay may overestimate insulin in non-insulin-dependent diabetics. Clin Endocrinol 1990; 32: 689–693.
[46] Nygren H, Stenberg AM. Immunochemistry at interfaces. Immunology 1989; 66: 321–327.

[47] Temple R, Clark PMS, Hales CN. Measurement of insulin secretion in type 2 diabetes: problems and pitfalls. Diabetic Medicine 1992; 9: 503–512.
[48] Gosling JP. A decade of development in immunoassay methodology. Clin Chem 1990; 36: 1408–1427.
[49] Boscato LM; Stuart MC. Incidence and specificity of interference in two-site immunoassays. Clin Chem 1986; 32: 1491–1495.
[50] Lookabaugh M, Biswas M, Krull IS. Quantitation of insulin injection by high-performance liquid chromatography and high-performance capillary electrophoresis. J Chromatography 1991; 549: 357–366.
[51] Linde S, Welinder BS. Non-ideal behaviour of silica-based stationary phases in trifluoroacetic acid-acetonitrile-based reversed-phase high-performance liquid chromatographic separations of insulins and proinsulins. J Chromatography 1991; 536: 43–55.
[52] Linde S, Røder ME, Hartling SG et al. Separation and quantitation of serum proinsulin and proinsulin intermediates in humans. J Chromatography 1991; 548: 371–380.
[53] Clark PMS, Ostrega D, Polonsky K et al. Measurement of proinsulin and intermediates: validation of immunoassay methods by high performance liquid chromatography. Proceedings of the ACB National Meeting 1993: 117–118.
[54] Cotes PM; Mussett VM, Berryman I et al. Collaborative study of estimates by radioimmunoassay of insulin concentrations in plasma samples examined in groups of five or six laboratories. J Endocrinol 1969; 45: 557–569.
[55] Shishiba Y, Takino H, Takagi A et al. The large 'kit to kit' variation in insulin radioimmunoassay is mainly due to the difference in standard concentration. Clin Chem 1982; 28: 2443–2444.
[56] Kruse V, Heding LG, Jørgensen KH et al. Human proinsulin standards. Diabetologia 1984; 27: 414–415.
[57] Frank BH, Pettee JM, Zimmerman RE et al. The production of human proinsulin and its transformation into insulin and C-peptide. In: Rich DH, Grosse E, eds. Peptides; Synthesis-Structure-Function. Proceedings of the Seventh American Peptide Symposium. Madison: WI Pierce Chemical Company, 1981; 729–738.
[58] O'Rahilly S, Burnett MA, Smith RF et al. Haemolysis affects insulin, but not C-peptide immunoassay. Diabetologia 1987; 30: 394–396.
[59] Livesy JH, Hodgkinson SC, Roud HR et al. Effect of time, temperature, and freezing on the stability of immunoreactive LH, FSH, TSH, growth hormone, prolactin and insulin in plasma. Clin Biochem 1980; 13: 151–155.
[60] Westgard JO, Groth T. Design and evaluation of statistical control procedures: applications of a computer "Quality control simulator" program. Clin Chem 1981; 27: 1536–1545.

Assessment of insulin production and secretion dynamics in health and disease, including diabetes

H. Tillil

Introduction

Most commonly, the peripheral concentrations of insulin or C-peptide, or both, are determined during fasting or after various stimuli in order to obtain a measurement of endogenous insulin secretion. Insulin and C-peptide, derived from the common precursor molecule pro-insulin by enzymatic cleavage, are co-secreted in equimolar concentrations into the portal circulation by the pancreatic β-cells [22]. While C-peptide traverses the liver without being extracted, in the basal state approximately 50% of the newly secreted insulin is extracted by the liver on the first pass [22]. Thus, the peripheral concentration of insulin more directly reflects post-hepatic insulin delivery rather than the secretion rate of insulin. Because of the higher peripheral C-peptide concentration as compared to the peripheral insulin concentration, measurement of C-peptide in the periphery seems to be a more suitable method for determination of insulin secretion. In addition, interpretation of the peripheral insulin concentration is difficult because of variable hepatic insulin extraction and variable insulin clearance from plasma. Clearance of endogenous insulin is diminished after marked stimulation of insulin secretion with larger doses of oral or intravenous glucose and shows evidence of saturation even at physiologic peripheral insulin concentrations [38, 39]. However, due to its relatively long half-life of approximately 30 min, as compared to the relatively short half-life of insulin (approximately 5 min), C-peptide does not adequately reflect rapid changes of insulin secretion, e. g. first-phase insulin secretion during IVGTT [28] or hyperglycaemic clamp [38]. Routine measurement of insulin concentrations in the portal vein is not feasible and limited to experimental situations [34].

A solution for these problems is the measurement of the pancreatic insulin secretion rate. Using C-peptide kinetic data derived by Faber et al. [9], Eaton et al. [8] have described a method for the measurement of the pancreatic C-peptide secretion rate which, in view of the equimolar secretion of insulin and C-peptide, is equal to the insulin secretion rate. By mathematical analysis

Offprint from
Research Methodologies in Human Diabetes – Part 1

of the peripheral plasma C-peptide concentrations using a two-compartment, open model [10, 17] of C-peptide distribution, the C-peptide secretion rate can be calculated [8]. With the availability of sufficient quantities of biosynthetic human C-peptide (BHCP) for experimental use in humans, this method has been validated by Polonsky et al. [15, 21, 22]. Beside the equimolar secretion of C-peptide and insulin, C-peptide fulfils further necessary conditions for the modelling process (Table 1): it is not extracted by the liver, and

Table 1 Validation of C-peptide as marker of insulin secretion

1. Equimolar co-secretion of insulin and C-peptide into the portal circulation by the pancreatic B-cells.
2. Absent (or negligible) hepatic extraction of insulin under physiologic conditions.
3. Constant metabolic clearance rate (MCR) of C-peptide from peripheral plasma at physiologic and supraphysiologic concentrations and under non-steady state conditions.

its plasma clearance is constant at physiologic and supraphysiologic plasma concentrations as well as under non-steady state conditions [21, 22]. C-peptide clearance from plasma is not affected by ingestion of a mixed meal or by changes in the plasma glucose concentration [15]. Note that the model refers to C-peptide and not to insulin itself.

Measurement of the pancreatic insulin secretion rate

The measurement of the insulin secretion rate is performed in two steps. Firstly, the kinetic model parameters of C-peptide are determined after bolus intravenous injection of BHCP. These parameters are then applied to the peripheral plasma C-peptide concentrations measured on a separate occasion, e. g. during OGTT, in order to derive the pancreatic C-peptide secretion rate.

Two-compartment, open model of C-peptide distribution

A two-compartment, open model of C-peptide distribution and degradation as proposed by Eaton et al. [8] is applied (Fig. 1). This model assumes that C-peptide distributes itself into a central (accessible) compartment which consists of the plasma space and tissues in rapid equilibrium with plasma and from which sampling occurs, and into a peripheral extravascular compartment. C(t) corresponds to the amount of C-peptide in the central and Y(t) in the peripheral compartments at time t. k_1 and k_2 are the (first-order)

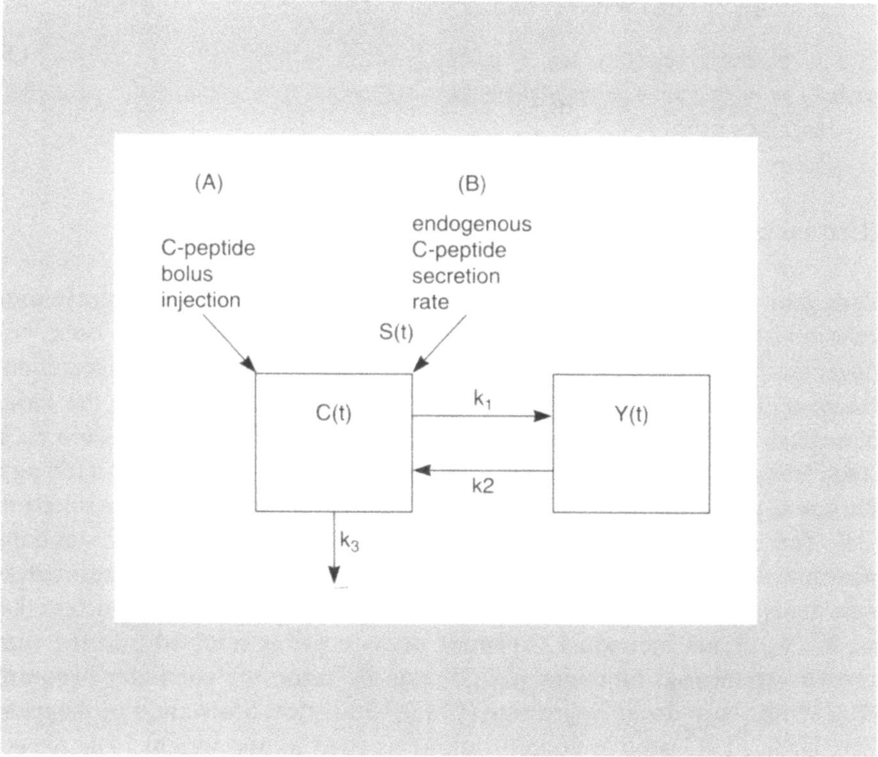

Fig. 1 Open two-compartment model of C-peptide distribution and degradation used in estimating the parameters of C-peptide kinetics (A) and in deriving the pancreatic C-peptide or insulin secretion rate (B). S(t), pancreatic C-peptide secretion rate; C(t), amount of C-peptide in the central compartment (C = plasma C-peptide concentration . volume of distribution of the central compartment); Y(t), amount of C-peptide in the peripheral compartment (at time t)

fractional kinetic rate constants which describe the C-peptide movement between the two compartments. k_3 is the (first-order) fractional rate constant which describes the irreversible metabolism of C-peptide from the central compartment. V_d denotes the volume of distribution of the central compartment. BHCP is injected into the central compartment, and the model representation used in estimating the parameters of C-peptide kinetics (Fig. 1) can be described by two differential equations:

$$\frac{dC}{dt} = -(k_1 + k_3)\,C(t) + k_2\,Y(t) \tag{1}$$

$$\frac{dY}{dt} = k_1\,C(t) - k_2 Y(t) \tag{2}$$

The solution of equations (1) and (2) for C(t) is

$$C(t) = p_1 \exp[-p_2(t - t_0)] + p_3 \exp[-p_4(t - t_0)] \quad (3)$$
$$\text{with } k_2 = -(p_1 p_4 + p_3 p_2)/(p_1 + p_3), \quad (4)$$
$$k_3 = p_2 p_4/k_2, \quad (5)$$
$$k_1 = -p_2 - p_4 - k_2 - k_3. \quad (6)$$

Bolus intravenous injection of biosynthetic human C-peptide

Endogenous C-peptide secretion is inhibited by a primed (50 µg) intravenous infusion of somatostatin (500 µg/h) for 4 hours. During the first hour, endogenous C-peptide is measured to document suppression of insulin secretion. Glucose (20%) is infused at a variable rate in order to maintain the basal plasma glucose concentration. After one hour of somatostatin infusion each study subject receives an intravenous bolus injection of BHCP (150 µg). Plasma C-peptide concentrations are frequently measured after bolus injection [21]. The individual C-peptide decay curves are then analysed by standard pharmacokinetic methods (iterative weighted non-linear least-squares regression analysis) in order to derive the C-peptide kinetic model parameters (k_1, k_2, k_3, V_d). Each individual C-peptide decay curve is resolved into the sum of two exponential functions (eq. 3), e. g. by using the computer program BMDP 3R: Non-linear Regression (BMDP Statistical Software, Los Angeles, CA, USA). 1/(C-peptide concentration)^2 is used as the weight [44]. As explained in detail by Gibaldi and Perrier [10], the two coefficients p_1 and p_3 and the two exponents p_2 and p_4 of the biexponential function yield the fractional kinetic rate constants k_1, k_2, k_3 (eq. 4–6). The volume of distribution (V_d) is calculated as the dose of BHCP in the bolus divided by ($p_1 + p_3$). The intravenous bolus injection technique also allows the determination of the metabolic clearance rate (MCR; dose of C-peptide in the bolus divided by the area under the C-peptide decay curve, integrated to

Table 2 Metabolic and kinetic C-peptide parameters in 14 normal subjects (data from ref. [39])

MCR ($ml.kg^{-1}.min^{-1}$)	3.75	±	0.1
($ml.m^{-2}.min^{-1}$)	135.7	±	3.8
$T_{1/2}$ short (min)	5.2	±	0.4
$T_{1/2}$ long (min)	34.4	±	1.4
k_1 (min^{-1})	0.0560	±	0.0068
k_2 (min^{-1})	0.0489	±	0.0041
k_3 (min^{-1})	0.0618	±	0.0068
V_d (ml/kg)	64.1	±	4.6
(ml/m^2)	2299.0	±	140.6

infinity) as well as the short ($\ln 2/p_2$) and long ($\ln 2/p_4$) half-lives ($T_{1/2}$) of C-peptide. The metabolic and kinetic data of 14 normal subjects [39] are given in Table 2. The fractional kinetic rate constants are in the order of 5–6%/min.

Calculation of the pancreatic insulin secretion rate

The fractional kinetic rate constants and the distribution volume of the central compartment are then applied to the peripheral plasma C-peptide concentrations, e. g. during OGGT, in order to derive the pancreatic C-peptide secretion rate. The model representation used in deriving the C-peptide secretion rate (Fig. 1) can be described by two differential equations:

$$\frac{dC}{dt} = S(t) - (k_1 + k_3)\,C(t) + k_2\,Y(t) \tag{7}$$

$$\frac{dY}{dt} = k_1\,C(t) - k_2\,Y(t) \tag{8}$$

The solution of these equations for S(t) yields the pancreatic C-peptide secretion rate which is equal to the insulin secretion rate [8]:

$$S(t) = -k_1\,C(t_0)\exp[-k_2(t - t_0)] - k_1 k_2 \int_{t_0}^{t_1} C(s)\exp[-k_2(t - s)]\,ds + \frac{dC}{dt} + (k_1 + k_3)\,C(t) \tag{9}$$

S(t) only depends on the fractional kinetic rate constants (k_1, k_2 and k_3) and on the amount of C-peptide in the central compartment (C) which is obtained by multiplying the C-peptide concentration by the volume of distribution of the central compartment (V_d). The mathematical procedure by which the secretion rate of a peptide or hormone is derived from its peripheral plasma concentrations and the kinetic model parameters is termed deconvolution analysis. A robust locally weighted regression procedure described by Cleveland [6] has been used to obtain a smooth representation of plasma C-peptide concentrations before performing the deconvolution procedure [27, 28, 31, 39]. In other studies smoothing has been performed by fitting a least-squares cubic spline to the discrete C-peptide concentrations [11, 21] or by using a two-point moving average filter [37].

One- or two-compartment model for C-peptide kinetics?

It has been suggested that one-compartment kinetics are sufficient to describe C-peptide clearance and that a two-compartment model of C-peptide cannot be resolved in a substantial number of subjects [7]. However, in a comparison study between one- and two-compartment models for C-peptide clearance, Van Cauter et al. [44] reported that failure to fit a two-compartment model did not occur in any of the 200 decay curves analysed. With frequent sampling over a 180-min period after a bolus injection of C-peptide during suppression of endogenous C-peptide secretion by somatostatin, the two-compartment model produced much better fits of the data than a one-compartment model [44] or a three-compartment model [22]. The residual sum of squares was 15-fold higher with the one-compartment model than with the two-compartment model [44]. Somatostatin has no effect on the clearance of C-peptide from peripheral plasma [21].

Calculation of the insulin secretion rate using the MCR of C-peptide

The C-peptide or insulin secretion rate can also be determined without relying on a model of C-peptide distribution by multiplying the peripheral plasma C-peptide concentration by the MCR of C-peptide [12, 13, 16]. Thus the basal insulin secretion rate is determined as the basal plasma C-peptide concentration multiplied by the MCR of C-peptide. The amount of insulin secreted, e. g. in response to an oral glucose stimulus, can be calculated as the area under the peripheral plasma C-peptide concentration curve multiplied by the MCR of C-peptide, because C-peptide kinetics are linear.

Urine C-peptide excretion

The measurement of the urinary excretion of various hormones has been used as a measure of the production rate of these hormones, and this approach has also been suggested for the quantitation of insulin secretion by the urinary excretion of C-peptide, because insulin and C-peptide are co-secreted equimolarly and a fraction of the secreted C-peptide is excreted in the urine [16]. The availability of pancreatic insulin secretion rates and the simultaneous measurement of C-peptide excretion in urine allowed a revaluation of urine C-peptide as quantitative measure of insulin secretion. Tillil et al. [40] reported a high intersubject variability as well as a low reproducibility (intrasubject variability) of urine C-peptide clearance and of fractional C-peptide excretion (percentage of secreted C-peptide that is excreted in the urine) in non-diabetic subjects and in patients with type 2 (non-insulin-dependent) diabetes on a mixed diet over a 24-hour period. The 24-hour insulin secretion rate correlated more closely with the fasting insulin secretion rate, the fasting C-peptide and insulin concentrations than with the 24-hour urine C-peptide excretion. Thus the most reliable method for quantitation of insulin secretion seems to be the application of a two-compartment model on the peripheral plasma C-peptide concentrations. This method is advantageous if rapid changes in insulin secretion are being studied or if an accurate quantitation of insulin secretion is needed. If this method is not available, the fasting C-peptide or fasting insulin concentrations can be used both of which correlate well with the daily insulin secretion rate. This is especially true for the fasting C-peptide which is not influenced by changes in hepatic extraction as is fasting insulin in obesity [23]. Although the daily urine C-peptide excretion correlates significantly with the daily insulin secretion rate, the high inter- and intrasubject variability of fractional C-peptide excretion limits the value of urine C-peptide as quantitative measure of insulin secretion.

Application of the two-compartment model for C-peptide

The deconvolution method for the measurement of pancreatic insulin secretion rates using a two-compartment, open model of C-peptide distribution and individually derived kinetic model parameters has been applied by several investigators in normal volunteers [12, 21, 27–29, 38, 39, 45] in obese subjects [23, 24], in aged subjects [11], in patients with type 2 (non-insulin-dependent) diabetes [1, 25, 30, 31, 37, 40], in type 1 (insulin-dependent) diabetic patients after combined pancreas and kidney transplantation [3] in patients with liver cirrhosis [13] and in patients with thyrotoxicosis [19]. Insulin secretion rates

Table 3 Integrated incremental insulin secretion rates after increasing oral glucose loads (25, 50 or 100 g) in seven normal subjects (mean ± SEM). Integration was performed over 300 min (data from [39])

	Oral glucose dose		
	25 g	50 g	100 g
Glucose ($g.dl^{-1}.min$)	2.2 ± 0.6	6.2 ± 0.9	10.5 ± 1.0
Insulin ($nmol.l^{-1}.min$)	15.4 ± 2.5	27.1 ± 2.7	85.2 ± 16.5
C-peptide ($nmol.l^{-1}.min$)	93.2 ± 15.9	187.4 ± 23.5	384.7 ± 27.2
Insulin secretion (nmol)	20.9 ± 4.8	42.4 ± 4.9	81.6 ± 4.0

The basal insulin secretion rate was 83.2±4.4 pmol/min. To convert nmol (insulin) to U, multiply by 0.145.

in normal subjects after increasing oral glucose doses (25, 50 and 100 g) are given in Table 3.

Standard C-peptide parameters

The proposed method for the quantitation of pancreatic insulin secretion rates is laborious and time-consuming, and BHCP is not always readily available. However, after the analysis of 200 C-peptide decay curves, Van Cauter et al. [44] suggested that it is possible to estimate insulin secretion rates from plasma C-peptide levels with standard parameters for C-peptide clearance, rather than individually derived parameters, without significant loss of accuracy. Van Cauter et al. [44] described a procedure to obtain standard parameters for C-peptide clearance in normal and obese subjects and in patients with type 2 (non-insulin-dependent) diabetes. However, as the authors pointed out, the approach with standard parameters is not applicable in conditions in which renal function is altered, because the kidney is the predominant site of C-peptide clearance. Standard parameters cannot be used in patients with thyrotoxicosis (enhanced clearance of C-peptide) [19] or in type 1 (insulin-dependent) patients with combined kidney-pancreas transplantation (reduced clearance of C-peptide) [3].

Alternative methods for the measurement of insulin secretion rates

Several other approaches have been proposed for the measurement of insulin secretion rates in human subjects from peripheral or hepatic vein C-peptide concentrations. Waldhäusl et al. [48] measured arterial and hepatic vein C-peptide concentrations in normal human subjects and, by assuming that its hepatic extraction was negligible, used this value together with splanchnic blood flow measurements to calculate splanchnic insulin production. They estimated an insulin secretion of 1.35 U per 12 g of ingested glucose, a value that is in close agreement with the value of 1.40 U per 12 g of glucose estimated with the two-compartment method by Tillil et al. [39]. Using a one-compartment model for C-peptide and insulin distribution, Volund et al. [47] suggested a combined model of insulin and C-peptide kinetics for the calculation of insulin secretion rates without using individually derived parameters. Also, the minimal model approach for C-peptide and insulin kinetics has been applied for the measurement of insulin secretion and hepatic insulin extraction [7].

Dynamics of insulin secretion

Several reviews are available on the dynamics of insulin secretion regarding the first and second phases of secretion, non-glucose stimuli or the glucose potentiation of insulin secretion [4, 49]. This review only deals with the pulsatile nature of insulin secretion.

Rapid pulses of insulin secretion

That insulin is secreted in a pulsatile fashion was first demonstrated in humans by Lang et al. [14]. Since then, a large number of studies on this issue have been performed and recently summarised [50]. These rapid pulses of insulin secretion with a periodicity of 8–15 min are probably generated in the pancreas and are independent of nerve control mechanisms [20]. In view of a higher amplitude of the rapid pulses in the portal as compared to the peripheral circulation these pulses are likely to be involved in the regulation of hepatic glucose production and in the regulation of insulin receptors [20]. Irregular oscillatory insulin secretion has been suggested to be an early feature of type 1 (insulin-dependent) diabetes [2] as well as of type 2 (non-insulin-dependent) diabetes [20].

Slow oscillations of insulin secretion

In addition, ultradian oscillations of insulin secretion with a greater periodicity (80–150 min) than the rapid pulses have recently been identified in humans during continuous enteral nutrition [32], during constant glucose infusion [29] and in response to meals [24, 25, 30, 33]. Circadian rhythms shorter than 24 hours have been termed "ultradian". Using accurately quantitated pancreatic insulin secretion rates these ultradian oscillations of insulin secretion have been shown to occur independently from food ingestion [29, 31] and intact innervation of the pancreas [3]. The rapid pulses are superimposed on the slow oscillations of insulin secretion [32]. It has been suggested that the insulin/glucose feedback mechanism plays an important role in generating and regulating the slow ultradian oscillations [35, 36]. The frequency of the ultradian oscillations of insulin secretion, the rate of concomitance of oscillations of insulin secretion with oscillations in glucose levels and the relative amplitudes of both the insulin and glucose oscillations were similar in fasting patients with type 2 (non-insulin-dependent) diabetes and in non-diabetic subjects [37]. Spectral analysis demonstrated a slowing of the glucose oscillations without a similar slowing of the oscillations in insulin secretion in these patients consistent with previous observations of sluggish and irregular glucose oscillations in patients with type 2 (non-insulin-dependent) diabetes receiving mixed meals [25]. This partial dissociation between the oscillatory patterns of insulin secretion and glucose levels has been suggested to reflect a breakdown of the insulin-glucose feedback loop in type 2 (non-insulin-dependent) diabetes [37].

Two major methods for the analysis of pulsatile hormone secretion are available: peak detection analysis and time series analysis (spectral analysis) [5, 26, 41, 42, 43].

Peak detection procedures

Several computer programs for the analysis of pulsatile hormonal secretion are available, e. g. "DETECT" from Oerter, Guardabasso and Rodbard [18], "CLUSTER" from Veldhuis and Johnson [46] and "ULTRA" from E. Van Cauter [43]. These programs have recently been compared [42]. ULTRA, a computer algorithm for identification and quantitative estimation of pulses of hormonal secretion, should be described briefly. The general principle of this algorithm is the elimination of all peaks for which either the increment (difference between the peak and the preceding trough) or the decrement (difference between the peak and the next trough) does not exceed a certain threshold related to measurement error. The output is a "clean" profile in which all temporal changes are significant with respect to assay precision. Simulation studies have indicated that a threshold twice the intra-assay coefficient of variation (IACV) generally minimises false-positive (type I) and false-negative (type II) errors [43]. However, because deconvolution involves an amplification of measurement error, a more conservative threshold of three times the IACV of C-peptide has been used in several studies to detect pulses of insulin secretion [24, 25, 29, 30]. Prior smoothing with a two-point moving average reduces the measurement error by a factor $\sqrt{2}$ [37]. For each significant pulse, the absolute amplitude is defined as the difference between the peak level and the level at the preceding trough. In view of the relatively long half-life of glucose in plasma, changes in either glucose production or utilisation, or both, may not be reflected as significant pulses in the peripheral glucose concentration curve. Therefore glucose "shoulders" have been defined, i. e. peaks in glucose for which either the increment or the decrement (but not both) do not exceed the threshold for significance [29, 35, 37]. The program ULTRA includes five major steps: data input, data preparation, elimination of non-significant peaks ("clean" series), identification of significant pulses and calculation of statistics for pulse parameters. For each pulse, the ascending portion, the declining portion, the total duration, the absolute and relative increment, the absolute and relative decrement and the apparent half-life are calculated. ULTRA has been applied in a number of studies of the pulsatile nature of insulin secretion in normal man [24, 29, 35, 45], in obese subjects [24], in patients with type 2 (non-insulin-dependent) diabetes [25, 30, 31, 37] and in type 1 (insulin-dependent) diabetic patients after combined kidney-pancreas transplantation [3].

Analysis of time series

In this review only the most important procedures can be mentioned. One major tool for the analysis of time series (i. e. a sequence of measurements made at regular time intervals) is the autocorrelation function which helps to describe the evolution of a process through time. Inference based on the autocorrelation function is called an analysis in the time domain. The spectral density function describes how the variation in a time series may be accounted for by cyclic components at different frequencies. The procedure for the estimation of this function is called spectral analysis. Inference based on the spectral density function is called an analysis in the frequency domain. A short introduction into methods for the analysis of time series has been given by Chatfield [5].

A number of computer programs for time series analysis are available. Most general computer packages offer some time-series options, including MINITAB (Minitab Inc., State College, PA, USA), BMDP (program P1T: univariate and bivariate spectral analysis, program P2T: Box-Jenkins time series analysis; BMDP Statistical Software, Los Angeles, CA, USA) and SPSS (SPSS Inc., Chicago, IL, USA). A short overview on the analysis of time series is available e. g. in the BMDP Statistical Software Manual, p. 595 – 660 and p. 686 – 691.

Time series analysis has been applied in the analysis of the temporal organisation of insulin secretion in a number of studies (rapid pulses: e. g. [2, 14, 20, 34, 37, 50]; slow oscillations: e. g. [32, 33, 37]).

Acknowledgments: H. T. is supported by a grant from the Paul-Kuth-Stiftung Wuppertal. Original work of the author presented herein was supported by the Deutsche Forschungsgemeinschaft (DFG) and the Deutsche Diabetes-Gesellschaft (DDG).

References

[1] Beebe CA, Van Cauter E, Shapiro ET et al. Effect of temporal distribution of calories on diurnal patterns of glucose levels and insulin secretion in NIDDM. Diabetes Care 1990; 13: 748–755.
[2] Bingley PJ, Matthews DR, Williams AJK et al. Loss of regular oscillatory insulin secretion in islet cell antibody positive non-diabetic subjects. Diabetologia 1992; 35: 32–38.
[3] Blackman JD, Polonsky KS, Jaspan JB et al. Insulin secretory profiles and C-peptide clearance kinetics at 6 months and 2 years after kidney-pancreas transplantation. Diabetes 1992; 41: 1346–1354.
[4] Cerasi E, Nesher R. Assessment of insulin secretion dynamics. In: Methods in Diabetes Research. Vol. II: Clinical Methods. Clarke WL, Larner J, Pohl SL, eds. New York: Wiley, 1986: 77–90.
[5] Chatfield C. The analysis of time series. An introduction. 4th ed. London: Chapman & Hall, 1989.
[6] Cleveland WS. Robust locally weighted regression and smoothing scatterplots. J Am Stat Assoc 1979; 74: 829–836.
[7] Cobelli C, Pacini G. Insulin secretion and hepatic extraction in humans by minimal modeling of C-peptide and insulin kinetics. Diabetes 1988; 37: 223–231.
[8] Eaton RP, Allen RC, Schade DS et al. Prehepatic insulin production in man: kinetic analysis using peripheral connecting peptide behavior. J Clin Endocrinol Metab 1980; 51: 520–528.
[9] Faber OK, Hagen C, Binder C et al. Kinetics of human connecting peptide in normal and diabetic subjects. J Clin Invest 1978; 62: 197–203.
[10] Gibaldi M, Perrier D. Pharmacokinetics. 2nd ed., revised and expanded. In: Drugs and the Pharmaceutical Sciences, Vol. 15. Swarbrick J, ed. New York/Basel: Dekker, 1982; 84–88.
[11] Gumbiner B, Polonsky K, Beltz W et al. Effects of aging on insulin secretion. Diabetes 1989; 38: 1549–1556.
[12] Kruszynska YT, Home PD, Hanning I et al. Basal and 24-h C-peptide and insulin secretion rate in normal man. Diabetologia 1987; 30: 16–21.
[13] Kruszynska YT, Munro J, Home PD et al. Twenty-four hour C-peptide and insulin secretion rates and diurnal profiles of glucose, lipids and interdediary metabolites in cirrhosis. Clin Sci 1992; 83: 597–605.
[14] Lang DA, Matthews DR, Peto et al. Cyclic oscillations of basal plasma glucose and insulin concentrations in human beings. N Engl J Med 1979; 301: 1023–1027.
[15] Licinio-Paixao J, Polonsky KS, Given BD et al. Ingestion of a mixed meal does not affect the metabolic clearance rate of biosynthetic human C-peptide. J Clin Endocrinol Metab 1986; 63: 401–403.
[16] Meistas MT, Rendell M, Margolis S et al. Estimation of the secretion rate of insulin from the urinary excretion rate of C-peptide: study in obese and diabetic subjects. Diabetes 1982; 31: 449–453.
[17] Metzler CM. Usefulness of the two-compartment, open model in pharmacokinetics. J Am Stat Ass 1971; 66: 49–53.
[18] Oerter KE, Guardabasso V, Rodbard D. Detection and characterization of peaks and estimation of instantaneous secretory rate for episodic pulsatile hormone secretion. Comput Biomed Res 1986; 19: 170–191.
[19] O'Meara NM, Blackman JD, Polonsky KS. Alterations in kinetics of C-peptide and insulin secretion in hyperthyroidism (Abstract). 73rd Annual Meeting of The Endocrine Society, Volume of Abstracts, 1991; 468.
[20] O'Rahilly S, Turner RC, Matthews DR. Impaired pulsatile secretion of insulin in relatives with non-insulin-dependent diabetes. N Engl J Med 1988; 318: 1225–1230.
[21] Polonsky KS, Licinio-Paixao J, Given BD et al. Use of biosynthetic human C-peptide in the measurement of insulin secretion rates in normal volunteers and type I diabetic patients. J Clin Invest 1986; 77: 98–105.

[22] Polonsky KS, Rubenstein AH. Current approaches to the measurement of insulin secretion. Diab/Metab Rev 1986; 2: 315–329.
[23] Polonsky KS, Given BD, Hirsch L et al. Quantitative study of insulin secretion and clearance in normal and obese subjects. J Clin Invest 1988; 81: 435–441.
[24] Polonsky KS, Given BD, Van Cauter E. Twenty-four hour profiles and pulsatile patterns of insulin secretion in normal and obese subjects. J Clin Invest 1988; 81: 442–448.
[25] Polonsky KS, Given BD, Hirsch LJ et al. Abnormal patterns of insulin secretion in non-insulin dependent diabetes. N Engl J Med 1988; 318: 1231–1239.
[26] Royston JP. The statistical analysis of pulsatile hormone secretion data (Review). Clin Endocrinol 1989; 30: 201–210.
[27] Shapiro ET, Tillil H, Miller MA et al. Insulin secretion and clearance. Comparison after oral and intravenous glucose. Diabetes 1987; 36: 1365–1371.
[28] Shapiro ET, Tillil H, Rubenstein AH et al. Peripheral insulin parallels changes in insulin secretion more closely than C-peptide after bolus intravenous glucose administration. J Clin Endocrinol Metab 1988; 67: 1094–1099.
[29] Shapiro ET, Tillil H, Polonsky KS et al. Oscillations in insulin secretion during constant glucose infusion in normal man: relationship to changes in plasma glucose. J Clin Endocrinol Metab 1988; 67: 307–314.
[30] Shapiro ET, Van Cauter E, Tillil H et al. Glyburide enhances the responsiveness of the B-cell to glucose but does not correct the abnormal patterns of insulin secretion in noninsulin-dependent diabetes mellitus. J Clin Endocrinol Metab 1989; 69: 571–576.
[31] Shapiro ET, Polonsky KS, Copinschi G et al. Nocturnal elevation of glucose levels during fasting in noninsulin-dependent diabetes. J Clin Endocrinol Metab 1991; 72: 444–454.
[32] Simon C, Brandenberger G, Follenius M. Ultradian oscillations of plasma glucose, insulin and C-peptide in man during continous enteral nutrition. J Clin Endocrinol Metab 1987; 64: 669–674.
[33] Simon C, Follenius M, Brandenberger G. Postprandial oscillations of plasma glucose, insulin and C-peptide in man. Diabetologia 1987; 30: 769–773.
[34] Storch M-J, Rössle M, Kerp L. Pulsatile Insulinsekretion in die Pfortader bei Leberzirrhose. Dtsch med Wschr 1993; 118: 134–138.
[35] Sturis J, Van Cauter E, Blackman JD et al. Entrainment of pulsatile insulin secretion by oscillatory glucose infusions. J Clin Invest 1991; 87: 439–445.
[36] Sturis J, Polonsky KS, Mosekilde E et al. Computer model for mechanisms underlying ultradian oscillations of insulin and glucose. Am J Physiol 1991; 260: E801-E809.
[37] Sturis J, Polonsky KS, Shapiro ET et al. Abnormalities in the ultradian oscillations of insulin secretion and glucose levels in Type 2 (non-insulin-dependent) diabetic patients. Diabetologia 1992; 35: 681–689.
[38] Tillil H, Shapiro ET, Rubenstein AH et al. Reduction of insulin clearance during hyperglycemic clamp. Dose-response study in normal humans. Diabetes 1988; 37: 1351–1357.
[39] Tillil H, Shapiro ET, Miller MA et al. Dose-dependent effects of oral and intravenous glucose on insulin secretion and clearance in humans. Am J Physiol 1988; 254: E349-E357.
[40] Tillil H, Shapiro ET, Given BD et al. Reevaluation of urine C-peptide as measure of insulin secretion. Diabetes 1988; 37: 1195–1201.
[41] Urban RJ, Evans WS, Rogol AD et al. Contemporary aspects of discrete peak-detection algorithms. I. The paradigm of the luteinizing hormone pulse signal in men. Endocr Rev 1988; 9: 3–37.
[42] Urban RJ, Kaiser DL, Van Cauter E et al. Comparative assessment of objective peak-detection algorithms. II. Studies in men. Am J Physiol 1988; 254: E113-E119.
[43] Van Cauter E. Estimating false-positive and false-negative errors in analyses of hormonal pulsatility. Am J Physiol 1988; 254: E786-E794.
[44] Van Cauter E, Mestrez F, Sturis J et al. Estimation of insulin secretion rates from C-peptide levels. Comparison of individual and standard kinetic parameters for C-peptide clearance. Diabetes 1992; 41: 368–377.

[45] Van Cauter E, Shapiro ET, Tillil H et al. Circadian modulation of glucose and insulin responses to meals: relationship to cortisol rhythm. Am J Physiol 1992; 262: E467-E475.
[46] Veldhuis JD, Johnson ML. Cluter analysis: a simple, versatile, and robust algorithm for endocrine pulse detection. Am J Physiol 1986; 250: E486-E493.
[47] Volund A, Polonsky KS, Bergman RN. Calculated pattern of intraportal insulin appearance without independent assessment of C-peptide kinetics. Diabetes 1987; 36: 1195–1202.
[48] Waldhäusl W, Bratusch-Marrain P, Gasic S et al. Insulin production rate following glucose ingestion estimated by splanchnic C-peptide output in normal man. Diabetologia 1979; 17: 221–227.
[49] Ward WK, Beard JC, Porte D Jr. Islet β-cell function in human subjects. In: Methods in Diabetes Research. Vol. II: Clinical Methods. Clarke WL, Larner J, Pohl SL, eds. New York: Wiley, 1986; 3–14.
[50] Weigle DS. Pulsatile secretion of fuel-regulatory hormones (Review). Diabetes 1987; 36: 764–775.

Methodologies in characterization and classification of prediabetic states to non-insulin-dependent diabetes mellitus (NIDDM)

H. Beck-Nielsen

Introduction

In order to understand the methods used in exploration of NIDDM and prediabetic states, a basic knowledge of pathogenesis of this disease is fundamental. Therefore, I will concentrate on this before going into details on methods.

NIDDM has been shown to be phenotypically heterogenous and therefore this syndrome may not be explained by one simple patophysiological mechanism. There seems to be many different causes for development of hyperglycaemia in these subjects. In common, however, is insulin resistance and absolute or relative insulin deficiency [1]. The causes of these events have not yet been completely identified and it will take years before the patophysiology is completely understood. However, in recent years, investigations have clarified metabolic characteristics of both the diabetic and the prediabetic state, enabling us to subdivide the disease into phenotypically characteristic stages [2, 3, 4].

In this review will mainly concentrate on the most common form of NIDDM, namely the form linked to overweight, arterial hypertension, dyslipoproteinaemia and coronary heart disease (CHD) i. e., a disease most often diagnosed in elderly subjects [5]. This form of NIDDM seems to be growing epidemically world wide following the industrial development or the "coca-colanization", as it has been called [6]. Around 2–3% of the western world suffers from this disease, but between subjects beyond 60 years of age the prevalence is 5–20%. In certain ethnical, isolated populations the prevalence may be much higher (40–50%) . Thus, we face an enormous challenge with extreme economical, social and humanitary implications and it is therefore important to continue the research of the aethiology and pathophysiology to this disease – or this syndrome. However, our current knowledge is on a

Offprint from
Research Methodologies in Human Diabetes – Part 1

level which enables us to start intervention, even in a very early stage of the disease. As a result of this we may be able to prevent development of the complications. This intervention in lifestyle or by drug treatment may be based on metabolic characteristics of the prediabetic stages starting as early as in the youth or the childhood. Despite the fact that genetic basis of the disease is still unknown, it is not necessary to await further progress in this area before starting prevention, since our metabolic investigations are sufficient to characterize subjects at risk. The methodology behind these metabolic investigations is the basis for this review.

The results obtained up to now in treatment of hyperglycaemic NIDDM patients (often started at the age of 60 years) have been rather disappointing [1]. Furthermore, even properly treated NIDDM patients develop substantial complications, especially macroangiopathy. Coronary heart disease is the main cause of death in these patients and the overall mortality rate in NIDDM patients is 2–3 times higher than in controls [7]. Furthermore, several complications may already be present at the diagnosis of the disease, about 40% of the newly diagnosed patients suffer from clinical macroangiopathy, 50% from arterial hypertension whereas around 20–30% present with microangiopathy as retinopathy and albuminuria [8]. This indicates that the so-called complications may not be secondary to the diabetic state itself, but rather a part of the NIDDM phenotype i. e. that glucose intolerance, hyperinsulinaemia, arterial hypertension and dyslipoproteinaemia form a syndrome – the Insulin Resistance Syndrome [5, 10]. The inherited basis for this syndrome has been hypothesized to be insulin resistance specifically to glucose storage in skeletal muscles [2, 3]. If this is true, and there is good evidence in favour of the hypothesis, it is evident that it is too late to start treatment of NIDDM when it is clinically present i. e. when hyperglycaemia induces so many symptoms that the patients contact their doctors. Therefore, it seems obvious that this syndrome must be diagnosed in the prediabetic states before macroangiopathy has started or reached a clinical manifest level, in order to present the complications. In the future, large multicentre studies of young subjects prone to develop NIDDM must be performed in order to clarify how to prevent development of diabetes and the diabetic complications. But even before these have been carried out, clinicians must learn to know the natural history of NIDDM in order to advise and treat their patients properly. In this review therefore, we will discuss the metabolic and genetic background of NIDDM in order to describe the preclinical stages. Furthermore, methodologies used for characterization and classification of these stages will be discussed in the text and described in more detail.

A hypothetical model for the development of NIDDM

Current data suggest that insulin resistance, primarily impaired stimulation of glycogen formation in skeletal muscle, represents a primary defect in the pathogenesis of NIDDM. [1, 3, 4, 11], but this disease does not develop unless insulin secretion is also diminished [1].

The following model for the development of NIDDM can therefore be proposed. Two genetic defects are required, one causing impaired glycogen formation in skeletal muscle, the other causing insulin deficiency, i. e. inability to compensate for insulin resistance. Although they act jointly to cause diabetes, insulin resistance is the trigger which increases the insulin demands, thereby unmasking the defect in the β-cell. A normal β-cell would compensate for the insulin resistance by increasing the amount of insulin secreted. The "prediabetic" β-cell cannot compensate for the insulin resistance in the long term and hyperglycaemia ensues. In the following, I will mainly concentrate on the investigation of insulin resistance. Methods for studying insulin secretion will be described elsewhere.

Insulin resistance in skeletal muscles from patients with NIDDM: cellular defects

In obese newly diagnosed NIDDM patients, clamped overnight to keep blood glucose and FFA values near normal to eliminate the metabolic impact of these variables, we found a significant reduction of insulin-mediated glucose disposal in skeletal muscles compared with both lean and obese control subjects [12]. Several other groups [1, 13, 14] have also substantiated this finding. By use of two other different techniques, nuclear magnetic resonance phosphospectroscopy [15] and AV catheterization across the leg, it has been clearly established that the reduced R_d (glucose disposal) found during in vivo clamp studies is mainly due to a reduced insulin-mediated glucose uptake in skeletal muscles. Thus, we can conclude that skeletal muscles from obese NIDDM patients are insulin resistant when measured during euglycaemic-hyperinsulinaemic clamp.

The reason for the reduced disposal was a defect in both the non-oxidative and the oxidative pathways [12, 13, 14]. However, quantitatively the most important defect was in the non-oxidative pathway, i. e. in glycogenesis (storage), as also outlined by the nuclear magnetic resonance studies [15]. The effect of insulin on fat oxidation was also abnormal in patients with NIDDM, because fat oxidation was only partially suppressed during insulin infusion. Thus, the cause of insulin resistance in these patients seems to be

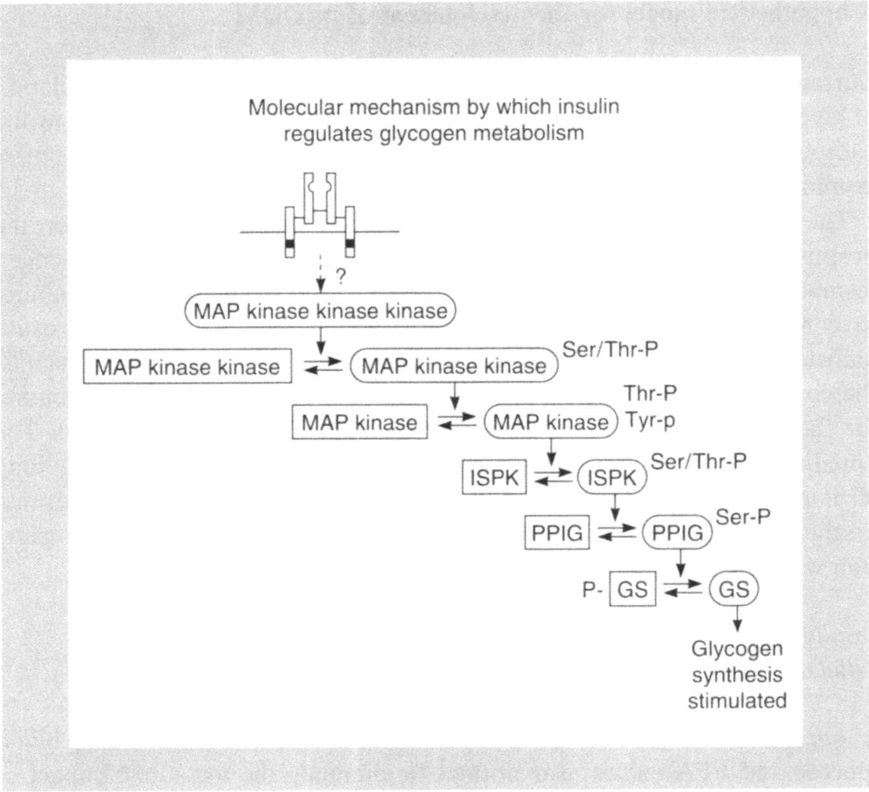

Fig. 1 Model for insulin signaling into skeletal muscle cells resulting in glycogen synthesis

multifactorial. To understand this, intracellular effect on insulin must be studied. Fig. 1 shows a model of the insulin signaling system in skeletal muscles, which results in glycogen synthesis.

Glycogen synthase (GS) activity: The glycogen synthase activities in lean and obese control subjects and in obese diabetic subjects during euglycaemic-hyperinsulinaemic clamp is shown in Fig. 2 [12]. In lean control subjects, insulin stimulated the fractional velocity of GS more than fourfold. However, in obese diabetic subjects, insulin was unable to increase GS activities. Thus, GS was determined to be completely resistant to insulin. Identical results were obtained when the enzyme activity was evaluated without G-6-P in the medium, indicating that the defect is independent of allosteric activation but is due to an abnormal covalent stimulation.

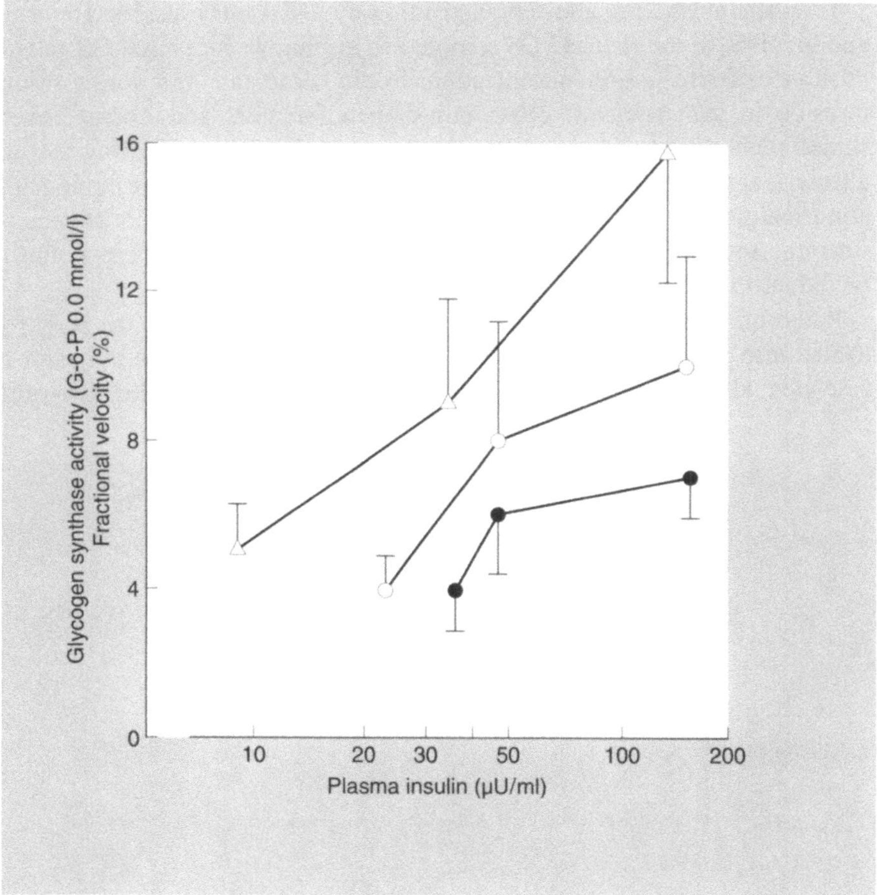

Fig. 2 Glycogen synthase activity, fractional velocities (%) when no glucose-6-phosphate (G6P) was added to the suspension. At the highest insulin level a significant difference was found between lean control subjects and obese diabetic patients ($p < 0.05$); △ Lean control subjects; ○ obese control subjects; ● obese diabetic patients

These results also support our hypothesis that the covalent regulation of the GS is the primary abnormality in obese diabetic subjects, a conclusion emphasized by the finding of reduced GS phosphatase activity and an increase of the cAMP-dependent protein kinase activity in skeletal muscles from obese diabetic subjects compared with non-diabetic subjects [17, 18]. Together these results clearly indicate that the reduced ability of insulin to stimulate GS phosphatases and to inhibit GS kinases may play an important role in reducing insulin-mediated glucose disposal in skeletal muscles.

To evaluate whether allosteric activation by G-6-P may also be abnormal and involved in the reduced GS response to insulin, we measured GS activity at three different G-6-P concentrations in the basal state and during insulin infusion in lean subjects, obese non-diabetic subjects and obese diabetic subjects. No difference in G-6-P activation was obtained, indicating that the allosteric activation is normal in insulin-resistant subjects, despite the covalent abnormalities [12]. However, all groups do not agree with this statement, since the total activity measured at G-6-P concentration has been found to be reduced in NIDDM patients [19].

Based on these data we conclude that the enzyme GS seems to be partly locked into its inactive G-6-P-dependent form, but the enzyme may still be activated allosterically by physiological concentrations of G6P. In other

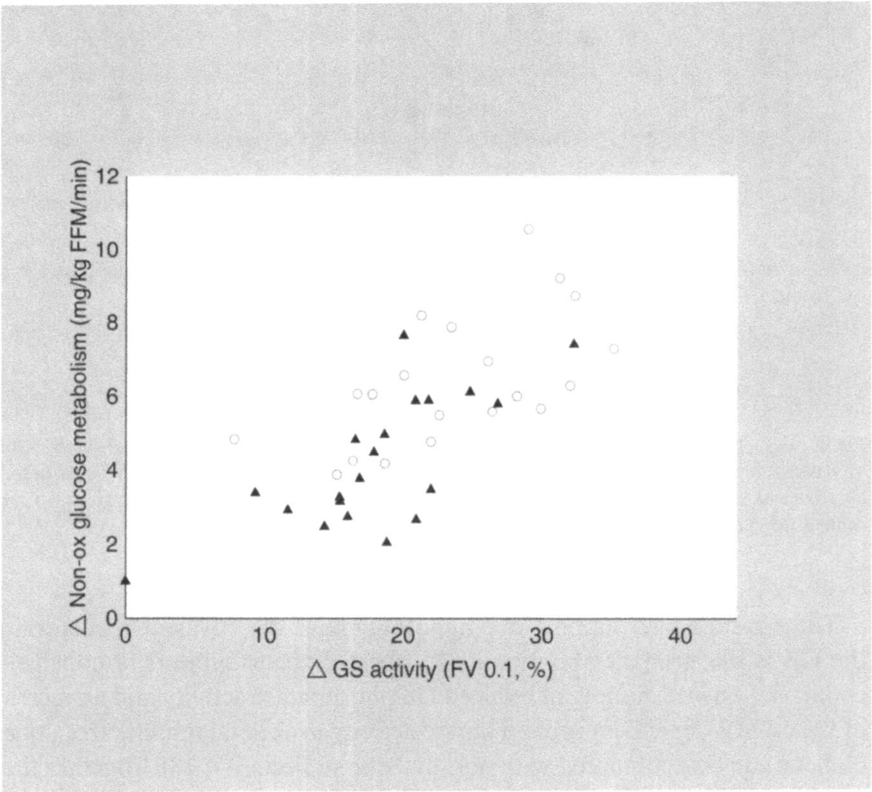

Fig. 3 Correlation between non-oxidative glucose metabolism and delta glycogen synthase activity in young, normoglycaemic relatives to NIDDM patients (reprinted from A. Vaag, JCI 1992; 89: 782–788)

words, an identical activity rate of GS may be obtained in diabetic subjects as in non-diabetic subjects, if the intracellular G-6-P concentration in diabetic subjects is sufficiently increased. Identical results were found both in a Danish and Finnish study of relatives, indicating that a defect in insulin stimulation of glycogen synthase and glycogen synthesis precedes the diabetic states and, therefore, is the candidate for the primary defect in the pathophysiology of NIDDM, see Fig. 3 [3, 20].
Insulin receptors: ^{125}I-labeled insulin binding to wheat germ agglutinin purified insulin receptors from rectus muscles isolated from severely obese subjects, with and without NIDDM, were found to be decreased because of a reduced number of receptors, as previously demonstrated in monocytes and adipocytes [21, 22]. However, this finding has not been generally confirmed.

Insulin receptor tyrosin kinase activity: The reduced ability of insulin to stimulate the consecutive phosphorylation of the three tyrosine residues of the β-sununit of the insulin receptor has been demonstrated in obese NIDDM patients [16]. Furthermore, transfer of phoshate from the receptor kinase to an external substrate, in this case GLU 4:Tyr 1, has been found to be reduced [23]. This defect, however, is identical in obese subjects with NIDDM and those without. Thus, covalent insulin signaling (Fig. 1) appears to be abnormal in skeletal muscles from obese subjects, but this does not explain why some obese subjects develop hyperglycaemia. A similar defect in insulin receptor tyrosin kinase activity was found in skeletal muscles from young normoglycaemic relatives to NIDDM patients, indicating that this defect could be of primary origin (unpublished data).

Glucose transporter activity: It is difficult to isolate skeletal muscle cells, but a new technique has recently been developed. Muscle fiber strips from rectus abdominis are isolated in toto and incubated in a buffer in vitro. This model demonstrated the ability of insulin to stimulate the glucose transport rate, in case 3-O-methylglucose, was reduced in strips from obese subjects [24]. However, there were no differences in the transport rates in obese subjects with diabetes and those without diabetes. Therefore, the insulin resistance of the GT-system is viewed as a characteristic feature of skeletal muscles from obese subjects, but the reduced GT activity may not alone explain why some obese individuals develop diabetes.

In conclusion: Metabolic defects in insulin-mediated glycogen synthesis may be of genetic origin and can be diagnosed 3–4 decades before frank diabetes occurs.

Prediabetic and diabetic stages of NIDDM

As stated above NIDDM starts much earlier than we thought up to now. Manifest diabetes rather represents the end of the spectrum, "the top of the iceberg", and at this stage, the patients usually have developed all the macroangiopathic complications typical for the disease. The metabolic derangements (insulin resistance and compensatory hyperinsulinism) responsible for NIDDM can be demonstrated years, probably decades, before the disease is diagnosed. The hyperglycaemic state or diabetic state may start up to ten years before the clinical presentation of the disease.This anticipation has recently been emphasized by a rather elegant study by Harris et al [25] by studying retinopathy. Prior to the hyperglycaemic, preclinical stage, a period, varying in length from 10 – 40 years, of normoglycaemia, but insulin resistance and compensatory hyperinsulinaemia takes place. This period may be divided into a period with impaired glucose tolerance (IGT), there always precedes frank diabetes, and a period with normal glucose tolerance (NGT). Each period or stage is phenotypically characterized by different degrees of the

Table 1 Prediabetic and diabetic states of the NIDDM syndrome. Natural history of the insulin resistance syndrom

	Prediabetic states		Diabetic states		
	−40 years NGT	−15 years IGT	−10 years Pre clin. state	t = 0 Diagnosis	+ 10−20 years Late diab. state
Fasting hyperglycaemia	−	−	+	+++	++
Fasting hyperinsulinaemia	+	+	++	+	(+)
Hypersecretion of insulin	++	(−)	−	−	−−
Insulin resistance	+	+ (+)	++	+++	++
Hypertriglyceridamia	(+)	+	++	+++	++
Elevated plasma NEFA	−	(+)	+	+++	++
Obesity (android)	+	+	++	+++	++
Arterial hypertension	(+)	+	+	++	+++
Macroangiopathy	(−)	+	+	++	+++
Microalbuminuria	(+)	+	+	+++	++
Nephropathy	−	−	−	+	+++
Retinopathy	−	−	+	+	+++

NGT = Normal oral glucose tolerance
IGT = Impaired oral glucose tolerance

insulin resistance syndrome and following variable degrees of macro- and microangiopathy as outlined in Table 1.

At the onset of the disease about 40% of diabetics present macroangiopathy, about 40% present micro- or macroalbuminuria, and about 50% suffer from hypertriglyceridaemia, whereas only 15% has retinopathy [8].

The division of the NIDDM syndrome into the better and less well defined stages, gives a better opportunity to predict, prevent and treat the disease. The different stages characterizing the prediabetic phases is outlined in Table 1 where the metabolic and clinical characteristics are indicated qualitatively. The subjects prone to develop NIDDM may be diagnosed as early as 15–40 years before the onset of the disease by familiar clustering and by the following phenotype: normoglycaemia, fasting hyperinsulinaemia, hypersecretion of insulin after a glucose challenge, elevated fasting plasma triglyceride, obesity or at least increased abdominal fat. If these characteristics are present in subjects from families with NIDDM clustering, insulin resistance measured during an euglycaemic hyperinsulinaemic clamp or measured by the minimal model may predict a relative risk of up to 80% for development of frank NIDDM within the next 10–25 years.

Prediction and prevention of NIDDM

Since the therapeutic results of treatment in NIDDM patients are rather poor, and since many patients already suffer from macroangiopathy at the onset of the disease, it is important to prevent the disease. In other words, it seems important to identify subjects at risk, i. e. subjects in the prediabetic NGT or IGT stages.

Of course genetic markers and/or characterized genetic defects would be the ideal way to identify subjects at risk, but neither the genes nor the markers for candidate genes are known at present, while other predictors may be used. In that respect, family history of NIDDM and metabolic variables seem to be the most appropriate tool [4].

As has been stated above, family history of NIDDM predispose to frank diabetes. Therefore, family history is the basis for screening in the prediabetic states. This may be supplemented with measurement of fasting plasma insulin, eventually combined with an OGTT measuring insulin responses. Of course the best prediction can be made on direct measurement of insulin resistance by euglycaemic clamp or by the minimal model test.

In non-familial disposed subjects an insulin resistant phenotype, i. e. glucose intolerance, arterial hypertension, hypertriglyceridemia and/or android obesity may also be the reason to investigate for clinically or non-clinically present NIDDM [5, 10].

In subjects with a high risk for development of NIDDM, prevention may be considered. But how and when? Only very few scientific data are available concerning this matter. Thus, until these data have been produced, prevention may be based on theoretical considerations. In that respect, the most important factor in order to prevent NIDDM, is to stay lean, since obesity has been shown to be able to provoke frank diabetes in subjects with inherited insulin resistance. Furthermore, prone subjects may be advised about the risk of hyperglycaemia during stress e. g., infectious diseases and pregnancy.

Measuring insulin sensitivity

Insulin sensitivity has been estimated by several different methods, which are reviewed in Table 2. They include high-dose glucose infusion (GIT) [26, 27], low-dose glucose infusion (CIGMA) [28, 29], the intravenous glucose tolerance test (IVGTT) [30, 31] and its subsequent analysis with the minimal model approach [4, 32, 33], the euglycaemic [2, 3] and hyperglycaemic clamp [34], a fixed infusion of glucose and insulin [35], and a combined infusion of somatostatin, insulin and – glucose or – insulin suppression test (IST) [36].

Several of these techniques (IVGTT, minimal model, GIT, CIGMA, hyperglycaemic clamp) also provide estimates of insulin secretion. The euglycaemic insulin clamp has been considered to be the "gold standard" for measuring insulin sensitivity, the major advantage being that, measurements are performed at a steady state of both insulin and glucose concentrations [37]. Another major advantage of the euglycaemic clamp is that it can be easily combined with the infusion of tritiated glucose (to allow measurements of hepatic glucose production and its sensitivity to insulin) and indirect calorimetry (to estimate intracellular glucose disposition, oxidation vs. storage). The hyperglycaemic version of the clamp, on the other hand, has gained a good reputation in the assessment of β-cell function, since it measures the insulin concentration response to a square wave of hyperglycaemia [37].

With regard to the methods that measure insulin sensitivity, they should satisfy at least five requirements.

First, the insulin levels achieved should be high enough to stimulate glucose metabolism and detect possibly small differences in sensitivity of glucose uptake to insulin. With the CIGMA method for example, the insulin concentrations achieved vary between 10–20 μU/ml (70–140 pmol/l). When using an exogeneous insulin infusion rate of 1 mU/min/kg (or 40 mU/min^1 m^2, 280 pmol/min/kg), it has been common experience that the sensitivity and reproducibility of the euglycaemic clamp are sufficient to pick up systematic differences upward of 10%.

Second, the test used should distinguish between peripheral and hepatic insulin sensitivity. Since these pathways may be affected differentially in the early stages of insulin resistance, their separate quantitation is crucial. A glance at the dose-response curve for stimulation of gucose uptake and suppression of hepatic glucose production (HGP) by insulin in non-diabetic and type 2 diabetic subjects, shows that significant differences in glucose metabolism between groups are not seen until the insulin concentrations have risen to levels of about 30–40 μU/ml (or 210–289 pmol/l). If suppression of HGP during the test is incomplete, the rate of glucose uptake is underestimated (see below).

Third, measurements should be made under steady-state conditions whenever possible. Many of the methods in Table 1 involve rapid perturbations of the glucose system, which are followed by changes in plasma glucose, insulin, and counterregulatory hormones. These all influence both insulin sensitivity and insulin secretion and their measurement. Available algorithms dealing with the non-steady state are intrinsically ill-suited. In, addition, counterregulatory hormonal responses can be triggered by rapid changes in plasma glucose even in the abscence of clinical hypoglycaemia. Although these problems may not be critical when studying large groups of subjects, they may dilute out small differences between study groups.

Fourth, the inevitable assumptions about the body glucose system must be physiologically sound. For example, the minimal model assumes that glucose kinetics are monocompartmental [33], and that insulin action takes place in a "remote" compartment. The former assumption is clearly untenable; the latter can possibly be defended for insulin effects on peripheral tissues, but is clearly wrong for hepatic insulin action.

Fifth, many of the tests result in a rise in plasma glucose levels with subsequent measurements of glucose uptake performed during hyperglycaemia. Glucose clearance is influenced by the plasma glucose level, especially at low insulin concentrations [38]. Therefore, hyperglycaemia may present a greater problem with methods detecting only modest increments in plasma insulin. Furthermore, the plasma glucose concentration is liable to rise more in glucose-intolerant than in glucose-tolerant individuals. Two sets of results illustrate this important point. (a) Activation of glycogen synthase by insulin is impaired in the offspring of parents with type 2 diabetes [2, 3]. This defect can, however, be overcome by raising the plasma glucose concentration. During euglycaemic hyperinsulinaemia, first-degree relatives of patients with type 2 diabetes with normal glucose tolerance show a 33% reduction in insulin-stimulated glucose metabolism as compared with healthy non-diabetic controls. During a hyperglycaemic clamp, on the other hand, the difference between relatives and controls is only 14%, and no longer reaches statistical significance. The interpretation of the latter result alone is equivocal. Are the relatives as insulin sensitive as are the controls, or is the hyperclycaemia somwhat more effective in the relatives (by mass action)? To further complicate the issue, endogenous plasma insulin concentrations are not clamped during a hyperglycaemic clamp, and in fact they were found to be higher in the insulin-resistant relatives than in the controls. Theoretically, dividing the glucose uptake rate by the plasma insulin concentration would correct this difference [15]. This operation, however, assumes that endogenous insulin levels are stable and that they are linearly related to glucose metabolism. Neither of these premises holds true. In response to square-wave hyperglycaemia, the pattern of endogenous insulin release resembles anything but a steady state. Furthermore, to the best of available information, the insulin dose-response for whole-body glucose uptake is sigmoidal, with a segment where it is linearly related to the log of peripheral plasma insulin concentrations. Thus, insulin sensitivity studies performed during hyperglycaemic conditions are more likely to miss small differences than euglycaemic methods. That the euglycaemic hyperinsulinaemic clamp is the "gold standard" to measure insulin sensitivity could be questioned on the grounds that the test creates non-physiological conditions which do not represent everyday life.

Table 2 Methods used to assess insulin sensitivity and insulin secretion

Method	Glucose infusion bolus $\mu mol\ kg^{-1}\ min^{-1}$	Glucose ($mmol\ l^{-1}$)	Insulin ($\mu U\ ml^{-1}$)	Time[1] (min)
Git	110	15–20	40–200	60
CIGMA	28	7–11	7–15	60
IVGTT (Minimal model)	2.8 $\mu mol\ kg^{-1}$ [2]	V[3]	15–50	B
Euglycaemic clamp	adjusted	1	50–80	120–180
Hyperglycaemic clamp	adjusted	10–12	30–100	120–180
IST	33	6–8	70–110	240
Glucose/Insulin	33	4–6	40–70	45

Abbreviations. GIT: glucose infusion test; CIGMA: continous infusion of glucose with model assessment; IVGTT: intravenous glucose tolerance test; IST: insulin suppression test; B: bolus; V: variable.

[1] Time of infusion; [2] given as intravenous bolus injection; [3] in patients with impaired insulin secretion, a bolus of insulin or tolbutamide is necessary; [4] endogenous insulin secretion suppressed by somatostatin.

This is certainly true, and this reservation applies to all the other methods in Table 2.

Specific problems in tracer methodology

When reviewing the literature of studies which measured HGP in type 2 diabetic subjects using the primed-^{3}H-glucose infusion technique, marked differences in glucose production rates were reported, ranging from normal up to 240% of normal [39,40]. In those studies which reported the highest elevation of HGP, a fixed priming dose of tritiated glucose was used, regardless of the basal blood glucose level present at the time of study. In contrast, in those studies which documented normal or near normal HGP values, the priming dose of tritiated glucose was adjusted to the prevailing fasting blood glucose concentration. In these latter studies, a constant level of plasma 3-^{3}H-glucose specific activity is approached after about one hour with the "adjusted" primary technique, whereas the tracer specific activity concentrations with the "fixed" priming method are still increasing after 6 hours. Only in the former adjusted priming technique is a plateau steady state situation reached which therefore permits glucose turnover to be calculated from the simple ratio of tracer infusion rate and the specific activity in plasma [39,40]. With the fixed prime, an ongoing rise in tracer specific activity in plasma occurs and plasma specific activities remain low, which together leads to the calculated glucose turnover rates being too high. This error will be greater in those studies with the highest fasting blood glucose level; it is not surprising that in these latter situations, the level of glucose turnover (HGP) will correlate positively with the fasting blood glucose level. An additional source of error in the majority of previous studies is the assumption that glucose appearance and glucose disappearance are equal in the fasting post absorptive state in type 2 diabetic subjects. This is incorrect since plasma glucose declines in time over 6 hours, at a rate of 0.52 mmol/l per hour [39,40,41]. Therefore, if HGP is calculated by dividing the tracer infusion rate with the specific activity of the tracer (i. e. assuming a steady state situation), an overstimate of HGP will also arise. On the other hand, if Steele's non-steady state equations are employed, a lower estimate of HGP will result [39,40]. In Figure 4, we have shown the correlation between fasting plasma glucose values and glucose turnover calculated by using the steady state equation (upper panel) and HGP as calculated using Steele's non steady state equation (lower panel), respectively. Results from the adjusted and the fixed priming method are also given. The data clearly show that HGP in type 2 diabetic subjects is normal or near normal, when measured using an adjusted prime and Steele's non-

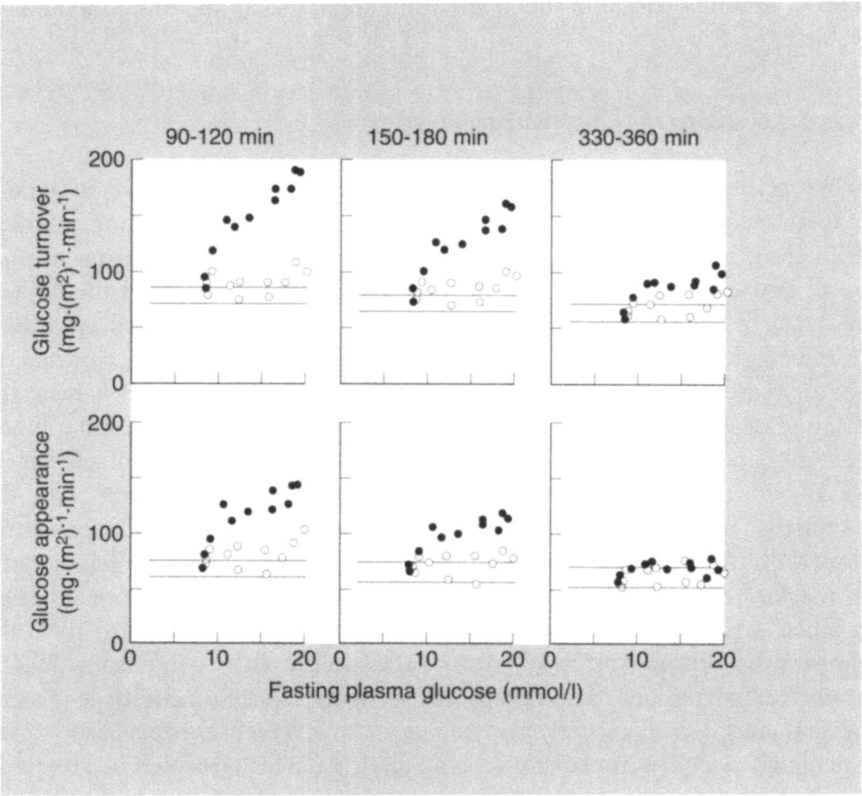

Fig. 4 Correlation between plasma glucose concentration and glucose turnover rate (GT) (upper panel) or glucose appearance rate calculated using Steele's equation (lower panel) after 90–120, 150–180 and 330–360 min tracer infusion in 11 type 2 (non-insulin-dependent) diabetic patients using fixed (●) or adjusted (○) primed-continous 3^3H-glucose infusion. Mean ± SD of seven non-diabetic control are indicated by horizontal lines. Using fixed priming the correlation of both glucose turnover (GT) and glucose appearance rate (Ra) to plasma glucose concentration decreased in time (GT: $r = 0.97, 0.97, 0.86$, all $p < 0.01$, Ra: $r = 0.91, 0.88$, both $p < 0.01$, and $r = 0.49, 0.51, 0.46$, Ra: $r = 0.47, 0.31, 0.14$, all $p =$ NS). Reprinted with permission from [39]

steady state equations. Furthermore, there is no tendency to a positive correlation between HGP and fasting blood glucose values at fasting blood glucose levels of < 15.0 mmol/l. This was confirmed in both obese and lean subjects. Thus, we may conclude that HGP may have been overestimated in most previous studies to a varying degree. The correlation observed between fasting blood glucose and HGP, which has been used to emphasize the importance of the overproduction of glucose by the liver in the development of hyperglycaemia should be seriously questioned. Admittedly, when significant glycosuria develops (in those patients at plasma glucose levels of about 12 – 15 mmol/l), HGP may rise to compensate for the glucose spillover.

Euglycaemic clamp employing the infusion of unlabelled "cold" glucose in combination with a tracer infusion has traditionally been used to measure rates of glucose production and utilisation in response to insulin. It has, however, been clearly documented that with this conventional approach of constant tracer and unlabelled glucose infusions, rates of glucose appearance are underestimated [42,43]. As a consequence, insulin stimulation of glucose utilisation has been *underestimated* and insulin suppression of glucose production *overestimated.* Because previous studies have used unlabelled glucose infusates it is therefore likely that glucose utilisation is more sensitive to insulin, and glucose production less sensitive than previously assumed. Furthermore, as errors are greater the greater the glucose infusion rate, mistakes may have been greatest in normal control subjects requiring large glucose infusions and smaller in resistent type 2 diabetic patients requiring smaller glucose infusions [3]. This means that previous studies may have underestimated peripheral insulin resistance and overestimated hepatic insulin resistance in patients with type 2 diabetes. Thus, to adequately assess glucose turnover rates during combined infusions of glucose, insulin and tracer, future studies will require maintenance of unchanged plasma specific activities by the co-infusion of labelled glucose ("hot" glucose) during the clamps [43,44]. The well known but often overlooked problem of negative HGP values during the infusion of cold glucose will thereby be resolved.The methodology behind this new approach is described in detail by Hother-Nielsen [43].

Measuring glucose and lipid oxidation (indirect calorimetry)

Indirect calorimetry can be performed using a computerized flowthrough canopy gas analyzer system (Deltatrac, Datex, Helsinki, Finland). Briefly, air is suctioned at a rate of 40 l per minute through a canopy placed over the head of the subject. Samples of inspired and expired air are analyzed for oxygen concentration using a paramagnetic differential oxygen sensor and for carbon dioxide using an infrared carbon dioxide sensor. Signals from the gas analyzers are processed by the computer and oxygen consumption and carbon dioxide production are calculated and recorded once a minute. After an equilibration period of 10 minutes, the average gas exchange rates recorded over the two 30-minute steady state periods are used to calculate rates of glucose oxidation, lipid oxidation and energy expenditure as previously described [45]: glucose oxidation (grams per minute) $= 4.55 \times VCO_2 - 3.21 \times VO_2 - 2.87 \times n$, and lipid oxidation (grams per minute) =

$1.67 \times VO_2 - 1.67 \times VCO_2 - 1.92 \times n$, where VCO_2 equals CO_2 production in litre per minute, VO_2 equals O_2 consumption in litre per minute, and n equals grams of excreted urinary nitrogen per minute. The protein oxidation rate is corrected for changes in pool size [152]. The mean coefficients of variation of the precisely determined VO_2-consumption and VCO_2-production rates average 7% and 6%, respectively.

It should be noted that erroneous calculations of glucose and lipid oxidation rates may arise from gaseous exchange rate measurements during situations with elevated rates of de novo lipogenesis, glyconeogenesis from alanine, ketogenesis and ketone body oxidation [45]. Thus, during situations with a substantial de novo lipogenesis, the rate of glucose oxidation may be overestimated, whereas during situations with elevated rates of glucoeogenesis from alanine, the rate of glucose oxidation may be underestimated. Ketone body formation may also cause an underestimation of the glucose oxidation rate, whereas ketone body oxidation may cause an overestimation of the glucose oxidation rate. The quantitative influence of these metabolic processes are generally considered to be of minor importance for indirect calorimetry measurements of glucose- and lipid oxidation rates in normal humans.

In vitro methods

Muscle biopsy

Muscle biopsies can be performed using a modified Bergström needle (including suction) under local anaesthesia. The biopsies must be rapidly (within 10–15 s) frozen and stored in liquid nitrogen for later analysis. Before the biochemical analysis, the muscle samples should be freeze-dried and dissected free of visible connective tissue, fat and blood. The freeze-dried and microdissected muscle samples are stored at − 80° C until the biochemical analyses are performed.

Glycogen and metabolite concentrations in muscle biopsies

Glycogen can be measured as glucose residues after hydrolysis of the muscle samples, in 1M HCL at 100° C for two hours [47]. Glucose, glucose 6-phosphate and lactate is measured flourometrically on neutralized perchloric acid extracts [47]. The intracellular concentrations of free glucose, G-6-P and lactate are calculated as millimoles per litre intracellular water, assuming an extracellular water content in the biopsies of 0.3 l/kg dry weight and an intracellular water content of 2.8 l/kg dry weight [48]. Intracellular concentrations of free glucose and lactate were corrected for extracellular concentrations using the above assumptions of intracellular and extracellular water content in the biopsies. The intra-assay coefficients of variations are 3% for glucose, 5% for G-6-P, 3% for lactate, and 3% for glycogen (total amount of glucose residues) [3].

A major limitation of the measurements of free glucose and lactate concentrations in muscle biopsies is that the extracellular and intracellular water contents of the muscle biopsies are assumed from published data obtained by other investigators in other groups of study subjects. This means that the measurements (and calculations) of intracellular substrate concentrations may only provide crude estimates of the true intracellular muscle concentrations, and that any differences in muscle glucose or lactate contents demonstrated between subjects, or in subjects in response to any experimental manipulations, could in theory be due to changes in both intra- and extracellular substrate concentrations. Another problem in measuring all of the above substrate concentrations in skeletal muscle biopsies is that the muscle biopsy procedure may, to varying degrees, induce an increased rate of glycogenolysis in the muscle cell. This may cause an artificial increase, especially in the muscle G-6-P content, which in turn may obscure real in vivo differences in muscle G-6-P contents between different experimental study situations or study subjects.

Muscle enzyme activities

Extraction of muscle samples and assays for glycogen synthase (GS), pyruvate dehydrogenase (PDH) and phosphofructokinase (PFK) activities can be performed as previously described by Mandarino and Beck-Nielsen [49]. The frozen muscle samples are weighed and immediately thereafter homogenized for 2 × 30 seconds in a polytron homogenizer. The buffer consists of 20 mM sodiumflouride (to inhibit PDH phosphatase and thereby to maintain PDH in its in situ phosphorylation state), 2 mM dithiothreitol (DTT), 20 mM EDTA, and 50 mM potassium phosphate, H 7.4, 0.1 ml buffer per mg dry weight muscle. The crude extract is then centrifuged at 15.000 rpm at 4° C for 20 minutes. Thereafter, the supernatant (containing the enzymes GS and PFK) is removed and stored at − 80° C for later determination of GS and PFK activities. The pellet, containing essentially all of the PDH activity, is divided into two portions. One portion of the pellet is resuspended in the same homogenization buffer for assay of active PDH (PDH_a), and the other portion is resuspended in the homogenization buffer without sodium fluoride for assay of total PDH (PDH_t). The two "pellet suspensions" are centrifuged

(15000 rpm, 4° C, 20 min), whereafter the supernatant is removed. The pellets are then rehomogenized in the polytron homogenizer for 5 seconds in Triton X-100 containing (0.2%) buffers with (PDH_a) and without (PDH_t) fluoride addition.

The assay for determination of PDH activity is then performed as described below by a modification of the method of Hagg et al. [50], based on the technique of Blass et al. [51]. For determination of PDH_t activity, 75 μl of the solubilized pellet, extracted as described above without fluoride added to the extraction buffers, is preincubated with 25 μl of a solution consisting of 0.5 mM calcium, 20 mM magnesium, 2 mM DTT, and 50 mM potassium phosphate, pH 7.4. The rationale behind the addition of high calcium and magnesium concentrations is that, in the absence of fluoride, these ions should activate the PDH phosphatase, thereby dephosphorylating and fully activating the PDH complex. For determination of PDH_a activity, 75 μl solubilized pellets prepared with fluoride present are preincubated with 25 μl of a solution containing final concentrations of 0.05 mM calcium, 0.05 mM magnesium, 2 mM DTT, and 50 mM potassium phosphate, pH 7.4. The reaction is started by addition of 25 μl of a mixture of substrates and cofactors such that the final concentrations were as follows: B-NAD+; 5 mM, coenzyme A; 1 mM, DTT; ^{14}C-pyruvate, 0.2 μCi; unlabelled pyruvate 4 m; and 50 mM potassium phosphate; pH 7.4. The tubes are immediately capped with a rubber stopper through which is suspended a plastic well containing a small roll of filter paper. After 20 min the reactions are stopped by injecting 0.2 ml of 3 mM H_2SO_4 through the rubber stopper into the reaction mixture. $^{14}Co_2$ is collected for 30 min by injecting 0.2 ml hyamine hydroxide through the rubber stopper onto the filter paper in the centre well. Blank values are determined by using boiled tissue extracts under the same assay conditions as above. All samples (filters) are counted for radioactivity in a liquid scintillation counter. PDH activity is expressed as picomoles of pyruvate oxidized per minute per milligram extract protein. The fractional activity of PDH is defined as the proportion of total enzyme which is active (PDHa/PDHt). This measure has been used as a measure of the extent of activation of PDH in vivo. The mean intraassay coefficient of variation as obtained in our laboratory was 23% for both PDHa and PDHt.

Glycogen synthase (GS) can be assayed by a modification of the method of Thomas et al. [52]. The supernatant extracted from muscle samples as described above is diluted 1:5 in a buffer consisting of 20 mM EDTA, 25 mM sodium fluoride, and 50 mM Tris-HCl. The reactions are started by addition of 30 μl aliquots of cell extracts to 60 μl of a reaction mixture composed of the buffer as described for the dilution procedure, 1% glycogen, 0.7 μCi ^{14}C-uridine diphosphate glucose (UDPG), and unlabelled UDPG, so that the total UDPG concentration in the reaction mixture (^{14}C-uridine + cold UDPG) is 0.31 mM. GS activity is assayed in the presence of a near physiological concentration of glucose-6-phosphate (G-6-P, 0.1 mM) and in the presence of a high concentration of G-6-P (10 mM) to determine maximum enzyme activity. Reactions are allowed to proceed for 15 min at 30° C and are terminated by precipitating 75-μl aliquots of the reaction mixture on 2x2 cm squares of filter paper immediately dropped into cold 66% ethanol. After 30 min of washing, the filter papers are washed twice for 20 min each in cold 66% ethanol, dried and counted for radioactivity in a liquid scintillation counter. GS activity is expressed as nanomoles of UDPG incorporated into glycogen per minute per milligram extract protein. Fractional velocity that is thought to reflect the proportion of total GS present that is active in vivo is calculated as the ratio between GS activity assayed at 0.1 mM G-6-P and 10 mM G-6-P. The mean intra assay coefficients of variation as obtained in our laboratory are 4% for GS activity determined at 0.1 mM G-6-P and 3% for GS activity determined at 10 mM G-6-P.

The enzymes PDH and GS are both activated in vivo through a dephosphorylation reaction of the enzyme. These dephosphorylation reactions are assumed to be caused by specific phosphatases for each of the enzymes. However, when biopsies are performed from skeletal muscles it cannot be excluded that a spontaneous dephosphorylation reaction of the enzymes may take place, which in turn may cause an artificially high activity ratio of the enzymes as determined in the in vitro assays. This may especially be a problem for the PDH assay, and may therefore to some extent explain some of the great variations in the assays obtained.

Partial purification of insulin receptors

Receptors are isolated in parallel from biopsies obtained in the basal and in the insulin stimulated state. Insulin receptors are partially purified essentially as described in [53]. Fifteen-50 mg of freeze-dried muscle, corresponding to around 60–200 mg of wet weight, is homogenized on ice with a polytron, max speed, for 2 x 15 s in 5 ml of 40 mM Hepes, pH 7.6, 1% Triton X-100 (w/v), 900 kallikren inhibiting units/ml Trasylol, 5mM EDTA, 10 mM NaF, 10 mM Na-pyrophosfate, 1.5 mg/ml Benzamidine, 2mM PMSF and 1 mM Na-vanadate. The homogenate is centrifuged 8000xG, 8 min, 4° C followed by solubilization in the cold room, end-over-end rotation, for 30 min. After centrifugation at 200,000xG for 60 min., 4° C, the supernatant is passed over a 1 ml WGA-sepharose column three times followed by washing with 50 ml of 40 mM Hepes, pH 7.6, 0.1% Triton X-100, 150 mM NaCl, and the partially purified insulin receptors are eluted in 1.5 ml of 40 mM Hepes, 7.6, 150 mM NaCl, 0.1% Triton X-100 (w/v) and 0.3 M N-acetylglucosamine. Protein concentrations of the eluates are determined according to the method of Bradford using the Bio-Rad assay. PMSF (1mM) and Trasylol (900 KIE/ml) were added and the preparations were stored at – 80° C until assayed.

Insulin binding

Fifty μl of WGA-eluate is incubated overnight with ^{125}I(TyrA14)-insulin (3×10^{11} M final) without or with various concentrations of unlabeled insulin (10^{10} – 10^{6} M final) in a buffer consisting of 25 mM Hepes, pH 7.6, 5 mM $mgSO_4$ and 0.5% BSA at 4° C. Bound and free insulin are separated using dextrancoated charcoal.

Receptor kinase activity towards poly(Glu–r(4:1))

Aliquots of partially purified insulin receptors are incubated without or with increasing concentrations of insulin (10^{10} – 10^{6} M final) for one hour at room temperature. Poly(Glu,–Tyr(4:1)) (1.3 mg/ml) is added and after 20 min the phosphorylation reaction is initiated by addition of 1mM Na-canadate and 50 μM gamma^{32}P-ATP (2 μCi per vial), 10 mM $MgCl_2$ and 5 mM $MnCl_2$. The reaction is stopped after 30 min by spotting aliquots on Whatman 3MM filter paper and precipitating in ice-cold 10% TCA containing 10 mM Na-pyrophosfate followed by washing, drying and counting in a β-scintillation counter.

References

[1] DeFronzo RA: The Triumvirate. β-Cell, Muscle, Liver. A collusion responsible for NIDDM. Diabetes 1983, 37: 667–687.

[2] Eriksson J, Franssila-Kallunki A, Ekstrand A et al. Early metabolic defects in persons at increased risk for non-insulin dependent diabetes mellitus. New Engl J Med 1989; 321: 337–343.

[3] Vaag A, Henriksen JE, Beck-Nielsen H. Decreased insulin activation of glycogen synthase in skeletal muscles in young nonobese Caucasian first-degree relatives of patients with non-insulin-dependent dibates mellitus. J Clin Invest 1992; 89: 782–788.

[4] Martin BC, Warram JH, Krolewski AS et al. Role of glucose and insulin resistance in development of type 2 diabetes mellitus: results of a 25-year follow-up study. Lancet 1992; 340: 925–929.

[5] Reaven GM. Banting Lecture 1998. Role of insulin resistance in human disease. Diabetes 1988; 37: 1595–1607.

[6] Sereantson SW, Zimmet P. Genetics of non-insulin dependent diabetes mellitus in 1990. Bailliére's Clinical Endocrinology and Metabolism 1991; 5: 477–493.

[7] Jarret K: Risk factors for coronary heart disease in diabetes mellitus. Diabetes 1992; 41 (suppl 2): 1–3.
[8] Personal communication with N. Olivarius. University of Copenhagen.
[9] Gall M-A, Skøtt P, Damsbo P et al. Prevalence of micro- and macroalbuminuria, arterial hypertension, retinopathy and large renal disease in non-insulin dependent diabetes mellitus. Diabetologia 1991; 34: 655–661.
[10] Modan M, Halkin H, Almog S et al. Hyperinsulinemia. A link between hypertension, obesity, and glucose intolerance. J Clin Invest 1975; 75: 809–817.
[11] Lillioja S, Mott DM, Howard BV et al. Impaired glucose tolerance as a disorder of insulin action. Longitudinal and crossectional studies in Pima Indians. New Engl J med 1989; 321: 337–343.
[12] Damsbo P, Vaag A, Hother-Nelsen O. et al. Reduced glycogen synthase activity in skeletal muscle from obese patients with and without Type 2 (non-insulin dependent) diabetes mellitus. Diabetologia 1991; 34: 239–245.
[13] Bogardus C, Lillioja S, Howard SV et al. Relationship between insulin secretion, insulin action, and fasting plasma glucose concentration in nondiabetic and noninsulindependent diabetic subjects. J Clin Invest 1984; 1238–1246.
[14] Felber JP, Ferrannini JPE, Golay et al. Role of lipid oxidation in pathogenesis of insulin resistance of obesity and type II diabetes. Diabetes 1987; 36: 1341–1350.
[15] Schulman GI, Rothman DL, Jue T et al. Quantitation of muscle glycogen synthesis in normal subjects and subjects with non-insulin dependent diabetes by ^{13}C nuclear magnetic resonance spectroscopy. New Engl J Med 1990; 322: 223–228.
[16] Wright KS, Beck-Nielsen H, Kolterman OG et al. Decreased activation of skeletal muscle glycogen synthase by mixed meal ingestion in NIDDM. Diabetes 1988; 37: 436–440.
[17] Kida Y, Puente AE-D, Bogardus C et al. Insulin resistance is associated with reduced fasting and insulin-stimulated glycogen synthase phosphatase activity in human skeletal muscle. J Clin Invest 1990; 85: 476–481.
[18] Kida Y, Nyomba BL, Bogardus C et al. Defective insulin response of cyclic adenosine monophosphate-dependent protein kinase in insulin-resistant humans. J Clin Invest 1990; 87: 673–679.
[19] Thorburn AW, Gumbiner B, Bulacan F et al. Multiple defects in muscle glycogen synthase activity contribute to reduced glycogen synthesis in non-insulin dependent-diabetes mellitus. J Clin Invest 1992; 87: 489–495.
[20] Shalin-Jäntti C, Härkönen M, Groop L. Impaired activation of glycogen synthase activity in people at increased risk for developing NIDDM. Diabetes 1992; 41: 598–604.
[21] Beck-Nielsen H. Insulin receptors in man. The monocyte as model for insulin receptor studies (Thesis). Dan Med Bull 1980; 27: 173–193.
[22] Caro J, Sinha MK, Raju SM et al. Insulin receptor kinase in human skeletal muscle from obese subjects with and without moninsulin dependent diabetes. J Clin Invest 1987; 1330–1337.
[23] Häring HU, Mehnert H. Pathogenesis of Type 2 (non-insulin-dependent) diabetes mellitus: candidates for a signal transmitter defect causing insulin resistance of the skeletal muscle. Diabetologia 1993; 36: 176–182.
[24] Dohm GL, Tapscott EB, Pories WJ et al. An in vitro human muscle preparation suitable for metabolic studies. – Decreased insulin stimulation of glucose transport in muscle from morbidly obese and diabetic subjects. J Clin Invest 1988; 82: 1–9.
[25] Harris MI, Klein R, Welborn TA et al. Onset of NIDDM occurs at least – 7yr before clinical diagnosis. Diabetes Care 1992; 15: 815–819.
[26] Cerasi E, Luft R. The plasma insulin response to glucose infusion healthy subjects and in diabetes mellitus. Acta Endocrinol 1967; 55: 278–304.
[27] Cerasi E, Luft R. Further studies on healthy subjects with low and high insulin response to glucose infusion. Acta endocrinol 1967; 305–329.
[28] O'Rahilly SP, Nugent Z, Rudenski AS et al. Beta-cell dysfunction, rather than insulin-insensitivity, is the primary defect in familial type 1 diabetes. Lancet 1986; 2: 360–364.

[29] Hosker JP, Matthews DR, Rudenski AS et al. Continuous infusion of glucose with model assessment: measurement of insulin resistance and B-cell function in man. Diabetologia 1985; 28: 401–411.
[30] Warram JH, Martin BC, Krolewski AS et al. Slow glucose removal rate and hyperinsulinemia precede the development of Type II diabetes in the offspring of diabetic parents. Ann Intern med 1990; 113: 909–915.
[31] Skarfors ET, Selinus KI, Lithell HO. Risk factors for developing non-insulin dependent diabetes: a 10 year follow-up of men in Uppsala. Brit Med J 1991; 303: 755–760.
[32] Osei K, Cottrell DA, Orabella MM. Insulin sensitivity, glucose effectiveness, and body fat distribution pattern in nondiabetic offspring of patients with NIDDM. Diabetes Care 1991; 14: 890–896.
[33] Bergman RN, Ider YZ, Bowden CR et al. Quantitative estimation of insulin sensitivity. Am J Physiol 1979; 236: E667–E667.
[34] Pimenta W, Mitrakou A, Capani F et al. β-cell dysfunction with normal insulin sensitivity in glucose tolerant first-degree relatives of Caucasian NIDDM patients. Diabetes 1992; 41 (suppl 1): 143A.
[35] Leslie RDG, Ganash A, Volkmann HP et al. Insensitivity to insulin in offspring of non-insulin dependent diabetic patients. Diab Nutr Metab 1988; 3: 235–237.
[36] Ho LT, Chang ZY, Wang JT et al. Insulin insensitivity in offspring of parents with Type 2 diabetes mellitus. Diabetic Medicine 1990; 7: 31–34.
[37] DeFronzo RA, Tobin JD, Andres R: Glucose clamp technique: a method for quantifying insulin secretion and resistance. Am J Physiol 1979; 237: E214–E223.
[38] DeFronzo RA, Ferrannini E. Influence of plasma glucose and insulin concentration on plasma glucose clearance in man. Diabetes 1982; 31: 683–688.
[39] Hother-Nielsen O, Beck-Nielsen H. On the determination of basal glucose production rate in patients with Type 2 (non-insulin-dependent) diabetes using primed-continuous 3-^{3}H-glucose infusion. Diabetologia 1990; 33: 603–610.
[40] Hother-Nielsen O, Beck-Nielsen H. Basal glucose metabolism in type 2 diabetes. A critical review. Diabete & Metabolisme (Paris); 17: 136–145.
[41] Chen Y-DI, Swislocki ALM, Jeng C-Y et al. Effect of time on measurement of hepatic glucose production. J Clin Endocrinol Metab 1988; 67: 1084–1088.
[42] Finegood DT, Bergman RN, Vranic M. Estimation of endogenous glucose production during hyperinsulinemic-euglycemic glucose clamps. Comparison of unlabeled and labeled exogenous glucose infusates. Diabetes 1987; 36: 914–924.
[43] Hother-Nielsen O, Mengel A, Møller J et al. Assessment of glucose turnover rates in euglycaemic clamp studies using primed-constant (3-^{3}H) glucose turnover infusion and labelled or unlabelled glucose infusates. Diabetic med 1992; 9: 840–849.
[44] Proitto J, Alford FP, Dudley FJ. The mechanism of carbohydrate intolerance of cirrhosis. J Clin Endocrinol Metab 1980; 51: 1030–1036.
[45] Frayn KN. Calculation of substrate oxidation rates in vivo from gaseous exchange. J Appl Physiol 1983; 55(2): 628–634.
[46] Tappy L, Owen OE, Boden G. Effect of hyperinsulinemia on urea pool size and substrate oxidation rates. Diabetes 1988; 37: 1212–1216.
[47] Lowry OH, Passoneau JV. A flexible system of enzymatic analysis. New York: Academic Press, 1972.
[48] Sjøgaard G, Adams RP, Saltin B. Water and ion shifts in skeletal muscle of humans with intense dynamic knee extension. AM J Physiol 1985; 248 (Regulatory Integrative Comp. Physiol. 17): R190–R196.
[49] Mandarino L, Wright K, Verity L et al. Effects of insulin infusion on human skeletal muscle pyruvate dehydrogenase, phosphofructokinase and glycogen synthase. J Clin Invest 1987; 80: 655–663.
[50] Hagg, SA, Taylor SI, Ruderman NB. Glucose metabolism in perfused skeletal muscle. Pyruvate dehydrogenase activity in starvation, diabetes and exercise. Biochem J 1976; 158: 203–210.

[51] Blass JP, Avigan J, Uhlendorf BW. A defect in pyruvate decarboxylase in a child with an intermittent movement disorder. J Clin Invest 1970; 49: 423–432.
[52] Thomas J, Schlender K, Larner J. A rapid filter paper assay for UDP-C-glucose-glucogen glucosyltransferase, including an improved biosynthesis of UDP-^{14}C-glucose. Anal Biochem 1968; 25: 486–499.
[53] Bass A, Brdicka D, Eyer P et al. Metabolic differentiation of distinct muscle types at the level of enzymatic organization. J Biochem 1969; 10: 198–206.
[54] Lowry OH, Rosebrough NJ, Farr AL et al. Protein measurements with Folin phenol reagent. J Biol Chem 1951; 193: 265–272.

Research methodologies in hypoglycaemia: counterregulation phenomena and nerve/brain dysfunction

A. Maran, S. A. Amiel

Introduction

Hypoglycaemia, literally low blood glucose, occurs when the rate of glucose utilisation by the body exceeds the rate of glucose entry into the circulation. Normally it does not occur. As blood glucose falls, a number of neurohumoral responses occur which act both to restimulate hepatic glucose production and produce a symptom complex which alerts the individual to eat. If these protective responses fail and blood glucose continues to fall, cerebral function, which is exclusively dependent on an adequate glucose supply, is impaired, leading to irritability, loss of concentration, confusion and eventually unconsciousness. The effector arm of the protective mechanisms has been relatively well studied but much remains to be done to elucidate the mechanisms by which it is brought into play.

Insulin is the major hypoglycaemic hormone. Clinically significant hypoglycaemia is seen almost exclusively in treated diabetes mellitus; where insulin levels are sustained artificially by exogenous insulin or by sulphonylureas, and in rare cases of tumours secreting insulin or insulin-like growth factors. Most of our knowledge of hypoglycaemia has come from studies of insulin-induced hypoglycaemia, although there have been some attempts to examine glucose counterregulation in prolonged fasting or after vigorous exercise. We know that as blood glucose falls, the release of endogenous insulin is suppressed and that of glucagon stimulated. The sympathetic system is activated and adrenaline and later growth hormone and cortisol levels rise. These processes activate glycogenolysis, stimulate and provide substrates for gluconeogenesis and inhibit glucose utilisation by peripheral insulin sensitive tissues, tending to correct the falling glucose levels and direct the available glucose to the brain. The associated symptoms encourage eating. Other parts of the neurohumoral responses with a less well defined role in counterregulation include pancreatic polypeptide, ADH and prolactin. Some of the

Offprint from
Research Methodologies in Human Diabetes – Part 1

components of the glucoregulatory responses fail in diabetes mellitus, increasing the risk of more profound hypoglycaemia with impairment of brain function. This chapter will deal with the practical issues of quantitating hypoglycaemia clinically and documenting responses to hypoglycaemia both as encountered in daily life and as investigated in a laboratory setting.

The documentation of hypoglycyaemia in daily life

Quantitative

Hypoglycaemia in diabetes is generally categorised as "mild" or "severe". By definition, "severe" hypoglycaemia is that in which cognitive function is so disturbed the subject requires external assistance for recovery [1]. "Mild" is all episodes treated by the patient him/her self. The prevalence of mild hypoglycaemia is difficult to assess because patients readily forget it. Recall of severe episodes is usually better and estimates quoted in the literature are

Table 1

Patient hypoglycaemic record

Please try and fill in one of these questionnaires each time you feel hypo and bring them with you at your next visit.

Please record even the mildest of hypos.

If possible, please do a blood sugar on these occasions – thank you.

Patient ID: .... Date: .... Time: ....

Who noticed you were hypo?

Yourself   Another Person

If yourself, what did you notice?

(Please describe your feelings and symptoms)

....

If another person, who? ....

What did they notice? ....

....

What was your blood sugar?

Was there any reason for the hypo?

Missed Meal   Late Meal   Heavy Exertion   No obvious Reason

Other, specify:

....

Please tick whichever of the following best describes the outcome?

1. No action taken or had normal meal within 15 minutes
2. Took some extra carbohydrate
3. Friend or relative had to give extra carbohydrate
4. Required glucagon and or doctor or hospital treatment

a little less variable [2]. Even in prospective studies where patients know they are collecting data on frequency of hypoglycaemia, recall over two months does not precisely match figures gained by records made at the time and collected at intervals of a week or two. Thus to quantify hypoglycaemia in a study setting, glucose diaries are essential with frequent review. We use simple record forms which patients are asked to complete at the time of every hypo (Table 1).

A substantial number of diabetic patients lose awareness of hypoglycaemia or underreport for other reasons. For a true estimate of hypoglycaemia experience, a spouse or close acquaintance of a patient should always be questioned.

Qualitative

For characterization of metabolic control, patients with diabetes mellitus participating in research studies are encouraged to maintain record of home glucose monitoring, the results of which can be verified by collection of simultaneous blood samples in capillary tubes for later measurement in a laboratory and the use of glycosylated haemoglobin and/or protein.

Laboratory studies of hypoglycaemia

Understanding of the mechanisms of counterregulation and investigations of the factors that influence responses to hypoglycaemia require the production of hypoglycaemia in a controlled environment during which responses can be measured. This means inducing hypoglycaemia in human subjects in a laboratory setting, most commonly by administering exogenous insulin. To follow the glucose response to the insulin, frequent measurements of blood or plasma glucose must be made. If samples are not measured frequently, important information (e.g. the depth of the glucose nadir or the time at which it was reached) may be missed. The frequency of the sampling requires placement of an intravascular cannula for painless blood sampling. Cannulae should be placed under strict aseptic technique, usually using local anaesthetic, in the form of intradermal 1–2% lignocaine or topical lignocaine gel. Lines are best kept patent during studies with slow infusion of sterile physiological saline or with intermittent flush of heparinised saline. Sampling can then be done through a three way tap but the initial 0.5 ml of blood must be discarded each time because it will be diluted by the saline. Except in the insulin tolerance test, separate lines are needed for infusion and sampling, to prevent both contamination of samples by infusates and interruption of infusions by sampling.

The siting of the cannulae is important. For infusion of test substances a large vein, often the antecubital, is used. This is especially important if hyperosmolar substances are to be used. For sampling one would ideally use an arterial line. Especially in the insulin stimulated state, the arterio-venous difference in glucose concentration may be significant [3] and venous sampling is not adequate. This is especially true in the investigation of the mechanisms of response to hypoglycaemia, where the glucose supply to the tissues (and perhaps especially to the brain) is important. One wants to measure what the brain is seeing i. e. the arterial glucose content. Because of the discomfort and increased risk of arterial vs venous cannulation, however, it is usually preferable to sample arterialised venous blood. For this the cannula is placed retrogradely in as distal a vein as possible, ideally on the back of the hand, so as to drain the smallest possible volume of metabolically active tissue. The hand is rested in a box of air pre-heated to and maintained at 55–60 °C, to accelerate flow and facilitate blood sampling. It is probably preferable to measure the glucose concentration of plasma rather than blood during hypoglycaemic clamping. Analysers using the glucose oxidase technique (for hypoglycaemic studies, reflectance meters are not accurate enough at low glucose levels) perform better on repeated sampling using plasma and the effects of a change in haematocrit during prolonged studies is avoided.

It is important to minimise risk of injury to the research volunteer. Hypoglycaemia is a major stress and can produce significant vasomotor responses. If blood glucose drops low enough, unconsciousness and seizures may develop. Research subjects should be screened to exclude people with ischaemic heart disease, epilepsy, hypertension, hypoadrenalism and in diabetic subjects, unstable diabetic retinopathy. Studies involving radiolabels should only be done in men or in non-pregnant women in the first 10 days of a menstrual cycle. Ideally men and women should not be mixed into a single group – there are differences in their responses to hypoglycaemia [4]. Posture may also affect counterregulatory responses [5], so subjects should remain either recumbent or semi-recumbent (or standing) throughout and care must be taken in quantitative application of results from studies thus conducted to the clinical situation. At the end of any study, the insulin infusion is stopped. If glucose is being infused, its rate should be then reduced gradually as the effect of the insulin wanes. The subject should eat a meal and if diabetic should receive a subcutaneous insulin dose immediately before the meal. Glucose monitoring should not be discontinued until stable euglycaemia is maintained spontaneously.

The insulin tolerance test

One of the first techniques used to evaluate glucose counterregulation in vivo was the insulin tolerance test (ITT) [6, 7]. With this technique, soluble insulin (0.05 to 0.1 U/kg body weight) is injected intravenously as a rapid bolus; blood, ideally arterialised venous, is measured at 5 minute intervals thereafter. The rate of glucose fall, the glucose nadir and the pattern of glucose recovery are determined (Fig. 1).

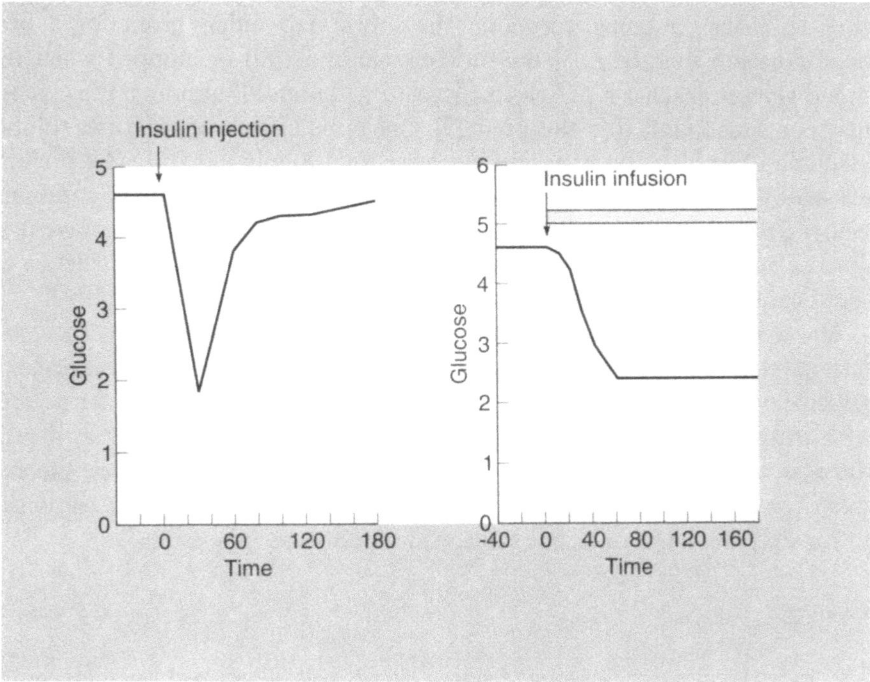

Fig. 1 Schematic representations of plasma glucose responses to an intravenous insulin bolus (left) and an intravenous insulin infusion (right). Note that glucose recovery can be examined in the former — in the latter, the slower glucose decline may allow identification of glucose levels triggering particular responses and a recovery phase could be observed after the insulin infusion is stopped

The initial plasma glucose fall results from the inhibition of hepatic glucose production and the stimulation of glucose uptake in peripheral tissues. The initial rate of decline in blood glucose concentration is taken as a measure of whole body insulin sensitivity to the injected insulin, the glucose nadir and the rate of recovery as a measure of the body's ability to counterregulate.

The ITT has been used to measure the components of the body's responses to hypoglycaemia. Additional blood samples are taken at 10–20 minute intervals for the measurement of the hormones of glucose counterregulation and physiological parameters (e. g. heart rate, blood pressure, sweating, skin and core temperature) and symptom scores can be assessed at regular intervals throughout. Some authorities time data collection from the glucose nadir, others from the time of the symptomatic autonomic reaction. It is sometimes useful to compare these two events.

The glucose fall in an ITT is fast, uncontrolled and may be very profound. A modification of the original protocol uses an infusion of soluble insulin (Fig. 1), rather a bolus injection. The infusion is either given for a predetermination time (e. g. 30 mU/m^2 for one hour [8]) or stopped when the blood glucose reaches a preselected level (e. g. 2 mmol/l) although the glucose may continue to fall after this point [9]. One popular technique infuses soluble insulin at 0.04 U/kg body weight per hour for 100 minutes [10]. The subjects are said to be unable to counterregulate if the plasma glucose fall continues below 2 mmol/l or if confusion is observed. In all these studies, intravenous glucose must be available to be infused if the subject shows evidence of significant cognitive dysfunction or becomes excessively uncomfortable.

The unopposed insulin infusion is a useful test of overall ability to counterregulate. Unless pharmacological doses of insulin are used it also perhaps approximates to hypoglycaemia as experienced in the daily life of the patient with treated diabetes mellitus. However, the hypoglycaemic stimulus it produces is not uniform – especially in the case of the ITT, where the glucose nadir can be very variable. This makes simple direct comparisons of responses to hypoglycaemia in different subjects or conditions impossible.

Clamps

The hyperinsulinaemic-hypoglycaemic clamp was developed as a means of applying a controlled and entirely reproducible hypoglycaemic stimulus in man. It is a modification of the euglycaemic clamp technique [11]. Soluble insulin is infused and the hypoglycaemia controlled by means of an adjustable infusion of exogenous glucose.

The insulin infusion is "primed" so as to achieve the desired hyperinsulinaemia rapidly (note that conventional priming regimens [11] produce an initial overshoot; also note that the full effect of the insulin will be manifest approximately 20 minutes later and continue slightly to increase thereafter). Exogenous glucose (usually 20%) is infused from 4 minutes after the start of the insulin infusion and its rate adjusted thereafter on the basis of a plasma

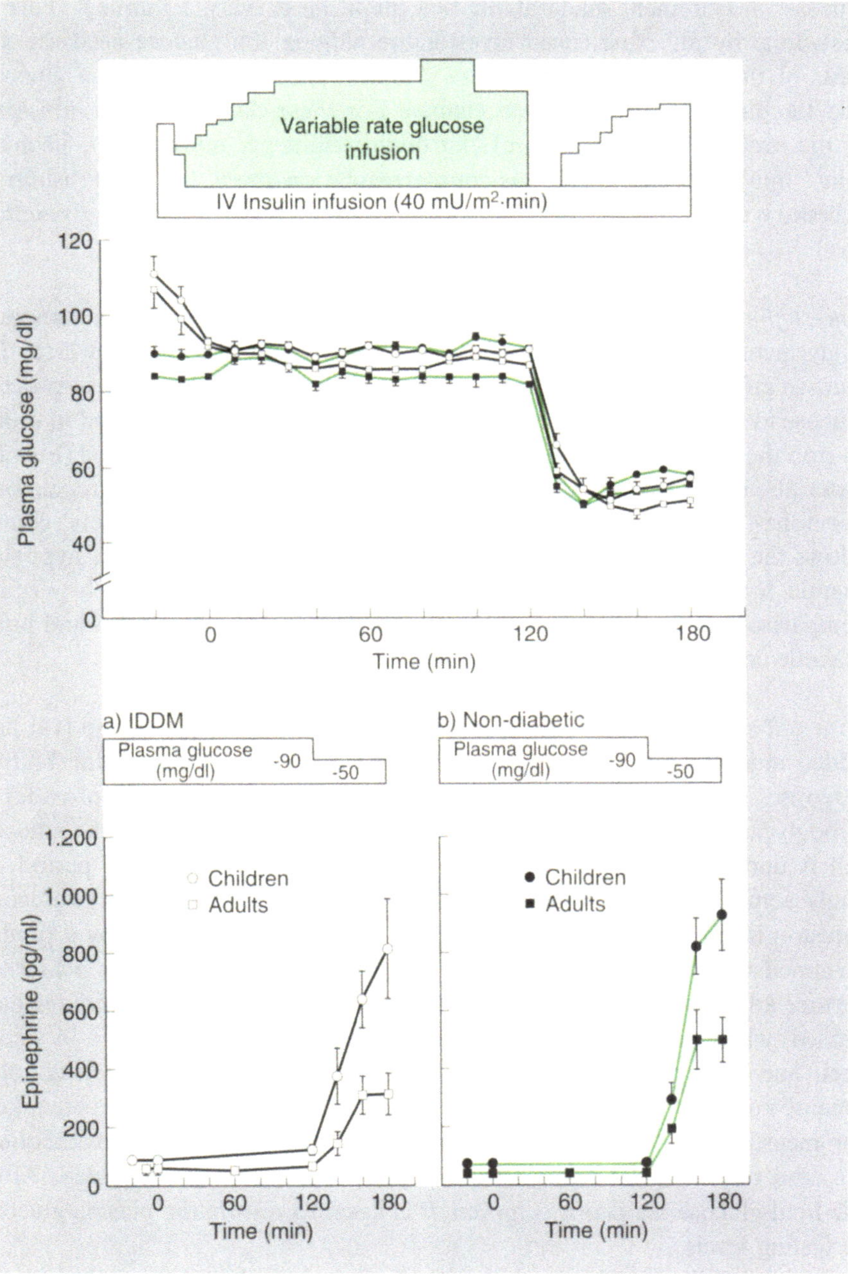

Fig. 2 Single-step euglycaemic hypoglycaemic clamp. Hyperinsulinaemia is induced by insulin infusion (open bar) and plasma glucose is controlled by exogenous glucose infusion (shared area). Reproduced by kind permission of the editors of the Journal of Pediatrics

glucose measurement made at the bedside at least every 5 minutes. This is best done by an experienced investigator judging the glucose need on the basis of the desired plasma glucose (the aims), the current plasma glucose and the direction of the glucose change. For these clamps, insulin infusions of the order of at least 1 – 2 mU/kg body weight per minute (40 – 80 mU/min^2 · min) are needed, since as counterregulation starts, the extra insulin is necessary to be able to hold the glucose down at the desired hypoglycaemic level.

One-step euglycaemic-hypoglycaemic clamp: With this technique, a standard euglycaemic clamp is performed for a set period at the end of which the glucose infusion is briefly interrupted [12]. There is a rapid decline in plasma glucose to hypoglycaemic levels and the glucose infusion is re-started in order to stop the fall and then maintain the hypoglycaemic level is required (Fig. 2). Arterialised venous blood is collected for estimation of counterregulatory hormones every 10 to 20 minutes. The euglycaemic-hypoglycaemic clamp allows the investigator to provide a reproducible [13] fixed level of hypoglycaemia for a predetermined time and an identical stimulus which permits comparisons between diabetic patients with different characteristics and non-diabetic controls.

Slow-fall stepped hypoglycaemic clamp: This variation of the clamp [14] has added much to our understanding of the factors that influence the body's responses to hypoglycaemia in patients with diabetes mellitus. It provides a hypoglycaemic stimulus in which the rate as well as the depth of the glucose fall is under the investigator's control. The clamp starts with a period of euglycaemia, usually maintained for 40 to 60 minutes. Thereafter, the glucose infusion is cut back slightly to allow the plasma glucose to fall by a predetermined value – for example 0.4 mmol/l. Once the new value is achieved, further adjustment is made to maintain the new level until 40 minutes had passed, when the process is repeated. The glucose is thus reduced in steps, each one lasting 30 to 60 minutes (Fig. 3). At the time of achieving each glucose goal and just before the next step, additional blood samples are taken for measurement of counterregulatory hormones, intermediary metabolites etc, and physiological parameters and symptom scores are recorded. After the final glucose plateau is achieved, it is usual to restore the plasma glucose to fasting levels.

The slow-fall stepped hypoglycaemic clamp is the only technique that allows the investigator to determine precisely the plasma glucose level at which any given response is initiated (sometimes referred to as the glucose threshold)

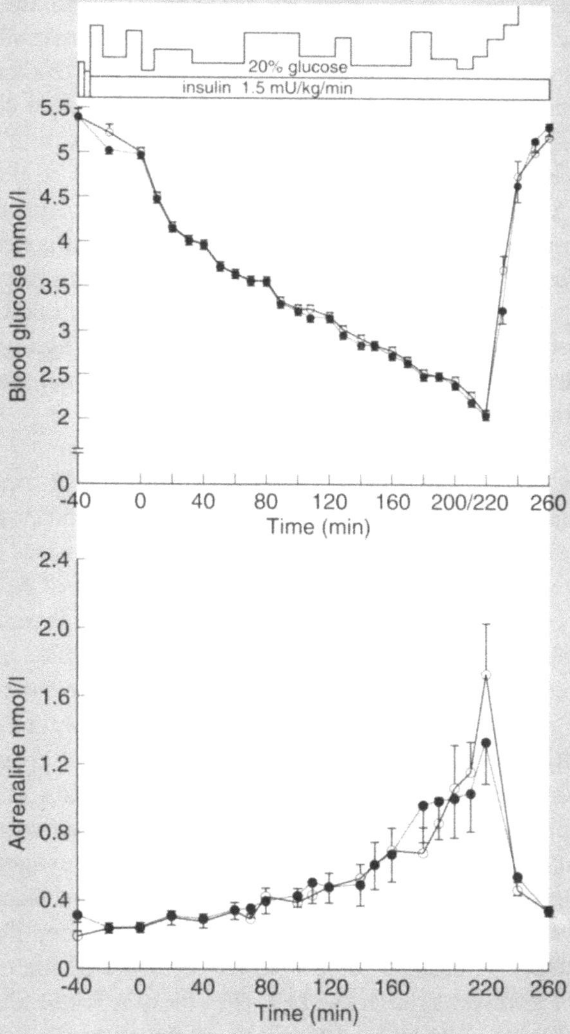

Fig. 3 The stepped hypoglycaemic clamp. The slow rate of glucose fall allows identification of the glucose level at the onset of any given response. Reproduced by kind permission of the editors of the British Medical Journal

[14]. Repeated observations made during the restoration of euglycaemia at the end of the study confirms that the changes are due to the low plasma glucose. The technique allows comparison of glucose thresholds within the same subject and between different subjects [15, 16]. Despite the differences between the rate of glucose fall between the slow fall and the single step hypoglycaemic clamps, there are no differences in the magnitude of the counterregulatory hormone responses to the hypoglycaemic challenge in either normal or insulin-dependent diabetic subjects [14]. The major limitation of the clamp technique is the non-physiological nature of the stimulus; although the plasma glucose is lowered, exogenous glucose may still be being infused. Furthermore, it is possible that the relatively high levels of insulin required to achieve and maintain the desired hypoglycaemia may influence the results [17, 18]. The effects of prolonging a hypoglycaemic stimulus have only been studied partially [19]. Despite these limitations, clamp studies have been invaluable in determining the hierarchy of responses to hypoglycaemia in different circumstances but the data should be applied qualitatively rather than the quantitatively to the clinical situation.

Low-dose insulin infusion: A low dose insulin infusion [20], unopposed by exogenous glucose goes some way to combining the advantages of an insulin injection with a slow fall clamp study and perhaps approximates most closely to a clinical hypoglycaemic episode. A continuous infusion of soluble insulin (dose 0.3 to 0.5 mU/kg body weight per minute) is applied intravenously for 180 minutes [21]. Priming, if done at all, must be modified to avoid all possibility of overshooting – running the infusion at twice the planned rate for the first five minutes achieves this. In healthy male volunteers using the lower dose results in a decline in plasma glucose over 60 to 80 minutes to a nadir of approximately 3.3 mmol/l, followed by stabilisation at 3.8 mmol/l. This technique produces only moderate hyperinsulinaemia (within the therapeutic range) and does not involve the administration of exogenous insulin during the hypoglycaemia (except in people with significant failure of counterregulation) [20]. The glucose fall is sufficiently slow to identify with some accuracy the glucose thresholds for particular elements of the counterregulatory response. However, as with the ITT, the stimulus is not identical in all cases. For example, there may be differences in the glucose profile between healthy men and women [4].

Subcutaneous insulin administration: A gradual hypoglycaemic stimulus has been achieved by the administration of subcutaneous insulin, either as a bolus (e. g. 0.15/kg will lower plasma glucose to a nadir of 3.5 mmol/l in about three hours, with recovery by 9 to 10 hours in normal volunteers [22]) or, for gradual and prolonged hypoglycaemia, by subcutaneous infusion (e.g. 15 mU/m^2 per minute, which reduces plasma glucose to 2.0 mmol/l for about 12 hours [23]). The balance of the hormonal responses to such prolonged hypoglycaemia may be different from those of acute episodes and so both techniques are valid but not the same [24].

Equipment and infusions

For intravenous insulin infusions, soluble (regular) insulin is always used, made into a solution the concentration of which is calculated for each subject so as to allow an adequate rate of delivery (e.g. 10 mls/hour). Insulin may bind to the plastics of the infusion devices so it is best made up either in a 4% solution of the subject's own blood in 0.9% physiological saline or in Gelofusin or in a saline solution of human albumin. All delivery lines should be flushed through with the insulin solution to saturate binding sites. Strict aseptic technique must be observed. We usually deliver insulin with a syringe pump. Doses are calculated individually to raise plasma insulin by a specific amount. Calculations based on body surface area are probably best, although this is less important in studies of hypoglycaemia than in measurement of insulin sensitivity. In non-diabetics, the effect of suppression of endogenous insulin must not be forgotten. Some assessment of its magnitude can be gained from measurements of C-peptide. Glucose solutions are best given from a pump with an infinitely variable of delivery rate and a completely constant and linear delivery pattern. We use a peristaltic finger pump (IVAC Corp., Basingstoke, Hampshire, U.K.) because this allows unlimited delivery of glucose – with practice, litre bags of glucose solution can be changed without interrupting delivery. All pumps should be tested for accuracy, constancy and linearity of flow before use and calibrated by timing delivery of measured volumes of solution about once every fifty clamps. If multiple infusions are to be made into a single cannula, the glucose infusion should be closest to the vein, the tracer infusion most distal (so its flow is not interrupted by changes in the glucose infusion rate). If any infusion is to be interrupted (e.g. the glucose) the line must be closed AT the infusion point first and on re-starting, the pump should be turned on before the line is opened at the subject end.

It should be remembered that potassium falls as insulin and glucose are infused. Some groups replace this in the infusate or monitor serum potassium or ECG.

Preparation of subjects with diabetes mellitus for hypoglycaemic studies

When studying subjects with diabetes mellitus it is important to exclude any hypoglycaemic event in the preceding 24 hours, since there is evidence to suggest that hypoglycaemia can diminish the responses to a subsequent episode [25, 26]. Studies should be postponed if there is significant hypoglycaemia within 48 hours. The evidence would suggest that recurrent hypoglycaemia separated by at least one week does not have this effect [13] so that serial studies should be separated by at least this period.

In order to achieve hypoglycaemic stimuli of identical magnitude, it is also important to ensure that subjects with diabetes mellitus are normoglycaemic at the time of starting the study, avoiding hyperglycaemia and also avoiding (especially if a low dose insulin infusion is planned) significant hyperinsulinaemia. If studies are planned to start in the morning, these requirements are usually met by admitting patients the night before the study. The subject is asked to take his/her usual pre-evening meal soluble insulin but to withhold only intermittent insulin injection. Blood glucose is controlled overnight (between 4 and 7 mmol/l) by means of an intravenous insulin infusion, adjusted on the basis of at least hourly blood glucose measurements [10]. Some groups prefer to admit subjects early in the morning, establish euglycaemia during the morning and start the study itself in the afternoon. If this approach is taken, care must be taken to ensure an adequate euglycaemic plateau at baseline to rule out the possibility that the study in some subjects is simply the final part of an uninterrupted glucose fall from morning hyperglycaemia. Control studies must also be done in the afternoon because of the diurnal pattern of some hormone responses. This may also influence studies of very prolonged hypoglycaemia.

An extreme example of the effect of diurnal rhythms on counterregulatory responses is seen with nocturnal hypoglycaemia. If one wishes to examine hypoglycaemia at night, the studies must be done at night [27]!

Measurements during hypoglycaemic studies

Glucose kinetics

Tracer techniques for the measurement of glucose kinetics and gluconeogenesis are discussed elsewhere in this volume. They have been applied in many studies of hypoglycaemia to examine the underlying mechanisms of counterregulation. In measurements of glucose kinetics, if exogenous glucose is to be infused, it should be labelled to achieve the same specific activity (or enrichment) as is anticipated for the steady state labelling of plasma glucose at baseline.

Identification of the starting point of a counterregulatory response

The threshold at which a counterregulatory response begins is defined as the glucose level at which a significant response begins. There have been several methods of defining a significant change – some authorities use a change in excess of 2 standard deviations over the mean of at least 5 basal values individually for each subject [14, 19, 28, 29]. Others have used the standard deviation of all measurements made during a euglycaemic study of the same duration [30]. The optimal but most labour intensive method is to perform a euglycaemic control study in all subjects and define the point at which the two curves differ [31], but counterregulatory response elements are very stable during euglycaemia, so this is not always necessary. An alternative method is to decide what level of response may be of clinical relevance and identify the glucose level at which this is first observed [14].

Measurements of symptoms during hypoglycaemic clamp studies

Subjective awareness of hypoglycaemia is assessed by questionnaires listing the symptoms of hypoglycaemia and including a few "dummy" symptoms unrelated to hypoglycaemia which the patient ranks on a linear or linear analogue scale. In the latter, symptoms can be ranked from 0 (not at all) to 6 (very severe) [32, 33]. Questionnaires are completed at baseline and at intervals throughout the studies and include autonomic symptoms (sweating, palpitations, feeling warm, anxiety, tingling and trembling) and neuroglycopenic symptoms (confusion, inability to concentrate, tiredness, drowsiness, weakness, blurred vision, irritability) [33]. The threshold for autonomic and neuroglycopenic symptoms is defined as a rise of 2 points or more over the score at euglycaemia for two or more consecutive readings [27]. The validity of this approach has recently been confirmed [33]. It has been suggested that symptom severity may diminish with prolonged hypoglycaemia although catecholamine levels may continue to rise [19]. This does not occur with continued fall in glucose as in the stepped-clamp or low dose infusion.

Cognitive function during hypoglycaemia

One of the earliest measurable parameters of cerebral function known to be affected during hypoglycaemia was the cortical electroencephalogram (EEG).

Slowing in EEG activity as blood glucose falls below 2 mmol/l was first described in insulin shock therapy [35]. Quantitative analysis from a single occipital lead as a measure of cognitive dysfunction during insulin-induced hypoglycaemia is much more recent [36]. During intravenous insulin infusion, a decrease in alpha activity and an increase in theta activity has been demonstrated in subjects with insulin-dependent diabetes mellitus at a blood glucose level of 2 mmol/l [37]. As blood glucose is lowered further, bursts of slow delta waves are seen. Because these are transient, automatic sampling techniques which usually perform frequency analyses over time and produce an average may miss them. All these changes are symmetrical and diffuse over the cortex, suggesting that they are reflections from lower centres rather than activation of pre-existing focal abnormalities. The changes are not specific for hypoglycaemia and may also occur in other metabolic encephalopathies such as hypoxia. Some may even occur in normal sleep so care must be taken to make measurements only from awake subjects. Moreover, cognitive function tested by other means (see below) have been shown to occur at glucose levels well above the 2 mmol/l required for substantial EEG changes [38, 39], making the EEG a relatively crude measure. A more sensitive measure of cerebral function is represented by changes in the latency of cortical electrical potentials evoked by specific stimuli. The P300 wave is the most prominent component of event related potentials and reflects active cognitive processing of the stimulus; its generation implies both perception and cognition of task-related stimuli, which can be acoustic, visual or somatosensory; its latency reflects the time required for the complete processing of the stimulus. Recording can be made from as few as three electrodes, with a reference electrode on the mastoid process and a further electrode to monitor and exclude blinking artifacts [40]. Frequent identical stimuli (e. g. 1000 Hz pips into earphones) are interrupted by rare different stimuli (e. g. 2000 Hz pips) and the subject counts the rare events. The P300 potential can be collected from the signals generated at the count and analysed for its latency (time from stimulus) and amplitude. During hypoglycaemia, a significant delay in the P300 has been reported with a fall in plasma glucose of as little as 0.5 mmol/l [41], although others have not described changes until hypoglycaemia becomes more severe, e. g. 2.8 mmol/l [42–44].

Recording of P300 and indeed of full cortical EEG requires specialised equipment and knowledge. Interference with the recordings from other pieces of equipment essential to the study such as the hot box many complicate analyses. The proper placing of electrodes is mildly uncomfortable, since many experts prefer to use mild skin scarification to achieve good electrical contact, especially if the subject is going to sweat during hypoglycaemia.

Most importantly, the interpretation of P300 requires a large reference sample of data collected by each group of investigators on their own equipment. Finally, although the relevance of the P300 to cognitive function is well investigated, it remains an indirect measure of ability to perform. For these reasons, some investigators prefer to use tests that directly measure cognitive function.

There are a variety of cognitive function tests now being used in hypoglycaemia studies. One problem in such studies is that the test must be repeated many times in relatively short periods of time. Learning effects (improvement by practice) can be eliminated by familiarising the subject with the test before making him/her hypoglycaemic by having him/her perform the test until a stable performance is achieved. The effects of boredom or tiredness can only be ruled out by euglycaemic control studies of similar duration or by repeating the tests after restoration of euglycaemia to ensure that all changes attributed to hypoglycaemia reverse. Trail making [45], in which a subject has to connect a series of numbered circles (or numbered and lettered circles alternately) and is timed for accuracy is a popular test and can be applied repeatedly if mirror images are made of the test sheets to eliminate the possibility of a learning effect. Measuring the time taken to complete serial subtractions [46] of 3 (easy) or 7 (difficult) from a different starting number each time or counting the number of words a subject can recall in one minute starting with B, F, L, M, (easy) or A, C, D, G, P (difficult) have also been used. Some of the tests e. g. the Stroop test [47, 48] in which the subject is asked to name coloured ink in which the name of a different colour is written can create stress and elevate catecholamine levels themselves! The full range of possible measures is beyond the scope of this manuscript. Many workers in the field prefer to use a battery of tests and create "scores" based on the variation from the mean to be able to add the results together. One problem with these tests is the time they take. It is essential to have a properly trained observer to apply the tests, while others concentrate on the management of the hypoglycaemic stimulus.

One test which is gaining in popularity is the reaction time test [49]. Simple reaction time, i. e. the time taken for a subject to respond to a single stimulus seems to correlate well with P300 [43, 50] and deteriorates at plasma glucose levels of between 3.5 to 2.6 mmol/l. The four choice reaction time appears to be as a strong indicator of cerebral dysfunction; in this, a computer screen is divided into quadrants and a signal is generated in one quadrant at a time in random order. The subject has to clear the signal by pressing the corresponding button on a adapted key pad and another signal then appears and must be cleared. The number and the speed of the responses is measured and a deterioration in either the percentage of correct responses made or the time taken to make a correct response is taken as evidence of deteriorating cognitive function.

Reaction time tests are a direct measure of psychomotor function and their relevance to the subject's ability to perform complex tasks is evident. One group have gone even further to devise a measure of cognitive function during hypoglycaemia that gives information on how hypoglycaemia might affect performance in daily life by using a driving simulator and measuring performance on that while creating hypoglycaemia in a controlled setting [51]!

Measurement of cerebral metabolism during hypoglycaemia

Impaired cognitive function during hypoglycaemia is presumed to be due to failure of adequate substrate supply for cerebral metabolism. It is thought that not only cognition is affected in this way but also that the detection of a falling blood glucose and the initiation of the protective counterregulatory responses is due to a fall in the metabolic rate in a glucose "sensing" area of the brain. In animals, maintenance of euglycaemia in the cerebral circulation by selective catheterisation during hypoglycaemia in the periphery abolishes the counterregulatory response to the peripheral hypoglycaemia. In man, selective catheterisation is too invasive a technique for general application, although arterio-venous differences across the brain have been used to record cerebral use of ketones as a metabolic fuel in starvation [52]. More recently, the technique has been resurrected to examine glucose utilisation across the brain [53] but this is a technique for highly specialised centres. Less invasive studies of cerebral metabolism during hypoglycaemia have been performed using the latest imaging techniques, such as single photon emission computed tomography (SPECT) [54] and positron emission tomography (PET) [55]. SPECT has limited application, being mostly used to infer facts about regional cerebral metabolism from measurements of cerebral blood flow; PET, which can measure rates of tissue glucose uptake using radiolabelled tracers such as fluro-deoxyglucose [56] and C-O-methylglucose, has also been used. Difficulties with the mathematical modelling for calculating metabolic rates from measurements of plasma and tissue radio-activity occur with the upset of steady state that occurs during hypoglycaemia and particularly during hypoglycaemic clamping, but useful information has been published already and these methods stand a good change of providing further information about cerebral dysfunction during hypoglycaemia and the initiation of the responses that should protect against it.

References

[1] Epidemiology of severe hypoglycaemia in the diabetes control and complications trial. The DCCT Research Group. Am J Med 1991; 90: 450–459.
[2] Amiel S. Glucose counter-regulation in health and disease: current concepts in hypoglycaemia recognition and response. Q J Med 1991; 80: 707–727.
[3] Liu D, Moberg E, Kollind M et al. Arterial, arterialized venous, venous and capillary blood glucose measurements in normal man during hyperinsulinaemic euglycaemia and hypoglycaemia. Diabetologia 1992; 35: 287–290.
[4] Amiel SA, Maran A, Powrie JK et al. Gender differences in counterregulation to hypoglycaemia. Diabetologia 1993; (in press).
[5] Hirsch IB, Heller SR, Cryer PE. Increased symptoms of hypoglycaemia in the standing position in insulin-dependent diabetes mellitus. Clin Sci 1991; 80: 583–586.
[6] Garber AJ, Cryer PE, Santiago JV et al. The role of adrenergic mechanisms in the substrate and hormonal response to insulin-induced hypoglycaemia in man. J Clin Invest 1976; 58: 7–15.
[7] Gerich J, Cryer PE, Rizza RA. Hormonal mechanisms in acute glucose counterregulation: the relative roles of glucagon, epinephrine, norepinephrine, growth hormone and cortisol. Metabolism 1980; 29: 1164–1175.
[8] De Feo P, Bolli G, Pierriello G et al. The adrenergic contribution to glucose counterregulation in type 1 diabetes mellitus. Dependency on A-cell function and mediation through beta 2-adrenergic receptors. Diabetes 1983; 32: 887–893.
[9] Rosenfalck AM, Bendtson I, Jorgensen S et al. Nasal glucagon in the treatment of hypoglycaemia in type 1 (insulin-dependent) diabetic patients. Diabetes Res Clin Pract 1992; 17: 43–50.
[10] White NH, Skor DA, Cryer PE et al. Identification of type 1 diabetic patients at increased risk for hypoglycemia during intensive therapy. N Engl J Med 1983; 308: 485–491.
[11] De Fronzo RA, Tobin JD, Andres R. Glucose champ technique: a method for quantifying insulin secretion and resistance. Am J Physiol 1979; 237: E214–E223.
[12] Simonson DC, Tamborlane WV, De Fronzo RA et al. Intensive insulin therapy reduces counterregulatory hormone responses to hypoglycaemia in patients with type 1 diabetes. Ann Intern Med 1985; 103: 184–190.
[13] Maran A, Macdonald IA, Amiel SA. The euglycaemic-hypoglycaemic clamp: a reliable tool for the investigation of responses to hypoglycaemia. Diabetes 1991; 40 suppl 1: 543A (Abstract).
[14] Amiel SA, Simonson DC, Tamborlane WV et al. Rate of glucose fall does not affect counterregulatory hormone responses to hypoglycemia in normal and diabetic humans. Diabetes 1987; 36: 518–522.
[15] Bolli G, De Feo P, Perriello G et al. Role of hepatic autoregulation in defense against hypoglycemia in humans. J Clin Invest 1985; 75: 1623–1631.
[16] Vea H, Jorde R, Sager G et al. Reproducibility of glycaemic thresholds for activation of counterregulatory hormones and hypoglycaemic symptoms in healthy subjects. Diabetologia 1992; 35: 958–961.
[17] Davis SN, Goldstein RE, Jacobs et al. The effects of differing insulin levels on the hormonal and metabolic responses to equivalent hypoglycemia in normal humans. Diabetes 1993; 42: 263–272.
[18] Diamond MP, Hallarman L, Starick Zych K et al. Suppression of counterregulatory hormone response to hypoglycemia by insulin per se. J Clin Endocrinol Metab 1991; 72: 1388–1390.
[19] Kerr D, Macdonald IA, Tattersall RB. Patients with type 1 diabetes adapt acutely to sustained mild hypoglycaemia. Diabetic Med 1991; 8: 123–128.
[20] Amiel SA, Tamborlane WV, Simonson DC et al. Defective glucose counterregulation after strict glycemic control of insulin-dependent diabetes mellitus. N Engl J Med 1987; 316: 1376–1383.

[21] Saccà L, Sherwin RS, Hendler R et al. Influence of continuous physiologic hyperinsulinemia on glucose kinetics and counterregulatory hormones in normal and diabetic humans. J Clin Invest 1979; 63: 849–857.
[22] Bolli GB, Gottesman IS, Cryer PE et al. Glucose counterregulation during prolonged hypoglycemia in normal humans. Am J Physiol 1984; 247: E206–E214.
[23] De Feo P, Perriello G, Torlone E et al. Contribution of cortisol to glucose counterregulation in humans. Am J Physiol 1989; 257: E35–E42.
[24] De Feo P, Perriello G, De Cosmo S et al. Comparison of glucose counterregulation during short-term and prolonged hypoglycemia in normal humans. Diabetes 1986; 35: 563–569.
[25] Heller SR, Cryer PE. Reduced neuroendocrine and symptomatic responses to subsequent hypoglycemia after 1 episode of hypoglycemia in nondiabetic humans. Diabetes 1991; 40: 223–226.
[26] Widom B, Simonson DC. Intermittant hypoglycemia impairs glucose counterregulation. Diabetes 1992; 41: 1597–1602.
[27] Bendtson I, Gade J, Theilgaard A et al. Cognitive function in type 1 (insulin-dependent) diabetic patients after nocturnal hypoglycaemia. Diabetologia 1992; 35: 898–903.
[28] Maran A, Lomas J, Archibald HR et al. Double blind clinical and laboratory study of hypoglycaemia with human and porcine insulin in diabetic patients reporting hypoglycaemia unawareness after transferring to human insulin. BMJ 1993; 306: 167–171.
[29] Amiel SA, Sherwin RS, Simonson DC et al. Effect of intensive insulin therapy on glycemic thresholds for counterregulatory hormone release. Diabetes 1988; 37: 901–907.
[30] Boyle PJ, Schwartz NS, Shah SD et al. Plasma glucose concentrations at the onset of hypoglycemic symptoms in patients with poorly controlled diabetes and in nondiabetics. N Engl J Med 1988; 318: 1487–1492.
[31] Mitrakou A, Ryan C, Veneman T et al. Hierarchy of glycemic thresholds for counterregulatory hormone secretion, symptoms, and cerebral dysfunction. Am J Physiol 1991; 260: E67–E74.
[32] Hepburn DA, Deary IJ, Frier BM. Classification of symptoms of hypoglycaemia in insulin-treated diabetic patients using factor analysis: relationship to hypoglycaemia unawareness. Diabet Med 1992; 9: 70–75.
[33] Hepburn DA, Deary IJ, Frier BM et al. Symptoms of acute insulin-induced hypoglycemia in humans with and without IDDM. Factor-analysis approach. Diabetes Care 1991; 41: 949–957.
[34] Cox DJ, Gonder-Fredrich L, Antoun B et al. Perceived symptoms in the recognition of hypoglycemia. Diabetes Care 1993; 16: 519–527.
[35] Himwick HE, Hadidian Z, Fazekas JF et al. Cerebral metabolism and electrical activity during insulin hypoglycemia in man. Am J Physiol 1939; 125: 578–585.
[36] Harrad RA, Cockram CS, Plumb AP et al. The effect of hypoglycemia on visual function: a clinical and electrophysiology study. Clin Sci 1985; 69: 673–679.
[37] Pramming S, Thorsteinsson B, Stingsby et al. Glycaemic threshold for changes in electroencephalograms during hypoglycaemia in patients with insulin dependent diabetes. BMJ 1988; 296: 665–667.
[38] Amiel SA, Pottinger RC, Archibald HR et al. Effect of antecedent glucose control on cerebral function during hypoglycemia. Diabetes Care 1991; 14: 109–118.
[39] Pramming S, Thorsteinsson B, Theilgaard A et al. Cognitive function during hypoglycaemia in type 1 diabetes mellitus. BMJ 1986; 292: 647–650.
[40] Tamburrano G, Lala A, Locuratolo N et al. Electroencephalography and visually evoked potentials during moderate hypoglycemia. J Clin Endocrinol Metab 1988; 66: 1301–1306.
[41] De Feo P, Gallai V, Mazzotta G et al. Modest decrements in plasma glucose concentration cause early impairment in cognitive function and later activation of glucose counterregulation in the absence of hypoglycemic symptoms in normal man. J Clin Invest 1988; 82: 436–444.
[42] Tallroth G, Lindgren M, Stenberg et al. Neurophysiological changes during insulin-induced hypoglycaemia and in the recovery period following glucose infusion in type 1 (insulin-dependent) diabetes mellitus and in normal man. Diabetologia 1990; 33: 319–323.

[43] Blackman JD, Towle VL, Sturis et al. Hypoglycemic thresholds for cognitive dysfunction in IDDM. Diabetes 1992; 41: 392–399.
[44] Jones TW, McCarthy G, Tamborlane WV et al. Mild hypoglycemia and impairment of brain stem and cortical evoked potentials in healthy subjects. Diabetes 1990; 39: 1550–1555.
[45] Boll T, Barth J. Neuropsychology of brain damage in children. In: Filskov S, Boll T, eds. Handbook of Clinical Neuropsychology. New York: Wiley, 1981; 418–452.
[46] Lezak M. Neuropsychological assessment. New York: Oxford University Press, 1983.
[47] Golden C. Stroop color and word test. Chicago: Stoelting, 1978.
[48] Widom B, Simonson DC. Glycemic control and neuropsychologic function during hypoglycemia in patients with insulin-dependent diabetes mellitus. Ann Intern Med 1990; 112: 904–912.
[49] Herold KC, Polonsky KS, Cohen RM et al. Variable deterioration in cortical function during insulin-induced hypoglycemia. Diabetes 1985; 34: 677–685.
[50] Blackman JD, Towle VL, Lewis GF et al. Hypoglycemia thresholds for cognitive dysfunction in humans. Diabetes 1990; 39: 828–835.
[51] Cox DJ, Gonder-Frederich L, Clarke W. Driving decrements in type 1 diabetes during moderate hypoglycemia. Diabetes 1993; 42: 239–243.
[52] Grill V, Gutniak M, Bjorkman O et al. Cerebral blood flow and substrate utilization in insulin-treated diabetic subjects. Am J Physiol 1990; 258: E813–E820.
[53] Nagy RJ, O'Connor A, Boyle PJ. Modest hypoglycaemia impairs brain glucose utilization before onset of symptoms. Diabetes 1992; 41 suppl 1: 69A (Abstract).
[54] Tallroth G, Ryding E, Agardh C-D. Regional cerebral flow in normal man during insulin-induced hypoglycemia and in the recovery period following glucose infusion. Metabolism 1992; 41: 717–721.
[55] Shapiro ET, Cooper M, Chen CT et al. Change in hexose distribution volume and fractional utilization of [18F]-2-deoxy-2-fluoro-D-glucose in brain during acute hypoglycemia in humans. Diabetes 1990; 39: 175–180.
[56] Huang S-C, Phelps ME, Hoffmann EJ et al. Noninvasive determination of local cerebral metabolic rate of glucose in man. Am J Physiol 1980; 238: E69–E82.

Methods in evaluating lipoprotein and triglyceride metabolism in diabetes

M.-R. Taskinen

Alterations of serum lipids, lipoproteins and apoproteins are frequent in diabetes. This is recognised by the advocation that annual measurements of serum cholesterol, triglycerides and HDL cholesterol should be obligatory for each diabetic patient. The clinical utility of these measurements serves to estimate CAD risk and the degree of metabolic control. It is well established that the concentration and metabolism of plasma lipoproteins and apoproteins in diabetes is modulated by several factors specific to the diabetic state: type of diabetes, glycaemic control, degree of insulin resistance, diabetic kidney disease and the mode of therapy [1]. Consequently, the concentration of an individual lipoprotein or apoprotein can be highly variable and is completely different in the two types of diabetes. In chronically insulin treated IDDM patients, the lipoprotein pattern is anti-atherogenic. The concentrations of serum and VLDL triglyceride and serum and LDL cholesterol are normal or even subnormal, whereas that of HDL cholesterol is commonly increased [1]. In contrast, NIDDM patients have elevations of serum and VLDL triglycerides and decreases of HDL cholesterol which are considered to be atherogenic changes [1]. Until recently, most studies have only focused on the measurement of the concentrations of serum lipids and lipoproteins in diabetes. However, there is substantial evidence to indicate that the composition and structure of lipoproteins in diabetes can be abnormal even when the concentration is within the normal range. Consequently, more sophisticated methodology is required to analyse disturbances of lipoprotein metabolism in diabetes in detail. Apolipoprotein quantitation is rapidly increasing as well as gradient gel electrophoresis (GGE) to separate subclasses of LDL and HDL. Lipoprotein turnover studies provide a research tool to study the VLDL-IDL-LDL cascade. These techniques have been used to define the metabolic disorders of lipoproteins in diabetes and to evaluate the pathophysiological basis of these disorders. Modern techniques of molecular biology have extended our understanding on the genetic variation of lipoprotein responses to diabetes.

Offprint from
Research Methodologies in Human Diabetes – Part 1

Evaluation of the lipid profile

Evaluation of the basic lipid profile should be performed at the time of diagnosis of diabetes and thereafter annually. Analysis should always include chemical measurements of fasting serum triglyceride and cholesterol and HDL cholesterol. The concentration of LDL cholesterol can be calculated using the Friedewald equation [2] in which:

$$\text{LDL cholesterol mmol/l} = \text{Total cholesterol} - \text{HDL cholesterol-}\\ \text{Triglycerides x 0.45}$$

Of note, the estimated concentration of LDL includes also relative contributions of IDL and Lp(a). This means that the value may be erroneously high compared to that obtained after separation of LDL by ultracentrifugation. The accuracy to estimate LDL concentrations also fails in hypertriglyceridaemia, i. e., if serum triglyceride value exceeds 4.0 mmol/l [3]. A wide variety of methods have been developed to measure the concentration of LDL cholesterol, but they are not commonly used in clinical laboratories [4]. Although lipid analyses are common procedures, the accuracy and precision of these measurements have not, until recently, become satisfactory [5–7]. This has required the creation of reliable reference materials and careful standardisation to minimise the analytical error.

Analysis of cholesterol

Increased demand for cholesterol testing has resulted in better standardisation of cholesterol measurements. In guidelines given by the NCEP (National Cholesterol Education Program) laboratory standardisation panel requests the accuracy for cholesterol measurement to be $\pm$ 3% and coefficient of variation (CV) to be $<3\%$ [6]. Overall, the standardisation of cholesterol measurements has succeeded well and the majority of clinical laboratories are able to fulfil these analytical requirements. Recently, possible pre-analytical error has been recognised as a major source of variation and it constitutes about 60% of the total error [8]. Alterations in life-style of the subjects and sampling procedures compose the major sources of pre-analytical errors. It is well-established that cholesterol levels vary with behavioural factors like diet, exercise, alcohol intake and smoking whereas serum-plasma differences, posture of sampling and storage constitute the error of sampling factors [8]. Consequently, the next guidelines will provide recommendations to minimise errors due to biological variation and sampling techniques and storage.

Recent development in technology allows cholesterol screening to take place by using compact analysis systems in diabetic clinics [9, 10]. This alternative is rapid and allows the immediate feedback to the patient, individualised counselling and regular follow-up of therapy. A variety of instruments are available and, normally, easy to operate and provide acceptable precision, but accuracy can still vary due to defective calibration and the errors of non-professional operators [10]. The use of this new technology for cholesterol testing is rapidly growing in the diagnosis and management of dyslipidaemias.

Analysis of serum triglycerides

Elevation of serum triglyceride levels is the most frequent lipid abnormality in diabetes [1]. There is rapidly growing evidence that, in diabetes hypertriglyceridaemia, per se, is associated with increased CHD risk [11]. Consequently, the annual analysis of serum triglycerides should be mandatory in each diabetic patient. The measurement of triglyceride concentration is also needed to estimate LDL cholesterol [2, 4]. Fasting for 10 to 12 hours is essential for a reliable measurement of serum triglycerides which rapidly increase after eating. The concentration of triglycerides in post-prandial state reflects that of chylomicron, VLDL and their remnants and can be highly variable, whereas the major component of fasting triglycerides is VLDL. If visual inspection of plasma sample reveals clear turbidity or milky appearance, this signifies severe hypertriglyceridaemia which is diagnostic of "diabetic hyperlipidaemia" [1]. It is well documented that the variability of triglyceride measurement is much greater than that of cholesterol; day-to-day variation being about 20% [12, 13]. This fact is mainly due to biological intraindividual variability, but, in addition, considerable interindividual variation also exists [12, 13]. Consequently, a single measurement of triglycerides is not a reliable parameter of CHD risk and the confidence intervals are wide [12]. The great variability of triglyceride measurements probably have biased the epidemiological database and led to underestimation of triglyceride levels as CHD risk factor [14]. Current targets for accuracy of triglyceride measurement is $\pm$ 5% and CV $<$ 5% in the recent guidelines by NCEP [6]. These criteria are stringent and require careful standardisation and the use of glycerol blanking system [6]. Triglycerides can also be measured in compact analysis systems concurrently or separately with cholesterol. However, to obtain an acceptable accuracy requires a careful minimisation of pre-analytical sources of errors and adequate quality-control procedures.

Analysis of HDL cholesterol

Since low HDL cholesterol is an independent predictor of CHD risk, the measurement of HDL cholesterol should be mandatory for each diabetic patient. The gold standard for the measurement of HDL cholesterol is to separate HDL by ultracentrifugation [15]. However, this method is too tedious for routine clinical use and requires special equipment. Most commonly, HDL cholesterol in plasma or serum is measured by different precipitation techniques in which apo B-containing particles are precipitated by use of a divalent cation and HDL cholesterol is measured in the supernatant [16, 17]. Nowadays, most clinical laboratories use the phosphotungstate method which seems to give less variability among laboratories than the other methods [16, 18]. Noteworthy, is that this method slightly underestimates the true HDL cholesterol concentration determined by ultracentrifugation. The requirements for reliable HDL cholesterol measurement are the specificity of the separation step for HDL cholesterol and good precision of cholesterol assay at low levels [6]. Proposed guidelines by NCEP request the accuracy and precision CV to be < 5% for measurement of HDL cholesterol. Of note is that errors in the quantitation of HDL are reflected in the calculated LDL value.

Measurements of apoproteins

Lipoprotein particles constitute of lipid and apoprotein components. Different apoproteins have specific functions as ligands for receptors or as enzyme activators and they play important roles in the metabolism of lipoproteins

Table 1 Major apoproteins and their functions in lipoprotein metabolism

Apolipo-protein	Chromo-some	Lipoprotein	Metabolic function
Apo AI	11		LCAT activator
Apo AII	1	HDL, chylomicrons	Stuctural protein for HDL
Apo AIV	11		Transfer of apo's between HDL and chylomicrons?
Apo(a)	6	Lp(a)	Interaction with fibrinolysis?
Apo B-48	2	Chylomicrons	Structural protein for chylomicrons
Apo B-100	2	VLDL, IDL, LDL	Ligand for binding to LDL receptor
Apo CI	19		Inhibitor for lipoprotein binding to LRP?
Apo CII	19	Chylomicrons, VLDL, IDL, HDL	Activator of LPL
Apo CIII	11		Inhibitor of LPL
Apo E	19	Chylomicrons, VLDL, IDL, HDL	Ligand for binding of lipoproteins to LDL receptor and to remnant receptor(?)

LCAT = lecithin-cholesterol acyl transferase, LRP = LDL receptor-related protein, LPL = lipoprotein lipase

(Table 1). Apo A-I and A-II are the major apoproteins of HDL whereas apo B is the structural protein of LDL and triglyceride-rich particles (VLDL, IDL). The development of specific and sensitive immunological assays to measure apoproteins have provided new tools to study the regulation of lipoprotein metabolism. Turbidimetric and nephelometric assay are increasingly used to quantitate apo B, apo A-I and A-II because these techniques are easy to automate [19]. Note that considerable transfer and exchange of lipids occurs between circulating lipoprotein particles. Therefore, measurements of apo A-I and apo B levels in conjunction with respective lipid values can reveal compositional changes of particles. Consequently, the ratios of HDL cholesterol/apo A-I + A-II and LDL cholesterol/apo B have been used as indices of particle composition [20, 21]. There is growing evidence that the measurements of apoproteins (apo B, apo A-I and A-II) may be useful as predictors of CHD [22–24]. The question if in diabetic patients apo B and/or apo A-I are better discriminators for CHD than LDL cholesterol or HDL cholesterol is open and remains to be established in prospective studies. So far, the clinical utility of apoprotein measurements have been limited because of lack of reliable reference methods and materials. Recently, international reference material for the assay of apo A-I and apo B has been introduced and the standardisation efforts have reduced the CVs below 5% [25, 26] among laboratories. Consequently, apolipoprotein quantitation will be commonly used in prospective studies also.

Recently, apoprotein components have been used to classify sub-populations of lipoprotein particles [27]. HDL constitutes of particles containing apo A-I but no apo A-II (LpA-I) and those containing both apo A-I and apo A-II (LpA-I: A-II)[27]. Similarly, apo B-containing particles can be separated into those containing only apo B (Lp B), apo B and apo C (LpB/C) and apo B, apo C and apo E (Lp B/C/E). Recent data indicate that the regulation and metabolic fate of different sub-populations is divergent and the particles also differ in their atherogeneity. So far, no data exists on the distribution of these particles in diabetic patients. Recognition of Lp(a) as an independent CHD risk factor [28, 29] has raised wide interest in the quantitation of Lp(a) in diabetes. The unique nature of Lp(a) with multiple apo(a) isoforms which determine Lp(a) plasma concentrations, poses specific problems to the assay procedures and their standardisation. Although reliable commercial assay systems are available, their standardisation is not yet optimal [30].

Recently, the genes coding for the major apolipoproteins have been characterised and this has allowed to define genetic defects behind abnormalities of lipoprotein metabolism. Genetic polymorphism occurs in several apoproteins and the structural variation in the genes of apo B and apo E contribute to the variability of LDL cholesterol at population level [31, 32, 33]. Several of the polymorphisms have also been associated with dyslipidaemias and with the risk of atherosclerosis. Question whether genetic variance of apoprotein genes alters the response of lipoproteins in the diabetic state is unresolved. Development of analytical techniques especially the polymerase chain reaction (PCR) facilitates the genetic and epidemiological studies in the future.

Separation and quantitation of lipoproteins

Lipoproteins are routinely subgrouped into four major categories: very low density lipoproteins (VLDL), intermediate density lipoproteins (IDL), low density lipoproteins (LDL) and high density lipoproteins (HDL). All major lipoproteins are highly heterogeneous with respect to size, density, electrical charge and apoprotein content. A number of procedures are available for quantitation of lipoproteins in human plasma. Traditionally lipoproteins (VLDL, IDL, LDL and HDL) have been separated according to their density by analytical ultracentrifugation, which is the gold standard for lipoprotein classification [34]. In general, lipoprotein fractions are isolated by sequential ultracentrifugation [15]. The different components (cholesterol, free cholesterol, triglycerides, phospholipids and proteins) in each lipoprotein fraction can be measured. These procedures allow to detect possible compositional abnormalities of lipoproteins in addition to the quantitation of lipoprotein masses. Noteworthy is that lipoprotein classes vary in response to metabolic changes in vivo and also have different atherogeneity. Interestingly, in both NIDDM and IDDM, lipoproteins demonstrate compositional changes, although their concentration may be within a normal range [1]. Ultracentrifugation procedures are tedious and not applicable in the clinical laboratories, but useful and valuable in research. Other common methods used to separate lipoproteins include gel filtration, chemical precipitation, agarose gel electrophoresis and affinity chromatography [35].

Quantitation of LDL and HDL subfractions

Both LDL and HDL particles vary in their size, density and composition [36, 37]. Recognition that individual subclasses of both LDL and HDL differ with respect to CHD risk has created the need for analysis of LDL and HDL subclasses. Growing evidence indicate that a preponderance of small dense LDL is associated with increased risk of CHD [38]. Interestingly, small dense LDL is accompanied by other atherogenic changes of lipoprotein profile, i. e., increases in plasma triglycerides, apo B and IDL and lowering of HDL cholesterol [39]. LDL size is closely correlated with plasma triglycerides [40]. Interestingly, recent data indicate that small dense LDL is a component of insulin resistance syndrome [39]. Both genetic and environmental factors influence LDL subclasses but, so far, their interaction is not well established. In the future, analyses of LDL subclasses will probably be included to estimate CHD risk for NIDDM patients and in insulin resistance syndrome.

The presence of polydisperse LDL pattern was initially detected by analytical ultracentrifugation [34]. Recently, gradient gel electrophoresis (GGE) has become the most common technique to examine particle size of LDL subclasses [41, 42]. GGE may be performed by using plasma with lipid staining of gels or isolated LDL with lipid or protein staining. Application of GGE allows LDL size to be easily assessed in a large number of samples and it is, therefore, a useful tool for epidemiological studies. In general, 3–5 distinct LDL subclasses can be visualised by scanning the stained gels [42]. Two major LDL patterns have been defined as pattern A and B [38]. In pattern A, large boyant LDL (with the peak at a particle diameter of 25.5 nm or greater) is preponderant, whereas in pattern B, small dense LDL is predominant. Another way to express the data is to calculate the mean particle diameter of the major LDL peak [41, 42]. Dense and light fractions of LDL can also be isolated by gradient ultracentrifugation which allows for the determination of their masses and the analysis of their composition [37, 43].

The two major subclasses of HDL are HDL2 (d 1.063–1.125 g/ml) and HDL3 (d 1.125–1.210 g/ml) which can be separated by sequential ultracentrifugation or by gradient ultracentrifugation [34].

The fact that the HDL2 subclass is more variable than the HDL3 and also seems to be a better predictor of CHD risk necessitated the development of more practical alternatives to measure HDL subclasses. In general, sequential precipitation procedures have been used in epidemiological studies to quantitate the HDL2 and HDL3 [16, 17]. Application of GGE can also be used to assess HDL subclasses [36]. Overall, five distinct HDL subclasses can be defined: HDL3c (7.2–7.8 nm), HDL3b (7.8–8.2 nm), HDL3a (8.2–8.8 nm), HDL2a (8.8–9.7 nm) and HDL2b (9.7–12 nm). These specific types of HDL subclasses are influenced by genetic and environmental factors [44–46]. Although clear alterations of the HDL concentration occur in both IDDM and NIDDM [1], so far no data exist on the distribution HDL subclasses.

Metabolic studies of lipoproteins

Chylomicrons are synthesised in the intestine during absorption of exogenous fat. Apo B-48 distinguishes chylomicrons and their remnants from other

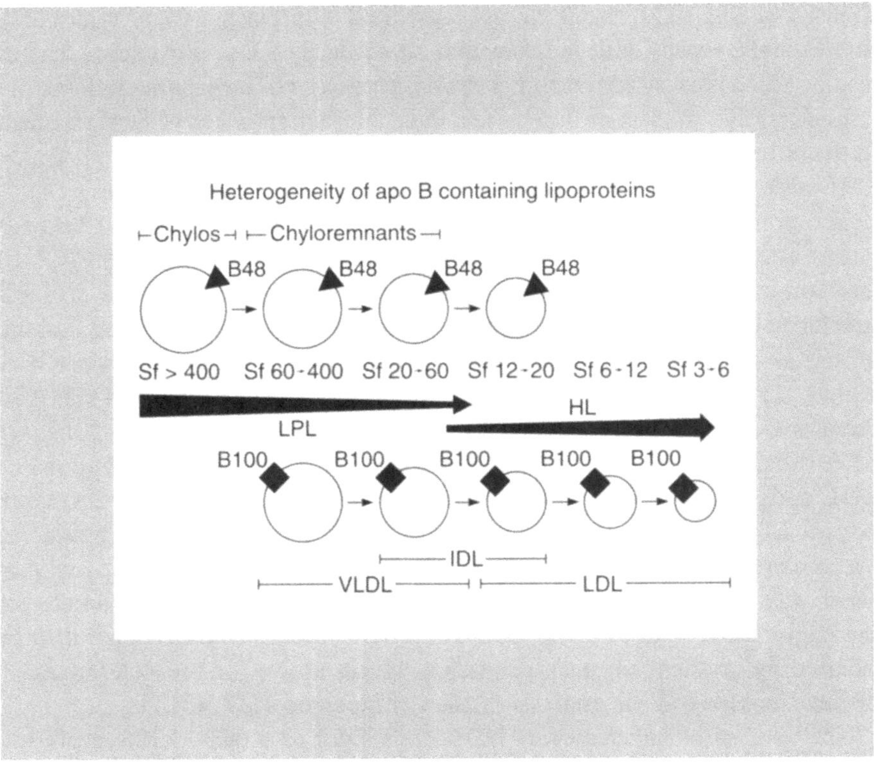

Fig. 1 Flux of apo B containing lipoproteins through exogenous pathway and endogenous pathway. Intestinal triglyceride-rich particles contain apo B-48 as a specific marker. Triglyceride-rich particles released from liver contain apo B-100. Sf denotes Svedberg flotation unit. LPL = lipoprotein lipase, HL = hepatic lipase. The arrows indicate the role of lipases in the metabolic procedures

triglyceride rich particles (Fig. 1). Lipoprotein lipase hydrolyses triglycerides into chylomicrons which are converted into remnant particles. Apo E acts as a ligand for receptor mediated uptake of chylomicron remnants in the liver. There is growing evidence to indicate that post-prandial remnant particles are highly atherogenic [47, 48, 49, 50]. The quantitation of post-prandial responses requires a challenge of triglyceride transport capacity. In general, changes of plasma triglyceride concentration after a mixed meal or an oral fat load are used to assess post-prandial lipaemia. The follow up of the metabolic fate of remnant particles requires the determination of apo B-48 in isolated lipoprotein fractions [49] or use of a marker like vitamin A [51]. Preliminary data indicate that NIDDM patients display alterations in the metabolism of chylomicron remnants [52, 53].

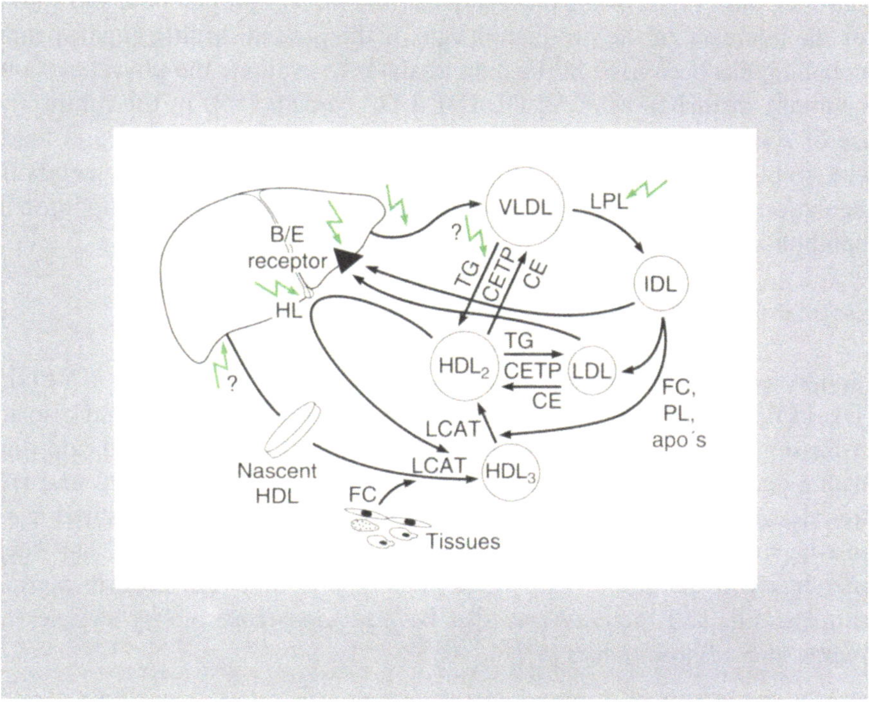

Fig. 2 Endogenous pathways of VLDL-IDL-LDL cascade and HDL metabolism. The arrows indicate possible sites of insulin action on lipoprotein metabolism

CETP = cholesterylester transfer protein
LCAT = lecithin cholesterol acyl transferase
LPL = lipoprotein lipase
HL = hepatic lipase

VLDL particles released from liver contain one apo B-100 molecule which is pertained in the particle during its flux through delipidation cascade (Fig. 1). Since insulin has multiple sites of action on VLDL-IDL-LDL cascade and HDL metabolism diabetes, per se, can cause severe disturbances of lipoprotein metabolism (Fig. 2). Notably, significant transfer and exchange of lipids occurs between circulating lipoprotein particles and these procedures modulate the composition and metabolic fate of lipoproteins. The measurement of apoprotein and lipoprotein metabolism in human has conventionally involved the use of in vitro radioactive iodine labelled lipoproteins or apoproteins [54]. Lipoproteins have been isolated from blood samples, trace-labelled by iodination and reinjected into a subject. Frequent, timed blood sampling allows to follow the plasma radioactivity decay curve and to calculate the fractional catabolic rate (FCR) of the protein. Determination of plasma pool size allows for the inference of the production rate of the protein. Multicompartmental modelling has been used in the data analyses to evaluate the physiology and metabolic disturbances of VLDL-IDL-LDL cascade [55]. In the future, the use of simultaneous endogenous labelling of several apoproteins and lipids with stable isotopes will be a powerful research tool to study the metabolic regulation of lipoproteins and will extend our understanding of lipoprotein metabolism [55, 56].

Enzymes involved in lipoprotein metabolism

Lipoprotein lipase (LPL) and hepatic lipase (HL) play a crucial role in VLDL-IDL-LDL cascade and in HDL metabolism [57]. LPL activity and also its expression at tissue level is regulated by insulin. Recent data indicate that insulin may also influence on hepatic lipase activity [58]. Both LPL and HL are released by heparin into plasma and their activity can be measured from post-heparin plasma samples [57]. Recently, an ELISA method has been introduced to quantitate LPL mass in both pre- and post-heparin plasma samples [59]. LPL activity can also be measured from biopsy samples of muscle and adipose tissues [57].

Measurements of lipoprotein modifications

Growing evidence indicate that modification of lipoproteins by glycosylation and oxidation occurs in diabetes. The glycosylation reaction involves the non-enzymatic binding of glucose to reactive amino groups on lysine side chain. Consequently, chronic hyperglycaemia may cause excessive glycation of all apoproteins. Glycosylation of VLDL, LDL and HDL interferes with their metabolic functions [60]. Moreover glycosylation may increase the susceptibility of lipoproteins to oxidation. However, no simple techniques exists to evaluate the glycosylation of lipoproteins. Borate affinity chromatography can be used to measure LDL glycosylation [61, 62]. Trinitrobenzenesulfonic acid (TNBS) reacts specifically with free amino groups and it can be used to quantitate the loss of free lysine and NH2-terminal amino groups in glycated proteins [61, 62]. In diabetes several factors enhance oxidation of lipoproteins, particularly that of LDL. No appropriate method is available to evaluate the oxidation of lipids and lipoproteins. Measurements of TBARS (thiobarbituric acid reactive substances) is commonly used as an index of lipoprotein oxidation in vivo. However, it should be recognised that the assay contains several pitfalls and is non-specific [63, 64].

Summary

Numerous methodologies for the study of lipoproteins and apoproteins are available in research and clinical laboratories. However, many of these techniques are cumbersome and require specialised instrumentation. In recent years, the complex nature of lipoprotein metabolism in diabetes has been recognised and this has presented a challenge for researchers. Consequently, traditional approaches have become insufficient and new methodologies have been required. The advantages and disadvantages of these methodologies must be evaluated to establish the clinical implications of different methodologies. Accurate laboratory measurement of serum lipids, lipoproteins and apoproteins has become a challenge to every clinician working in a diabetes clinic.

References

[1] Taskinen M-R. Quantitative and qualitative lipoprotein abnormalities in diabetes mellitus. Diabetes 1992; 41 (suppl 2): 12–17.
[2] Friedewald WT, Levy RI, Fredrickson DS. Estimation of concentration of low density lipoprotein cholesterol in plasma without use of the ultracentrifuge. Clin Chem 1972; 18: 449–502.
[3] McNamara JR, Cohn JS, Wilson PWF et al. Calculated values for low-density lipoprotein cholesterol in the assessment of lipid abnormalities and coronary disease risk. Clin Chem 1990; 36: 36–42.
[4] Rifai N, Warnick GR, McNamara JR et al. Measurement of low-density-lipoprotein cholesterol in serum: a status report. Clin Chem 1992; 38: 150–160.
[5] Bachorik PS, Cloey TA, Finney CA et al. Lipoprotein-cholesterol analysis during screening: accuracy and reliability. Ann Intern Med 1991; 114: 741–747.
[6] Bachorik PS. Developing guidelines for reliable triglyceride, high-density lipoprotein cholesterol and low-density lipoprotein cholesterol measurement. Current Opinion in Lipidology 1991; 2: 349–354.
[7] Cooper GR, Myers GL, Smith J et al. Blood lipid measurements; variations and practical ulitity. JAMA 1992; 267: 1652–1660.
[8] Cooper GR, Sampson EJ, Smith SJ. Preanalytical, including biological, variation in lipid and apolipoprotein measurements. Current Opinion in Lipidology 1992; 3: 365–371.
[9] Warwick G, Packard CJ, Shepherd J. Plasma lipid measurement. Current Opinion in Lipidology 1990; 1: 500–507.
[10] Naughton MJ, Luepker RV, Strickland D. The accuracy of portable cholesterol analyzers in public screening programs. JAMA 1990; 263: 1213–1217.
[11] Fontbonne A, Eschwège E, Cambien F et al. Hypertriglyceridaemia as a risk factor of coronary heart disease mortality in subjects with impaired glucose tolerance or diabetes. Diabetologia 1989; 32: 300–304.
[12] Brenner H, Heiss G. The intraindividual variability of fasting triglyceride-challenge for further standardization. Eur Heart J 1990; 11: 1054–1058.
[13] Bookstein L, Gidding SS, Donovan M et al. Day-to-day variability of serum cholesterol, triglyceride, and high-density lipoprotein cholesterol levels. Arch Intern Med 1990; 150: 1653–1657.

[14] Austin MA. Plasma triglyceride as a risk factor for coronary heart disease. Am J Epidemiol 1989; 129: 249–259.
[15] Havel RJ, Eden HA, Bragdon JH. The distribution and chemical composition of ultracentrifugally separated lipoproteins in human serum. J Clin Invest 1955; 34: 1345–1354.
[16] Warnick GR, Nguyen T, Albers JJ. Comparison of improved precipitation methods for quantitation of high density lipoprotein cholesterol. Clin Chem 1985; 31: 217–222.
[17] Wiebe DA, Warnick GR. Measurement of high density lipoprotein cholesterol concentration. In: Methods for Clinical Laboratory Measurement of Lipid and Lipoprotein Risk Factors,Rifai N, Warnick GR eds Washington DC: AACC Press, 1991; 61–74.
[18] Assmann G, Schriewer H, Schmitz G et al. Quantification of high-density-lipoprotein cholesterol by precipitation with phosphotungstic acid/$MgCl_2$. Clin Chem 1983; 29: 2026–2030.
[19] Labeur C, Shepherd J, Rosseneu M. Immunological assays of apolipoproteins in plasma: methods and instrumentation. Clin Chem 1990; 36: 591–597.
[20] Sniderman AD, Silberberg J. Is it time to measure apolipoprotein B? Arteriosclerosis 1990; 10: 665–667.
[21] Brinton EA, Eisenberg S, Breslow JL. Increased apo A-I and apo A-II fractional catabolic rate in patients with low high density lipoprotein-cholesterol levels with or without hypertriglyceridemia. J Clin Invest 1991; 87: 536–544.
[22] Miller NE. Associations of high-density lipoprotein subclasses and apolipoproteins with ischemic heart disease and coronary atherosclerosis. Am Heart J 1987; 113: 589–597.
[23] Hamsten A. Apolipoproteins, dyslipoproteinaemia and premature coronary heart disease. Acta Med Scand 1988; 223: 389–403.
[24] Kwiterovich PO, Coresh J, Smith HH et al. Comparison of the plasma levels of apolipoproteins B and A-I, and other risk factors in men and women with premature coronary artery disease. Am J Cardiol 1992; 69: 1015–1021.
[25] Cooper GR, Henderson LO, Smith SJ et al. Clinical applications and standardization of apolipoprotein measurements in the diagnostic workup of lipid disorders. Clin Chem 1991; 37: 619–620.
[26] Albers JJ, Marcovina SM, Kennedy H. International federation of clinical chemistry standardization project for measurements of apolipoproteins A-I and B. II. Evaluation and selection of candidate reference materials. Clin Chem 1992; 38: 658–662.
[27] Fruchart JC, Bard JM. Lipoprotein particle measurement: an alternative approach to classification of lipid disorders. Current Opinion in Lipidology 1991; 2: 362–366.
[28] Sandkamp M, Funke H, Schulte H et al. Lipoprotein(a) is an independent risk factor for myocardial infarction at a young age. Clin Chem 1990; 36: 20–23.
[29] Scanu AM, Lawn RM, Berg K. Lipoprotein(a) and atherosclerosis. Ann Intern Med 1991; 115: 209–218.
[30] Labeur C, Rosseneu M. Methods for the measurement of lipoprotein (a) in the clinical laboratory. Current Opinion in Lipidology 1992; 3: 372–376.
[31] Utermann G. Apolipoprotein E polymorphism in health and disease. Am Heart J 1987; 113: 433–439.
[32] Davignon J, Gregg RE, Sing CF. Apolipoprotein E polymorphism and atherosclerosis. Arteriosclerosis 1988; 8: 1–21.
[33] Abbey M. The influence of apolipoprotein polymorphism on the response to dietary fat and cholesterol. Current Opinion in Lipidology 1992; 3: 12–16.
[34] Lindgren FT, Jensen LC. The isolation and quantitative analysis of serum lipoproteins. In: Blood lipids and lipoproteins: quantitation, composition and metabolism, Nelson GJ., ed. John Wiley & Sons, 1972; 180–217.
[35] Warnick GR, Dominiczak MH. Separation and quantitation of lipoproteins. Current Opinion in Lipidology 1990; 1: 493–499.
[36] Blanche PJ, Gong EL, Forte TM et al. Characterization of human high-density lipoproteins by gradient gel electrophoresis. Biochim Biophys Acta 1981; 665: 408–419.

[37] Krauss RM, Burke DJ. Identification of multiple subclasses of plasma low density lipoproteins in normal humans. J Lipid Res 1982; 23: 97–104.
[38] Austin MA, Breslow JL, Hennekens CH et al. Low-density lipoprotein subclass patterns and risk of myocardial infarction. JAMA 1988; 260: 1917–1921.
[39] Austin MA. Genetics of low-density lipoprotein subclasses. Current Opinion in Lipidology 1993; 4: 125–132.
[40] McNamara JR, Jenner JL, Li Z et al. Change in LDL particle size is associated with change in plasma triglyceride concentration. Arterioscler Thromb 1992; 12: 1284–1290.
[41] McNamara JR, Campos H, Ordovas JM et al. Gradient gel electrophoretic analysis of low density lipoproteins. American Biotechology Laboratory, 1988.
[42] Krauss RM, Blanche PJ. Detection and quantitation of LDL subfractions. Current Opinion in Lipidology 1992; 3: 377–383.
[43] Griffin BA, Caslake MJ, Yip B et al. Rapid isolation of low density lipoprotein (LDL) subfractions from plasma by density gradient ultracentrifugation. Atherosclerosis 1990; 83: 59–67.
[44] Williams PT, Vranizan KM, Austin MA et al. Familial correlations of HDL subclasses based on gradient gel electrophoresis. Arterioscler Thromb 1992; 12: 1467–1474.
[45] Williams PT, Krauss RM, Vranizan KM et al. Associations of lipoproteins and apolipoproteins with gradient gel electrophoresis estimates of high density lipoprotein subfractions in men and women. Arterioscler Thromb 1992; 12: 332–340.
[46] Williams PT, Krauss RM, Vranizan KM et al. Effects of weight loss by exercise and by diet on apolipoprotein A-I and A-II and the particle size distribution of high density lipoproteins in men. Metabolism 1992; 41: 441–449.
[47] Groot PHE, Stiphout WAHJ, Krauss XH et al. Postprandial lipoprotein metabolism in normolipidemic men with and without coronary artery disease. Arterioscler Thromb 1991; 11: 653–662.
[48] Patsch JR, Miesenböck G, Hopferwieser T et al. Relation of triglyceride metabolism and coronary artery disease. Arterioscler Thromb 1992; 12: 1336–1345.
[49] Karpe F, Bard J-M, Steiner G et al. HDLs and alimentary lipemia. Arterioscler Thromb 1993; 13: 11–22.
[50] Miesenböck G, Patsch JR. Postprandial hyperlipidemia: the search for the atherogenic lipoprotein. Current Opinion in Lipidology 1992; 3: 196–201.
[51] Chen Y-DI, Reaven GM. Intestinally-derived lipoproteins: metabolism and clinical significance. Diabetes/Metabolism Reviews 1991; 7: 191–208.
[52] Chen Y-DI, Swami S, Skowronski R et al. Differences in postprandial lipemia between patients with normal glucose tolerance in noninsulin-dependent diabetes mellitus. J Clin Endocrinol Metab 1993; 76: 172–177.
[53] Syvänne M, Hilden H, Taskinen M-R. Exaggerated postprandial lipemic response in patients with non-insulin-dependent diabetes (NIDDM) in the presence and absence of CAD. Ninth International Symposium on Atherosclerosis 1991; 302A.
[54] Gaw A, Packard CJ, Shepherd J. Lipoprotein turnover and metabolism. In: Lipoprotein Analysis, A Practical Approach Converse CA, Skinner ER, eds. Oxford: IRL Press 1992; 119–144.
[55] Gaw A, Packard CJ, Shepherd J. VLDL and LDL turnover: methods and clinical application. Current Opinion in Lipidology 1992; 3: 384–388.
[56] Schaefer JR, Rader DJ, Brewer HB. Investigation of lipoprotein kinetics using endogenous labeling with stable isotopes. Current Opinion in Lipidology 1992; 3: 227–232.
[57] Taskinen M-R, Kuusi T. Enzymes involved in triglyceride hydrolysis. Baill Clin Endocrinol Metab 1987; 1: 639–666.
[58] Baynes C, Hendersen AD, Anyaoku V et al. The role of insulin insensitivity and hepatic lipase in the dyslipidaemia of type 2 diabetes. Diabetic Medicine 1991; 8: 560–566.
[59] Antikainen M, Holmberg C, Olivecrona T et al. Changes in biological activity and immunoreactive mass of lipoprotein lipase in congenital nephrosis: relationship to hypertriglyceridemia. Eur J Clin Invest 1993; 23: 368–374.

[60] Lyons TJ. Lipoprotein glycation and its metabolic consequences. Diabetes 1992; 41: 67–73.

[61] Snyder SL, Sobocinski PZ. An improved 2,4,6-Trinitrobenzenesulfonic acid method for the determination of amines. Anal Biochem 1975; 64: 284–288.

[62] Lyons TJ, Baynes JW, Patrick JS et al. Glycosylation of low density lipoprotein in patients with Type 1 (insulin-dependent) diabetes: correlations with other parameters of glycaemic control. Diabetologia 1986; 29: 685–689.

[63] Chait A. Methods for assessing lipid and lipoprotein oxidation. Current Opinion in Lipidology 1992; 3: 389–394.

[64] Esterbauer H, Jürgens G. Mechanistic and genetic aspects of susceptibility of LDL to oxidation. Current Opinion in Lipidology 1993; 4: 114–124.

Research methodologies in the evaluation of intestinal glucose absorption and the concept of glycaemic index

K. Hermansen

Introduction

Digestion and absorption of starch

Starch is digested in the gastrointestinal tract by the action of several enzymes, including amylase and disaccharidases. The digestion leads to complete hydrolysis of the starch constituents to free glucose. Glucose is actively transported through the brush border membrane by Na+ dependent carrier mechanisms. After leaving the epithelial cell layer of the small intestine, glucose is transported to the portal blood and then distributed into the circulation resulting in an increase in blood glucose levels and enhanced secretion of insulin from the pancreas.

Different carbohydrate foods produce different glycaemic responses, despite an apparent lack of difference in macronutrient composition. The systematic classification of carbohydrate foods according to their glycaemic responses was first done by Moskowitz [1] and Otto and co-workers [2, 3], who after testing individual foods allowed their incorporation into the diabetic diet in proportion to their glycaemic responses. In this way, the glycaemic impact of the diet could be kept constant, regardless of the variety of the carbohydrate food used. Crapo et al. [4, 5] postulated that the magnitude of the glycaemic and insulinaemic responses to starchy foods are influenced mainly by their rates of digestion in the small intestine. Jenkins and co-workers [6, 7] confirmed that the rates of digestion of starchy foods were strongly related to the glycaemic responses in both normal and diabetic subjects.

Glycaemic index

During the last 10 years, many tests of single food and mixed meals have been carried out in both normal and diabetic subjects. Due to lack of

Offprint from
Research Methodologies in Human Diabetes – Part 1

standardisation of methods, the results of different studies are not always directly comparable. In 1981, the glycaemic index (GI) was proposed by Jenkins and co-workers [8] as a method of assessing and classifying the glycaemic responses to foods. It was hoped that this would allow foods to be compared more readily. By indexing results against a common standard, the results of tests done by different subjects could be compared, and the experience of different investigators pooled. Initially glucose was used as the standard, but this proved to be less acceptable for routine use than white bread (WB) of known composition. The GI of the food was therefore defined as: incremental blood glucose area after food/corresponding area after equi-carbohydrate portion of white bread x 100. By applying this approach to data from different groups of subjects and different centers, it has been possible to classify the glycaemic responses of a substantial number of foods (Table 1). Foods that have been shown to have low glycaemic responses include pasta [8–11], whole-grain cereals [12–14] and legumes [15].

Variation of glycaemic responses

Important variables that affect the glycaemic responses to a test meal include: method of area calculation; length of observation time; subject characteristics e. g., sex, age, weight; type of diabetes (IDDM or NIDDM); preprandial blood glucose level; food factors (food portions; eating time; nature of starch; content of fat, protein and fiber; anti-nutrients; food processing and storage). Although the treatment and degree of control may have important impact on the size of the large individual variation (intra- and interindividual variation) of the glycaemic responses obtained, the standardisation introduced with the GI values should be able to reduce the influence on this variability.

Methods of calculation of glycaemic responses

Blood glucose area under the curve (AUC): Various methods have been used for calculating the glycaemic responses and GI which has made comparison between studies difficult. A common method applied to calculate the area under the glycaemic response curve [16] gives the total area under the curve (TAUC) i. e., the area under the blood glucose curve and above the blood glucose value of zero. Approximately 80% of variation of TAUC can be explained by the basal blood glucose value [17]. Since TAUC, however, is largely dependent upon the fasting blood glucose level, it is not a sensitive method for detecting differences between postprandial glycaemic responses to different meals. In contrast, the area termed incremental area under the

Table 1 Glycaemic index values of different foods

Food	GI (Mean (Range))	Number of studies
Breads		
Rye (whole grain)	71 (58–77)	3
Wheat (white)	100 (Defined)	–
Wheat (wholemeal)	100 (93–106)	9
Pasta		
Spaghetti (white)	60 (46–88)	8
Cereal grains		
Barley	36 (31–41)	2
Rice (polished)	81 (68–104)	8
Rice (parboiled)	67 (58–78)	5
Sweat corn	80 (66–90)	6
Breakfast cereals		
Cornflakes	121 (107–139)	4
Root vegetables		
Potatoes (white/new)	80 (66–90)	6
Legumes		
Green peas (frozen)	65 (55–74)	2
Kidney beans (dried)	43 (27–65)	6
Lentils (red, dried)	38 (25–45)	6
Fruit		
Apple	49 (40–57)	4
Banana (ripe/unripe)	76 (43–99)	6
Orange	55 (44–73)	4

curve (IAUC) defines the area beneath the blood glucose response curve above the level of fasting blood glucose. Any area below the fasting blood glucose concentration is ignored. About 80% of the changes in IAUC can be ascribed to the rise in blood glucose [17], which consequently should be applied also for calculation of GI.

Length of observation time: Gannon and Nuttall [18] have looked at the effect of the length of observation time on the glycaemic area. Usually, blood glucose responses are measured for 2–4 hours in normal subjects and 3–5 hours in diabetic patients. Because the GI and glycaemic responses are calculated from the area under the glycaemic curve, ignoring the area under the baseline, measurements need only to be continued until the blood glucose response returns to baseline. Extending measurements any longer tend to reduce the differences in glycaemic responses and GI between foods. For normal subjects, 2 hours, and for diabetic subjects, 3 hours can be applied as a compromise between what is ideal (i. e., to allow the blood glucose responses to return to baseline) and what is practical for subjects testing many foods.

Methods of blood sampling: Glycaemic responses in capillary blood are greater that those in venous blood or plasma and, therefore, may allow smaller differences in glycaemic responses to different foods to be detected [19]. In diabetic subjects, this will possibly play only a minor role.

Intra-individual variation

Day-to-day variation: Day-to-day variation of blood glucose responses can be determined by repeating the same food tests in the same subjects. The variation can be expressed as the coefficient of variation (CV) i. e., the standard deviation expressed as per cent of the mean. The average CV

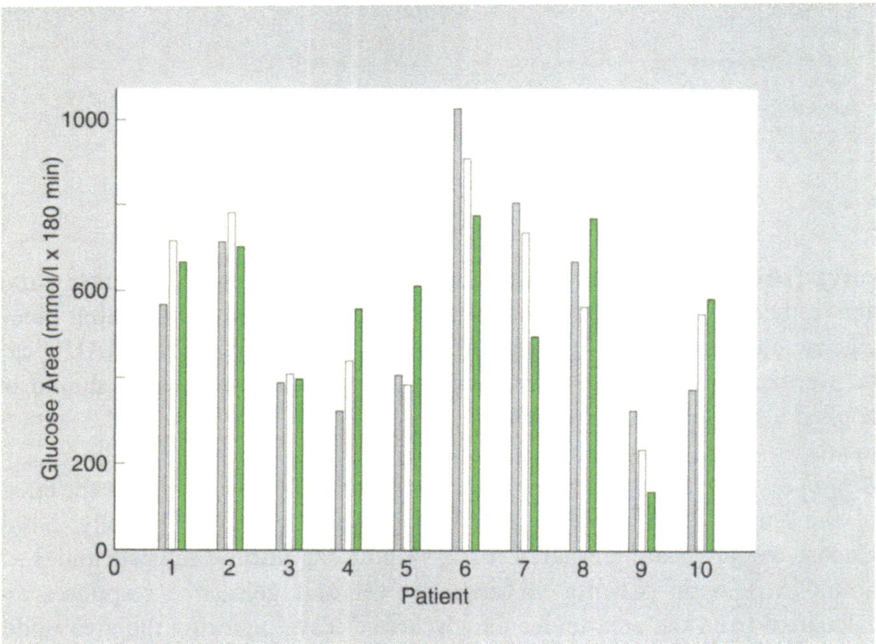

Fig. 1 Individual blood glucose response areas (above basal) to 3 test meals of 90 g white bread in 10 NIDDM subjects (Reprinted with permission of Diabetes Care (22).)

constituted 22–25% in normal subjects [20, 21], 15–19% in NIDDM [20, 22] and 29% in IDDM [20]. We found, that the intraindividual variation of glycaemic responses in NIDDM made up only 25% of the total variance of response areas [22] (Fig. 1). Due to low within-person variation, a good estimate of the glycaemic response to starch-rich food in NIDDM subjects were obtained after a single meal [22]. In contrast, subjects with IDDM have very variable insulin and glucose levels as well as glycaemic responses from day-to-day [20, 23].

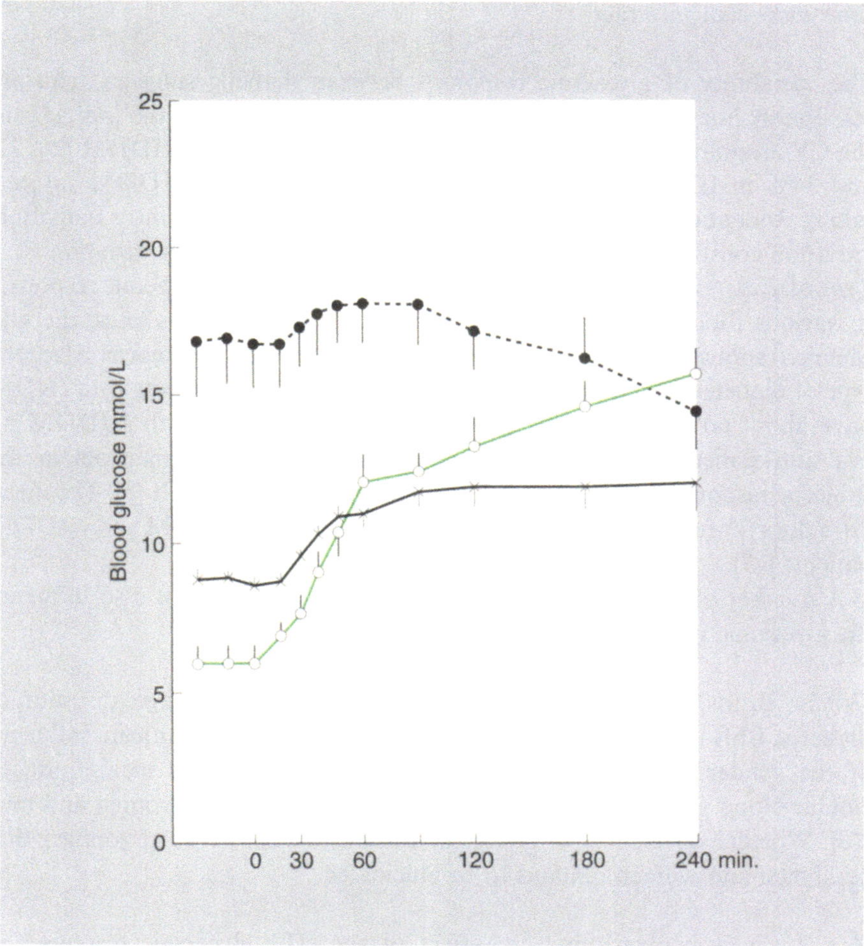

Fig. 2 Blood glucose responses to 50 g parboiled rice in 7 IDDM subjects who had achieved pre-prandial blood glucose levels of 6,9 and 17 mmol/l (mean ± SE) (Reprinted with permission of Am. J. Clin. Nutr. American society for Clinical Nutrition [24].)

Preprandial blood glucose level: Interestingly, we demonstrated a negative correlation (r = −0,94) between preprandial blood glucose concentration and glycaemic response [24] (Fig. 2), i. e., a reduction in blood glucose increments is seen at rising preprandial blood glucose concentrations in IDDM [24]. To circumvent this problem in IDDM, blood glucose levels can be normalised and blood insulin levels stabilised by using the artificial pancreas before tests of foods are performed [25, 26]. However, it would be difficult to carry out as a routine investigation in large scale due to the expense and subject time involved.

Inter-individual variation

The variability of glycaemic responses between diabetic subjects, who are reasonably homogenous, is larger that the variability within the individuals, the CV attaining 26% in normal subjects [20], 23−34% in NIDDM [20, 22] and 34% in IDDM [20]. Blood glucose responses in 10 NIDDM subjects taking 3 identical meals are shown in fig. 1. The inter-and intra-individual variation constituted 75% and 25%, respectively, of the total variation.
Type of diabetes: It is not reliable to compare the absolute glycaemic responses to various food tested in different groups of subjects. In diabetes, the glycaemic response areas may be 5−10 times that of normal subjects. Also, the type of diabetes influences the glycaemic responses, i. e., subjects with IDDM have about 60% greater glycaemic responses than those with NIDDM on oral anti-diabetic drugs and/or diet. In order to overcome this problem, the subjects' responses can be indexed to a standard such as the GI [8]. The mean GI-values for foods have been found to be very similar in IDDM and NIDDM patients [27].

A number of factors such as gender, age and weight might also influence the glycaemic responses.

Gender: In middle-aged subjects with NIDDM matched for age, duration of diabetes, BMI and metabolic control, we could not detect significant influence of the gender [28]. Thus, two different, carbohydrate-rich meals induced similar blood glucose and insulin responses in middle-aged women and men [28]. Whether differences in glycaemic responses exist between younger diabetic men and women remains to be elucidated.

Age: Little is known about the effect of age. The glycaemic responses in IDDM subjects of respectively 46 years or 11 years in average were similar to bread and lentils [29].

BMI: Whether obese diabetic subjects respond differently than non-obese subjects to different meals is unknown.

Food factors

An understanding of the carbohydrate content of foods remains necessary but the glycaemic response to food might be governed by many factors other than simply the carbohydrate content. They include: the content of fat, protein and dietary fiber; the nature of starch; anti-nutrients; food form, processing and storage of food; eating time and water content; and the meal frequency.

Fat, protein and dietary fiber: Fat delays gastric emptying and, usually, blunts the rate of increase in blood glucose to a meal [30]. This is important to realise, since fat-rich foods can appear in falsely favourable light if only the acute glycaemic response is considered.

Although protein stimulates insulin secretion in NIDDM, the glycaemic response is diminished only after addition of larger amounts of protein [31, 32]. In contrast, coingestion of protein causes an augmentation in blood glucose responses in IDDM rather than a reduction [33]. The use of high fiber foods is encouraged as a means of suppressing the rate of absorption of glucose from the gastrointestinal tract. No simple correlation exists, however, between the fiber content of foods and the glycaemic responses. Different types of dietary fiber have different effects. Viscous fibers which are found in fruit, barley and vegetables (especially legumes) can lower the blood glucose response [34], presumably by slowing the digestion of carbohydrate and reducing the rate of glucose towards the absorptive mucosal surface. Fruits such as orange and apple have low GI of 44 and 40, respectively [35]. The low glycaemic response to orange and apple may, however, be ascribed to the high content of fructose which is rapidly cleared and metabolised by the liver without elevating the blood glucose. In contrast, insoluble fibers as cereal fiber as such has little or no effect [34]; no difference in blood glucose responses is detected between white bread and wholemeal bread (graham bread) [36] as well as between white and brown rice. In some foods, fat-starch and protein-starch interactions may play a significant role for the flat glycaemic response. Thus, starch forms molecular complexes with lipids and protein which render it less susceptible to amylolytic digestion.

Type and amount of starch: Food starches are composed of variable ratios of amylose and amylopectin. Both are polymeres of glucose, amylose only having glucose molecules linked by α – 1,4-glucosidic linkage while amylopectin, a much larger molecule, in addition to $\alpha - 1,4$ linkages also has $\alpha - 1,6$ linkage branch point. The bioavailability of a particular starch is highly dependent on the degrees of gelatinisation and the extent of retrogradation. Amylose is less readily gelatinised and more easily retrograded than amylopectin, thereby being more resistant to enzymatic degradation and consequently eliciting lower glycaemic responses. Legumes starches are characterised by relatively high amylose contents, generally above 29%, which may in part explain the low GI and glycaemic responses to beans and lentils [37].

The question arises whether the GI of a food depends on the amount of starch. In other words, if smaller amounts of food than 50 g carbohydrate behave in a similar way with respect to the GI. We found, that the GI of parboiled white rice corresponding to 25 and 50 g carbohydrate were similar: 55 and 60, respectively [38]. However, whether the GI of other foods is always constant, regardless of the amount of carbohydrate is not known.

Antinutrients: Lectins and phytates are antinutrients, examples on compounds that decrease the bioavailability of starch and consequently cause a reduction in GI of starchy foods. Lectins inhibits the access of starch to the active site of amylase due to binding of the lectin, either to the enzyme or to the starch, while phytate acts by complexing with metal ions that are necessary for amylase activity.

Food form, processing and storage: The use of whole grains in whole meal bread is associated with a significant lower glycaemic response [36, 39]. Furthermore, whole rice produces lower glucose responses than does grounded rice.

Raw starch granules are digested slowly by amylases. Cooking causes granular disorganisation and gelatinisation i. e. swelling of starch granules in the presence of heat and water, which facilitates the enzymatic digestion of starch. A larger rise in blood glucose has been found after ingestion of cooked as opposed to raw potatoes [40], rice [41] and legumes [37]. Increased cooking is, however, not associated with increased glycaemic responses in pasta [9], carrots [40] or rolled oats [42].

Recently, we found that ripening of banana has a profound impact on the GI [43]. In the under-ripe bananas, starch accounted for 91%, versus 13% of the carbohydrate content in over-ripe bananas [43]. The GI of the under-ripe and over-ripe bananas was 43 and 74, respectively [43]. The low glycaemic response to under-ripe bananas may be explained by the relative high content of "resistant starch", which is only slowly hydrolysed by amylase. Potatoes

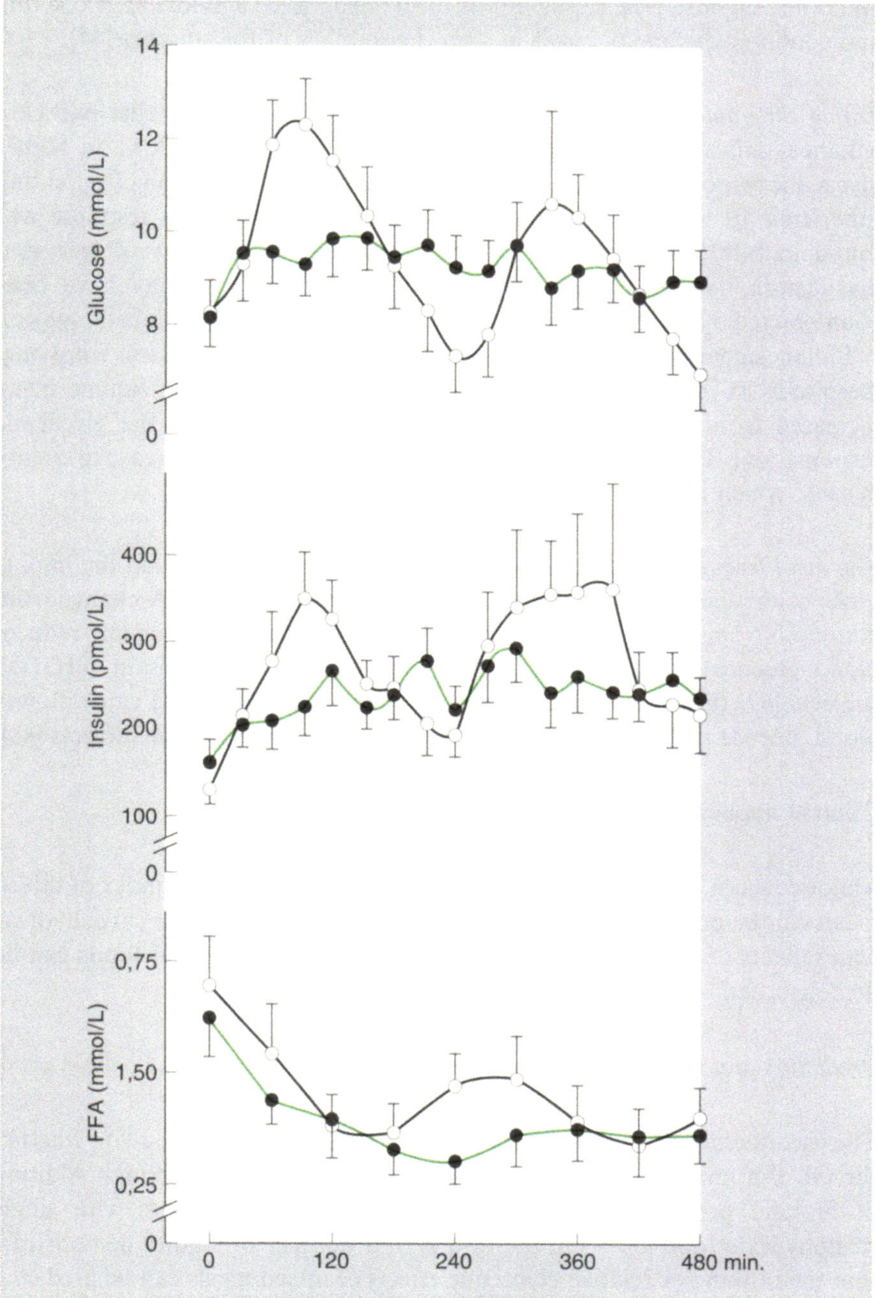

Fig. 3 Blood glucose, insulin and FFA levels in 12 NIDDM patients after isocaloric diets taken as 6 meals (●) or 2 meals (○) (mean ± SE) (Reprinted with permission of Diabetes Care [47].)

and other amylose-rich starchy foods form retrograded amylose after cooking and cooling, which may result in slow digestibility of the starches [44].

Eating time and water content: Chewing breaks foods into smaller particles, enhances salivation and mixes it with salivary amylase resulting in higher glycaemic responses in normal subjects [45]. Despite an extension of the eating time from 10 to 30 minutes, no effect on the blood glucose response was found in NIDDM [46]. The potential hyperglycaemic effect of increased mastication induced by an extension of the eating time may have been counteracted by the effect of a delayed gastric emptying in the diabetic subject.

Enhancement of the meal volume increases the rate of gastric emptying. Despite a six-fold increase of water volume (i. e. total meal volume being increased from 265 to 775 ml), there was no influence on the glycaemic response [46]. The reason for this may be the concomitant decrease in energy density, which is known to cause a delay in gastric emptying.

The meal frequency: National diabetes associations have debated the importance of the temporal distribution of ingested carbohydrates. A change from 2 large to 6 small meals during a 8 hours observation period acutely reduces blood glucose fluctuations and lowers average insulin levels in NIDDM subjects [47] (Fig. 3). Also, a diet of 13 snacks (nibbling diet) causes lower blood glucose and insulin levels than a 3-meal diet in NIDDM subjects [48].

Clinical application of the glycaemic responses and GI

Major concern, however, still exists, whether (1) the glycaemic index of mixed meals can be predicted from the blood glucose responses to the carbohydrate components of the latter, and (2) long-term benefits of low GI foods can be demonstrated.

Prediction and ranking of glycaemic responses

The usefulness of the glycaemic index approach depends first of all on whether the GI of a mixture of foods in a meal can be predicted. Although addition of fat and protein alter the glycaemic impact of challenges with single carbohydrate food [30–33], the results of a number of studies demonstrate that the ranking or relative glycaemic effects of mixed meals can be predicted from the GI and blood glucose responses to the carbohydrate components in both IDDM [20, 25–27] and NIDDM patients [11, 20, 49, 50]. However, some studies fail to show the expected difference in glycaemic response to mixed meals [51, 52]. In these studies [51, 52], the foods used were not tested individually before incorporation into the mixed meal, i. e., the GI of all the individual foods were not known for certain. Furthermore, the high content of monosaccharide in the test meals [51, 52] might have diluted any potential difference. It should be stressed that incremental rather than total areas should be applied to compare post-prandial responses, as previously discussed.

Longitudinal studies

Another of the major questions concerning the fractional use of the glycaemic index and responses is whether low glycaemic index/response meals are beneficial in the long term. Few studies have tested the long-term effects on carbohydrate and lipid metabolism. Low glycaemic index foods have been shown to give a modest improvement in the glycaemic control after 3 and 5 weeks treatment in IDDM subjects [53, 54] and after 2 [55], 5 [54] and 12 weeks treatment [56] in NIDDM subjects. While low GI diets reduce insulin secretion in NIDDM [55], the impact on the insulin requirement in IDDM is more dubious [53, 54]. In normolipidaemic diabetic subjects, low GI diets cause little suppression of triglyceride and cholesterol [53, 55] or no effect on the circulating lipids [54]. In a group of hyperlipidaemic non-diabetics patients, however, a reduction in triglyceride, total and LDL-cholesterol was seen, while no change in HDL-cholesterol appeared with a low GI-diet [57]. Recent studies [55] indicate that a low GI-diet reduces the urinary creatinine and urea output. Whether this, in the light of the concept of dietary protein inducing renal hyperperfusion and renal damage, may involve a beneficial effect by reducing amino acid fluxides remains speculative.

The application of the GI to therapeutic diets should be in the context of the overall nutrient composition of the diet. The GI does not take into account the energy content of foods e. g., high-fat foods may have a low GI and may not be prudent to recommend to the majority of diabetic patients who are overweight. It may, however, be possible to incorporate into a patient's diet, specific foods with low GI which have the desired nutritional profile e. g., pasta, parboiled rice, beans, barley, lentils, bulgur, pumpernickel bread, under-ripe banana etc. Most people find at least some of these low GI foods acceptable and, thus, allow an expansion of the number of foods which the patient may choose to use. Any more systematic application to long-term use will require a better understanding of nutrient interactions in food and meals if the therapeutic potential of this manoeuver is to be realised.

References

[1] Moskowitz E. Der Einfluss vegetabiler Nahrungsmittel auf den Blutzucker bei Diabetikern. Z Klin Med 1937; 131: 648–659.
[2] Otto H, Bleyer G, Pennartz M et al. Kohlenhydrataustausch nach biologischen ækvivalenten. In Otto H, Spaethe R (ed): Diætetik bei Diabetes Mellitus. Bern: Huber 1973, 41–50.
[3] Otto H, Niklas L. Differences d'action sur la glycemie d'alimentes constant des hydrates de carbone. Consequences pour le traitment dietique du diabete sucre. Med Hyg 1980; 38: 3424–3429.
[4] Crapo PA, Reaven GM, Olefsky J. Plasma glucose and insulin responses to orally administered simple and complex carbohydrates. Diabetes 1977; 26: 1178–1183.
[5] Crapo PA, Kolterman OG, Waldec N et al. Postprandial hormonal responses to different types of complex carbohydrate in individuals with impaired glucose tolerance. Am J Clin Nutr 1980; 33: 1723–1728.
[6] Jenkins DJA, Ghafari H, Wolever TMS et al. Relationship between the rate of digestion of foods and postprandial glycaemia. Diabetologia 1982; 22: 450–455.
[7] Jenkins DJA, Wolever TMS, Thorne MJ et al. The relationship between the glycaemic response, digestibility, and factors influencing the dietary habits of diabetics. Am J Clin Nutr 1984; 40: 1175–1191.
[8] Jenkins DJA, Wolever TMS, Tailor RH et al. Glycaemic index of foods: A physiological basis for carbohydrate exchange. Am J Clin Nutr 1981; 34: 362–366.
[9] Jenkins DJA, Wolever TMS, Jenkins AL et al. Glycaemic response to wheat products: reduced response to pasta but no effect of fiber. Diabetes Care 1983; 6: 155–159.
[10] Wolever TMS, Jenkins DJA, Kalmusky J et al. Glycaemic response to pasta: effect of food form, cooking and protein enrichment. Diabetes Care 1986; 9: 401–404.
[11] Rasmusen O, Winther E, Arnfred J et al. Comparison of blood glucose and insulin responses in non-insulin-dependent diabetic patients. Europ J Clin Nutr 1988; 42: 953–961.
[12] Heinonen L, Korpela R, Mantere S. The effect of different types of Finnish bread on postprandial glucose responses in diabetic patients. Hum Nutr App Nutr 1985; 39 A: 108–113.
[13] Jenkins DJA, Wolever TMS, Jenkins AL et al. Low glycaemic response to traditionally processed wheat and rye products: bulgur and pumpernickel bread. Am J Clin Nutr 1986; 43: 516–520.
[14] Rasmussen O, Winther E, Hermansen K. Glycaemic responses to different types of bread in insulin-dependant diabetic subjects (IDDM): Studies at constant insulinaemia. European J of Clin Nutr 1991; 45: 97–103.
[15] Jenkins DJA, Wolever TMS, Taylor RH et al. Exeptionally low blood glucose response to dried beans: comparison with other carbohydrate foods. Br Med J 1980; ii: 578–580.
[16] Wolever TMS, Jenkins DJA, Jenkins AL et al. The glycaemic index: methodology and clinical implications. Am J Clin Nutr 1991; 54: 846–854.
[17] Le Floch JP, Escuyer P, Baudin E et al. Blood glucose area under the curve. Methodological Aspects. Diabetes Care 1990; 13: 172–175.
[18] Gannon MC, Nuttall FQ. Factors affecting interpretation of postprandial glucose and insulin in areas. Diabetes Care 1987; 10: 759–763.
[19] Wolever TMS, Jenkins DJA, Collier GR et al. Metabolic response to test meals containing different carbohydrate foods. 1. Relationship between rate of digestion and plasma insulin response. Nutr Res 1988; 8: 573–581.
[20] Wolever TMS, Nuttall FQ, Lee R et al. Prediction of the relative blood glucose response of mixed meals using the white bread glycaemic index. Diabetes Care 1985; 8: 418–428.
[21] Wolever TMS. The glycaemic index: A physiological basis for carbohydrate exchange; PhD thesis, University of Toronto, 1986.

[22] Rasmussen O, Gregersen S, Sørup J et al. Day-to-day variation of blood glucose and insulin responses in NIDDM subjects after a starch-rich meal. Diabetes Care 1992; 4: 542–545.
[23] Schmidt MI, Hadji-Georgopoulos A, Rendell M et al. The dawn phenomenon, an early morning glucose rise: implications for diabetic intraday blood glucose variation. Diabetes Care 1981; 4: 579–585.
[24] Rasmussen O, Hermansen K. Preprandial blood glucose values and glycaemic responses in insulin-dependent diabetes mellitus at constant insulinemia. Am J Clin Nutr 1991; 53: 520–523.
[25] Hermansen K, Rasmussen O, Arnfred J et al. Differential glycaemic effects of potato, rice and spaghetti in type 1 (insulin-dependent) diabetic patients at constant insulinaemia. Diabetologia 1986; 29: 358–361.
[26] Hermansen K, Rasmussen O, Arnfred J et al. Glycaemic effects of spaghetti and potato consumed as part of mixed meal on IDDM patients. Diabetes Care 1987; 10: 401–406.
[27] Wolever TMS, Jenkins DJA, Josse RG et al. The glycaemic index: similarity of values derived in insulin-dependent and non-insulin-dependent diabetic patients. J Am Coll Nutr 1987; 6: 295–305.
[28] Rasmussen O, Gregersen S, Dørup J et al. Blood glucose and insulin responses to different meals in non-insulin-dependent diabetic subjects of both sexes. Am J Clin Nutr 1992; 56: 712–715.
[29] Wolever TMS, Jenkins DJA, Collier GR et al. The glycaemic index: effect of age in insulin-dependent diabetes mellitus. Diabetes Res 1988; 7: 71–74.
[30] Collier G, O'Dea K. The effect of coingestion of fat on the glucose, insulin and gastric inhibitory polypeptide responses to carbohydrate and protein. Am J Clin Nutr 1983; 37: 941–944.
[31] Nuttall FQ, Mooradian AD, Gannon MC et al. Effect of protein ingestion on the glucose and insulin response to a standardized oral glucose load. Diabetes Care 1984; 7: 465–470.
[32] Gulliford MC, Bicknell EJ, Scarpello JH. Differential effect of protein and fat ingestion on blood glucose responses to high- and low-glycaemic-index carbohydrates in noninsulin-dependent diabetic subjects. Am J Clin Nutr 1989; 50: 773–777.
[33] Simpson RW, McDonald J, Walqvist ML et al. Macronutrients have different metabolic effects in nondiabetics and diabetics. Am J Clin Nutr 1985; 42: 449–453.
[34] Jenkins DJA, Leeds AR, Gassull MA et al. Unabsorbable carbohydrates and diabetes: decreased postprandial hyperglycaemia. Lancet 1976; ii: 172–174.
[35] Gregersen S, Rasmussen O, Larsen S et al. Glycaemic and insulinaemic responses to orange and apple compared with white bread in non-insulin-dependent diabetic subjects. Eur J Clin Nutr 1992; 46: 301–303.
[36] Rasmussen O, Winther E, Hermansen K. Glycaemic responses to different types of bread in insulin-dependant diabetic subjects (IDDM): Studies at constant insulinaemia. Eur J Clin Nutr 1991; 45: 97–103.
[37] Tovar J. Bioavailability of starch in processed legumes: importance of physical inaccessibility and retrogradation. Scand J Nutr 1992; 36: 164–172.
[38] Rasmussen O, Gregersen S, Hermansen K. Influence of the amount of starch on the glycaemic index to rice in non-insulin-dependent diabetic subjects. Br J Nutr 1992; 67: 371–377.
[39] Arends J, Ahrens K, Lubke D et al. 1 factors influencing the blood glucose response to different breads in type II diabetic patients. Klin Wochenschr 1987; 65: 469–474.
[40] Vaaler S, Hanssen KE, Aagenaes O.: The effect of cooking upon the blood glucose response to ingested carrots and potatoes. Diabetes Care 1984; 7: 221–223.
[41] Wolever TMS, Jenkins DJA, Kalmusky J et al. Comparison of regular and parboiled rices: explanation of discrepancies between reported glycaemic responses to rice. Nutr Res 1986; 6: 349–357.
[42] Rasmussen O, Winther E, Hermansen K. Postprandial glucose and insulin responses to rolled oats ingested raw, cooked or as a mixture with raisins in normal subjects and type 2 diabetic patients. Diabetic Medicine 1989; 6: 337–341.

[43] Hermansen, K, Rasmussen O, Gregersen S et al. Influence of ripeness of banana on the blood glucose and insulin response in type 2 diabetic subjects. Diabetic Medicine 1992; 9: 739–743.
[44] Englyst HN, Cummings JH. Digestion of polysaccharides of potato in the small intestine of man. Am J Clin Nutr 1987; 45: 423–431.
[45] Read NW, Welch I McL, Austen CJ et al. Swallowing food without chewing: a simple way to reduce postprandial glycaemia. Br J Nutr 1986; 55: 43–47.
[46] Gregersen S, Rasmussen O, Winther E et al. Water volume and consumption time: influence on the glycaemic and insulinemic responses in non-insulin-dependent diabetic subjects. Am J Clin Nutr 1990; 52: 515–518.
[47] Bertelsen J, Christiansen C, Thomsen C et al. Effect of meal frequency on blood glucose, insulin, and free fatty acids in NIDDM subjects. Diabetes Care 1993; 16: 4–7.
[48] Jenkins DJA, Ocana A, Jenkins AL et al. Metabolic advantages of spreading the nutrient load: effects of incrased meal frequency in non-insulin-dependent diabetes. Am J Clin Nutr 1992; 55: 461–467.
[49] Collier GR, Wolever TMS, Wong GS et al. Prediction of glycaemic response to mixed meals in noninsulin-dependent diabetic subjects. Am J Clin Nutr 1986; 44: 349–352.
[50] Bornet FRJ, Costagliola D, Rizkalla SW et al. Insulinemic and glycaemic indexes of six starch-rich foods taken alone and in a mixed meal by type 2 diabetics. Am J Clin Nutr 1987; 45: 588–595.
[51] Laine DC, T homas W, Levitt MD et al. Comparison of predictive capabilities of diabetic exchange lists and glycaemic index of foods. Diabetes Care 1987; 10: 387–394.
[52] Coulston AM, Hollenbeck CB, Swislocki ALM et al. Effect of source of dietary carbohydrate on plasma glucose and insulin responses to mixed meals in subjects with NIDDM. Diabetes Care 1987; 10: 395–400.
[53] Fontvieille AM, Acosta M, Rizkalla SW et al. A moderate switch from high to low glycaemic-index foods for 3 weeks improves the metabolic control of Type 1 (IDDM) diabetic subjects. Diab Nutr Metab 1988; 1: 139–143.
[54] Fontvieille AM, Rizkalla SW, Penfornis A et al. The use of low glycaemic index foods improves metabolic control of diabetic patients over five weeks. Diabetic Medicine 1992; 9: 444–450.
[55] Wolever TMS, Jenkins DJA, Vuksan V et al. Beneficial effect of a low glycaemic index diet in type 2 diabetes. Diabetic Medicine 1992; 9: 451–458.
[56] Brand JC, Colagiuri S, Corssman S et al. Low-glycaemic index foods improve long-term glycaemic control in NIDDM. Diabetes Care 1991; 14: 95–101.
[57] Jenkins DJA, Wolever TMS, Kalmusky J et al. Low-glycaemic index diet in hyperlipidemia: use of traditional starchy foods. Am J Clin Nutr 1987; 46: 66–71.

Evaluation of cardiac autonomic neuropathy by heart rate variability

H. Mølgaard, K. Hermansen

Introduction

The autonomic nervous system is an important control system which influences the function of many organs. Dysfunction of the autonomic system is commonly encountered in both type 1 and type 2 diabetes mellitus, and is designated the diabetic autonomic neuropathy. The aetiology to this complication is unclear. As demonstrated by clinical testing, 17–40% of diabetic patients have signs of dysfunction [1–5]. The natural history is not fully elucidated. The prevalence of positive tests for autonomic neuropathy increases by increasing duration of the disease [2, 3]. However, aspects regarding a possible reversibility, in particular in the early stages, has not been sufficiently addressed. The presence of severe autonomic neuropathy can indicate increased mortality [6–8]. The independent pathophysiological impact of the neuropathy has, however, not been investigated. This is important because the neuropathy may itself contribute to the development of other complications [9] and the pathophysiology of the increased mortality rates [4, 10]. Impaired vagal function has proved to be of importance for the genesis of arrhythmic death, both in experimental and clinical studies [11, 12]. In coronary heart disease, cardiac autonomic imbalance is an important predictive factor for sudden cardiac death [13–15].

Symptoms of autonomic neuropathy are non-specific. Autonomic function has traditionally been evaluated by a battery of "bed-side" tests, which mainly rely on the heart rate response to various procedures. However, new analysis techniques of the heart rate variability [16–18] and new methodologies based on 24-hour heart rate variability, seem to be more sensitive, and to improve the evaluation of autonomic function [4, 19–22]. This chapter will elucidate the background for estimation of autonomic function by means of heart rate variability measurement, and focus on the deep breathing test and methodologies based on 24-hour ECG recordings.

Offprint from
Research Methodologies in Human Diabetes – Part 1

Autonomic nervous system

For more than 200 years it has been recognised that heart rate and blood pressure undergo periodic oscillations [23]. These spontaneous oscillations are due to neural control mechanisms mediated through the autonomic nervous system [17]. This nervous system consists of dual pathways – the sympathetic and parasympathetic efferents. Their regulating centres are both located in the medulla [24] and are probably connected directly to the respiratory centre. The afferent input to the vasomotor centre is very complex and not yet sufficiently investigated. The basic knowledge is based on direct [25] and indirect [16, 26, 27] measurements of efferent nervous activity in the two pathways during defined cardiovascular circumstances, and through surgically or pharmacologically selective denervation. Direct measurements of nervous activity require anaesthetised open chest preparations. This is difficult, and may also interfere with motor neuron activity, and in particular with the coupling of heart rate changes to respiratory pattern. Non-invasively, the sinus node has been used as target organ, as the response – heart rate changes, are very easy to measure in the conscious, spontaneously breathing man.

Heart rate and heart period variability

In clinical use, heart rate (HR) means the average heart rate for a given time period, i. e., 1 minute. Instantaneous HR is HR calculated from one RR interval (the distance between two heart beats). For identical HR, the variations in instantaneous HR can be quite different, depending on the actual autonomic balance (Fig. 1). HR variability is a quantification of the variations in instantaneous HR. HR also varies in relation to a number of circumstances. HR variability also expresses how these changes in instantaneous HR takes place. The unit for HR is beats per minute (b.p.m.). However, measurements are often kept in time periods (RR intervals), which are denoted heart period (HP) (unit = millisecond (ms)). The relationship between HR and HP (RR intervals) is non-linear ($y = 1/x$). This is important because identical changes in i. e., instantaneous HP (ms), up to levels of mean HP above and below 1000 ms, do not correspond with identical changes in absolute values when measured in HR.

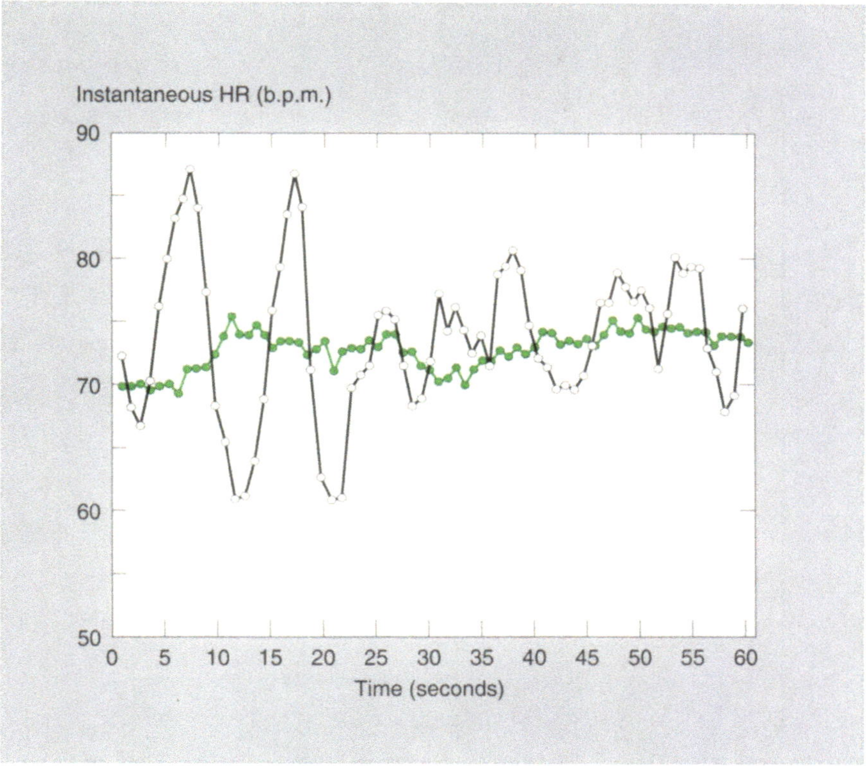

Fig. 1 Variation in instantaneous heart rate (HR) in a person with normal (o) and low (•) HR variability, during a one minute period. The average HR is for both persons 73 beats per minute (b.p.m.), whereas HR variability (the standard deviation) is 69 ms and 18 ms, respectively. Instantaneous HR is HR calculated from one RR interval and converted to b.p.m.

Components of heart period variability

Vagal activity causes a decrease in HR [28]. Changes in vagal activity are associated with immediate changes in HR within 1 to 2 beats, whereas changes in sympathetic activity are associated with more gradual and slower changes in HR. Recordings of instantaneous HP variations during spontaneous respiration contains certain systematic oscillations (Fig. 2A, 3A). A high frequency oscillation which has a cycle-time of approximately 4 seconds (0.25 Hz) (Fig. 2A). This component is dominant during resting conditions and in the supine position [16, 20] or during sleep (Fig. 6A) [20]. It disappears by pharmacological vagotomy, independent of body position [16]. Its amplitude is unchanged by intravenously beta blockage during resting conditions. This

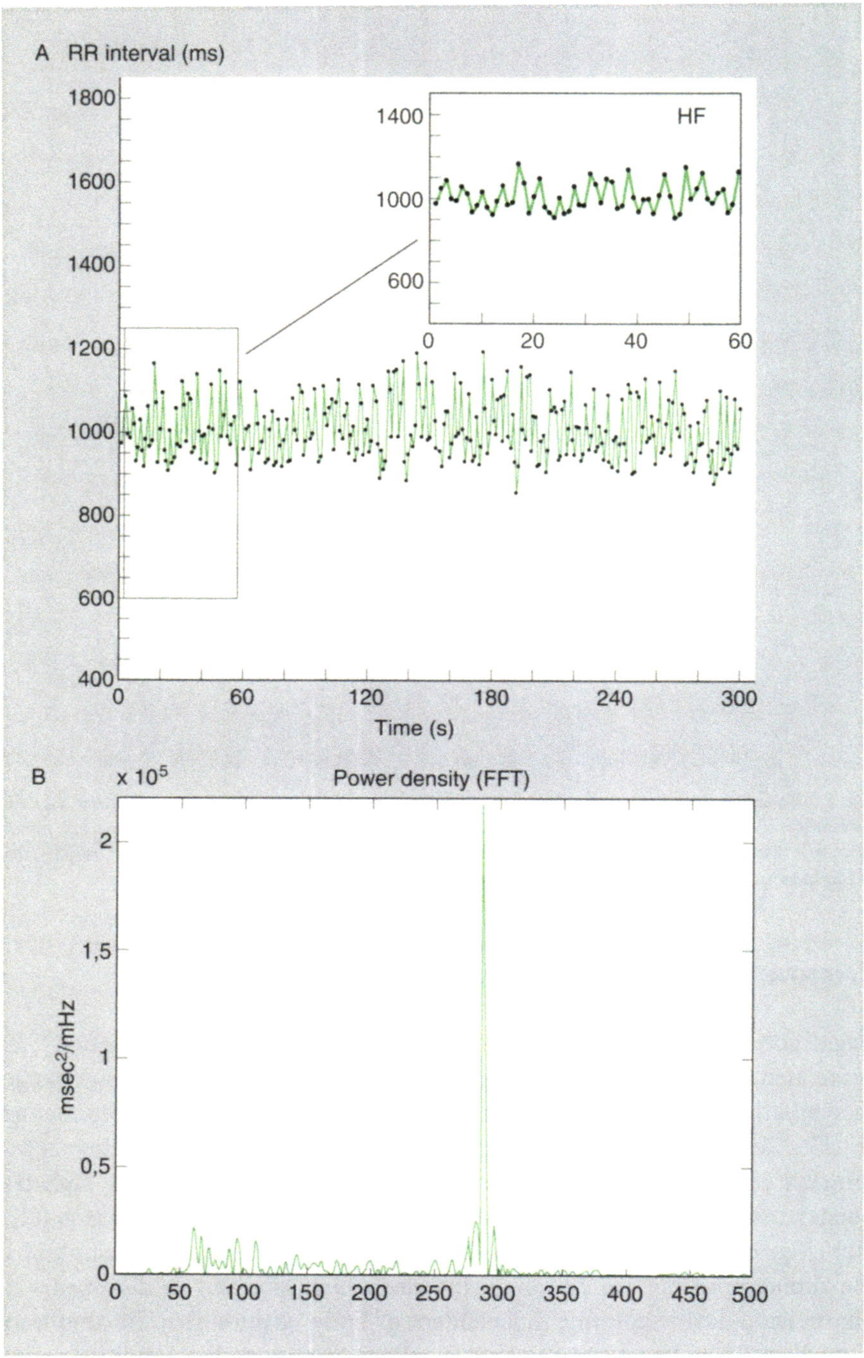
A RR interval (ms)
1800
1600
1400
1200
1000
800
600
400
0
60
120
180
240
300
Time (s)
1400
HF
1000
600
0
20
40
60
B
x 10^5
Power density (FFT)
2
1,5
1
0,5
0
msec²/mHz
0
50
100
150
200
250
300
350
400
450
500

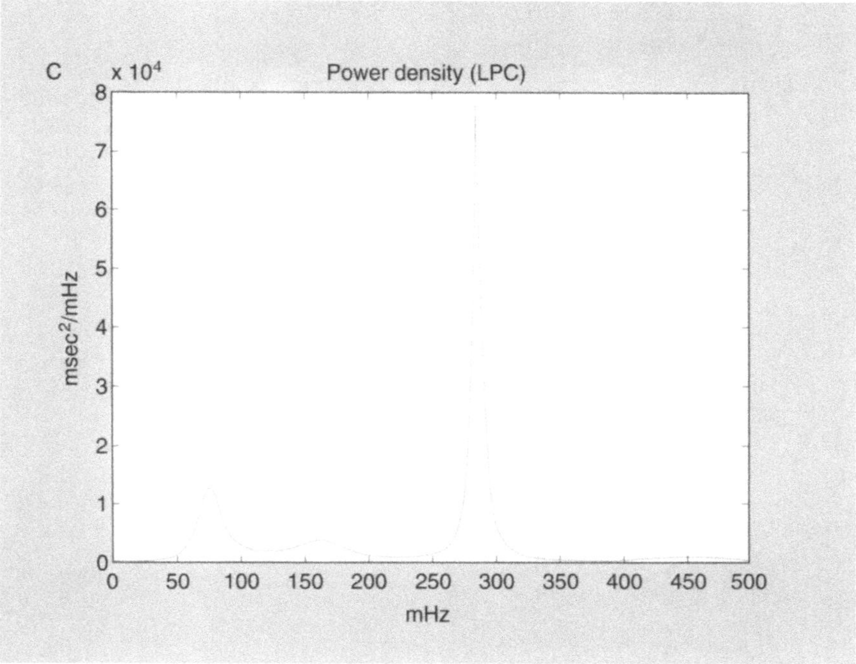

Fig. 2 A: RR interval variations in a healthy subject during sleep. The RR interval variations are dominated by a high frequency (HF) oscillations as shown in the insert. This is the respiratory-dependent vagally-mediated sinus arrhythmia. B and C show the result of a spectral analysis based on the time series shown in A. In B, an FFT technique has been used, and in C, an autoregressive technique (LPC). Both power density curves identify a large peak at 0.25 – 0.35 Hz (HF component). Additionally a low frequency oscillation (centre frequency 0.06 – 0.1 Hz), but of much less power, is identified

is the so-called respiratory dependent sinus arrhythmia which is completely mediated by vagal activity. The intensity, or amplitude, of this component is linearly related to vagal tone. In the frequency domain description of HP oscillations, this component is designated the high frequency component (HF). Its centre frequency is around 0.25 Hz (0.15 – 0.40 Hz), cross correlating to the respiratory frequency (15 cycles/min = 0.25 Hz) [29, 30]. The second short-term variability component is a relatively low frequency oscillation, initially called the Mayer wave [31], now designated the LF component. It has an average cycle-time of approximately 10 seconds (0.1 Hz) (Fig. 3A). This component is mediated by an interaction of sympathetic and vagal activity and is dependent on baroreceptor reflex activity [16, 19]. In the supine position, it is mostly mediated by vagal activity, whereas in the upright

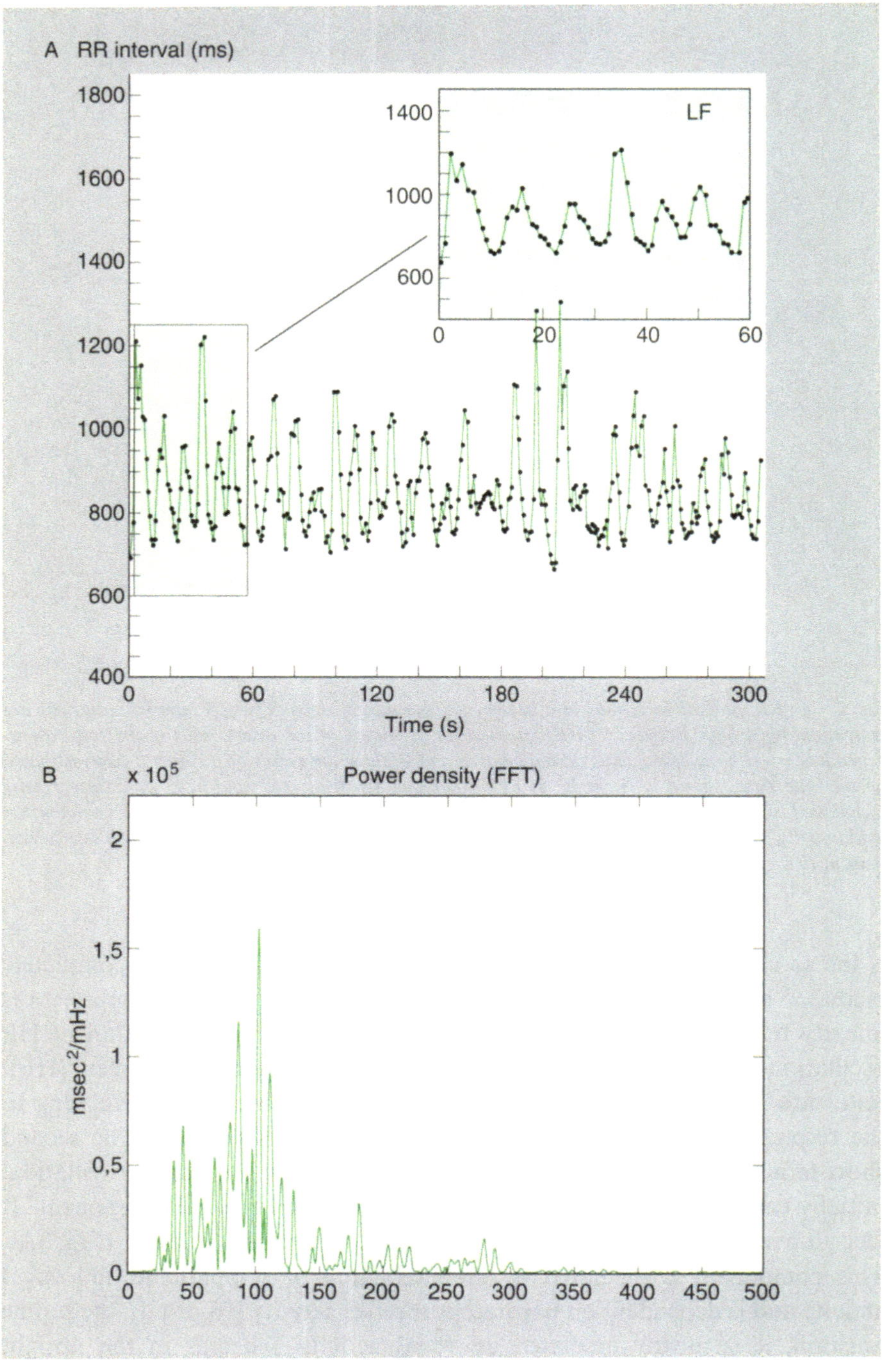
A RR interval (ms)
1800
1600
1400
1200
1000
800
600
400
0
60
120
180
240
300
Time (s)
1400
LF
1000
600
0
20
40
60
B
x 10^5
Power density (FFT)
msec^2/mHz
2
1,5
1
0,5
0
0
50
100
150
200
250
300
350
400
450
500

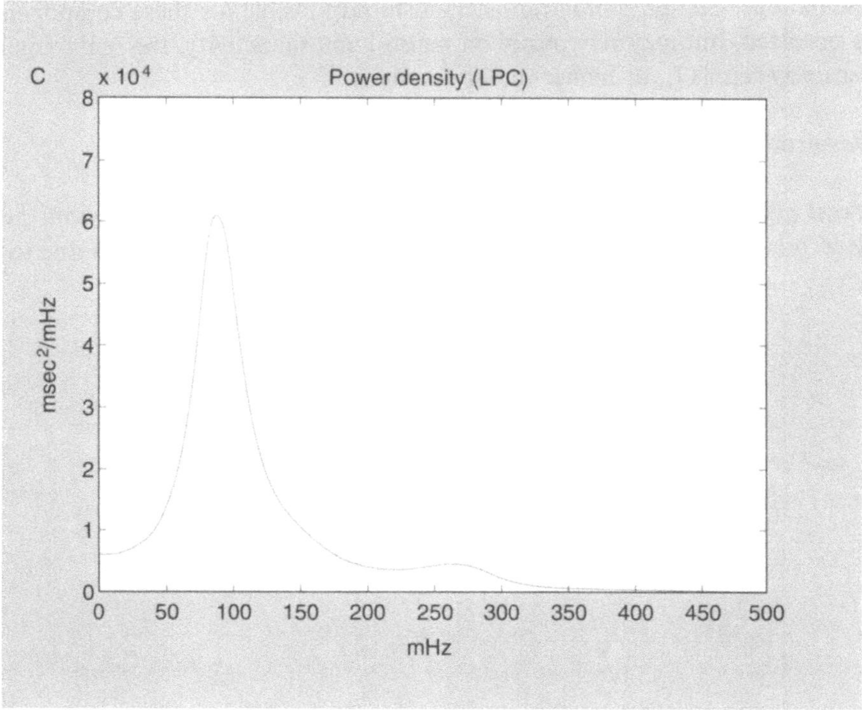

Fig. 3 A: RR interval variations for a 5-minute period, in a healthy subject during daytime. The insert shows the typical low frequency oscillation (LF), which is dominating. B and C show the result of a spectral analysis based on the time series shown in A. In B, an FFT technique has been used, and in C, an autoregressive technique (LPC). Both power density curves show a large peak around 0.1 Hz (LF component), whereas only the autoregressive density curve identifies a significant high frequency component (0.25 Hz)

position, its intensity is highly reduced by intravenously beta blockage, indicating its dependence on sympathetic activity [19]. Sympathetic activity only mediates HP variations in the frequency-band of 0.0 – 0.15 Hz, but isolation of a parameter which estimates pure sympathetic activity has not been accomplished so far.

The above two components can be measured reliably in HP recordings of 5 minutes in length. In recordings of longer duration (up to 24 hours), more low frequency components with cycle-times of minutes to hours (<0.04 Hz) can be identified (32 – 34). They are arbitrarily described as very low frequency (VLF; 0.04 – 0.003 Hz) and ultra low frequency (ULF; <0.0033 Hz) [34]. The general circadian variation in mean HP level (the difference between day and night in mean HP) makes an important contribution to these ULF oscillations. The physiological mechanism responsible for these components is unsolved, but may rely partly on neuro-humoral activity, the renin-angiotensin system [17], or higher cerebral activity.

Respiration and HP variability

Vagal efferent activity is linked to respiration [26, 29]. In spontaneous and deep breathing, the increase in HR during the inspiratory phase, is due to a

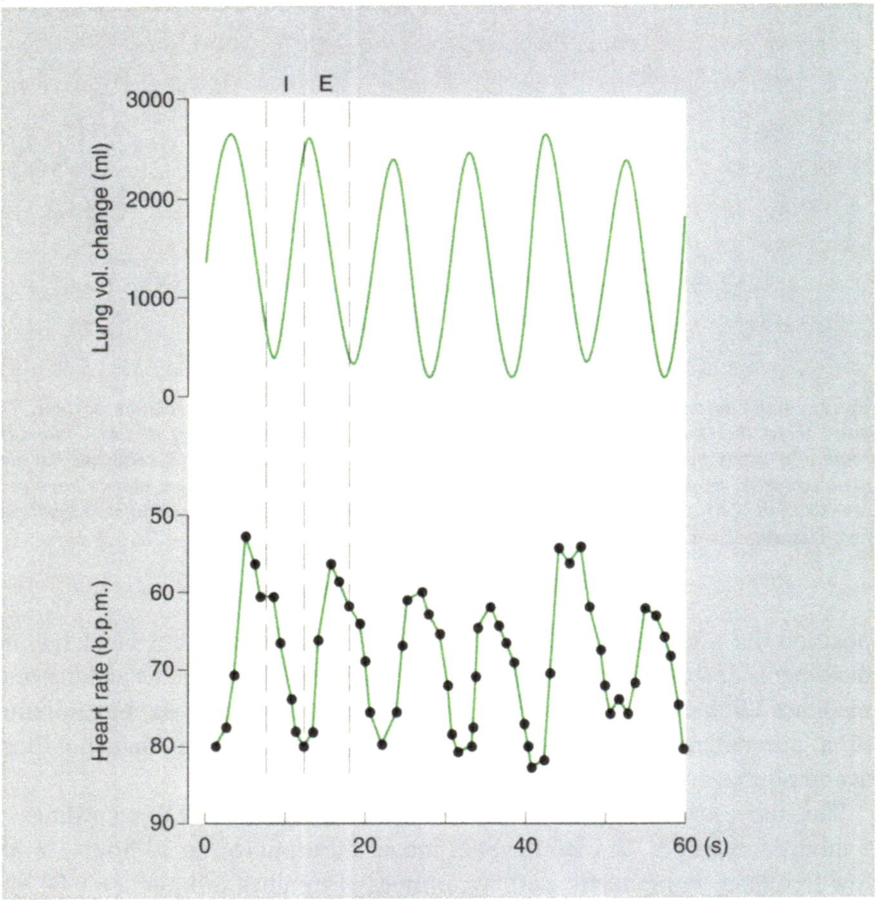

Fig. 4 Relationship between the respiratory phases (inspiration(I) and expiration (E)) and heart rate variations during deep breathing (6/min), in a healthy subject. Lung volume change is calculated according to breast and abdominal movements (Re-drawn from Lawrence et al; Br Heart J 1992 [47])

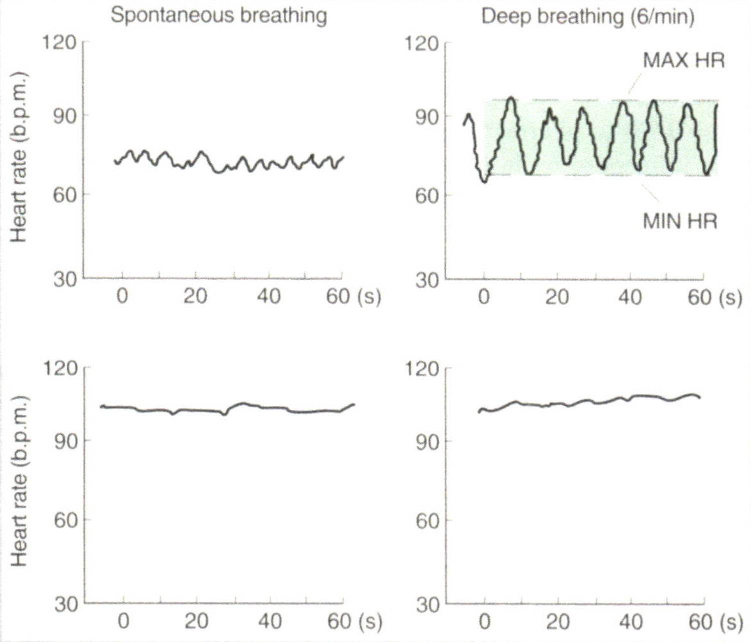

Fig. 5 Heart rate variability during spontaneous-and deep-breathing in two diabetic patients of similar age and diabetes duration. The patient in the upper panel has normal vagal function whereas the patient in the lower panel has severe vagal neuropathy. Vagal function is estimated by the IE difference = maximum HR − minimum HR, during deep breathing. (Re-drawn from Masaoka et al; Diabetes Care 1985 [49])

cessation of vagal activity [25, 35]. Vagal firing takes place in the expiratory phase. The decrease in HR is relatively abruptly and starts early in the expiratory phase and may continue within the following inspiratory phase (Fig. 4, 5). This is usually seen most clearly during deep breathing. Cooling of the vagal nerve or blocking the muscarinic receptor by atropine abolishes the respiratory-dependent sinus arrhythmia completely [26] Maximal efferent vagal activity is obtained at slow respiratory frequencies. In healthy subjects, maximal peak-valley HR (Fig. 4, 5) is observed at respiratory rates of 6/

minute. However, in patients maximal values may be observed at a lower respiratory rate [36]. The tidal volume is less important than the respiratory rate [26].

Vagal tone can be quantitated by measuring the effect of total pharmacological vagotomy – that is, the difference in mean HP before and after completely blockade by atropine [35, 37, 38]. However, peak valley variation in instantaneous HP during fixed spontaneous respiration correlates very highly (r = 0.95) to pharmacologically determined vagal tone. This association is not influenced by intravenously beta blockage [37]. Therefore, vagal tone can be estimated non-invasively by quantitating the degree of sinus arrhythmia. During standardised resting circumstances, this may be accomplished by measuring the difference in maximal and minimal HR within a respiratory cycle [38] (Fig. 4, 5). This is the background for the most often used bed-side test, the inspiratory-expiratory (IE) difference during deep breathing (Fig. 5). Other indexes which quantitate the sinus arrhythmia in the time- and frequency-domain, also correlates highly with vagal tone [38].

ECG sampling techniques

Recordings of short ECG segments (1 – 5 minutes) for deep breathing test, tilt testing or resting conditions, may rely on ordinarily ECG amplifiers. Uni- or bipolar leads may be used. Leads which generally have a high mono-phasic R-wave is preferable. Electrodes should be placed anteriorly on the shoulders, which reduces muscular noise during breathing test. The ECG should be digitally sampled to a computer at 1000 Hz. The QRS detection algorithm should be insensitive to baseline shifts and changes in amplitude of the QRS complex, which occur during deep breathing. In this way, RR intervals may be detected with a precision of 1 – 2 ms. Omission of segments containing ectopic beats or AV block is mandatory. Ideally, the recorded RR intervals should visualised in time (Fig. 5). This allows easy identification of i. e., missed or ectopic beats. For the deep breathing test, the HP fluctuations for each respiratory cycle may be compared in order to assure that a homogeneous respiratory pattern was followed. Most investigators produce their own software for sampling, editing and calculation; this is relatively simple. The analysis system should be tested by artificially produced QRS complexes with known HP, and/or by manual comparison of recorded RR intervals and measured RR intervals in a simultaneous high speed ECG printout.

24-hour ECG recordings offer the advantage of studying autonomic function during ambulatory conditions, and its circadian variation [20, 39]. Standardised conditions can be obtained by investigation of separate sleep-time. The 24-hour RR interval files may be investigated in toto [32–34], however, most investigators divide the file into consecutive 5 minutes segments which are analysed separately.

Only tape-based, 24-hour Holter recording systems have been used so far for 24-hour HP variability analysis. Although these systems have some drawbacks compared to solid state systems (tape speed problems) [32, 40], their basic QRS algorithms etc., have been extensively validated. HP variability is based on files of normal RR intervals which have been produced by ordinary Holter recording and QRS detection systems. The final editing and variability analysis is performed by nearly all research groups using their own software. Holter systems consists of a tape recorder, replay- and QRS detection/classification-unit. Replay is performed at around 60 times real time. Acquisition of RR interval data may be accomplished in several ways: (1) Direct analog-digital conversion of the recorded ECG signal [20]. This, however, requires development of software for subsequent QRS and arrhythmia detection. (2) Sampling of triggers for identified QRS complexes and arrhythmias as detected by the Holter analyser, and subsequent classification, supplementary editing, and measurement of RR intervals [15, 34, 40]. 3) Complete HP variability analysis by a commercially available Holter system [13, 14, 41]. For simple HP variability indexes, such as the St. George index [14] and the Ewing index for vagal activity [21, 42], this is a reliable method, because these indexes are relatively insensitive to artefacts. However, for other measurements of HP variability, it is not recommended.

Measurements are based on sinus rhythm-related RR intervals. RR intervals associated with arrhythmias, artefacts, and tape speed errors must, therefore, be identified and discharged. This is a key point to high quality variability data, since missed ectopic beats and dropped beats may impose a considerable error in variability calculations [32, 40]. All tapes must be preprocessed in order to identify the lead having the best signal quality. Furthermore, non-usable segments, due to artefacts or sustained arrhythmias, must be identified, and trigger levels must be optimally adjusted with regard to classification of ventricular and supraventricular ectopic beats. The prematurity index is often highly individual. After sampling, the classified RR intervals may be re-edited, particularly the longest and shortest intervals. During sampling or in the re-editing phase, simple algorithms should be used to remove RR intervals related to misclassified ectopic beats and missed beats: Discharge of RR intervals deviating more than -20 to -35% and $+20$ to $+65\%$ from the preceding interval. In young healthy subjects and diabetic patients nearly all beat to beat variations are within $+35\%$ to -65%, whereas in patients with overt heart disease, a cut-off threshold of +/−20% may be more appropriate [15, 43].

Correct determination of RR interval length and HP variability calculations also depends on overall and short-term speed stability of the recorder and replay unit [40]. This is important when dealing with the high frequency components of HP variability. Recording speed of tape recorder systems are only adjusted approximately. Instead, a timing track of 16−160 Hz [20, 32, 40] generated by a crystal, is recorded onto the tape. This signal is phase-locked with a similar signal in the replay unit in order to continuously adjust speed to i. e., 60 times real time. This ensures a mean recorded RR level very close to true mean RR [40]. However, as these systems are dependent on mechanical systems which corrects replay speed, some short-term speed variability is inevitable. Ideally, these variations can be omitted by sampling of the RR intervals together with the timing track, and then correcting each interval accordingly [32]. This is, however, complicated. The addition of a speed surveyor system, which provides an error signal when the phase-locked-loop can not adjust appropriately, is sufficient [20, 40]. It's recommended to test the overall accuracy of RR interval detection of the recorder and analysis system used by analysis of 24-hour test tapes, into which artificially QRS complexes with known RR interval durations have been fed [40].

Deep breathing test

This test estimates vagal function during standardised conditions. The circumstances during which the test is performed and control of respiratory rate is important. Interpretation of the result must take into account age, physical training level, and the presence of coronary heart disease and its complications.

The test should be performed in the morning between eight and ten a.m., during a period of stable glucose control in a quiet non-stressed atmosphere after 10−15 minutes of resting. Whether or not breakfast and insulin may influence the result has not been separately addressed. It is suggested that the test be performed 1 hour after eating. The patient, however, should be fasting with regard to smoking and caffeine, which may cause an increased catecholamine level. Infusion of isoproterenol increases mean heart rate and reduces HP variability significantly [44]. Drugs which may affect autonomic balance should be withdrawn before testing (oral beta blockers [45], ACE-inhibitors, cardiac glucosides, anticholinergics, sympathomimetics). The patient should have stable sinus rhythm and no history suggestive of sinus node disease.

Theoretically, vagal activity should be highest in the lying position. However, results obtained in the sitting position are not significantly different, separating diabetics patients equally well and having identical reproducibility [46, 47]. The sitting position is more practical, as the patient can observe a screen displaying the required respiratory pattern. A respiratory rate of 6 respiratory cycles per minute (5 seconds inspiration and 5 seconds expiration) is associated with maximal HR difference [26, 36], and is widely used [46–49). However, maximum HR difference may be obtained in some patients with evident autonomic neuropathy at lower respiratory rates [36]. Ideally, the individual's optimum respiratory rate should be identified. The respiratory cycles to be used can be displayed on a screen [44, 47]. Deep breathing should be performed for one minute, and the calculation based on these 6 respiratory cycles. Deep breathing for longer than 1 minute may feel uncomfortable, and reduce compliance. Although shorter periods may not give significantly different results, in some studies [50], one minute of data allows discharge of invalid respiratory cycles. The test should be performed twice with a 10-minute rest in between, and the highest value of the 2 tests used as result. Variability in respiratory pattern is a main source of poor reproducibility [47]. Therefore, careful instruction is important. Compliance may be tested by displaying the measured RR interval series in time [49].

The highest and lowest HR or HP in each respiratory cycle is measured and the mean difference of 6 cycles calculated, expressed as either the mean inspiratory-expiratory (IE) difference, in b.p.m., or the expiratory-inspiratory difference, in ms. The IE difference is used most often. Large data bases of normal values in healthy subjects and diabetic patients exist for reference [48, 49]. The reproducibility (coefficient of variation) of the test is 10–15% [44, 47]. Each laboratory should establish its own reproducibility data. This facilitates the identification of poor test or analysis procedures.

The IE difference decays by increasing age [48]. Other indexes of vagal function are highly dependent on physical training level. Physically trained individuals have higher basic vagal activity during rest and sleep [39]. This association should also be considered when applying the deep breathing test. In diabetic patients with overt heart disease, differences in IE difference may well be caused by the heart disease. Coronary heart disease is associated with a generally reduced vagal function [43, 51]. Patients who have survived a myocardial infarction have disturbed autonomic balance for at least 3 months after the infarction [12, 52], and severe heart failure is associated with reduced vagal activity [53].

24-hour HP variability

This method allows evaluation of components of autonomic function other than vagal activity. Measurements are based on spontaneously HP variations during ambulatory conditions. Basically, the techniques used to estimate autonomic activity, both in the time- and frequency-domain, are identical to those used in short ECG segments, during standardised conditions [18, 19]. Comparison of 24-hour indices of vagal activity and ordinary batteries of bed-side tests, including the deep breathing test, strongly indicate that the 24 hour measurements are more sensitive in detecting the early diabetic autonomic neuropathy [4, 21, 22, 54]. Additionally, the method allows investigation of changes in the circadian modulation of the sympathovagal balance [4, 20, 39, 54]. This may prove important for the understanding of the temporal onset of cardiovascular disease in diabetic patients [4, 54]. The prognostic value of HP variability in relation to sudden cardiac death is associated to indices of 24-hour overall variability [13–15, 34].

Recordings should take place during stable glucose control. Information regarding smoking and leisure-time physical activity are important since these factors significantly influence HP variability [39, 55, 56]. Information regarding sleeping time is needed, because this part may be analysed separately. As for the deep breathing test, the impact of drugs must be omitted.

Quantification of HP oscillations is done by two different methods. The first of these is a simple model which measures variations in the time-domain. Most of these parameters are resistant to sampling errors and easy to calculate. The second method uses an advanced model which looks at the instantaneous HP oscillations in the frequency domain, by which the frequency and intensity of the dominant HP oscillations are determined. Theoretically, these measurements are more directly related to nervous activity [57]. So far, there is no consensus on precise sampling standards and calculation algorithms, which makes direct comparisons of data between various research groups difficult. Its is, therefore, recommended to establish one's own reproducibility data and normal values. A summary of the most frequently used parameters and their relation to autonomic function is given in Table 1.

Time domain characteristics are statistical descriptions of the variations in instantaneous HP. The prognostic value of HP variability for patients with coronary disease with regard to arrhythmic death, is related to overall variability during a 24-hour period [14, 15, 34]. Overall variability is measured by the 24-hour standard deviation. This is a broad-band measure of auto-

Table 1 Definitions of commonly used time-and frequency-domain measures of 24-hour heart period variability and their relation to autonomic activity. Figures shown in brackets refer to references containing more detailed describtion

Variable	unit	A. A.	Definition
Time-domain			
24-hour SD (43,39)	ms	S/PS	Standard deviation of all normal RR intervals in the entire 24-hour recording around mean RR.
24-hour HPV index (St. George C) (41,13)	none	S/PS	Baseline width of main modus of RR interval distribution curve on discrete time scale. (Total number of normal RR intervals/number in peak column)
Day-night difference (39)	ms	S/PS	The difference between mean RR day and mean RR night.
RMSSD	ms	PS	Root mean square of successive differences in consequtive RR intervals.
% DIF50 (42,21)	%	PS	Percent successive RR interval differences exceeding 50 ms. May also be given as a count. Count should be related to number of RR interval differences to account for differences in analysed time.
% DIF6 % (42,21)	%	PS	Percent succesive RR interval differences exceeding 6%. May also be given as a count as % DIF50.
*Frequency-Domain**			
Total power (33,34)	ms^2	S/PS	The total energy in the heart period power spectrum from 0.0 – 0.4 Hz (Area under curve). Its squared value corresponds to the 24-hour SD.
Low frequency (LF) power(16,19)	ms^2	S/(PS)	The energy in the heart period power spectrum between 0.04 and 0.15 Hz. The Mayer wave.
High frequency (HF) (16,19)	ms^2	PS	The energy in the heart period power spectrum from 0.15 to 0.40 Hz. The respiratory dependent sinus arrhythmia.
Coefficient of component variance of LF (38)	%	S/(PS)	Low frequency power divided by mean RR. (squareroot of LF power/mean RR).
Coefficient of component variance of HF (38)	%	PS	High frequency power divided by mean RR (squarerrot of HF power/mean RR).
Normalized LF power(19,38)	%	?	(LF power / total power – the DC component) *100. DC-components = Power of spectral components < 0.04 Hz.
Normalized HF power (19,38)	%	?	(HF power / total power – the DC component) *100.

Spectral power can be measured both by *autoregressive [19, 38] and Fast Fourier Transform (FFT) [16, 33] analysis. A.A.: type of Autonomic activity estimated by variable. S = Sympathetic activity. PS = Parasympathetic activity

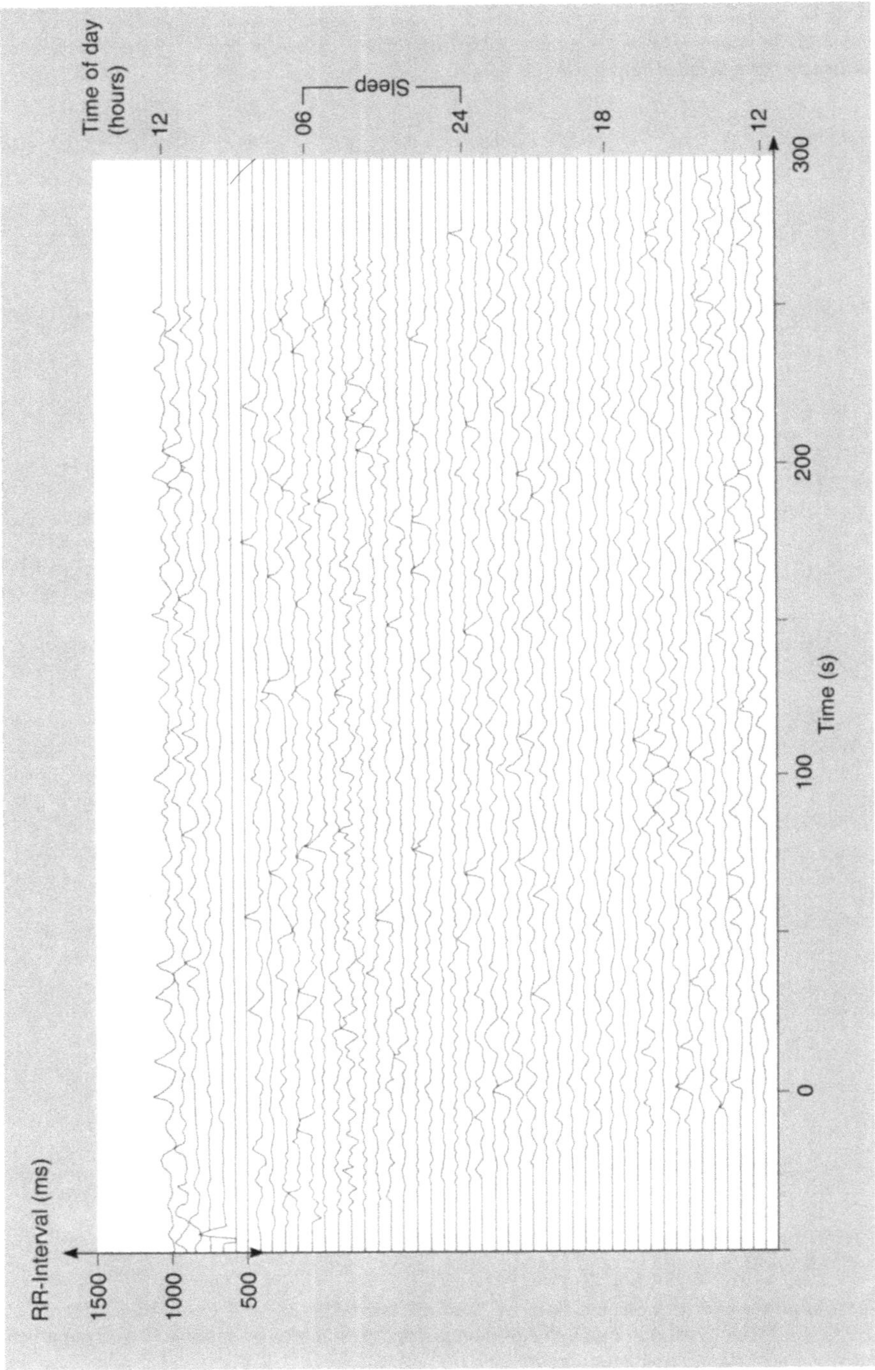
RR-Interval (ms)
1500
1000
500
Time of day (hours)
12
06
24
18
12
Sleep
0
100
200
300
Time (s)

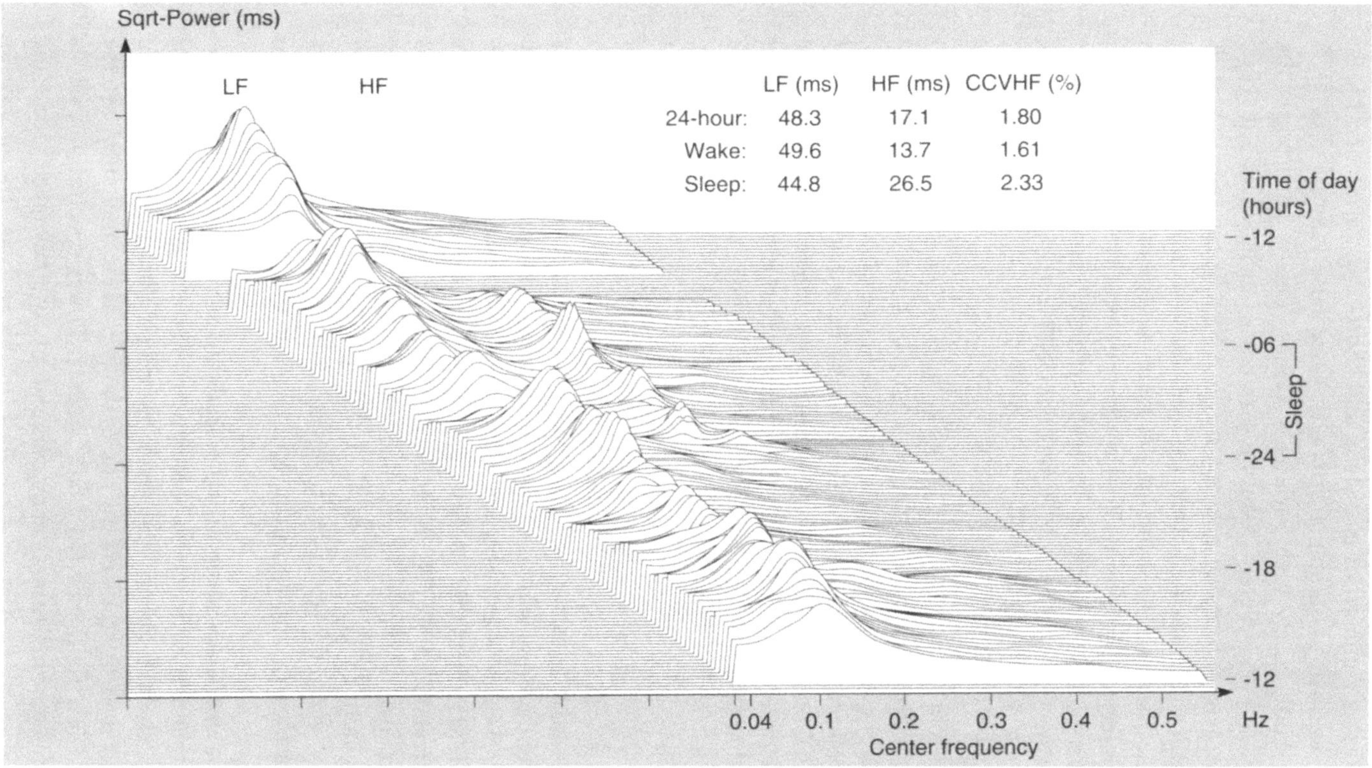

Fig. 6 Frequency domain characteristics of RR interval variability during a 24-hour period in a healthy subject A: 24-hour RR interval variations, shown for consecutive 300-second segments. For practical reasons, only 300-second RR interval variations (one horizontal curve) for each half hour, is shown. The time of day is indicated on the right y-axis from 12:00 (noon) to 12:00 the next day. During sleep, vagal-dependent high frequency oscillations (HF, 0.25 Hz) become prominent. The low frequency oscillation (LF, 0.1 Hz) is dominant during daytime. The RR interval series shown has been pre-processed for spectral analysis (time equidistant sampled, interpolated, removal of DC component, etc.). B: The result of the spectral analysis (autoregressive), showing the dynamic changes in power (squaewroot) of the HF and LF component throughout the 24 hours. The vagal-dependent HF component has peak values in the early morning hours, whereas the sympathetic-dependent LF component has peak values before midday

nomic activity, as it summarises both long and short-term variability. Measurements are sensitive to sampling artefacts, since false long or short RR intervals may cause falsely high variability values. This is particularly the case for patients with severely reduced variability, such as i. e., diabetic patients with severe autonomic neuropathy. The St. George indices [41] of overall variability is, however, generally insensitive to sampling artefacts. They determine the baseline width of the main modus in the distribution curve of RR intervals. Index C [13, 41], which is most frequently used, is, additionally, very easy to calculate. Several parameters estimate pure vagal activity: The RMSSD and threshold counts. RMSSD – the root mean square of successive RR interval differences, is insensitive to trends in mean RR. However, values are very sensitive to sampling errors, because the error is squared. Threshold counts were first introduced by Ewing [42]. These counts quantitate vagal-dependent short-term variability by measuring the incidence of larger changes (> 50 ms, or relatively > 6%) in successive RR intervals. A relative threshold is preferable since it makes the count independent of mean RR level. Counts should be given as percentage of available RR interval differences, in order to correct for differences in recording length. Recent data indicate that threshold counts are more sensitive than ordinary batteries of bed-side tests to detect early diabetic autonomic neuropathy [4, 21, 42], because 20–30% of patients with normal cardiovascular tests have count values below normal limits for healthy subjects. Additionally, all patients with abnormal bed-side tests have very low counts. Threshold counts are easy to measure and relatively insensitive to artefact. The interindividual variation is very large ranging from 0.01% in diabetic patients with severe autonomic neuropathy to 50% in young healthy physically well-trained subjects [4, 39]. Values of RMSSD, threshold counts and the power of the high frequency component correlate closely [58]. Additionally, these parameters may be used to monitor circadian variation in vagal activity as they may be computed in 5 minutes to 1 hour ECG segments [4, 21, 22]. The intraindividual variation or day to day variation (coefficient of variation) is 7% for the 24-hour standard deviation [59] and approximately 15% for threshold counts.

Frequency domain characteristics of HP variability are measurements of the frequency content in the RR interval oscillations. The analysis (power spectral analysis) does basically identify the main "melodies" (centre frequency) and quantitate their intensity (power). In Fig. 6, the two main "melodies" are the high (HF) and low frequency (LF) components. Power spectral analysis is based on complicated mathematical models and involves advanced processing of the RR interval time series to make them fit the analysis. The processing can be performed several ways [16, 19, 38] and contains many pitfalls. No commercially available software has been sufficiently validated and there are no agreed recommendations. Accordingly, most research groups have developed their own techniques in close collaboration with technological institutions.

High-quality RR interval files are important. Invalid RR intervals due to artefacts and ectopic beats are interpolated [60]. Interpolation of more than 20–30% of a 5-minute segment may interfere with the power spectrum [60, 61]. Spectral analysis requires that time series data are equidistantly sampled along the time axis. RR interval data inherently lack this equidistant character because each datum occurs whenever an QRS complex is detected. Files of RR intervals must, therefore, be time-equidistant sampled at 2–4 Hz. Several additional steps, including removal of the DC component, antialiasing, downsampling, high-pass filtering and Hamming weighing, are needed before the file can be entered into the spectral analysis. Fig. 6A shows the processed RR interval file from a 24-hour ECG recording.

Spectral analysis can be based on autoregressive (parametric) and Fast Fourie Transform (FFT) (non-parametric) analysis [38]. Figures 2B, C and 3B, C show the power spectrum of the two methods. The autoregressive technique detects the centre frequencies more precisely and gives a smoother spectral estimation [19, 61]. Two spectral components are seen: The HF component (centre frequency 0.15–0.25 Hz) and the LF component (centre frequency 0.04–0.15 Hz). The intensity of the two components are given as power (ms^2/mHz). However, to improve the quantification of the HF component, which becomes affected early in the course of the neuropathy, many investigators use the square root of power (ms/mHz), which enhances small figures. The square root of the power of the HF component (area under curve) is proportional, linearly, to vagal activity [38]. The power of the LF oscillation is dependent on the sympathetic-vagal interaction [16].

In 5-minute RR interval segments it is only possible to measure components in the frequency band, 0.04–0.4 Hz. Spectral energy at frequencies < 0.03 Hz are considered DC components (noise). However, the 24-hour RR interval file may be analysed in toto [32, 33], allowing estimation of the very low frequency components – VLF (0.0033–0.04 Hz) and ULF (< 0.0033 Hz). The day/night difference in mean RR, in the time-domain, is a simple measure of very low frequency HP oscillations. The total power spectral energy within the whole frequency band (0.0 to 0.4 Hz) is a summarisation of ULF, VLF, LF and HF spectral energy. More than 80% of the energy is related to the ULF and VLF components. The square root of the total power spectral energy corresponds theoretically and practically to the 24-hour standard deviation. For mathematical reasons, the power of the HF and LF components in absolute values, will, to some degree, be dependent on mean RR level. The coefficient of component variance (square root of power of component/mean RR) corrects for this (Table 1). However, the sensitivity of this index in relation to vagal activity is poorer (small slope-vagal activity versus index) [38], and may make an overcorrection, since differences in mean RR level are also due to differences in vagal tone.

Investigations of the diabetic autonomic neuropathy by 24-hour heart period variability must take into account the effects of sex, age, smoking and physical training level [39, 56]. Furthermore, the influence of coronary heart disease and its complications on autonomic function, must be considered.

References

[1] Ewing DJ. Cardiac autonomic neuropathy. In: Jarrett, ed. Diabetes and heart disease. Elsevier Science Publishers B.V., 1984; 99–132.

[2] Dyrberg T, Benn J, Christiansen JS et al. Prevalence of diabetic autonomic neuropathy measured by simple bedside tests. Diabetologia 1981; 20: 190–194.

[3] O'Brien IAD, O'Hare JP, Lewin IG et al. The prevalence of autonomic neuropathy in insulin dependent diabetes mellitus: A controlled study based on heart rate variability. Quart J Med 1986; 61: 957–967.

[4] Mølgaard H, Christensen PD, Sørensen KE et al. Association of 24-hour Cardiac parasympathetic activity and degree of nephropathy in insulin-dependent diabetic patients. Diabetes 1992; 41: 812–817.

[5] Neil HA, Thompson AV, John S et al. Diabetic autonomic neuropathy: the prevalence of impaired heart rate variability in a geographically defined population. Diabetic Med 1989; 6: 20–24.

[6] Ewing DJ, Campbell IW, Clarke BF. Mortality in diabetic autonomic neuropathy. Lancet 1976; I: 601–603.

[7] Ewing DJ, Campbell IW, Clarke BF. Assessment of cardiovascular effects in diabetic autonomic neuropathy and prognostic implications. Ann Int Med 1980; 92: 308–311.

[8] Sampson MJ, Wilson S, Karagiannis P et al. Progression of diabetic autonomic neuropathy over a decade in insulin-dependent diabetics. Quart J Med 1990; 75: 635–646.

[9] Winocour PH, Dhar H, Anderson DC. The relationship between autonomic neuropathy and urinary sodium and albumin excretion in insulintreated diabetics. Diabetic medicine 1986; 3: 436–440.

[10] Page MMcB, Watkins PJ. Cardiorespiratory arrest and diabetic autonomic neuropathy. Lancet 1978; I: 14–16.

[11] Billman G, Schwartz PJ, Stone HL. Baroreceptor reflex control of heart rate: A predictor of sudden cardiac death. Circulation 1982; 66: 874–880.

[12] Bigger JT, Kleiger RE, Fleiss JL et al. Components of heart rate variability measured during healing of acute myocardial infarction. Am J Cardiol 1988; 61: 208–215.

[13] Cripps TR, Malik M, Farrell TG et al. Prognostic value of reduced heart rate variability after myocardial infarction: Clinical evaluation of a new analysis method. Br Heart J 1991; 65: 14–19.

[14] Farrell TG, Bashir Y, Cripps T et al. Risk stratification for arrhythmic events in postinfarction patients based on heart rate variability, ambulatory electrocardiographic variables and the signal averaged electrocardiogram. JACC 1991; 18: 687–697.

[15] Kleiger RE, Miller JP, Bigger JT et al. Decreased heart rate variability and its association with increased mortality after acute myocardial infarction. Am J Cardiol 1987; 59: 256–262.
[16] Pomeranz B, Macaulay RJB, Caudill MA et al. Assessment of autonomic function in humans by heart rate spectral analysis. Am J Physiol 1985; 248: H151-H153.
[17] Akselrod S, Gordon D, Andrew Ubel F et al. Power spectrum anaysis of heart rate fluctuation: A quatitative probe of beattobeat cardiovascular control. Science 1981; 213: 220–222.
[18] Bianchi A, Bontempi B, Cerutti S et al. Spectral analysis of heart rate variability signal and respiration in diabetic subjects. Med Biol Eng Comput 1990; 28: 205–211.
[19] Pagani M, Lombardi F, Guzzetti S et al. Power spectral analysis of heart rate and arterial pressure variabilities as a marker of sympatho-vagal interaction in man and conscious dog. Circ Res 1986; 59: 178–193.
[20] Furlan R, Guzzetti S, Crivellaro W et al. Continous 24-hour assessment of the neural regulation of systemic arterial pressure and RR variabilities in ambulant subjects. Circulation 1990; 81: 537–547.
[21] Ewing DJ, Neilson JM, Shapiro CM et al. Twenty four hour heart rate variability: Effects of posture, sleep, and time of day in healthy controls and comparison with bedside tests of autonomic function in diabetic patients. Br Heart J 1991; 65: 239–244.
[22] Malpas SC, Maling TJ. Heartrate variability and cardiac autonomic function in diabetes. Diabetes 1990; 39: 1177–1181.
[23] Hales S. Statistical essays. In: Haemastaticks. London: Innings and Manby, 1973:
[24] Kent KM, Cooper T. The denervated heart. A model for studying autonomic control of the heart. N Engl J Med 1974; 291: 1017–1021.
[25] Katona PG, Poitras JW, Barnett GO et al. Cardiac vagal efferent activity and heart period in the carotid sinus reflex. Am J Physiol 1970; 218: 1030–1037.
[26] Eckberg DL. Human sinus arrhythmia as an index of vagal cardiac outflow. J Appl Physiol 1983; 54: 961–966.
[27] Katona PG, Jih F. Respiratory sinus arrhythmia: noninvasive measure of parasympathetic cardiac control. J Appl Physiol 1975; 39: 801–805.
[28] Rosenblueth A, Simeone FA. The interrelations of vagal and accelerator effects on the cardiac rate. Am J Physiol 1934; 110: 42–55.
[29] Ahmed AK, Harness JB, Mearns AJ. Respiratory control of heart rate. Eur J Appl Physiol 1982; 50: 95–104.
[30] Bernardi L, Rossi M, Soffiantiono F et al. Cross correlation of heart rate and respiration versus deep breathing. Diabetes 1989; 38: 589–596.
[31] Penáz J. Mayer waves: History and methodology. Automedica 1978; 2: 135–141.
[32] Saul JP, Albrecht P, Berger RD et al. Analysis of long term heart rate variability: Methods, 1/f scaling and implications. Comput Cardiol 1987; 14: 419–422.
[33] Rottman JN, Steinman RC, Albrecht P et al. Efficient estimation of the heart period power spectrum suitable for physiological or pharmacological studies. Am J Cardiol 1990; 66: 1522–1524.
[34] Bigger JT, Fleiss JL, Steinman RC et al. Frequency Domain Measures of heart period variability and mortality after myocardial infarction. Circulation 1992; 85: 164–171.
[35] Katona PG, Felix JIH. Respiratory sinus arrhythmia: A noninvasive measure of parasympathetic cardiac control. J Appl Physiol 1975; 39: 801–805.
[36] Watkins PJ, Mackay JD. Cardiac denervation in diabetic neuropathy. Ann Int Med 1980; 92 (2): 304–307.
[37] Fouad FM, Tarazi RC, Ferrario CM et al. Assessment of parasympathetic control of heart rate by a noninvasive method. Am J Physiol 1984; 246: H838-H842.
[38] Hayano J, Skakibara Y, Yamada A et al. Accuracy of assessment of cardiac vagal tone by heart rate variability in normal subjects. Am J Cardiol 1991; 67: 199–204.
[39] Mølgaard H, Sørensen KE, Bjerregaard P. Circadian variation and influence of risk factors on heart rate variability in healthy subjects. Am J Cardiol 1991; 68: 777–784.

[40] Mølgaard H. Evaluation of the Reynolds Pathfinder II system for 24-hour heart rate variability analysis. Eur Heart J 1991; 12: 1153–1162.
[41] Malik M, Farrell T, Cripps T et al. Heart rate variability in relation to prognosis after myocardial infarction: selection of optimal processing techniques. Eur Heart J 1989; 10: 1060–1074.
[42] Ewing DJ, Neilson JMM, Travis P. New method for assessing cardiac parasympathetic activity using 24-hour electrocardiograms. Br Heart J 1984; 52: 396–402.
[43] Bigger JT, Fleiss JL, Steinman RC et al. Correlation among time and frequency domain variables two weeks after acute myocardial infarction. Am J Cardiol 1992; 69: 891–898
[44] Pfeifer MA, Cook D, Brodsky J et al. Quantitative evaluation of cardiac parasympathetic activity in normal and diabetic man. Diabetes 1982; 31: 339–345.
[45] Mølgaard H, Mickley H, Pless P et al. Effects of Metoprolol on heart rate variability in survivors of acute myocardial infarction. Am J Cardiol 1993; 71: 1357–1359.
[46] Ewing DJ, Borsey DQ, Bellavere DQ et al. Cardiac autonomic neuropathy in diabetes: Comparison of measures of R-R interval variation. Diabetologia 1981; 21: 18–24.
[47] Lawrence GP, Home PD, Murray A. Repeatability of measurements and sources of variability in tests of cardiovascular autonomic function. Br Heart J 1992; 68: 205–211.
[48] Wieling W, Van Brederode JFM, De Rijk LG et al. Reflex control of heart rate in normal subjects in relation to age: A data base for cardiac vagal neuropathy. Diabetologia 1982; 22: 163–166.
[49] Masaoka S, Lev-Ran A, Robert Hill L et al. Heart rate variability in diabetes: Relationship to age and duration of the disease. Diabetes Care 1985; 8: 64–68.
[50] Mustonen J, Länsimies E, Uusitupa M et al. Testing of autonomic cardiovascular regulation-methodological considerations. Clin Physiol 1989; 9: 249–257.
[51] Eckberg DL, Drabinsky M, Braunwald E. Defective cardiac parasympathetic control in patients with heart disease. N Engl J Med 1971; 285: 877–883.
[52] Bigger JT, Fleiss JL, Rolnitzky LM et al. Time course of recovery of heart period variability after myocardial infarction. JACC 1991; 18: 1643–1649.
[53] Coats AJS, Adamopoulos S, Radaelli A et al. Controlled trial of physical training in chronic heart failure. Circulation 1992; 85: 2119–2131.
[54] Bernardi L, Ricordi L, Lazzari P et al. Impaired circadian modulation of sympathovagal activity in diabetes. Circulation 1992; 86: 1443–1452.
[55] Hayano J, Yamada M, Sakakibara Y et al. Short- and long-term effects of cigarette smoking on heart rate variability. Am J Cardiol 1990; 65: 84–88.
[56] Mølgaard H, Hermansen K, Bjerregaard P. Spectral components of short term RR interval variability in healthy subjects and effects of risk factors. (Submitted 1993)
[57] Malliani A, Pagani M, Lombardi M et al. Cardiovascular neural regulation explored in the frequency domain. Circulation 1991; 84: 482–492.
[58] Bigger JT, Albrecht P, Steinman RC et al. Comparison of time- and frequency-domain measures of cardiac parasympathetic activity in holter recordings after myocardial infarction. Am J Cardiol 1989; 64: 536–538.
[59] Huikuri HV, Kessler KM, Terracall E et al. Reproducibility and circadian rhythm of heart rate variability in healthy subjects. Am J Cardiol 1990; 65: 391–393.
[60] Albrecht P, Cohen RJ. Estimation of heart rate power spectrum bands from real-world data: Dealing with ectopic beats and noisy data. Comput Cardiol 1988; 15: 311–314.
[61] Mølgaard H, Hermansen K, Assentoft JE. A new method for estimation of 24-hour dynamics in cardiac autonomic activity. Eur Heart J 1992; 13 suppl: P1987, abstract.

Methodologies in sodium-lithium countertransport as related to other cation transport systems in diabetes

P. A. Rutherford, T. H. Thomas

Introduction

It became apparent from *in vivo* and *in vitro* studies of psychiatric patients receiving lithium therapy that there was a distinct cell membrane transport system capable of transporting lithium in and out of cells [1]. An elegant series of experiments demonstrated a bicarbonate-independent lithium transporter in the erythrocyte [2, 3]. Further kinetic analysis [4–6] confirmed this transport system mediated the electroneutral 1 : 1 monovalent transfer of sodium and lithium – sodium-lithium countertransport (SLC). This was an active transport system and the electro-chemical gradient for sodium which exists across the erythrocyte plasma membrane was sufficient to supply the energy needs.

SLC follows "ping-pong" kinetics, in which one ion binds to the transporter, is transported across the membrane then dissociates before the countertransported ion binds and is then transported across to the opposite side of the membrane [6, 7]. It is believed that *in vivo* the SLC system functions as a sodium : sodium exchanger [8].

The clinical relevance of sodium-lithium countertransport activity

It is difficult to perceive how an *in vivo* sodium : sodium exchanger could have any pathophysiological effects and it might have been expected that interest in SLC would have waned. However, stimulated by the interest in other erythrocyte cation transport systems in essential hypertension, clinical studies then demonstrated that SLC activity was increased in a proportion of patients with essential hypertension [9, 10]. Subsequent studies showed that SLC activity was affected by changes in plasma lipids [11, 12] and was temporarily increased during normal pregnancy [13]. A great deal of interest was aroused when evidence emerged that SLC activity was increased in type 1

Offprint from
Research Methodologies in Human Diabetes – Part 1

diabetic patients with diabetic nephropathy [14–16]. It has been proposed that erythrocyte SLC activity could be a marker in early diabetes for the future development of nephropathy.

However, other studies [17–19] have failed to confirm the association of increased SLC activity with diabetic nephropathy. This controversy highlights a major problem in the previous studies of SLC activity. There have been very few studies aiming to understand the physiology of the SLC transporter and *in vitro* effects that may explain the clinical correlates. Instead attention has been focussed on the measurement of SLC activity in various selected clinical populations.

It is important to understand the basic methods for measuring SLC activity *in vitro*, the effect of variation in experimental conditions on SLC activity and the serious limitations in the interpretation of results obtained by this method.

Techniques to measure sodium-lithium countertransport activity

Techniques are available to measure SLC activity by two methods. The most commonly used method (see below) is to measure sodium-stimulated lithium efflux from erythrocytes loaded to a high intra-cellular lithium concentration [9]. The other method measures lithium-stimulated sodium efflux [20] from erythrocytes. As SLC follows "ping-pong" kinetics the rate of movement of transport ions may be different depending on the direction of transport [7]. Thus, SLC activity measured by sodium-stimulated lithium efflux is higher than activity measured by lithium-stimulated sodium efflux. The latter method will be less precise and its only merit is that it can be used in a combined assay to measure Na-K co-transport and the sodium pump.

Both methods require the assessment of the passive ion fluxes to calculate SLC activity and movement of ions by other transporters must be inhibited e. g. ouabain to inhibit the sodium pump. The measurement of passive ion fluxes is particularly important, ideally a complete inhibitor of SLC activity would be used but at present no such inhibitor is available. Phloretin has been used in some studies [6, 21] but inhibition of SLC by phloretin is only partial [22, 23] and it undoubtedly has generalised effects on the plasma membrane. In the most commonly used method to measure SLC activity, sodium-stimulated lithium efflux, passive lithium efflux is measured using sodium-free media. Initially a magnesium-based medium was generally used but now most investigators used a sodium-free medium, choline [19] or potassium [24]. There is evidence that magnesium ions are not "inert" when used in techniques to measure the activity of other cation transport systems [25] and are best avoided.

Other experimental conditions need to be carefully controlled. SLC activity is temperature sensitive and activity rapidly decreases below 37 °C [26] with changes in the underlying kinetic determinants [27]. It is also important to ensure that the pH of all incubation media is 7.4 since SLC activity is pH sensitive (unpublished observations). Erythrocytes act as a powerful buffer so it is particularly important to control the pH if a low haematocrit in the incubation media is used.

Two methods are available to lithium load the erythrocytes for the lithium efflux assay – a prolonged (3 hours) incubation with lithium chloride [9] or a shorter incubation with either a mixture of lithium chloride and 10 mmol/l lithium carbonate [10] or isotonic lithium carbonate [18, 24]. In the lithium carbonate method lithium rapidly enters the erythrocyte through the anion exchanger. Both lithium carbonate methods are valid and any induced pH changes rapidly equilibrate as the assay proceeds. Nystatin has been used in lithium loading but there are reservations about this technique (see below).

Method for the measurement of the standard sodium-lithium countertransport activity

This is the description of an assay for the measurement of SLC activity at the standard external sodium concentration of 150 mmol/l used in previous studies of diabetic and non-diabetic patients [9–18]. It must be emphasised that at this external sodium concentration SLC activity is *not* maximal.

1. The choline and sodium media detailed below are prepared and their osmolality adjusted to 280 mOsm/kg.

Choline medium – 139 mmol/l choline chloride, 1 mmol/l $MgCl_2$, 10 mmol/l glucose.

Sodium medium – 150 mmol/l NaCl, 1 mmol/l $MgCl_2$, 10 mmol/l glucose.

These solutions and Tris-MOPS (1 molar) are stored as stock solutions at 4 °C. Each day the stock Tris-MOPS is adjusted to a pH of 7.55 at 37 °C and 1 ml Tris-MOPS is added to 100 ml of the choline and sodium medium. The final pH of the buffered solutions is 7.4 at 37 °C.

2. Venous blood is collected into tubes containing lithium heparin, centrifuged (5 minutes at 2000 g) and the erythrocytes are washed once in choline medium.

3. After centrifugation the erythrocytes are incubated at a haematocrit of 30–40% in lithium-loading solution (140 mmol/l LiCl, 10 mmol/l Li_2CO_3,

10 mmol/glucose, 10 mmol/l Tris-MOPS, gassed with 95% O_2/5% CO_2, pH 7.5, 290 ± 2 mosmol/kg) for 1.5 h.

4. The erythrocytes are then washed once with $MgCl_2$ (288 ± 1 mosmol/kg) and twice with choline medium and then left for 10 minutes in choline medium at 37 °C. The erythrocytes are at a haematocrit of 30–40% throughout this period to ensure adequate removal of the background lithium. Washings are performed with centrifugation at 2000 g so that the packed cell volume of the packed cells is > 90%.

5. After the final washing, the packed cell volume of the erythrocytes is measured using a micro-haematocrit centrifuge.

6. Then, 0.225 ml of the packed erythrocytes are incubated in either 2.25 ml of choline medium or 2.25 ml of sodium medium. In each case 10^{-4} mol/l ouabain is added. Each mixture of media and cells is then split into three for separate incubations. This whole step is performed at 4 °C to ensure that the SLC transporter does not function until all of the mixing etc. is complete.

7. The triplicate samples are incubated for varying times – 40, 80 and 120 minutes at 37 °C.

8. After centrifugation of incubation mixtures at 2000 g for 3 minutes, the lithium concentration of the supernatant is measured. This can be measured either by flame photometry using caesium but not potassium as the internal standard or by atomic absorption spectrometry.

9. The rate of lithium efflux in the choline and sodium media is calculated by linear regression analysis and corrected for the measured packed cell volume. The SLC activity is determined as the difference between lithium efflux from erythrocytes in the sodium and choline media.

Transport kinetics

Transport proteins span the lipid bilayer of the membrane so that they are in contact with the aqueous phase on either side. Transport proteins may be a single molecule, such as the anion exchanger, or composed of sub-units, such as the Na-K ATPase pump. The movement of ions from one aqueous phase to the other across the lipid bilayer involves several steps. The transported ion must first bind to a specific site on the transporter. This is followed by translocation of the ion through the transporter protein across the lipid bilayer. The ion must then dissociate from its binding site. In countertransport systems the movement of an ion in one direction is coupled to the movement of an ion in the opposite direction. Nonetheless these systems commonly have a single ion binding site, as with the anion exchanger or sodium-lithium countertransport. This single binding site is then envisaged to shuttle backwards and forwards across the membrane and has been described as a "ping-pong" mechanism. It has some kinetic characteristics.

Each of the steps in ion transport: binding, translocation and dissociation, are reversible and have rate constants for each direction. Thus k + 1, k + 2 and k + 3 in the forward direction and k − 1, k − 2 and k − 3 in the reverse direction (Fig. 1). When the transporter is in steady state the ratio of the rate constants for the 1 and 3 steps gives the association/dissociation constants.

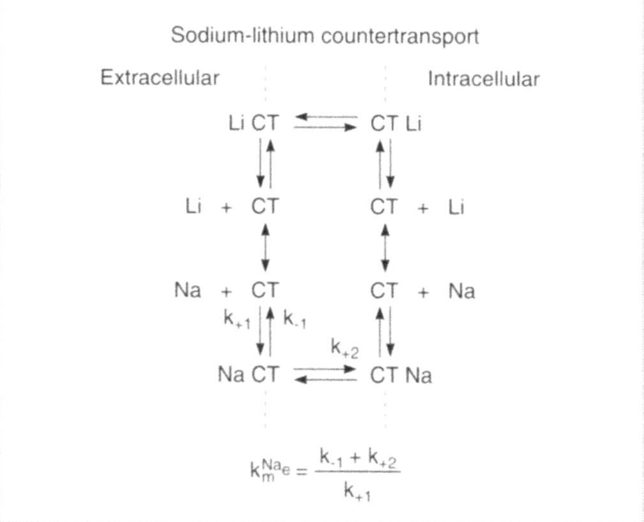

Fig. 1 The kinetic mechanism of sodium-lithium countertransport activity (CT = sodium-lithium countertransport)

The measurement of individual rate constants is difficult and rarely attempted but the measurement of the rate of movement of a transported ion from one side of the membrane to the other is affected by all of them and possibly also by the number of transporters in the membrane. The measurement of a simple transport rate, such as the standard SLC activity, gives a very poor level of scientific information to understand how a transport system is behaving.

The simplest assessment of transport kinetics is the measurement of the Michaelis-Menten constant (k_m) and the maximum velocity (Vmax) and it has been argued that this is the minimum that should be expected [28]. To measure k_m and Vmax, ion flux is measured at a range of ion concentrations and shows a generally parabolic curve relating the increase in ion flux with increasing ion concentration. There are slight variations in the shape of the curve depending for example on the number of ions transported at each cycle. The general equation is:

$$\text{flux} = \frac{\text{Vmax}}{(1 + \text{km}/[\text{ion}])^n}$$

where n is the number of ions transported at each cycle. In the case of SLC n = 1.

There are several well described methods for transforming this equation to a straight line form. The Lineweaver-Burke plot of 1/flux against 1/[ion] is the least satisfactory because of the skewed distribution that it gives to the data with heavy bias on the low fluxes at low ion concentration. The Hanes-Woolf plot of [ion]/flux against [ion] and the Eadie-Hofstee plot of flux/[ion] against flux give similar results for km and Vmax but the Hanes-Woolf plot gives optimistically high correlation coefficients since [ion] is on the x and y axes and varies over a wider range than the flux.

The Vmax and the k_m may not be independent and if Vmax changes greatly then caution should be exercised in the interpretation of k_m. This is because Vmax is affected by both the number of transporter units and also by their turnover rate i.e. k + 2. The k_m value may also be affected by k + 2 but is conventionally taken to reflect the association constant for ion binding; k + 1/k − 1. Obviously the extent to which this is true depends on the relative magnitude of k + 1 and k + 2 (Fig. 1).

SLC kinetics

There has only been one attempt at a detailed kinetic study of SLC and the analysis agreed with single ion movements on a single ion carrier site with the "ping-pong" mechanism obeying Michaelis-Menten kinetics [7]. In this study the k_m's for sodium and lithium were measured with the emphasis on intracellular sodium and extracellular lithium because of the assay technique used but the alternative k_m's were also estimated. The k_m values for lithium were much lower than those for sodium at both intra- and extracellular faces. The intracellular k_m for lithium was low enough to allow saturation of the transporter with this ion to be achieved easily. Similar k_m values for intracellular lithium have been found by other investigators [6, 29, 30]. However, if the k_m for intracellular lithium can be up to 2 mmol/l in some subjects, this is not compatible with the generally held view that an intracellular lithium of greater than 5 or even 3 mmol/l is enough to achieve saturation since in Michaelis-Menten kinetics a substrate concentration of 10 × km is required to give 90% saturation. This is probably a function of the ping-pong kinetics in which the ratio k_m/Vmax is constant. Therefore if intracellular lithium concentration is studie at an extracellular sodium concentration below saturation, as in the usual SLC assay, then an apparent k_m below the real k_m will be observed. An important methodological point is that the higher affinity for lithium means that this ion will quickly compete with sodium for the transporter as the assay progresses so that activity will be underestimated. This effect will be most severe where the activity is highest, such as at the higher sodium concentrations in an assay to measure k_m and Vmax. The result will be inaccurately low values for k_m and Vmax.

The value for k_m for extracellular sodium in the study of Hannaert and Garay [7] was high. This was surprising in view of the earlier study of Sarkadi et al. [6] using 4 normal subjects which found a much lower k_m for extracellular sodium. Hannaert and Garay [7] could not reconcile these results which appeared to exceed experimental variation. It is perhaps interesting to note that in concurrent work the investigators that found the low k_m [6] also found that SLC was inhibited by frusemide and quinidine [5] which has not been observed by any other workers.

As a general guide in biochemistry, to measure a value similar to Vmax a substrate concentration of at least 10 × k_m should be used. This would theoretically give a value 90% of Vmax. Even at the low k_m of 25 mmol/l reported by Sarkadi et al [6] this would not be achieved at 150 mmol/l sodium and with the Hannaert and Garay values [7] of more than 100 mmol/l activities of not much more than half of Vmax would be observed. Despite this the k_m was not further evaluated and values of activity at 150 mmol/l sodium were referred to as Vmax [9]. This is obviously scientifically unacceptable. There has been some misunderstanding of the basic tenets of Michaelis-Menten kinetics in that the k_m and Vmax are independent of the substrate (i.e. sodium) concentrations at which activity is measured. Only if there is co-operativity or substrate inhibition is the range of substrate concentration likely to affect the apparent k_m and Vmax values calculated using the Michaelis-Menten equations. The procedure to measure k_m and Vmax is quite simple. The SLC activity is measured as described above but activity is determined at a range of sodium concentrations in addition to 150 mmol/l [19]. However, in the case of SLC the passive lithium flux must be subtracted from each total lithium flux at each sodium concentration. The value of the passive flux can have a marked effect on the k_m and Vmax values subsequently calculated.

The use of nystatin [31] to allow the use of saturating sodium concentrations, as well as in lithium loading, should be treated with caution since nystatin causes marked increases in membrane fluidity (unpublished observations) and membrane fluidity is associated with an altered Vmax in hyperlipidaemia [32] and diabetes [33]. The interaction between membrane fluidity and SLC has analogies in observations of the interaction of membrane fluidity and the kinetics of other ion transporters in the erythrocyte [34].

Recent studies on much larger groups of normal subjects have found that the k_m for extracellular sodium is very variable with a mean or median value in the region of 100 mmol/l sodium [35, 36]. This would suggest that in the great majority of clinical studies measuring lithium efflux at a sodium of 150 mmol/l did not give a value for Vmax as had been claimed. Furthermore, the large variation in km values means that the flux values observed almost certainly had little relation to Vmax. This may be very important when studying membrane factors that affect the total available transporters or their turnover rate, such as membrane fluidity. In these cases the principal effect is likely to be on Vmax [32, 33].

Normal factors causing variation in sodium-lithium countertransport activity within and between subjects

Most of the information on SLC is of its activity at a sodium concentration of 130– 150 mmol/l. The widely held view is that this activity is below 0.4 mmol Li/hr × l rbc in normal subjects [37]. The mean value in a group of normal subjects is often in the region of 0.25 mmol Li/hr × l rbc with values between 0.1 and 0.3 (i.e. a 3 fold range) being common. Although there is a paucity of information on the variation of SLC within the individual, it seems likely that it can vary over a similar range.

The factors causing variation within the individual are not entirely clear. There is good evidence of a relationship of SLC activity with lipid status [11, 38]. This is easily evident in the pathological range of plasma lipids where the relationship between SLC activity and plasma triglyceride is most consistent and a treatment induced change in plasma triglyceride is associated with a change SLC activity [39]. This relationship is probably due to changes in the physical state of the plasma membrane lipid bilayer [21, 32] and the correlation coefficient with plasma lipids is usually low and sometimes lost in the variability caused by other factors. It seems likely that this influence will continue into the normal range of membrane lipids. There is some evidence that exercise training over a period will reduce SLC activity and this is most likely to be mediated by a change in lipid status [40].

The other within subject variable that has received some consideration is glucose/insulin status with feeding and fasting. However in a group of normal subjects there was no effect of feeding after an overnight fast on either the SLC activity as usually measured or the kinetics despite marked increases in plasma insulin [41]. Therefore the state of feeding appears to be irrelevant to SLC activity.

The variation in SLC activity between subjects is believed to be influenced most strongly by genetic factors [37]. Significant parent-offspring correlations of SLC activity have been found with no husband-wife correlation suggesting a genetic effect on SLC above any environmental effect [42, 43]. Greater concordance for SLC activity in mono-compared to di-zygotic twins has also been reported [44]. However, one study of more than 1000 subjects was unable to distinguish between a single genetic or environmental factor as the major effect on SLC and even then only 16–35% of SLC variability could be explained [45]. Another study in the general population found 50% polygenic inheritance [42]. A study of the inheritance of SLC in pedigrees with high cardiovascular risk found evidence for 34.4% a major gene locus and 49.5% polygenic inheritance [46]. SLC is also clearly higher in the normotensive first degree relatives of essential hypertensives [12, 47]. This picture could be explained by a subgroup of pedigree prone to essential hypertension in which SLC is a marker for the susceptibility gene. When probands were selected for an SLC greater than 0.4 mmol Li/hr x l rbc, 48% of first degree relatives had increased SLC but these subjects also had raised plasma lipids compared to the relatives with normal SLC [12]. Using SLC activity for such studies when it is affected by both k_m and Vmax, only one of which may be genetically controlled, is almost certain to lead to the sort of inconclusive results so far obtained. There appear to be differences in SLC activity with sex and body mass index but the effects are small and often do not reach significance. There is also a well defined racial difference with blacks having lower activity than caucasians [48, 49].

It therefore appears that genetic factors are important in determining SLC activity and a family history of hypertension should be excluded in normal control subjects. Lipid status is probably the largest environmental effect that should be considered in control groups but plasma lipids are a poor index of the effect on SLC activity.

Sodium-lithium countertransport and other cation transport systems in diabetes mellitus

The activity of other cation transport systems in diabetes have been assessed to determine if there are changes in their activity secondary to diabetes *per se* or as complications such as hypertension or nephropathy develop [50, 51]. However, the results of these studies in terms of the potential for clinical use, e. g. in the identification of patients at risk of nephropathy, has been disappointing. In contradistinction studies of SLC activity in diabetes have raised some intriguing hypotheses. However, whereas other cation transport systems have been measured in such a fashion to allow the calculation of the underlying kinetic determinants, k_m and Vmax, SLC activity has with the exception of our own work [19, 52] been simply measured as a single sub-maximal flux rate (still erroneously described as "Vmax"). This has undoubtedly led to problems in interpretation and comparison between studies. Many of the controversies in the literature regarding SLC activity, particularly in the studies of diabetic subjects, could have been avoided if SLC was routinely measured to allow the calculation of k_m and Vmax.

A separate problem is the relationship between erythrocyte SLC activity and Na-H exchange activity, generally measured in leucocytes. It would be tempting to link these two transport systems as being performed by the same transport protein, particularly since elevated Na-H exchange has been observed in diabetes [53]. The evidence for this link is minimal – the inhibitor profiles are different [54] and the kinetic mechanism of the SLC transporter ("ping-pong") is entirely different from the antiport system in Na-H exchange. Furthermore, two studies [55, 56] have failed to observe genetic linkage between the human Na-H exchange locus and SLC – in one case by an odds ratio of 1,000,000 : 1!

SLC activity has interesting links with diabetes mellitus and merits further study for both scientific and clinical reasons. It is important that in the future all studies of SLC measure its k_m and Vmax and look for other evidence of plasma membrane dysfunction in diabetes.

References

[1] Mendels J, Frazer A, Alterations in cell membrane activity in depression. Am J Physiol 1974; 131: 1240–1246.
[2] Haas M, Schooler J, Tosteson DC. Coupling of lithium to sodium transport in human red cells. Nature 1975; 258: 425–427.
[3] Duhm J, Eisenreid F, Becker BF et al. Studies on the lithium transport across the red cell membrane I. Li+ uphill transport by the Na+-dependent Li+ countertransport system of human erythrocytes. Pflug Arch 1976; 364: 147–155.

[4] Duhm J, Becker BF. Studies on the lithium transport across the red cell membrane II. Characterisation of ouabain-sensitive and ouabain-insensitive Li+ transport. Effects of bicarbonate and dipyridamole. Pflug Arch 1977; 367: 211–219.
[5] Pandey GN, Darkadi B, Haas, M et al. Lithium transport pathways in human red blood cells. J Gen Physiol 1978; 72: 233–247.
[6] Sarkadi B, Alifimoff JK, Gunn RB et al. Kinetics and stoichiometry of Na-dependent Li transport in human red blood cells. J Gen Physiol 1978; 72: 249–265.
[7] Hannaert PA, Garay RP. A kinetic analysis of Na-Li countertransport in human red blood cells. J Gen Physiol 1986; 87: 353–368.
[8] Duhm J, Becker BF. Studies on lithium transport across the red cell membrane V. On the nature of the Na+-dependent Li+ countertransport system of mammalian erythrocytes. J Memb Biol 1979; 51: 263–286.
[9] Canessa M, Adragna N, Solomon HS et al. Increased sodium-lithium countertransport in red cells of patients with essential hypertension. N Engl J Med 1980; 302: 772–776.
[10] Carr SJ, Thomas TH, Wilkinson R. Erythrocyte sodium-lithium countertransport in primary and renal hypertension. Eur J Clin Invest 1989; 19: 101–106.
[11] Corrocher R, Steinmayr M, Ruzzenente O et al. Elevation of red cell sodium-lithium countertransport in hyperlipidemias. Life Sci 1985; 36: 649–655.
[12] Carr SJ, Thomas TH, Laker MF et al. Elevated sodium-lithium countertransport: a familial marker of hyperlipidaemia and hypertension? J Hypertens 1990; 8: 139–146.
[13] Worley RJ, Hentschel WM, Cormier C et al. Increased sodium-lithium countertransport in erythrocytes of pregnant women. N Engl J Med 1982; 307: 412–416.
[14] Krowleski AS, Canessa M, Warram JH et al. Predisposition to hypertension and susceptibility to renal disease in insulin-dependent diabetes mellitus. N Engl J Med 1988; 318: 140–145.
[15] Mangili R, Bending JJ, Scott G et al. Increased sodium-lithium countertransport activity in red cells of patients with insulin-dependent diabetes and nephropathy. N Engl J Med 1988; 318: 146–150.
[16] Jones SL, Trevisan R, Tariq T et al. Sodium-lithium countertransport in microalbuminuric insulin-dependent diabetic patients. Hypertension 1990; 15: 570–575.
[17] Jensen JS, Mathieson ER, Norgaard K et al. Increased blood pressure and erythrocyte sodium/lithium countertransport are not inherited in diabetic nephropathy. Diabetologia 1990; 33: 619–624.
[18] Elving LD, Wetzels JFM, DeNobel E et al. Erythrocyte sodium-lithium countertransport is not different in type 1 (insulin-dependent) diabetic patients with and without nephropathy. Diabetologia 1991; 34: 126–128.
[19] Rutherford PA, Thomas TH, Taylor R et al. Changes in erythrocyte sodium-lithium countertransport kinetics in diabetic nephropathy. Clin Sci 1992; 82: 301–307.
[20] De La Sierra A, Coca A, Aguilera MT et al. Na+-Li+ countertransport in essential hypertension. J Hypertens 1988; 6 (11): 931–937.
[21] Engelmann B, Duhm J. Effect of cholesterol and dipalmitoyl phosphatidylcholine enrichment on the kinetics of Na-Li exchange of human erythrocytes. J Membrane Biol 1991; 122: 231–238.
[22] Morgan K, Spurlock G, Collins PA et al. Interaction of inhibition with the human erythrocyte Na+(Li+)i/Na+o exchanger. Biochim Biophys Acta 1989; 979: 53–61.
[23] Carr SJ, Thomas TH, Wilkinson R. Sodium-lithium countertransport activity and its sensitivity to inhibitors with erythrocyte ageing in man. Clin Chim Acta 1988; 128: 1–8.
[24] Gall MA, Rossing P, Jensen JS et al. Parving H-H. Red cell Na+/Li+ countertransport in non-insulin-dependent diabetics with diabetic nephropathy. Kidney Int 1991; 39: 135–140.
[25] Ellory JC, Flatman PW, Stewart GW. Inhibition of human red cell sodium and potassium transport by divalent cations. J Physiol 1983; 340: 1–17.
[26] Levy R, Zimlichman R, Keynan A et al. The erythrocyte membrane in essential hypertension: modified temperature-dependence of Li-efflux. Biochim Biophys Acta 1982; 685: 214–218.

[27] Rutherford PA, Thomas TH, Wilkinson R. The relationship between the temperature sensitivity and the kinetic characteristics of erythrocyte sodium-lithium countertransport activity (SLC). Clin Sci; (Abstract, accepted for publication).
[28] Aronson JK. Methods for expressing the characteristics of transmembrane ion transport systems. Clin Sci 1990; 78: 247–254.
[29] Siebers RWL, Maling TJB. Kinetics of sodium-lithium countertransport in normotensive and hypertensive subjects. J Cardiovasc Pharmacol 1990; 16 suppl 7: S59–S61.
[30] Duhm J, Becker BF. Studies on the lithium transport across the red cell membrane. IV. Inter-individual variations in the Na+-dependent Li+ countertransport system of human erythrocytes. Pflugers Arch 1977; 370: 211–219.
[31] Canessa M, Zerbini G, Laffel LMB. Sodium activation kinetics of red blood cell Na+/Li+ countertransport in diabetes: methodology and controversy. J Am Soc Nephrol 1992; 3 suppl 1: S41–S49.
[32] Dowd A, Thomas TH, Wilkinson R. Increased human erythrocyte sodium-lithium countertransport in hyperlipidaemic patients may indicate increased membrane lipid fluidity. Eur J Clin Invest 1993; 23: 102–107.
[33] Dowd A, Thomas TH, Wilkinson R. Erythrocyte sodium-lithium countertransport activity (SLC) is related to membrane fluidity in type 1 diabetes. Diab Med 1992; 9 suppl 2: S13.
[34] Giraud F, Claret M, Garay R. Interactions of cholesterol with the Na pump in red blood cells. Nature (London) 1976; 646: 1976.
[35] Rutherford PA, Thomas TH, Wilkinson R. Increased erythrocyte sodium-lithium countertransport activity in essential hypertension is due to an increased affinity for extracellular sodium. Clin Sci 1990; 79: 365–369.
[36] Hardman TC, Sandhu S, Irving F et al. Characterisation of the erythrocyte sodium-lithium countertransporter (SLC) by traditional and kinetic methodologies. Clin Sci 1993; 84 suppl 28: 26P.
[37] Rutherford PA, Thomas TH, Wilkinson R. Erythrocyte sodium-lithium countertransport: clinically useful, pathophysiologically instructive or just phenomenology? Clin Sci 1992; 82: 241–352.
[38] Rutherford PA, Thomas TH, Laker MF et al. Plasma lipids affect maximum velocity not sodium affinity of human sodium-lithium countertransport: distinction from essential hypertension. Eur J Clin Invest 1992; 22: 719–724.
[39] Carr SJ, Thomas TH, Laker MF et al. Lipid lowering therapy leads to a reduction in sodium-lithium countertransport activity. Arteriosclerosis 1991; 87: 103–108.
[40] Adragna N, Chang S, Morey M et al. Effects of exercise on cation transport in human red cells. Hypertension 1985; 7: 132–139.
[41] Rutherford PA, Thomas TH, Hardman TH et al. Sodium-lithium countertransport activity is not affected by acute insulin exposure in vivo or in a physiological medium in vitro. Metabolism; (in press).
[42] Boerwinkle E, Turner ST, Weinshilboum R et al. Analysis of the distribution of erythrocyte sodium lithium countertransport in a sample representative of the general population. Genet Epidemiol 1986; 3: 365–378.
[43] Kagamimori S, Naruse Y, Takata M et al. Familial aggregation of red blood cell cation transport systems in Japanese families. Am J Epidemiol 1985; 122: 386–390.
[44] Motulsky AG, Burke W, Billings PR et al. Hypertension and the genetics of red cell membrane abnormalities. Ciba Found Symp 1987; 130: 150–166.
[45] Rebbeck TR, Turner ST, Michels VV et al. Genetic and environmental explanations for the distribution of sodium-lithium countertransport in pedigrees from Rochester, MN. Am J Hum Genet 1991; 48: 1092–1104.
[46] Hasstedt SJ, Wu LL, Ash KO et al. Hypertension and sodium-lithium countertransport in Utah pedigrees: evidence for major-locus inheritance. Am J Hum Genet 1988; 43: 14–22.
[47] Woods JW, Falk RJ, Pittman AW et al. Increased red-cell sodium-lithium countertransport in normotensive sons of hypertensive parents. N Engl J Med 1982; 306: 593–595.

[48] Trevisan M, Ostrow D, Cooper RS et al. Sex and race differences in sodium-lithium countertransport and red cell sodium concentration. Am J Epidemiol 1984; 120: 537–541.
[49] Bunker CH, Mallinger AG, Adams LL et al. Red blood cell sodium-lithium countertransport and cardiovascular crisk factors in black and white college students. J Hypertens 1987; 5: 7–15.
[50] Baldini P, Incerpi S, Lambert-Gardini S et al. Membrane lipid alterations and Na+-pumping activity in erythrocytes from IDDM and NIDDM subjects. Diabetes 1989; 38: 825–831.
[51] Suhail M, Rizvi SI. Red cell membrane (Na-K)-ATPase in diabetes mellitus. Biochem Biophys Res Commun 1987; 148: 179–186.
[52] Rutherford PA, Thomas TH, Carr SJ et al. Kinetics of sodium-lithium countertransport activity in patients with uncomplicated type 1 diabetes. Clin Sci 1992; 82: 291–299.
[53] Ng LL, Simmons D, Frighi V et al. Leucocyte Na+/H+ antiport activity in type 1 (insulin-dependent) diabetic patients with nephropathy. Diabetologia 1990; 33: 371–377.
[54] Kahn AM. Difference between human red blood cell Na+-Li+ countertransport and renal Na+-H+ exchange. Hypertension 1987; 9 (1): 7–12.
[55] Lefton RP, Hunt SC, Williams RR et al. Exclusion of the Na+-H+ antiporter as a candidate gene in human essential hypertension. Hypertension 1991; 17 (1): 8–14.
[56] Dudley CRK, Giuffra LA, Raine AEG et al. Assessing the role of APNH, a gene encoding for a human amiloride sensitive Na+-H+ antiporter, on the interindividual variation in red cell Na+/Li+ countertransport. J Am Soc Nephrol 1991; 2 (4): 937–943.

Methods in the assessment of transcapillary escape rate of plasma proteins

H.-H. Parving

Introduction

Information concerning microvascular permeability to plasma proteins in man in health and in disease is rather sparse and, in many instances, probably also unreliable. This is mainly due to the use of qualitative, non-kinetic methods for studying a dynamic process, i. e., the escape of proteins from plasma to the interstitial fluid. The most commonly used method in the past has been: determination of proteins in spontaneous or experimentally induced oedema fluid [1], or observations of protein escape during application of severe venous congestion [2], a method which must be considered rather non-physiological.

However, information concerning the quantitative and dynamic aspects of the overall microvascular leakage of plasma proteins can be obtained by measuring the transcapillary escape rate of labelled plasma proteins [3]. Unfortunately, the quantitative results obtained in several of the early investigations were unreliable due to the use of partly denatured tracer albumin preparations containing a high amount of free radioactive iodine, and due to the lack of steady state during the investigation as discussed by Parving [4]. The shortcomings of the method have been eliminated and the technique for measuring transcapillary escape rate of plasma protein has been developed to yield quantitatively reliable results. This is mainly due to the tracer albumin preparation employed, which now warrants the basic assumption in tracer theory: the organism does not have to distinguish between tracer albumin and the endogenous albumin.

The present review will describe and discuss: the model for the dynamics of endogenous plasma albumin, determination and calculation of the transcapillary escape rate of albumin in the body and in a single tissue (skin), and finally present data obtained by these methods in patients with human diabetes mellitus. The albumin molecule will be used as a model for plasma proteins in general.

Offprint from
Research Methodologies in Human Diabetes – Part 1

Calculation of the transcapillary escape rate of albumin

Figure 1A depicts the assumed model for the dynamics of the endogenous plasma albumin: Newly synthesised albumin molecules enter the blood stream at the rate S and mix evenly with the intravascular mass (IVM). Molecules pass continuously from IVM to the interstitial space where they mix with the extravascular mass (EVM). In the steady state – which is assumed to pertain – the transfer from IVM to EVM occurs at the constant rate and can be expressed as a percentage of IVM escaping from the circulation per unit time: the transcapillary escape rate, (TER_{alb}). Extravascular albumin returns to the

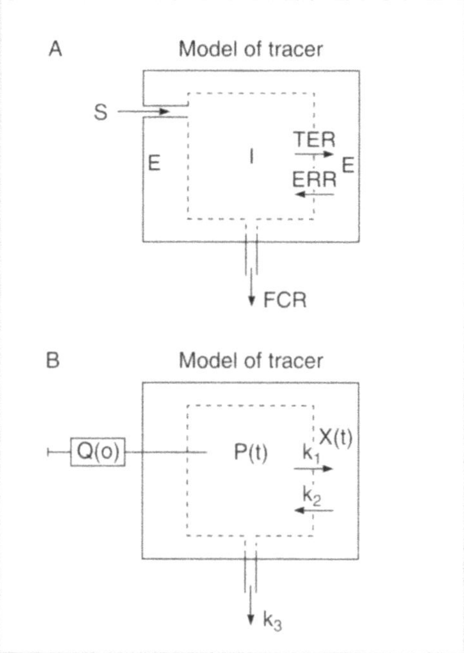

Fig. 1 Model for the dynamics of endogenous albumin in the organism (A) and the fate of the tracer albumin (B). Refer to the text

blood, that is to IVM, at an overall constant rate; this is labelled the lymphatic return rate (LRR) when expressed relative to EVM. Thus, expressed LRR also includes that presumably quite small fraction of the EVM which is transported back into the blood at the level of microcirculation. Normal catabolism of albumin occurs from the intravascular space, or in close relation to the intravascular space. The fraction of IVM catabolized per unit time is the fractional catabolic rate (FCR). In the steady state, the amount of albumin escaping from the circulation to the interstitial space and the amount returning to plasma from the extravascular mass through the lymph is equal; therefore $TER_{alb} * IVM = LRR * EVM$.

Fig. 1 B shows the fate of the tracer albumin studied. The tracer is suddenly injected into the blood, where it is mixed evenly with IVM. The intravascular tracer concentration P(t) will decrease with the time, because a constant fraction, k_1, of the intravascular tracer will pass across the microvascular wall per unit time to the extravascular tracer, X(t). Furthermore, P(t) decreases because of catabolism at the fractional rate, k_3. Since the intravascular tracer is mixed evenly with IVM from the moment of injection, k_1 equals TER_{alb} and k_3 equals FCR. Since the extravascular tracer is not mixed evenly in one homogeneous extravascular protein pool with a fixed LRR, the fraction of extravascular tracer returning per unit time k_2 is not constant. Thus

$$-dP(t)/dt = k_1 *P(t) + k_3 *P(t) - k_2 *X(t) \quad (1)$$

or, since $k_3 \ll k_1$

$$-dP(t)/dt = k_1 *P(t) - k_2 *X(t) \quad (2)$$

Initially, when X(t) is close to zero we can neglect $k_2 *X(t)$ and write

$$\left[-d\,P(t)/dt\right]_{t \to 0} = k_1 *P(t) \quad (3)$$

Since the intravascular tracer is mixed evenly with IVM from the moment of injection, k_1 equals TER_{alb}. Thus, TER_{alb} can be determined as the initial decrease in plasma activity as a function of time. The inherent approximations will be dealt with below.

Assumptions

The following assumptions must be fulfilled in order to calculate the transcapillary escape rate of endogenous albumin from the initial disappearance rate of radio-iodinated albumin: (1) the tracer will behave like the endogenous albumin; (2) a steady state with respect to albumin metabolism during the period of investigation (constancy of all masses and rates); (3) the disappearance of intravenously injected radio-iodinated albumin is a monoexponential function during the entire 60 min period following the injection, with a rate constant equal to that of time zero (no early back transport); and (4) the initial disappearance will reflect extravasation and not be influenced significantly by the rate of catabolism. Before discussing these assumptions, the method and the experimental procedure used for determination of TER_{alb} will be described in some detail.

Transcapillary escape rate of albumin (initial slope method)

We have described the experimental procedure and the theoretical basis for the calculation of TER_{alb} in detail previously [5]. Briefly, the subjects were studied in the morning after at least 12 h fasting and 1 h rest in the supine position; human serum albumin labelled electrolytically with ^{125}I or ^{131}I (code MIAK and MIMS, Institute for Atomic Energy, Kjeller, Norway) was used. These tracer preparations contain less than 1.0 per cent free radioactive iodide and have, in metabolic studies, been demonstrated to behave like endogenous albumin [6, 7]. Four to eight μCi of one of the tracers were injected in an arm vein, and eight venous blood samples of 6 ml each were drawn from the other arm at 10, 15, 20, 30, 40, 50, 55, and 60 min after the injection. The plasma radioactivity and total plasma protein concentration (refractometry) were determined in each sample in duplicate, and the radioactivity was expressed as cpm/g total plasma protein in all steady state (control) experiments, which implies constant total plasma protein mass. After logarithmic transformation of this ratio, the regression equation for the time-concentration curve was compiled by a computer. The TER_{alb} (% IVM/hour) was compiled from the slope of the regression equation. The outflux of albumin was calculated by multiplying the intravascular mass of albumin (IVM, g) by the TER_{alb} measurement. It was accepted only if the correlation coefficient for the time concentration curve exceeded 0.80. At least 10,000 counts were recorded.

In experiments involving non-steady state, the use of the specific activity (cmp/g total plasma protein) is not warranted. In such conditions the radioactivity was expressed as

$$\frac{\text{cpm} * (100 - \text{haematocrit} * 0.91)}{\text{haematocrit} * 0.91} \quad (4)$$

thereby eliminating the influence of plasma volume changes during the sampling period. This ratio is based on the relationship between plasma volume (PV) and erythrocyte volume (EV):

$$PV = \frac{EV * (100 - \text{haematocrit} * 0.91)}{\text{haematocrit} * 0.91} \quad (5)$$

The factor 0.91 was used to calculate the body haematocrit from the venous haematocrit. Assuming constant EV during the sampling period, we obtain a relative measurement of intravascular tracer using this approach.

Change in transcapillary escape rate of plasma proteins (intravascular mass reduction method)

The change in the transcapillary escape rate of plasma proteins, e. g., albumin during non-steady state, can also be calculated by determination of the intravascular mass of albumin before and during the non-steady state. The reduction in IVM/unit time was taken as a measure of the net increase in the transcapillary escape rate. This procedure, described in detail previously [8], can only be used during non-steady state in which a net transport of proteins from plasma to the interstitial space takes place. The method yields the true changes in the transcapillary escape rate if – and only if – the lymphatic return of the protein in question remains essentially unchanged during the period of measurement, as in control conditions.

Determination of plasma proteins, plasma volume, and intravascular mass

Plasma albumin concentration was measured according to Laurell's method [9]. The immunodiffusion method described by Mancini et al [10], was used in other studies for determination of albumin, IgG, and IgM.

PV was calculated from the radioactivity at time zero by retropolation of the initial plasma disappearance curve and the injected amount of radioiodinated albumin, measured by weighing the syringes before and after injection. IVM equals PC * plasma concentration of the protein in question.

Normal values and their variation

The normal values of the measured variables in healthy adults are given in Table I.

The reproducibility of the methods was calculated from two determinations carried out in four subjects under basal conditions, one immediately after the other, using two preparations of the same albumin labelled with ^{125}I and ^{131}I, respectively. The following results expressed as a coefficient of variation were; TER_{alb}: 8.5 per cent, albumin concentration: 1.4 per cent, PV: 1.5 per cent,

Table 1 Normal values of transcapillary escape rate of albumin (TER_{alb}), plasma albumin concentration, plasma volume and intravascular mass of albumin in healthy adults

	TER_{alb} (% IVM/h)	Albumin (g/l)	Plasma volume		IVM	
			(ml)	(ml/kg)	(g)	(g/kg)
Adults* (n = 28)						
Mean	5.4	38.2	3485	47.4	133	1.81
± SD	1.1	2.2	364	6.2	14	0.25

* Values from Parving et al [4]

and IVM: 2.2 per cent [4]. In each sample, the total protein concentration was read refractiometrically, in duplicate (coefficient of variation 0.5 per cent) with a T.S.-meter (American Optical Company). Due to the low coefficient of variation, this method is recommended, and used in all steady state studies to express specific activity.

Three determinations of the TER_{alb}, albumin concentration, PV, and IVM were made over a period of one year in five healthy subjects. The variation coefficients were below 5 per cent for all variables (albumin, IVM, PV) except for TER_{alb} (14.4 per cent). The good correlation between these variation coefficients and the above-mentioned ones for the reproducibility of the methods indicated that, over a period of one year, these variables are quite constant in the individual. These findings are in complete agreement with the results obtained by Rossing [11, 13], concerning the albumin metabolism.

Discussion of the method and the experimental procedure

The tracer

The prerequisite for correct results regarding the transcapillary escape rate of endogenous albumin is that the organism does not distinguish between labelled and endogenous albumin. The tracer albumin has been shown to be pure and metabolically non-denatured. The preparation is Human Albumin, 'trocken reinst' (Behringwerke, Germany) iodinated electrolytically, which is the gentlest procedure according to Katz and Bonorris [13]. The iodination degree was less than one iodine atom per molecule.

In all metabolic studies employing this preparation, we find a smaller fraction of the intravascular activity in the urine excreted during the first 24 h than subsequently. The transcapillary escape rate of albumin has been found to remain within the same range in normal subjects studied over a two-year period, which rules out the possibility of gross denaturation causing rapid uptake by the reticulo-endothelial system of any of the batches. In metabolic control studies in four normal subjects examined during the same period as my own studies, we found the fractional catabolic rate of albumin to be within the normal range found by Rossing [11, 12], with only one upper borderline value. This suggests that the metabolic behaviour of the albumin tracer is satisfactory.

The steady state

All subjects investigated were considered to be in the steady state, because of the experimental procedure (rest and fasting) and the finding of stable values for total plasma protein concentration and haematocrit during the investigation period.

The initial plasma disappearance

It is assumed that the plasma disappearance of radio-iodinated albumin during the first 60 min is a monoexponential function, at a constant rate equal to that at time zero. Theoretically, this assumption is not fulfilled because there is lymphatic return of tracer albumin (k_2 *X(t)) during the investigation period. However, the back-transport during this period is negligible because of the low lymph flow in a fasting, resting subject and the dilution of the tracer in the interstitial fluid. Also, the return of measurable amounts of tracer through the lymphatics is delayed 10 to 20 min, depending on the lymph flow rate. The following example illustrates the order of magnitude of the lymphatic return of tracer albumin within the initial 60 min: assuming instant extravascular mixing of tracer, a subject in a steady state (TER_{alb} *IVM = LRR *EVM) with an intravascular mass of albumin of 100 g, an extravascular mass of albumin of 125 g, a transcapillary escape rate of 5 percent/hour, and extravascular return rate of 4 percent/hour, and an influx of albumin of 5g/hour has a lymphatic return of tracer albumin of (5*4)/100 = 0.2 percent/hour.

The initial plasma disappearance of tracer albumin was found to be linear when plotted with the specific activity as the logarithmic ordinate versus time in linear scale, which is in accordance with the findings of several other investigations (Fig. 2). In order to evaluate how well the experimental data fit in with a logarithmic decrease, the correlation coefficient of the logarithmic regression of plasma activity versus time was calculated in each investigation. Only disappearance curves with a correlation coefficient above 0.8 was were

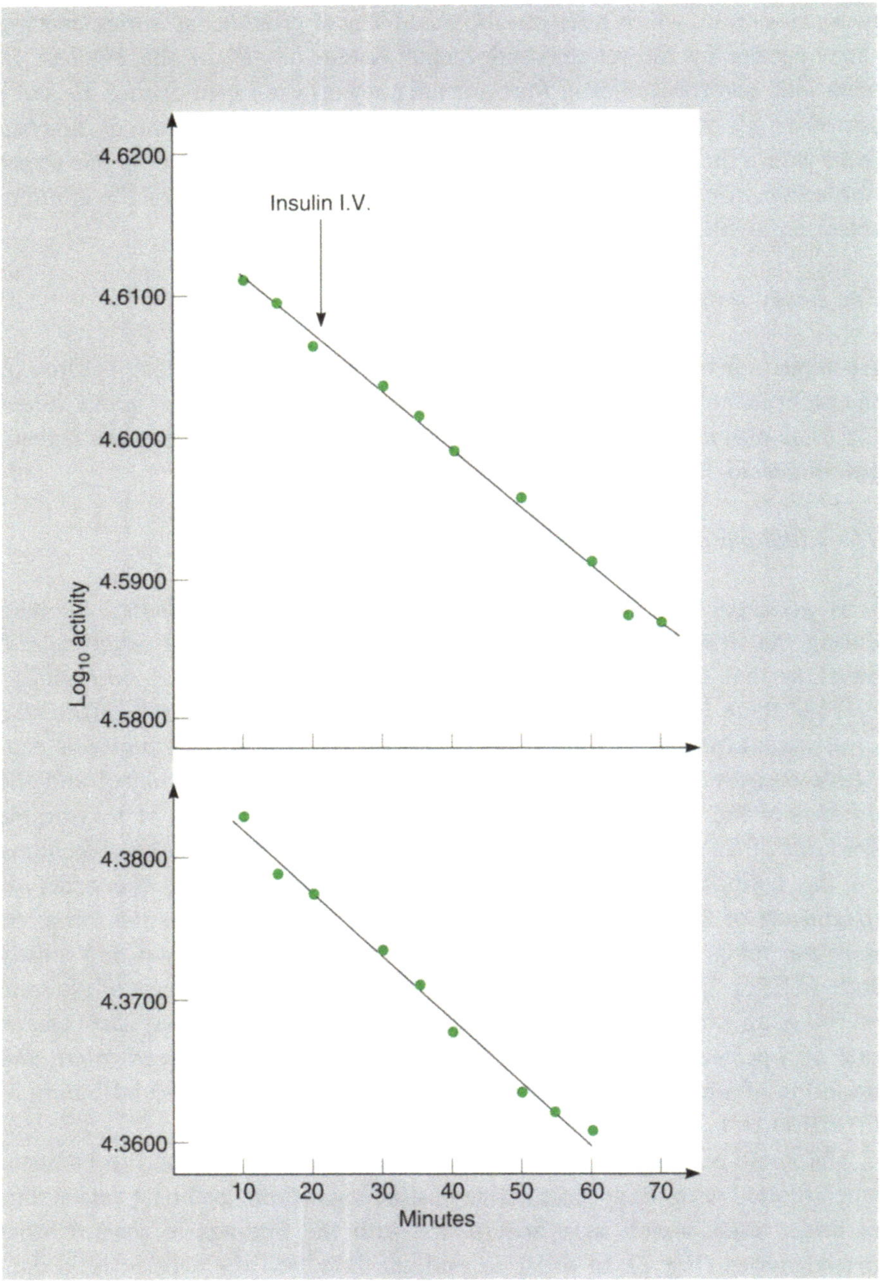

Fig. 2 A semi-logarithmic plot of the initial disappearance of tracer albumin (^{125}I) from plasma compiled from short-term IDDM patients (top), as compared to healthy controls (bottom). The observations fit a straight line

accepted. Except for the earliest investigations, the correlation coefficient was always above 0.9. This was probably due to the use of duplicate determination of plasma radioactivity and total plasma protein concentration in all the later studies.

The albumin catabolism

The decrease in plasma activity, P(t), due to albumin catabolism can be ignored; FCR is without quantitative importance over 60 min, since it is in the order of 8.5 percent of the IVM per 24 h, and, thus, only 0.35 percent of the IVM per hour, compared to the normal TER_{alb} of 5.4 percent of the IVM per hour. It should be stressed that even in conditions with a marked elevated FCR, e. g., essential hypertension, the catabolism is of little quantitative importance for the results of the TER_{alb}-determinations, as discussed by Parving et al [7]. Theoretically, the fractional catabolic rate should be subtracted from the transcapillary escape rate if catabolism occurs in the intravascular space. This point was made above (cf. equation (1) and (2)). However, it is likely, in my opinion, that the albumin molecules must leave the intravascular space prior to catabolic breakdown, e. g., catabolism might occur in the microvascular endothelium. If extravasation precedes catabolism, no such subtraction should be applied.

Pitfalls in measuring TER_{alb}

Determination of the specific radioactivity is strongly recommended in all steady state determination of TER_{alb}. Avoiding determination of plasma protein concentration is hazardous, since significant changes occur in approximately 20 percent of all TER_{alb} determinations, the changes consist of the following abnormalities: deviation in plasma protein concentration in one or two out of the eight samples, or a systematic raise or reduction in plasma protein concentration during the one hour investigation period. The most likely explanation for these fluctuations are changes in venous tonus. Originally, Ismail et al [14] described that the TER_{alb} measured during 3.5 hours was reduced in diabetics with and without late complications. Even more surprising, 8 out of 59 diabetic patients had practically no change in the blood radioactivity during the 3.5 hours of study, in other words, a TER_{alb} of zero. This finding is an artefact and can only be explained by a progressive haemoconcentration (raising plasma protein concentration), abolishing the decline in plasma radioactivity of albumin. Plasma protein concentration or haematocrit were not measured by Ismail et al [14]. Furthermore, Ismail and his colleagues used a commercial preparation of radio-iodinated serum albumin which is known to be metabolically denatured to a varying degree. The great reduction of intravascular radioactivity in their normal subjects during the period of investigation emphasises this point.

To determine whether insulin per se might increase vascular permeability, five non-diabetic men were studied by the hyperinsulinaemic-euglycemic clamp technique for 7 hours with and without (0.45 percent saline, control study) insulin infusion [15]. Identical fluid volumes were infused during the two sessions (1500–2000 ml/7 hours). At 7 hours of study, 10 μCi i. v. ^{125}I-labelled albumin was injected as bolus dose. Frequent blood samples were drawn during the next 70 min for determination of TER_{alb}. The TER_{alb} was greater in all five men after hyperinsulinemia than after saline infusion (18.3 ± 2.7 percent/h versus −2.8 ± 2.3 percent/h, $p = 0.01$). Three of the five subjects had a negative TER_{alb} during saline infusion. This artefact can only be explained by haemoconcentration following the prior plasma volume expansion, i. e., unsteady state. The artefact could have been avoided by applying the above mentioned valid technique for determination of TER_{alb} during non-steady state. Radioactivity should be corrected for haematocrit (Hct) by multiplying counts/min by (100-Hct)/Hct, thereby eliminating the influence of plasma volume changes during the investigation period.

Transcapillary exchange of proteins in the skin: Wick method and suction blister technique

Assumptions

The following assumptions must be fulfilled in order to obtain correct measurements of the subcutaneous interstitial protein concentration: 1) The sieving properties of the vascular endothelium must remain intact during the procedures; 2) the procedures per se must not enhance the microvascular escape rate of plasma proteins and thereby induce changes in the interstitial protein concentration; 3) the fluid collected by the two methods represent interstitial fluid (lymph); 4) correction for blood contamination can be performed by measurement of haemoglobin in the collected fluids and in the blood; and 5) local anaesthesia must not influence interstitial protein concentration.

Before discussing the above mentioned assumptions, the techniques and the experimental procedures used for determination of interstitial fluid protein concentration with the wick method and the suction blister method will be described in detail.

Wick method

A detailed description of the method has been presented by Poulsen [16]. After intracutaneous application on the forearm of a local anaesthetic, two tiny incisions were made 5 cm apart. A multifilament nylon wick with a diameter of 0.6 mm was sewn into the subcutaneous tissue through the incisions with a straight, round, and slightly blunted needle. Four wicks were placed at the forearm, each through its own pair of incisions. After an equilibration period of one hour, the wicks were individually removed. The two ends were cut (about 0.5 cm) and the middle part originating from subcutaneous tissue transferred to a previously weighted plasma test tube with a tight cover. The net weight of the wick was determined as the difference between the test tube weight after and before the added wick. The individual wick was eluted in the test tube with two ml saline (weighted) over 24 hours. The dry weight of the wick was measured after elution and drying for 2 hours at 100° C. Subtracting the dry weight from the wet weight, the wick fluid volume could be calculated by using specific gravity for saline to calculate volume for weight. The average fluid volume uptake per wick was 4 – 5 μl. Since the fluid uptake was small, the weighting procedure had to be performed with the utmost care. All weightings were done three times, the average weight being used in the further calculation. The albumin concentration of the eluate was determined according to Laurell [9]. In addition, the haemoglobin concentration was determined by means of a photometric benzidine method. Venous blood samples were drawn after at least 30 min in a resting position from all the investigated subjects for determination of haemoglobin concentration, haematocrit and plasma albumin concentration. These data were used to correct for contamination with albumin from plasma in the wick fluids. Thereafter, interstitial fluid albumin concentrations were calculated (the correction procedure is described in detail later).

Suction blister method

Interstitial fluid can be obtained by the suction blister device as described by Kiistala [17]. Sub-atmospheric pressure (200 mmHg) was obtained using an automatic pump device with one PVC suction cup applied on non-oedematous tissue (groin region). The suction cup was 50 mm in diameter and the inside of the cup was a concave PVC diaphragm. The adapter plate was perforated and had 5 round concentric holes, each 5 mm in diameter into which the blisters were produced. After 90 minutes, the blisters were punctuated with a thin needle and the fluid was collected in a heparinized glass capillaries. The fluids from the 5 blisters formed one sample of approximately 0.5 ml. The method is painless and requires no local anaesthesia.

Normal values and their variation

The normal values for different plasma proteins have been determined by Rossing and Worm [18], and are presented in table 2. The values obtained in normal skin by use of the wick method are usually slightly higher (0.6 – 0.65) for the interstitial/plasma albumin concentration ratio. Several studies have shown a close correlation between the interstitial plasma protein concentration measured by the two techniques. Due to the small volume of fluid collected by the wick method, we have no information on the other plasma proteins concentration. The precision of the whole method (wick implantation, determination of wick volume and albumin content) has been calculated, using analysis of variance on a large number of individual determinations of interstitial/plasma albumin concentration ratios. A variation coefficient of 10 – 12 percent has been demonstrated, both in healthy subjects and in insulin-dependent diabetic patients [16]. Data reflecting the coefficient of variation applying the blister suction method are still lacking.

*Table 2 Interstitial fluid/plasma protein concentration ratio in 10 normal subjects**

	Albumin	transferrin	IgG	α-macroglobulin
Mean	0.55	0.48	0.43	0.21
± SD	0.06	0.04	0.05	0.04

* Values from Rossing & Worm [18]

Discussion of the methods and the experimental procedures

Several studies have documented that the sieving properties of the vascular endothelium remained intact during the suction procedure [18, 19]. The same is true for the wick method if the duration of the wick implantation is less than 120 min. If more prolonged implantation is used, the concentration of albumin and, thereby, the oncotic pressure increases, probably due to inflammation. Therefore, 60 min has been chosen as standard wick implantation time in man [20].

It cannot be definitively excluded from protein tracer determinations that suction, per se, increases the microvascular escape rate. This confounding effect is not at hand when applying the wick method for less than 2 hours. However, the use of local anaesthetic might influence the subcutaneous albumin concentration if changes in blood flow and, thereby, changes in the permeability surface area product take place. In an attempt to avoid such an influence, injectable non-vasoconstricting 1% lidocain has been applied routinely. Furthermore, comparison between interstitial albumin concentration obtained with and without local anaesthesia has yielded the same results [16]. Whether or not pre-nodal lymph is identical to the free tissue fluid is still an unsettled question. Experimental studies have not revealed any statistically significant difference between lymph and subcutaneous wick fluid albumin concentration [20].

While blood contamination is extremely rare in using the suction blister method, it frequently occurs using the wick method. All wick fluids with a fractional haemoglobin concentration above 0.25, corresponding to more than 25% blood in the wick fluid are discarded owing to uncertainty in relation to validity of the correction procedure described above. The correction procedure has been carefully evaluated and found valid [16]. Actually, the study demonstrated a tendency to overcorrection at higher level of blood contamination.

Transcapillary escape of plasma proteins in diabetes mellitus

The term 'transcapillary escape rate' is used in the present review because this is conventional terminology. However, I realise that this term is something of a misnomer, since the rate is a measure of the leakiness of the microvasculature of which the capillaries are only a part. TER_{alb} reflects the overall leakage of albumin from the intravascular to the extravascular space. The leakage is determined by the following variables: the permeability surface area product of the microvasculature and hydraulic pressure in the microcirculation. The microvascular permeability is characterised by having both charge- and size-selective properties. Filtration in the form of sieving (ultrafiltration), and perhaps also in the form of simple convective outflow of plasma (bulk flow), is the classical mechanism that must be invoked to explain what essentially appears to be a unidirectional microvascular protein transport [21].

Originally, we found that the TER_{alb} was elevated in normotensive long-term IDDM patients with diabetic retinopathy [22]. We extended this observation by demonstrating an enhanced transcapillary escape rate of IgG [23]. Investigations in hypertensive long-term IDDM patients have revealed even more pronounced elevation in TER_{alb} [24]. Furthermore, a significant positive correlation between TER_{alb} and mean blood pressure ($r = 0.62$, $p < 0.01$) has been demonstrated in IDDM patients with diabetic nephropathy (Fig. 4). O'Hare et al [25] have confirmed and extended our results by demonstrating

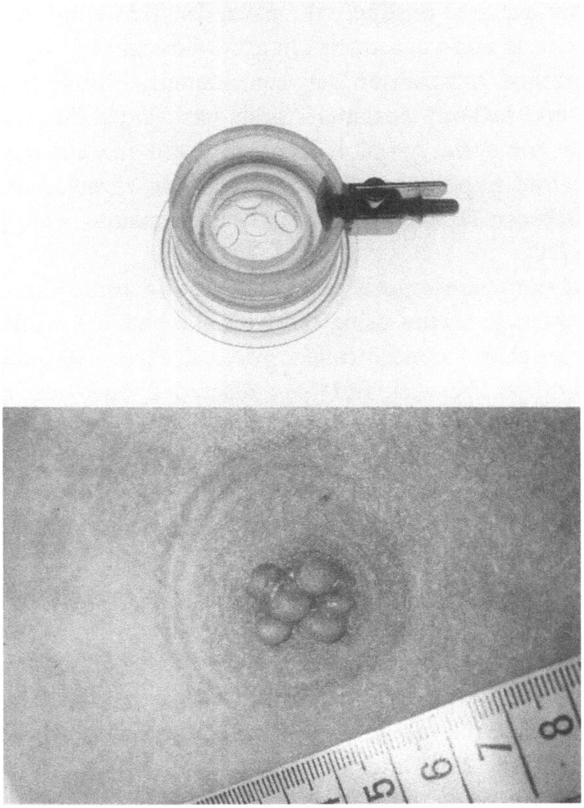

Fig. 3 Blister suction device (top) and blisters (bottom). Refer to the text

that metabolic control, hypertension, and the presence of microangiopathy independently enhance TER_{alb} in NIDDM and IDDM patients. Feldt-Rasmussen et al. [26] have demonstrated that long-standing diabetics without retinopathy have completely normal TER_{alb}, while elevated values were found in long-term IDDM patients with microalbuminuria and diabetic retinopathy (presenting 70%). TER_{alb} is increased in hypertension, while normal values have been reported in sufficiently-treated hypertensive subjects and in IDDM patients with borderline hypertension [2, 7].

Increased leakage of small and large molecules through the microvasculature has been demonstrated in newly diagnosed IDDM patients during poor metabolic control [28]. Improved metabolic control for only one week induced normalisation of the microvascular leakage. In contrast, the enhanced TER_{alb} observed in long-term IDDM patients with microalbuminuria is resistant to prolonged near-normal blood glucose control achieved by continuous subcutaneous insulin infusion [29]. Finally, note that intravenous insulin has no effect on TER_{alb}, unless hypoglycaemia is induced [30].

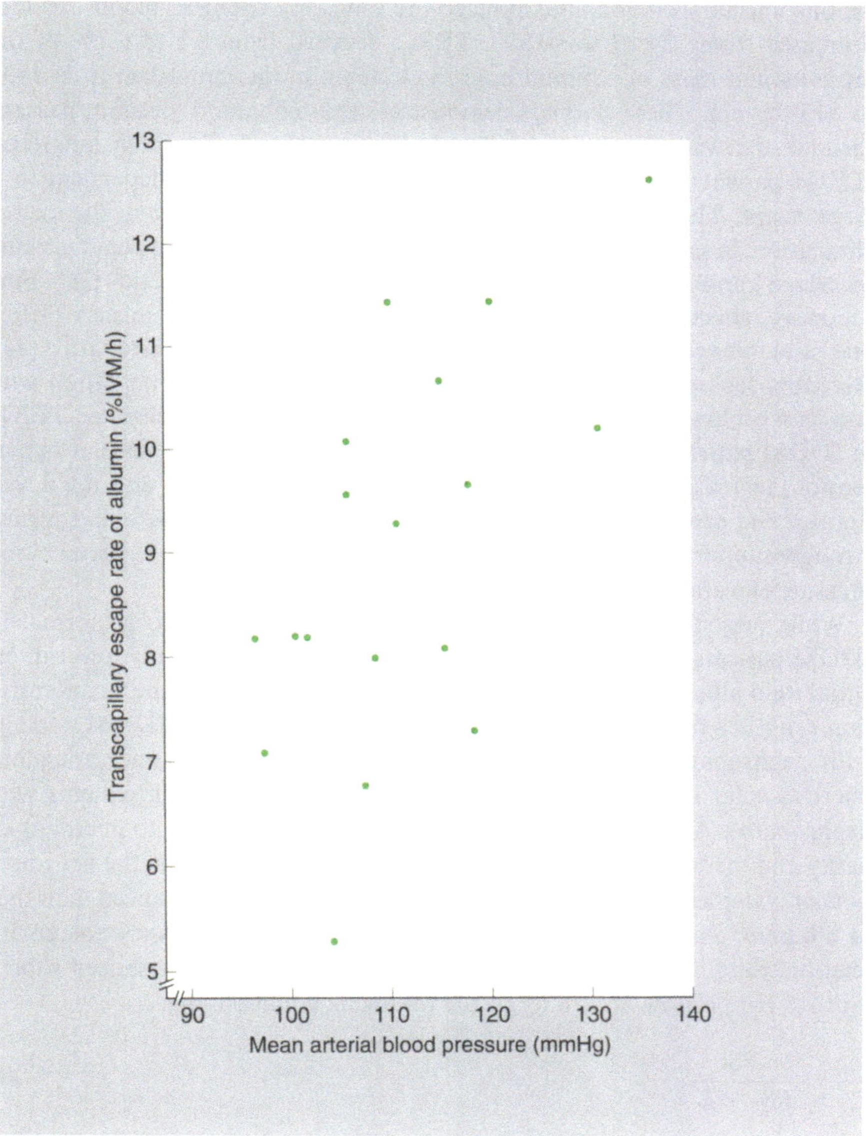

Fig. 4 Association between mean arterial blood pressure and TER_{alb} ($r = 0.62$, $p < 0.01$) in 18 IDDM patients with diabetic nephropathy. Parving et al [24]. By Diabetic Medicine

The link between microvascular hypertension, increased extravasation of plasma proteins, and the development and progression of diabetic microangiopathy has been suggested [31, 32]. To evaluate this haemodynamic concept, we assessed the effect of acute blood pressure reduction on TER_{alb} and albuminuria in normotensive IDDM patients with nephropathy [33]. Intravenous injection of clonidine induced the following changes: blood pressure decreased from 134/87 to 107/93, TER_{alb} declined from 8.1 to 6.7% of the intravascular mass of albumin/hour, and albuminuria diminished from 1434 to 815 μg/min. These findings demonstrate that enhanced albumin passage through the wall of microvasculature characteristically found in long-term IDDM patients with clinically microangiopathy is pressure-dependent to a large extent. This may be due to elevated hydrostatic pressure in the microcirculation. It should be stressed that direct measurements have demonstrated increased capillary pressure in the nail folds of human diabetics [34]. Furthermore, effective long-term anti-hypertensive treatment diminishes TER_{alb} and albuminuria in hypertensive IDDM patients with nephropathy [24]. Recently, Jensen et al [35] demonstrated that dietary supplementation with cod-liver oil lowers arterial blood pressure and the abnormal elevated TER_{alb} in IDDM patients with nephropathy. If a link between microvascular hypertension, increased microvascular leakage of plasma proteins, and the development and progression of diabetic microangiopathy exists, the above results strongly support the case for an early and effective treatment of arterial blood pressure elevation.

While interstitial fluid/plasma albumin concentration ratio is normal in IDDM patients without clinical microangiopathy, a significantly lower interstitial fluid albumin concentration and interstitial/plasma albumin concentration ratio has been documented by 3 independent groups in IDDM patients with nephropathy [16, 36, 37]. This finding is surprising, since enhanced microvascular leakage has been documented in long-standing patients with nephropathy. A conceivable explanation would be that owing to microangiopathy and increased hydraulic pressure in the microcirculation, the net transport of water across the capillary membrane is even more enhanced than that of albumin. The demonstration of reduced ratio between subcutaneous interstitial fluid and plasma albumin concentration indicates enhanced subcutaneous lymph flow according to the following equation [38]:

$$\frac{C_L}{C_P} = \frac{PS}{PS + L} \tag{6}$$

where C_L and C_P are protein concentration in lymph and plasma, respectively, PS the permeability-surface area product and L is lymph flow. It should be recalled, that the increased TER_{alb} is evidence of an overall enhanced lymph flow. Finally, it should be stressed that information on transcapillary escape of plasma proteins is lacking in NIDDM patients.

References

[1] Jones JH, Peters DK. Measurement of capillary permeability to plasma proteins by a gel-filtration technique. Clin Sci 1966; 31: 389–401.
[2] Landis EM, Jonas L, Augereine M et al. The passage of fluid and protein through the human capillary wall during venous congestion. J Clin Invest 1932; 11: 717–734,
[3] Parving H-H. Impact of blood pressure and antihypertensive treatment on incipient and overt nephropathy, retinopathy, and endothelial permeability in diabetes mellitus. Diabetes Care 1991; 14: 260–269.
[4] Parving H-H. Microvascular permeability to plasma proteins in hypertension and diabetes mellitus in man – on the pathogenesis of hypertensive and diabetic microangiopathy. Danish Med Bull 1975; 22: 217–233.
[5] Parving H-H, Gyntelberg F. Transcapillary escape rate of albumin and plasma volume in essential hypertension. Circ Res 1973; 32: 643–651.
[6] Rossing N, Jensen H. Metabolism of different albumin preparations. Clin Sci 1967; 32: 89–99.
[7] Parving H-H, Rossing N, Jensen HE. Increased metabolic turn-over rate and transcapillary escape rate of albumin in essential hypertension. Circ Res 1974; 35: 544–552.
[8] Parving H-H, Rossing N, Nielsen SL et al. Increased transcapillary escape rate of albumin, IgG and IgM after plasma volume expansion. Amer J Physiol 1974; 227: 245–250.
[9] Laurell C-B. Quantitative estimation of proteins by electrophoresis in agarose gel-containing antibodies. Anal Biochem 1966; 15: 45–52.
[10] Mancini G, Carbonara AO, Heremans JF. Immuno-chemical quantitation of antigens by single radial immunodiffusion. Immunochemistry 1965; 2: 235–254.
[11] Rossing N. Human albumin metabolism determined with radioiodinated albumin. Copenhagen: Munksgaard 1971: 45–48.
[12] Rossing N. The normal metabolism of ^{131}-I-labelled albumin. Clin Sci 1967; 33: 593–602.
[13] Katz J, Bonorris G. Electrolytic iodination of proteins with ^{126}I and ^{131}I. J Lab Clin Med 1968; 72: 966–970.
[14] Ismail AA, Khalifa K, Madwar KR. Capillary loss of radioiodinated serum albumin in diabetics. Lancet 1965; II: 810–813.
[15] Nestler JE, Barlascini CD, Tetrault GA et al. Increased transcapillary escape rate of albumin in non-diabetic men in response to hyperinsulinemia. Diabetes 1990; 39: 1212–1217.
[16] Poulsen HL. Subcutaneous interstitial fluid albumin concentration in long-term diabetes mellitus. Scand J Clin Lab Invest 1973; 32: 167–173.
[17] Hiistata U. Suction blister device for separation of variable epidermis from dermis. J Invest Dermatol 1968; 50: 129–137.
[18] Rossing N, Worm AM. Interstitial fluid: Exchange of macromolecules between plasma and skin interstitium. Clin Physiol 1981; 1: 275–284.
[19] Groth S, Staberg B. Suction blisters of the skin: a compartment with physiological, interstitium-like properties. Scand J Clin Lab Invest 1984; 44: 311–316.
[20] Noddeland H. Colloid osmotic pressure of human subcutaneous interstitial fluid sampled by nylon wicks: evaluation of the method. Scand J Clin Lab Invest 1982; 42: 123–130.
[21] Lassen NA, Parving H-H,Rossing N. Filtration as the main mechanism of overall transcapillary protein escape from the plasma. Microvasc Res 1974; 7: 1–4.
[22] Parving H-H, Rasmussen SM. Transcapillary escape rate of albumin and plasma volume in short- and long-term juvenile diabetics. Scand J Clin Lab Invest 1973; 32: 81–87.

[23] Parving H-H, Rossing N. Simultaneous determination of the transcapillary escape rate of albumin and IgG in normal and long-term juvenile diabetic subjects. Sand J Clin Lab Invest 1973; 32: 239–244.
[24] Parving H-H, Smidt UM. Hypotensive therapy reduces microvascular albumin leakage in insulin-dependent diabetic patients with nephropathy. Diabetic Med 1986; 3: 312–315.
[25] O'Hare JA, Ferries JB, Twomey B et al. Poor metabolic control, hypertension, and microangiopathy independently increase the transcapillary escape rate of albumin in diabetes. Diabetologia 1983; 25: 260–263.
[26] Feldt-Rasmussen B. Increased transcapillary escape rate of albumin in type 1 (insulin-dependent) diabetic patients with microalbuminuria. Diabetologia 1986; 29: 282–286.
[27] Norgaard K, Jensen T, Feldt-Rasmussen B. Transcapillary escape rate of albumin in hypertensive patients with Type 1 (insulin-dependent) diabetes mellitus. Diabetologia 1993; 36: 57–61.
[28] Parving H-H, Noer J, Deckert T, Evrin P-E et al. The effect of metabolic regulation on microvascular permeability to small and large molecules in short-term juvenile diabetics. Diabetologia 1976; 12: 161–166.
[29] Feldt-Rasmussen B, Mathiesen ER, Deckert T. Effects of two years of strict metabolic control on progression of incipient nephropathy in insulin-dependent diabetes. Lancet 1986; 2: 1300–1304.
[30] Parving H-H, Noer J, Deckert T et al. Intravenous insulin has no effect on transcapillary escape rate of albumin and on plasma volume in short-term juvenile diabetics. Diabetes 1979; 28: 282–286.
[31] Hostetter TH, Renneke HG, Brenner BM. The case for intrarenal hypertension in the initiation and progression of diabetic and other glomerulopathies. Am J Med 1982; 72: 375–380.
[32] Parving H-H, Viberti GC, Keen H et al. Hemodynamic factors in the genesis of diabetic microangiopathy. Metabolism 1983; 32: 943–949.
[33] Parving H-H, Kastrup J, Smidt UM. Reduced transcapillary escape rate of albumin during acute blood pressure-lowering in type 1 (insulin-dependent) diabetic patients with nephropathy. Diabetologia 1985; 28: 797–801.
[34] Sandeman DD, Shore AC, Tooke JE. Relation of skin capillary pressure in patients with insulin-dependent diabetes mellitus to complications and metabolic control. N Engl J Med 1992; 327: 760–764.
[35] Jensen T, Stender S, Goldstein K et al. Partial normalization by dietary cod-liver oil of increased microvascular albumin leakage in patients with insulin-dependent diabetes and albuminuria. N Engl J Med 1989; 321: 1572–1577.
[36] Hommel E, Mathiesen ER, Auckland K et al. Pathophysiological aspects of edema formation in diabetic nephropathy. Kidney Int 1990; 38: 1187–1192.
[37] Kofoed-Enevoldsen A, Bent-Hansen L, Deckert T. Transcapillary filtration of plasma protein in long-term type 1 (insulin-dependent) diabetic patients. Scand J Clin Lab Invest 1992; 52: 591–597.
[38] Garlick DG, Renkin EM. Transport of large molecules from plasma to interstitial fluid and lymph in dogs. Am J Physiol 1970; 219: 1595–1605.

Measurement of advanced glycosylation endproducts

R. Bucala, H. Vlassara, A. Cerami

Evidence to support the direct, a aetiological role of advanced glycosylation in the development of diabetic complications has increased substantially over the last few years. Both the tissue distribution and absolute level of protein advanced glycosylation endproducts (AGEs) correlate significantly with end-organ pathology. These pathological changes encompass both the macro- and microvascular complications of diabetes and include atherosclerosis, nephropathy, and retinopathy [1–4]. The recent development and clinical application of quantitative methods for the measurement of AGEs that form in vivo promises to further increase our understanding of the pathophysiology of advanced glycosylation [5–9].

Advanced glycosylation describes the chemical pathway that leads from early glycation products, such as Schiff bases and Amadori products, to more advanced protein-bound moieties that possess distinct fluorescence and cross-linking properties [10, 11]. Early glycation products result from the non-enzymatic addition of reducing sugars such as glucose to the primary amino groups of proteins. The N-terminal residues and the ε-amino group of lysine participate in the first stage of this reaction by forming freely reversible Schiff base adducts (Fig. 1). Protein-bound Schiff bases then slowly undergo rearrangement to produce Amadori products. These are more stable and achieve equilibrium in vivo over a period of 3–4 weeks. An increase in the formation of haemoglobin Amadori product accounts for the increased level of the minor haemoglobin species A_{1c} that is present in patients with diabetes mellitus. Because circulating levels of haemoglobin A_{1c} reflect average glycaemia over a preceding 3–4 week time period, clinical measurements of haemoglobin A_{1c} have achieved worldwide application as a method to assess long-term glucose control in diabetic patients [12, 13].

Over a time period of weeks to months, glucose-derived Amadori products undergo additional rearrangement reactions to produce the more "advanced" class of protein-bound moieties called advanced glycosylation endproducts or AGEs. Proteins with half-lives of greater than a few weeks are most suspectible to AGE-modification. As in the case of the early glycation products that form on haemoglobin and serum proteins, significant amounts of

Offprint from
Research Methodologies in Human Diabetes – Part 1

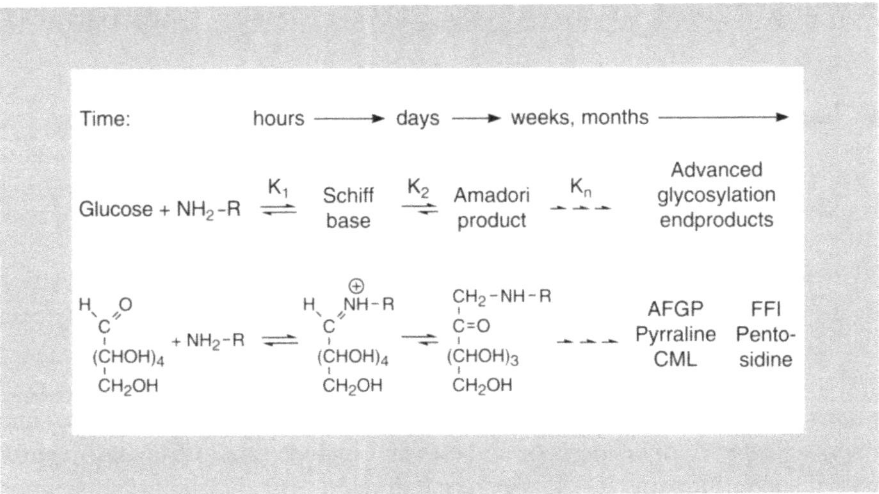

Fig. 1 Pathway of formation of protein-bound AGEs. Equilibrium levels of the reversible Schiff base and Amadori products are reached within hours and days respectively. AGEs are irreversibly attached and accumulate on long-lived proteins

AGEs form only on proteins within the non-insulin dependent tissue compartments that are exposed to high glucose levels.

AGEs alter the structural and functional properties of proteins, and many of these alterations have been linked to the pathophysiological changes that accompany both long-standing diabetes and normal aging. AGEs progressively crosslink connective tissue collagen for example, and increase connective tissue rigidity [14, 15]. This contributes to the vascular and ligamentous rigidity that occurs during normal aging and presumably, for the high prevalence of joint stiffness and cheirarthropathy that has been observed in patients with diabetes mellitus [16, 17]. Collagen-linked AGEs also act as reactive foci to covalently "trap" circulating serum proteins such as albumin, lipoproteins, and immunoglobulins [18, 19]. This accounts in part for the increase in protein deposition and in basement membrane thickening that occurs in the systemic and renal vasculature of patients with diabetes. Cell surface receptors that are specific for the recognition, uptake, and degradation of AGE-modified proteins have been identified to be present on monocytes, endothelial cells, and renal mesangial cells [20–22]. AGEs are chemotactic for monocytes, and the receptor-mediated uptake of AGE-modified proteins initiates cytokine-mediated processes that promote tissue remodelling [23]. Occupancy of endothelial cell receptors by AGEs leads to increased vascular permeability, down-regulation of the anticoagulant factor thrombomodulin, and increased synthesis of the procoagulant tissue factor [21]. Protein-bound AGEs also react with and chemically inactivate nitric oxide (endothelium-derived relaxing factor), thereby contributing to diabetes-related defects in vascular relaxation [24–26]. More recently, AGEs have been observed also to form on amine-containing phospholipids [27]. Once glucose attaches to phospholipids, intramolecular oxidation-reduction reactions occur that then initiate fatty acid oxidation. These reactions occur in situ on low-density lipoprotein (LDL), and readily explain the increased level of oxidized-LDL in diabetic plasma [27–29]. Since the oxidative modification of LDL has been proposed to play a central role in atherogenesis, the formation of AGEs on LDL may contribute significantly to the propensity of diabetic patients to develop early and severe cardiovascular disease.

For many years, investigation of the pathological sequelae associated with advanced glycosylation has been hampered by the lack of sensitive and specific methods to detect AGEs in vivo. This situation resulted in part from a lack of knowledge concerning the precise structures and pathway of formation of AGEs in vivo. Despite intensive efforts, early biochemical studies were successful only in revealing that AGEs are chemically heterogenous, present in low abundance, and labile to the conventional methods of protein hydrolysis and isolation necessary for structure elucidation. Initial methods for assessing advanced glycosylation consequently relied on measurements of protein-linked fluorescence. Although these studies were not strictly quantitative, it was established nevertheless that advanced glycosylation occurred in vivo, and that AGEs formed progressively on proteins as a function of tissue age and duration of diabetes [10, 11].

Within the last several years, several candidate AGEs have been isolated and structurally characterized (Fig. 2). These products were purified from model glucose-protein incubations or isolated directly from aged connective tissue proteins. The first AGE that was identified was furoyl-furanyl imidazole (FFI), a crosslink that appeared to result from the condensation of two lysine-derived Amadori products [30]. Later mechanistic studies suggested however that the greatest portion of FFI may form during purification [31]. Nevertheless, AGEs that are structurally similar to FFI appear to exist in vivo since anti-FFI antibodies crossreact with native, AGE-modified proteins [32, 33]. Pyrrole containing AGEs such as AFGP and pyrraline also have been isolated from model in vitro incubation mixtures [34, 35] and recent immunohistochemical studies suggest that these AGEs occur in vivo and accumulate on long-lived basement membrane and connective tissue proteins [33, 36, 37].

Sell and Monnier recently isolated an acid-resistant, fluorescent AGE from aged connective tissue collagen [38]. This compound, pentosidine, results from the covalent crosslinking of lysine to arginine by a five carbon sugar backbone. Postulated originally to arise from the reaction of pentoses with proteins, pentosidine subsequently was found to also form from glucose(hexose)-modified proteins [39]. Sensitive HPLC methods for the detection of pentosidine have been devised and have confirmed its presence in aged and in diabetic tissues. Quantitative considerations suggest however, that pentosidine constitutes only a small fraction (about 1 percent) of AGE-derived crosslinks. This fact, together with the requirement for specimens of connective tissue and subsequent chemical hydrolysis procedures, has limited somewhat the utility of pentosidine measurements to clinical investigation. Nevertheless, prospective and cross-sectional investigations of pentosidine levels in aged and diabetic tissue have affirmed basic features of the formation of this AGE in vivo. Collagen-linked pentosidine levels increase in connective tissue as a function of age and glycaemia and accumulate to very high levels in patients

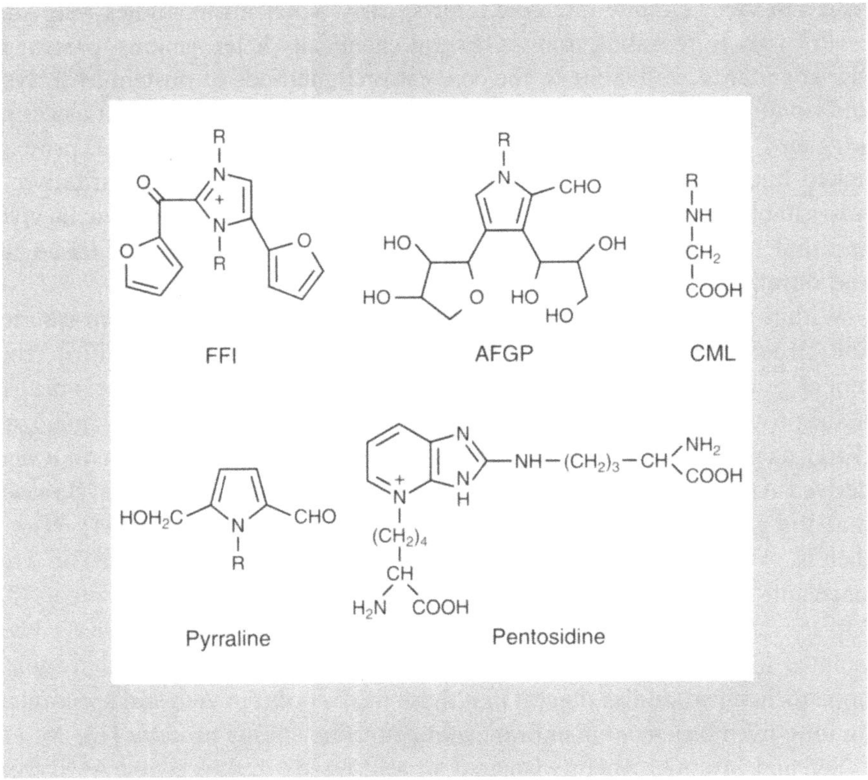

Fig. 2 Structure of AGEs. "R" denotes lysine carbon backbone

with chronic renal failure, in whom protein and amino acid excretion is impaired [40–42].

Research into the development of sensitive and specific immunochemical methods for the detection of the AGEs that form in vivo has been pursued for a number of years. Although antibody reagents for the detection of FFI, pyrraline, and AFGP have been developed, the low abundance of these particular AGEs in vivo continues to restrict the clinical applicability of these antibody detection methods [32, 33, 36, 43]. One successful approach for measuring the AGEs that form in vivo has exploited the specific binding activity of AGEs for receptors present on the monocyte cell line RAW 264.7 [7]. Standard radio-receptor techniques were applied to AGE measurements and detailed information about circulating serum levels, molecular size distribution, and the clearance rate of AGEs has been obtained in normal, diabetic, and renally-impaired patient populations [3].

Several years ago, we set out to develop antibodies that might react with the major class(es) of AGEs that exist in vivo. Although the dominant structural features of "native" AGEs remain unknown, it was reasoned that AGEs prepared in vitro under physiological conditions might share epitopes that also are present on proteins modified by AGEs in vivo. Test immunogens were prepared by incubating different proteins with glucose for long periods of time at 37° and at neutral pH. Glucose was selected as the glycosylating sugar because it is the major circulating sugar and it might be expected to produce epitopes that closely resemble those present on "native" AGE-modified proteins in vivo. Unfortunately, early immunization attempts were frustrated by poor reactivity of antisera to AGE epitope(s). These results generally were attributed to heterogeneity in the structure of the AGE epitope(s), a low epitope density, and self-tolerance to AGEs.

Within the last 2–3 years, modifications of conventional immunization protocols have led to the production of high-titre polyclonal, and monoclonal anti-AGE antibodies that have been applied successfully to the development of enzyme-linked immunosorbent assays (ELISA) [5, 6, 8]. In our laboratory, hyperimmunization techniques were employed to suppress the host response to common (peptide backbone) epitopes and enhance responsivity to the more rare AGE epitopes [44]. Optimal antibody responses also appeared to result from the utilization of ribonuclease as the carrier protein for the AGE epitope(s) in place of higher molecular weight (and generally more immunogenic) proteins such as BSA or KLH. Ribonuclease, in contrast to BSA for example, readily forms oligomers as a result of AGE-modification [45]. It was reasoned therefore, that AGE-modified ribonuclease may be relatively more enriched for the AGE crosslinking moieties that occur in vivo.

Detailed crossreactivity studies revealed several interesting features about the anti-AGE antibodies that ultimately were elicited and utilized for anti-AGE ELISA. The first and unexpected finding was the lack of reactivity of anti-AGE antibody with all of the known, structurally-defined AGEs such as FFI, AFGP, pyrraline, carboxymethyllysine, and pentosidine; even when these compounds were tested at a several log-fold molar excess compared to native AGE antigen (Table 1). These data suggested that the structurally-defined AGEs that have been described to date represent antigenically minor products when compared to the AGEs that are present in vivo [8].

The second important finding was the identification of an apparently major class of crossreactive AGE epitope(s) that are common to proteins modified

Table 1. Crossreactivity analysis of rabbit anti-AGE antibody with diverse AGE-proteins, chemically-modified proteins, model AGEs, and Amadori products. AGE-modified proteins were prepared by incubation with the sugar displayed in parenthesis. Percent crossreactivity (molar) was calculated relative to AGE-BSA (glucose) at the 50% inhibition point. Data compiled from ref. [8]

Antigen	Percent Crossreactivity (M)
Modified BSA	
AGE-BSA (glucose)	100.0
AGE-BSA (Glc-6-PO_4)	20.0
AGE-BSA (fructose)	6.0
FFI-BSA	< 0.004
Formyl-BSA	< 0.004
Maleyl-BSA	< 0.004
Malonyldialdehycle-BSA	< 0.004
Heterologous proteins	
AGE-HSA (Glc-6-PO_4)	18.0
AGE-LDL (glucose)	16.0
AGE-collagen IV (glucose)	0.4
HSA	< 0.004
LDL	< 0.004
Acetyl-LDL	< 0.004
Collagen IV	< 0.004
Ribonuclease	< 0.004
Model AGEs and Amadori products	
AGE-lysine (glucose)	24.0
AGE-lysine (Glc-6-PO_4)	7.0
FFI-hexanoic acid	< 0.004
Pyrraline	< 0.004
AFGP	< 0.004
Pentosidine	< 0.004
Carboxymethyllysine	< 0.004
Deoxypropylaminofructose	< 0.004
Deoxymorpholinofructose	< 0.004

Table 2 Representative values for collagen-linked AGEs in rats (A), total AGEs in human serum (B), and haemoglobin-AGE (Hb-AGE) (C) in selected patient populations. ELISA reactivity is expressed in AGE Units, calculated relative to a synthesized AGE-albumin standard (data compiled from refs. [8, 9])

A. Collagen-AGE levels in experimentally-induced diabetes		
	16 weeks	64 weeks
Non-diabetic rats:	2.5 ± 0.6 U/mg	4.3 ± 0.4 U/mg
Diabetic rats:	4.8 ± 0.5 U/mg	10.5 ± 1.8 U/mg
B. Serum AGE levels in human subjects		
Non-diabetic patients:	10.5 ± 1.3 U/ml	
Diabetic patients:	24.7 ± 2.4 U/ml	
Diabetic patients on haemodialysis:	79.4 ± 9.9 U/ml	
C. Haemoglobin-AGE levels in human subjects		
Non-diabetic patients:	4.3 ± 0.3 U/mg	
Diabetic patients:	7.7 ± 0.6 U/mg	

by advanced glycosylation in vitro and in vivo. Immunochemical analysis showed that crossreactive AGE epitopes form when glucose is incubated with different proteins, such as lysozyme, albumin, low density lipoprotein (LDL), and collagen. When in vivo specimens were studied, anti-AGE antiserum was found to react both with arterial collagen and with serum known to contain high levels of AGEs, as assessed by fluorescence or radio-receptor detection methods. In the case of arterial collagen obtained from rats with experimentally-induced diabetes, the level of AGEs detected by anti-AGE antibody increased with the duration of diabetes (Table 2). Smaller, age-related increases in collagen-bound AGEs also were observed. Circulating serum AGEs were detected in diabetic patients, and were highest in those patients undergoing haemodialysis, a group shown previously to have increased amounts of both circulating and collagen-bound AGEs [8].

Different glycosylating sugars such as glucose, glucose-6-phosphate (Glc-6-PO_4), and fructose were found to produce antigenically cross-reactive epitopes when incubated with albumin in vitro. These results provided additional evidence for the concept that a common immunological epitope forms as a result of the reaction of reducing sugars with proteins. Of note, immunoreactive AGE epitopes were found to be labile to standard acid hydrolysis conditions (6M HCl, 110°). Other albumin modifications that produce specific recognition signals for albumin uptake in vivo such as formylation, acetylation, or maleylation did not demonstrate any cross-reactivity with anti-AGE antibody. One important property of the antibody "reactive" AGE(s) was that its formation was inhibited by aminoguanidine, an agent currently under development as a pharmacological inhibitor of advanced glycosylation [8].

Anti-AGE ELISA is being applied to a variety of clinical investigations with the aim of specifically assessing the role of advanced glycosylation in diabetic and age-related complications. At the outset, it was considered that since Amadori products such as HbA_{1c} are AGE precursors, haemoglobin might similarly acquire and accumulate AGE modifications. In the same way as HbA_{1c} serves to integrate serum glucose concentration over a 3–4 week period, haemoglobin-AGE (Hb-AGE) could function as a readily measured, circulating index of tissue advanced glycosylation. Haemoglobin-linked AGEs in fact were detected to be present in red cells and, not surprisingly, higher amounts were found to be present in the diabetic group (Table 2) [9].

A significant correlation between the levels of red cell HbA_{1c} and Hb-AGE was observed (Fig. 3). This finding further verified the concept that protein-bound AGEs arise from Amadori product precursors. In vitro studies confirmed that Hb-AGE formed in a time- and concentration-dependent manner as a result of the incubation of glucose with haemoglobin. As expected, the addition of aminoguanidine, an inhibitor of advanced glycosylation, prevented the formation of haemoglobin-associated AGEs in vitro [9].

The identification of an AGE-modified haemoglobin is noteworthy for several reasons. First, AGEs generally have been considered to require a time course of months to years to form, even under hyperglycaemic conditions. Yet, Hb-AGE accounts for approximately $0.42 \pm 0.07\%$ of circulating haemoglobin, and was observed to increase to $0.75 \pm 0.08\%$ in the particular group of diabetic patients that were studied. These values are approximately one-tenth of the corresponding HbA_{1c} values for these two patient groups. The reason for the readily detected levels of AGE formation on haemoglobin within the 60 day half-life of the red cells is unknown, but may indicate an inherently enhanced rate of AGE formation on haemoglobin as a protein substrate.

The second important implication of these findings is that Hb-AGE may serve as a readily measured index of advanced glycosylation in vivo. To begin to address this question, we performed Hb-AGE measurements on blood specimens obtained from diabetic patients undergoing treatment with the advanced glycosylation inhibitor aminoguanidine. Blood samples were obtained before and after aminoguanidine therapy and the Hb-AGE levels measured by ELISA. The mean Hb-AGE value decreased significantly as a result of aminoguanidine therapy (13.8 ± 0.8 U/mg Hb at the initiation of therapy versus 10.0 ± 0.9 U/mg Hb after 28 days of therapy). HbA_{1c} values were not affected by aminoguanidine treatment, pointing to the specificity of aminoguanidine for inhibition of post-Amadori, advanced glycosylation reactions [9].

Previous in vitro and in vivo studies would indicate that the formation of Hb-AGE reflects a time integral of blood glucose concentration that is significantly longer than that established for HbA_{1c}, a slowly reversible adduct that reflects a blood glucose integral of only 30 days [12]. The precise temporal relationship between the formation of Hb-AGE and average glycaemia has yet to be established; however, 4-week pharmacological intervention with aminoguanidine lowered significantly (28%) the Hb-AGE levels in a treated diabetic population. Extrapolation of this rate suggests that in approximately 50% decrease in Hb-AGE would occur after 60 days, the time when one-half of the red cell mass had turned over. Hb-AGE measurement ultimately may replace $Hb\text{-}A_{1c}$ is a clinical marker of average glycaemia since it reflects the full 60 day half-life of the red cell. Hb-AGE measurements should facilitate a variety of clinical studies concerned with the pathophysiology of diabetic

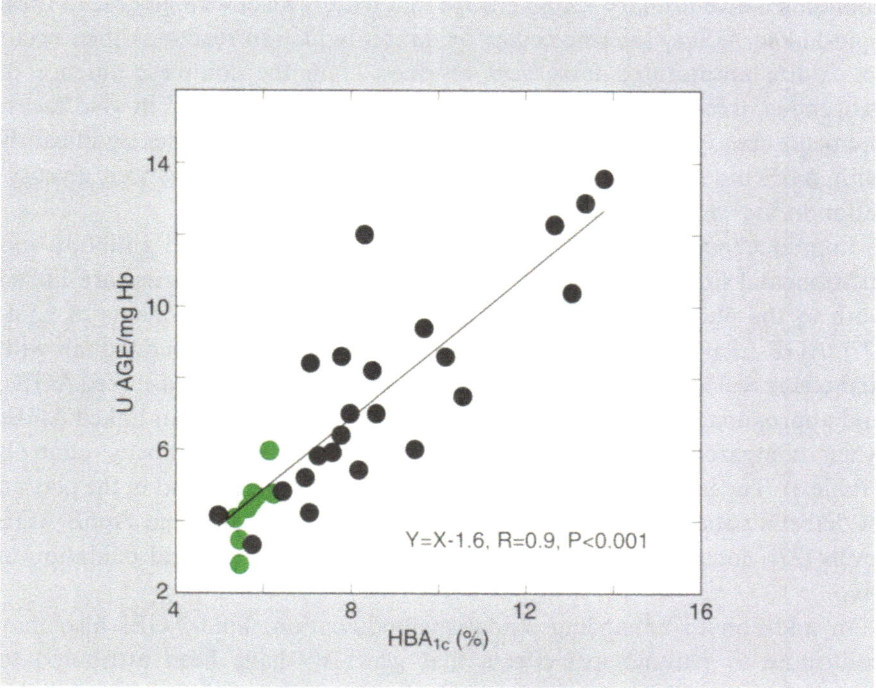

Fig. 3 Correlation between Hb-AGE and HbA_{1c} in 9 normoglycaemic (•) and 23 diabetic (•) individuals. From ref. [9]

complications, including those investigations aimed at elucidating the benefit of strict glucose control in preventing complications, and pharmacological studies of advanced glycosylation inhibitors.

The second area that we have applied the immunochemical detection of AGEs is in the study of the advanced glycosylation of lipoprotein [27]. Lipoprotein modification has been proposed to play a central role in atherogenesis and to contribute to the diverse vascular sequelae of diabetes and aging [46]. In particular, the oxidative modification of LDL has been shown to result in the loss of its recognition by cellular LDL receptors, and in the preferential uptake of oxidized-LDL (ox-LDL) by macrophage "scavenger" receptors [47]. The enhanced endocytosis of ox-LDL by vascular wall macrophages transforms them into the lipid-laden foam cells that characterize early atherosclerotic lesions. This is followed progressively by the development of fatty streaks and the complex, proliferative lesions that ultimately cause arterial insufficiency and occlusion [46].

In recent studies, we have obtained evidence that glucose-mediated advanced glycosylation reactions directly initiate lipid oxidation in vitro and in vivo. Phospholipids such as phosphatidylethanolamine or phosphatidylserine contain reactive primary amino groups that readily react with glucose to form lipid-linked AGEs. Intermolecular oxidation-reduction reactions then occur to oxidize unsaturated fatty acid residues – in the complete absence of exogenous, free-radical generating systems. Both in vitro and in vivo measurements demonstrate that the level of LDL oxidation correlates significantly with AGE modification, supporting the primary role of advanced glycosylation in the formation of ox-LDL [27].

Immunochemical analysis of purified LDL with anti-AGE antibody was instrumental in establishing the fact that in vivo, AGE moieties are linked both to the phospholipid and the apoprotein (ApoB) components of LDL [27]. AGE-ELISA analysis of LDL specimens obtained from individuals with diabetes revealed four-fold increases in the level of phospholipid-linked AGEs, and approximately two-fold increases in the level of apoprotein-linked AGEs when compared to LDL obtained from normal, non-diabetic controls (Table 3). The increased levels of oxidized-LDL that were found in the plasma of diabetic patients correlated significantly with both lipid- and ApoB-AGE levels [27], consistent with a mechanism of AGE-induced lipid oxidation in vivo.

In addition to enhancing oxidative modification, lipid-AGEs also may contribute to pathological effects that generally have been attributed to protein-linked AGEs. An increase in the subendothelial density of lipid-AGEs, as might occur in atherosclerotic plaque for example, would enhance

Table 3 Measurements of advanced glycosylation and oxidative modification of human LDL isolated from the plasma of 8 normoglycaemic, non-diabetic individuals and 16 patients with diabetes mellitus. Advanced glycosylation was measured in the ApoB and the lipid components of LDL. Oxidative modification (expressed as nmole malonyldialdehyde equivalents) was determined from measurements performed on intact LDL. Data from ref. [27]

	ApoB-AGEs	Lipid-AGEs	Oxidative Modification
Non-diabetic patients:	2.8 ± 0.6 U/mg	110 ± 30 U/mg	3.7 ± 1.3 nm/mg
Diabetic patients:	6.8 ± 4.0 U/mg	410 ± 25 U/mg	6.8 ± 1.2 nm/mg

protein deposition and crosslinking, stimulate macrophage-monocyte chemotaxis, and inactivate the vasodilatory effects of nitric oxide (endothelial-derived relaxing factor) [19, 21, 24]. Lipid-AGEs also could function to activate AGE-receptors that have been identified to be present on macrophages and endothelial cells. Additional effects might then ensue, such as a stimulation of local cytokine and growth factor release, and an enhancement of vascular permeability [21, 23]. Clinical measurement of lipid-linked AGEs may serve as a convenient, surrogate marker of oxidative modification in vivo. Quantitative assessments of AGE-modified LDL will help to delineate the relationship between LDL modification, lipid oxidation, and the abnormalities of lipoprotein clearance that contribute to diabetic and non-diabetic vasculopathy.

In conclusion, recent progress in the development of immunochemical techniques to quantitate AGEs in vivo promises to contribute substantially to our understanding of the biology and pathophysiology of advanced glycosylation. Clinical application of AGE-specific ELISAs will facilitate a variety of investigations aimed at assessing the precise role of advanced glycosylation in particular diabetic complications. The identification of Hb-AGE as a circulating marker of advanced glycosylation will assist in the clinical evaluation of recently developed pharmacological inhibitors of advanced glycosylation such as aminoguanidine. Furthermore, continued investigation into the formation of AGE-LDL, and its propensity to undergo oxidative modification, will enhance our understanding of atherogenic mechanisms in both diabetic and non-diabetic vascular disease.

References

[1] Monnier VM, Vishwanath V, Frank KE et al. Relation between complications of type 1 diabetes mellitus and collagen-linked fluorescence. N Eng J Med 1986; 314: 403–408.

[2] Brownlee M, Cerami A, Vlassara H. Advanced glycosylation endproducts in tissue and the biochemical basis of diabetic complications. N Eng J Med 1988; 318: 1315–1321.

[3] Makita Z, Radoff S, Rayfield EJ et al. Advanced glycosylation endproducts in patients with diabetic nephropathy. N Eng J Med 1991; 325: 836–842.
[4] Hammes HP, Martin S, Federlin K et al. Aminoguanidine treatment inhibits the development of experimental diabetic retinopathy. Proc Natl Acad Sci USA 1991; 88: 11555–11558.
[5] Nakayama H, Taneda S, Kuwajima S et al. Production and characterization of antibodies to advanced glycation products on proteins. Biochem Biophys Res Comm 1989; 162: 740–745.
[6] Horiuchi S, Araki N, Morino Y. Immunochemical approach to characterize advanced glycation endproducts of the Maillard Reaction. J Biol Chem 1991; 266: 7329–7332.
[7] Radoff S, Makita Z, Vlassara H. Radioreceptor assay for advanced glycosylation endproducts. Diabetes 1991; 40: 1731–1738.
[8] Makita Z, Vlassara H, Cerami A et al. Immunochemical detection of advanced glycosylation endproducts in vivo. J Biol Chem 1992; 267: 5133–5138.
[9] Makita Z, Vlassara H, Rayfield E et al. Hemoglobin-AGE: A circulating marker of advanced glycosylation. Science 1992; 258: 651–653.
[10] Njoroge FG, Monnier VM. The chemistry of the Maillard reaction under physiological conditions: a review. Prog Clin Biol Res 1989; 304: 85–107.
[11] Bucala R, Cerami A. Advanced glycosylation: chemistry, biology, and implications for Diabetes and Aging. Adv Pharmacol 1992; 23: 1–34.
[12] Koenig RJ, Peterson CM, Jones RL et al. Correlation of glucose regulation and hemoglobin A_{1c} in diabetes mellitus. N Eng J Med 1976; 295: 417–420.
[13] Larsen ML, Horder M, Mogensen EF. Effect of long-term monitoring of glycosylated hemoglobin levels in insulin-dependent diabetes mellitus. N Eng J Med 1990; 323: 1021–1025.
[14] Schnider SL, Kohn RR. Effects of age and diabetes mellitus on the solubility of collagen from human skin, tracheal cartilage and dura mater. Exp Geront 1982; 17: 184–194.
[15] Monnier VM, Kohn RR, Cerami A. Accelerated age-related browning of human collagen in diabetes mellitus. Proc Natl Acad Sci USA 1984; 81: 583–587.
[16] Rosenbloom AL, Silverstein JH, Lezotte DC et al. Limited joint mobility in childhood diabetes mellitus indicates increased risk for microvascular disease. N Eng J Med 1981; 305: 191–194.
[17] Fisher L, Kurtz A, Shipley M. Association between cheirarthropathy and frozen shoulder in patients with insulin-dependent diabetes mellitus. Br J Rheumatol 1986; 25: 141–146.
[18] Brownlee M, Pongor S, Cerami A. Covalent attachment of soluble proteins by nonenzymatically glycosylated collagen; role in the in situ formation of immune complexes. J Exp Med 1983; 158: 1739–1744.
[19] Brownlee M, Vlassara H, Cerami A. Nonenzymatic glycosylation products on collagen covalently trap low-density lipoprotein. Diabetes 1985; 34: 938–941.
[20] Vlassara H, Brownlee M, Cerami A. High-affinity receptor-mediated uptake and degradation of glucose-modified proteins: a potential mechanism for the removal of senescent macromolecules. Proc Natl Acad Sci USA 1985; 82: 5588–5592.
[21] Esposito C, Gerlach H, Brett J et al. Endothelial receptor-mediated binding of glucose-modified albumin is associated with incresaed monolayer permeability and modulation of cell surface coagulant properties. J Exp Med 1989; 170: 1387–1407.
[22] Skolnik EY, Yang Z, Makita Z et al. Human and rat mesangial cell receptors for glucose-modified proteins: Potential role in kidney tissue remodelling and diabetic nephropathy. J Exp Med 1991; 174: 931–938.
[23] Vlassara H, Brownlee M, Manogue K et al. Cachectin/TNF and IL-1 induced by glucose-modified proteins: Role in normal tissue remodeling. Science 1988; 240: 1546–1548.
[24] Bucala R, Tracey K, Cerami A. Advanced glycosylation products quench nitric oxide and mediate defective endothelium-dependent vasodilatation in experimental diabetes. J Clin Invest 1991; 87: 432–438.

[25] Hogan M, Cerami A, Bucala R. Advanced glycosylation endproducts block the antiproliferative effect of nitric oxide. J Clin Invest 1992; 90: 1110–1115.
[26] Vlassara H, Fuh H, Makita Z et al. Exogenous advanced glycosylation endproducts induce complex vascular dysfunction in normal animals: A model for diabetic and aging complications. Proc Natl Acad Sci USA 1992; 89: 12043–12047.
[27] Bucala R, Makita Z, Koschinsky T et al. Lipid advanced glycocylation: Pathway for lipid oxidation in vivo. Proc Natl Acad Sci USA 1993; 90: 6434–6438.
[28] Nishigaki I, Hagihara M, Tsunekawa H et al. Lipid peroxide levels of serum lipoprotein fractions of diabetic patients. Biochem Med 1981; 25: 373–378.
[29] Armstrong D, Abdell N, Salman A et al. Relationship of lipid peroxides to diabetic complications. J Diabetes Comp 1992; 6: 116–122.
[30] Pongor S, Ulrich PC, Bencsath FA et al. Aging of proteins: Isolation and identification of a fluorescent chromophore from the reaction of polypeptides with glucose. Proc Natl Acad Sci USA 1984; 81: 2684–2688.
[31] Njoroge FG, Fernandes AA, Monnier V. Mechanism of formation of the putative advanced glycosylation endproduct and protein cross-link 2-(2-furoyl)-4(5)-(2-furanyl)-1H-imidazole. J Biol Chem 1988; 263: 10646–10652.
[32] Chang JCF, Ulrich PC, Bucala R et al. Detection of an advanced glycosylation product bound to protein in situ. J Biol Chem 1985; 260: 7970–7974.
[33] Palinski W, Koschinsky T, Butler SW et al. Immunological evidence for the in vivo presence of advanced glycosylation endproducts: Development of antibodies specific for furoyl-furanyl-imidazole (FFI) or alkyl-furanyl-diglycosylpyrrole (AFGP)-conjugated proteins. Diabetes 1993; (in press).
[34] Njoroge FG, Sayre LM, Monnier V. Detection of D-glucose-derived pyrrole compounds during Maillard reaction under physiological conditions. Carbohydrate Res 1987; 167: 211–220.
[35] Farmar J, Ulrich P, Cerami A. Novel pyrroles from sulfite-inhibited Maillard reactions: insight into the mechanism of inhibition. J Org Chem 1988; 53: 2346–2349.
[36] Hayase F, Nagaraj RH, Miyata S et al. Aging of proteins: Immunological detection of a glucose-derived pyrrole formed during Maillard reaction in vivo. J Biol Chem 1989; 264: 3758–3764.
[37] Miyata S, Monnier V. Immunohistochemical detection of advanced glycosylation end products in diabetic tissues using monoclonal antibody to pyrraline. J Clin Invest 1992; 89: 1102–1112.
[38] Sell DR, Monnier VM. Structure elucidation of a senescence cross-link from human extracellular matrix. J Biol Chem 1989; 264: 21597–21602.
[39] Grandhee S, Monnier VM. Mechanism of formation of pentosidine: ribose, glucose, fructose and ascorbate as pentosidine precursors. J Biol Chem 1991; 266: 11649–11653.
[40] Sell DR, Monnier VM. End-stage renal disease and diabetes catalyze the formation of a pentose-derived crosslink from aging human collagen. J Clin Invest 1990; 85: 380–384.
[41] Odetti P, Fogarty J, Sell DR et al. Chromatographic quantitation of plasma and erythrocyte pentosidine in diabetic and uremic subjects. Diabetes 1992; 41: 153–160.
[42] Sell DR, Lapolla A, Odetti P et al. Pentosidine formation in skin correlates with severity of complications in individuals with long-standing IDDM. Diabetes 1992; 41(10): 1286–1292.
[43] Smith PR, Somani HH, Thornalley PJ et al. Evidence against the formation of 2-amino-6-(2-formyl-5-hydroxymethyl-pyrrol-l-yl)-hexanoic acid ("pyrraline") as an early-stage product or advanced glycation end product in non-enzymic protein glycation. Clin Sci 1993; 84: 87–93.
[44] Bucala R, Cerami A. Characterization of antisera to the addition product formed by the nonenzymatic reaction of 16α-hydroxyestrone with albumin. Mol Immunol 1983; 20: 1289–1292.

[45] Eble AS, Thrope SR, Baynes JW. Nonenzymatic glycosylation and glucose-dependent cross-linking of proteins. J Biol Chem 1983; 258: 9406–9412.
[46] Witztum JL, Steinberg D. Role of oxidized low density lipoprotein in atherogenesis. J Clin Invest 1991; 88: 1785–1792.
[47] Sparrow CP, Parthasarathy S, Steinberg D. A macrophage receptor that recognizes oxidized LDL but not acetylated LDL. J Biol Chem 1989; 264: 2599–2604.

Research methodologies in the evaluation of home glucose monitoring

B. Willms

Introduction

Home glucose monitoring (or self-monitoring of blood glucose, which is used synonymously with the former in this article) has become an important tool in the management of individuals with diabetes mellitus for more than ten years. It is a major technical advance which provides both the diabetic patient and the health-care team with vital clinical information that was previously unattainable. It is now possible for the diabetic patient and health-care personnel to measure and record blood glucose levels frequently with the use of reagent-impregnated strips, which are visually read or analyzed by a portable glucose meter. Physicians can adjust insulin dosages after reviewing previously recorded self-monitored blood glucose values at the time of patient's visits. Diabetic patients themselves, using algorithms [19] or past experience, often vary the content of individual insulin injections in response to home glucose monitoring.

Individuals with diabetes mellitus, as well as health-care professionals involved with their care, must be trained to understand the purpose of home glucose monitoring, use the technique accurately, and record and make appropriate use of the results. Home glucose monitoring is essential for any insulin-injecting diabetic patient [7].

Numerous systems have been developed and upgraded in an effort to facilitate the ease and accuracy of patient-generated glucose values. Extensive published research attests to the accuracy of these systems both in the laboratory and during observed patient use [8, 12, 13, 17, 18, 20, 21]. However, the evaluation of methods for home glucose monitoring is done using very different methods. There is no internationally accepted agreement concerning a standardized procedure for the technical and clinical evaluation of methods for self-monitoring of blood glucose [11].

Offprint from
Research Methodologies in Human Diabetes — Part 1

Requirements for self-monitoring of blood glucose

In November 1986, the American Diabetes Association sponsored a consensus conference on self-monitoring of blood glucose. This panel of experts stated in a consensus statement [1] that the goal of all future self-glucose monitoring systems should be to achieve a variability (system plus user) of $< 10\%$ at glucose concentrations of 30–400 mg/dl 100% of the time. However, the panel was also aware that the accuracy for clinical management had not been rigorously defined. It has been argued that this goal for home blood glucose monitoring is an ideal, but unrealistic approach [11].

Furthermore, the expert committee endorsed the position of the Joint Commission of Accreditation of Hospitals (JCAH) that self-monitoring of blood glucose by non-laboratory personnel must meet for following minimum standards:

- Personnel performing the test must be qualified through training. Training must be documented.
- There should be written procedures and policies for test performance, quality control, standardization and calibration of instruments, and reagent acquisition and storage.
- Quality control must occur daily and be documented.
- A basic accession record to include patient name, test, and date should be maintained to correlate with documented quality control results.

With current systems, self-monitoring blood glucose measurements should be within 15% of the results of the reference measurement.

Technical evaluation of home glucose monitoring

Prerequisites

Methods for home glucose monitoring should give an accurate measurement of the blood glucose value across the entire range of the clinically relevant blood glucose concentration in diabetes, that is hypoglycaemia, euglycaemia, and hyperglycaemia. The American Diabetes Association proposes the range of 30–400 mg/dl. To cover this field $\sim$ 100 single independent measurements are adequate. Koschinsky [11] choses a minimum of 30 independent values with a log-homogeneous sample distribution over the blood glucose range as $n \geq 5$ for 25–40, 40–65, 65–100, 100–160, 160–250, and 250–400 mg/dl. To simplify this procedure, we would suggest that the three clinically relevant areas, such as hypoglycaemia ($<$ 70 mg/dl), euglycaemia (70–180 mg/dl) and hyperglycaemia (180–400 mg/dl), be covered with sufficient measurement-points.

Since methods for self-glucose monitoring are at least derived from laboratory methods, they should be evaluated technically according to the standards of clinical chemistry using the concept of accuracy and precision. Only a small degree of deviation from the true value is acceptable from the standpoint of the clinical chemist. However, because most methods for home glucose monitoring deviate so much more from the true value than a clinical laboratory, an additional clinical evaluation is necessary to determine the clinically acceptable degree of deviation within the clinically relevant blood glucose range. However, no clear distinctions exist between demarcations of acceptable and unacceptable blood glucose values within a clinically relevant range.

The blood glucose measurements obtained from the self-monitoring systems should be compared with the measurements determined using a laboratory method acknowledged as "gold standard" or "true" measure of blood glucose. This is normally the hexokinase method for determining the glucose concentration. Blood should be taken from capillary blood by finger or ear pricking. The blood for the measurements should be taken from the same prick at the same time, within the same minute.

Accuracy and precision

The deviation of the self-monitored blood glucose values from the "true" values are viewed as errors in the self-monitoring system and may be due to random factors (chance variation), systematic factors (bias), or a combination of random and systematic factors. Random error increases the imprecision of the measurements, while systematic error (either constant or proportional) increases the inaccuracy of the measurements.

To detect a systematic deviation, $\sim$ 100 measurements with a home glucose monitoring system should be compared with the reference glucose method and the deviation calculated in mg/dl as well as percentage. Both figures should be given for the entire blood glucose range as well as for the three relevant areas hypo-, eu- and hyperglycaemia.

If qualified laboratory personnel perform these measurements, a systematic deviation of the home glucose monitoring system may be detected, e. g., that a certain device underestimates hypoglycaemic values and/or overestimates hyperglycaemic values or vice versa. Continuous overestimation as well as continuous underestimation also occurs with self-glucose monitoring system.

As is the case for any laboratory method, the precision of a home glucose monitoring system has to be evaluated. Precision or reproducibility of a method describes how multiple measurements of the same probe agree with each other

- as in precision in the run, that is under identical conditions on the same day
- as in precision within runs, that is precision from day to day.

About 20 measurements should be taken from an artificial blood (EDTA blood) or a standardized control solution. Mean value, standard deviation (SD) and coefficient of variation ($CV\ \% = \frac{SD}{\bar{x}} \cdot 100$) are calculated. The standard for precision is the coefficient of variation which is aimed for blood constituents to be $< 5\%$.

Correlation and regression

The correlation coefficient (r) and the linear regression technique are statistical methods which tell us to which extent pairs of measurements, that is, the values of home glucose monitoring and the reference glucose method, correlate to each other.

A r value of 1 means that the two variables are completely dependent on each other, and the two regression lines y and x are identical. If the correlation coefficient tends to zero, the two variables do not correlate well to each other and may be completely independent from each other (at r = zero). Correlation coefficients of $r = 0.98$ and more are considered as an excellent association of two methods.

The ideal linear regression curve would be $y = x$ (y = tested home glucose monitoring system, x = reference blood glucose method). The real (calculated) regression line $y = ax + b$, where a is the slope of the regression line and b is the y-intercept, may vary from the ideal curve. The deviation of the regression curve represents the systematic deviation (inaccuracy) of the tested versus the reference method, whereas the correlation coefficient r provides information about the random error (imprecision) influencing the system.

Examples are given in Fig. 1 and Fig. 2. Fig. 1 gives the method comparison by professional laboratory personnel, whereas Fig. 2 gives the comparison of the same device by 10 diabetic patients. The linear regression line is very similar in both experiments, the correlation coefficient is better in the tests by the professional personnel [21].

However, it has been pointed out [6], that under certain conditions these statistics may provide misleading estimates of the amount of error present in the self-monitoring system. A correlation coefficient (r) of 1.00 does not necessarily mean that the measurements from the self-monitoring system are the same as those from the laboratory reference method. The r is a statistic designed to measure the extent to which pairs of measurements are associated,not the extent to which measurements agree with each other. Association represents the extent to which pairs of measurements go together according to some mathematical rule or function, while agreement represents the extent to which pairs of measurements are identical. The implication of this fact is that if measurements from a self-monitoring system differ from a reference (laboratory measurement) by a proportional amount (e.g. a systematic error of 350%) or a constant amount (e.g. a systematic error of 350 units) the correlations will be 1.00 because these measurements, although not identical, will exhibit perfect association. This association, however, does not mean that there is an absence of error in the self-monitoring system.

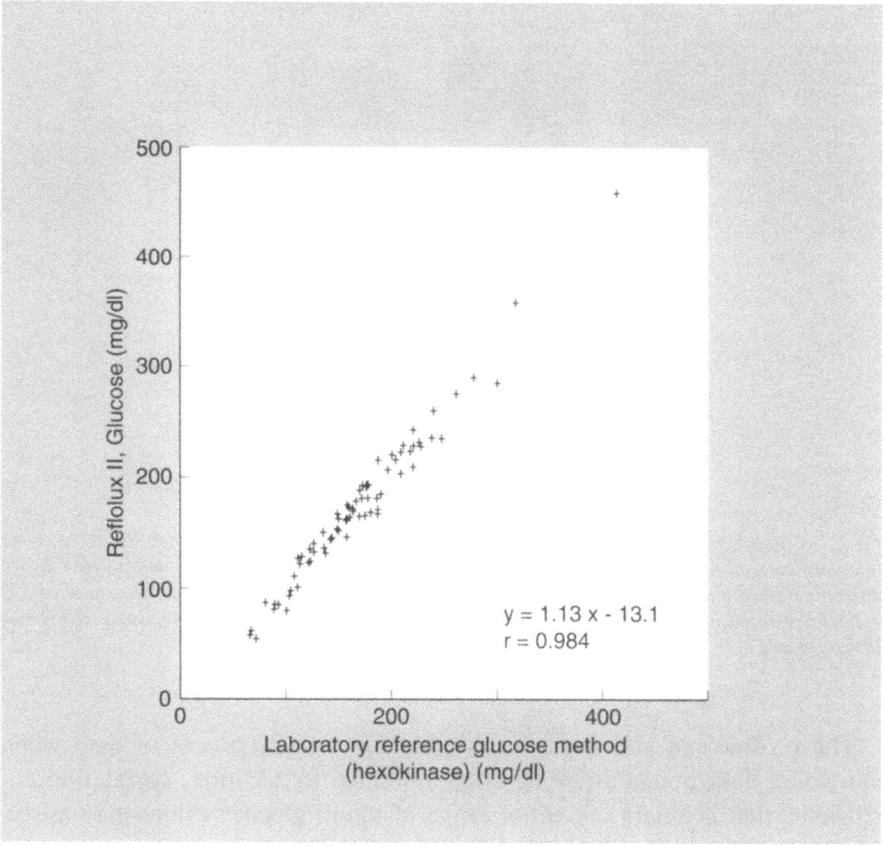

Fig. 1. Comparison of a home glucose monitoring system (Reflolux II, Accuchek BG II) with the reference method hexokinase (Gluco-quant Boehringer Mannheim, after deproteinization) by professional laboratory personnel. 80 measurements from different diabetic patients. Reflolux II is the German name for Accuchek BG. From Willms et al. [21]

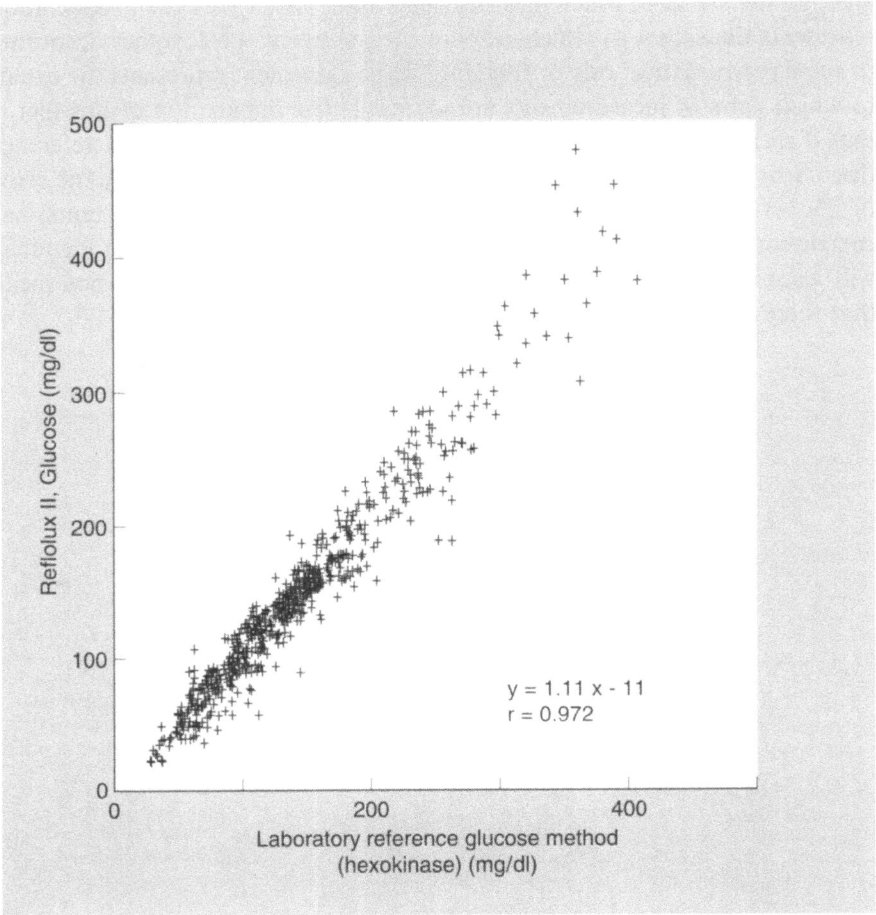

Fig. 2. Comparison of a home glucose monitoring system (Reflolux II, Accuchek BG II) with the reference method hexokinase (Gluco-quant Boehringer Mannheim, after deproteinization) by 10 different trained and educated diabetic patients. The regression curve is made from a total of 523 patient-generated blood glucose values. Reflolux II is the German name for Accuchek BG. From Willms et al [21]

The r value can also be close to unity for very large sets of data when individual data points differ by large amounts. In addition, correlation coefficients that evaluate the entire range of blood glucose values may misrepresent the true relationship between subset of data, e. g. in the hypoglycaemic or hyperglycaemic range.

The same can be true for the linear regression line. A slope of 1.0 and an y-intercept of zero do not necessarily mean that the measurements from the self-monitoring system are identical with the measurements obtained using a laboratory method.

In order to obtain a more complete description of the errors influencing the self-monitoring system it would be necessary to compute the standard error of estimate for the regression line, in addition to determining the slope and y-intercept. The standard error of estimate is the standard deviation of the points around the regression line and provides a quantitative estimate of the amount of random error influencing the self-monitoring system.

In any case, these more theoretical criticisms of correlation and regression do not mean that these statistical methods should not be used in the process of evaluation of a home glucose monitoring system, but

1. that the results of this statistical evaluation has to be interpreted with the necessary caution, and
2. that an additional clinical evaluation of a home glucose monitoring system has to be performed.

Clinical evaluation

An evaluation of a home glucose monitoring system may give unacceptable technical results, which may be irrelevant from the clinical standpoint of view and thus be clinically acceptable.

What a practitioner needs – in addition to the technical evaluation of a home glucose monitoring system – is an evaluation that describes the clinical significance of the potential error of a self-glucose monitoring system. The criteria for this clinical evaluation depend on the consensus of interested physicians, and varied opinions can be expected due to variable clinical needs.

Various procedures have been proposed for clinical evaluation of a home glucose monitoring system:

1. the precision index from Halle et al [9],
2. the error grid analysis from Clarke et al [3],
3. the proficiency score from Pollard et al [16],
4. and the acceptance analysis from Koschinsky et al [11].

In this paper, only the error grid analysis is described because it is very simple to understand and to perform, and used by several other authors [2, 4, 8, 10, 12–15, 17].

Error grid analysis

The error grid analysis (Fig. 3) also uses the y-axis for the values generated by the home glucose monitoring system and the x-axis for the reference

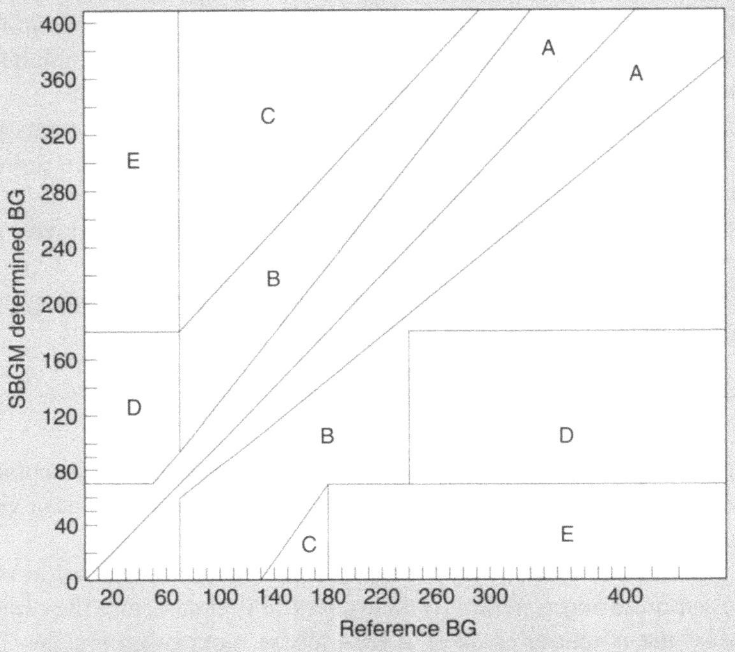

Fig. 3 Error grid analysis for evaluation of clinical implications of patient-generated blood glucose values. SBGM = self-monitoring of blood glucose; BG = blood glucose. From Clarke et al [3]

glucose method. The diagonal represents perfect agreement between the two, with data points above and below representing overestimates and underestimates, respectively. This method is based on the following assumptions:

1. the target blood glucose range or the range of glucose values which should be attained and maintained by the diabetic patient is between 70 and 180 mg/dl,
2. patients will attempt to correct blood glucose readings that are above or below the target range but not those readings that are within the target range,

3. corrective treatment on the patient's part is inappropriate if such treatment results in blood glucose values outside of the target range, and
4. failure to treat blood glucose values < 70 or > 240 mg/dl is inappropriate. (A value of 240 rather than 180 mg/dl is arbitrarily used in the last assumption, because lowering a blood glucose value slightly greater than the target might frequently result in a blood glucose value outside of the target zone.)

Based on these assumptions, the grid is divided into five zones of varying degrees of accuracy and inaccuracy of glucose estimations. Zone A (acceptable zone) represents glucose values that deviate from the reference by no more than 20% or are in the hypoglycaemic range (< 70 mg/dl) when the reference is also in the hypoglycaemic range. Values falling within this range are clinically accurate in that they would lead to clinically correct treatment decisions. Upper and lower zone B (benign errors) represents values that deviate from the reference by > 20% but would lead to benign or no treatment based on the assumptions. Zone C (correlation errors) values would result in overcorrecting acceptable blood glucose levels; such treatment might cause the actual blood glucose to fall below 70 mg/dl or rise above 180 mg/dl. Zone D (detection errors) represents "dangerous failure to detect and treat" errors. Actual glucose values are outside of the target range, but patient-generated values are within the target range. Zone E is an "erroneous treatment" zone. Patient-generated values within this zone are opposite to

Table 1 Methodologies for evaluation of a home glucose monitoring system

1	~ 100 samples should be tested
2	3 areas (< 70, 70–180, > 180 mg/dl) should be adequately covered
3	Separate evaluation by laboratory personnel and by diabetic patients
Technical evaluation	
4	Mean difference (mg/dl) (to reference method)
5	Mean difference (%)
6	% values which differ > 10% (ADA recommendation)
7	Precision a) in the run b) within runs
8	Correlation coefficient (r)
9	Linear regression line (y = ax + b)
Clinical evaluation	
10	Error grid analysis

Nos. 4–9 to be considered separately according for the hypo-, eu- and hyperglycaemic range (cf. No. 2)

the reference values, and corresponding treatment decisions would therefore be opposite to those called for.

In summary, values in zones A and B are clinically acceptable, whereas values in zones C, D, and E are potentially dangerous and, therefore, are clinically significant errors.

Cox et al. [5] recommend a home glucose monitoring system be considered acceptable if at least 95% of the tests fall into the A zones and 0% fall in the C – E zones.

The error grid analysis is a current useful means for quantifying and describing clinically acceptable and dangerous blood glucose determinations by a home glucose monitoring system.

A summary of an evaluation scheme of a home glucose monitoring system is given in Table 1.

References

[1] American Diabetes Association. Consensus Development Panel. Consensus statement on self-monitoring of blood glucose. Diabetes Care 1987; 10: 95 – 99.

[2] Atkin SH, Dasmahapatra A, Jaker MA et al. Fingerstick glucose determination in shock. Ann Intern Med 1991; 114: 1020 – 1024.

[3] Clarke WL, Cox D, Gonder-Frederick LA et al. Evaluating clinical accuracy of systems for self-monitoring of blood glucose. Diabetes Care 1987; 10: 622 – 628.

[4] Clarke WL, Levandovski LA, Prusinski EA et al. Evaluation of a new system for self glucose monitoring. Diabetes Res Clin Pract 1988; 4: 209 – 213.

[5] Cox DJ, Richards FE, Gonder-Frederick LA et al. Clarification of Error-Grid Analysis. Diabetes Care 1989; 12: 235 – 236.

[6] Dedrick RF, Davis WK: What do statistics really tell us about the quality of the data from self-monitoring of blood glucose? Diabetic Med 1989; 6: 267 – 273.

[7] Deutsche Diabetes-Gesellschaft: Verwendung von Geräten zur Blutglukose-Selbstkontrolle. Med Klin 1991; 86: 331.

[8] Gonder-Frederick LA, Snyder AL, Clarke WL. Accuracy of blood glucose estimation by children with IDDM and their parents. Diabetes Care 1991; 14: 565 – 570.

[9] Hallé JP, Lambert J, Renaud E et al. A precision index for evaluation of techniques for self-monitoring of blood glucose. Diabetes Care 1986; 9: 319 – 320.

[10] Hunt JA, Alojado NC. A new, improved test system for rapid measurement of blood glucose. Diabetes Res Clin Pract 1989; 7: 51 – 55.

[11] Koschinsky T, Dannehl K, Gries FA. New approach to technical and clinical evaluation of devices for self-monitoring of blood glucose. Diabetes Care 1988; 11: 619 – 629.

[12] Matthews DR, Burton SF, Bown E et al. Capillary and venous blood glucose measurements using a direct glucose-sensing meter. Diabetic Med 1991; 8: 875 – 890.

[13] Mühlhauser I, Heinemann L, Karingergananmatton J et al. Accuracy of blood glucose self monitoring in elderly insulin treated diabetic patients. Diabete Metab 1991; 17: 476 – 482.

[14] Nurick MA, Johnson SB. Enhancing blood glucose awareness in adolescents and young adults with IDDM. Diabetes Care 1991; 14: 1 – 7.

[15] Odenthal C. Evaluation of an electro-enzymatic system (Satellite G) for blood glucose monitoring in hospital use. Diabete-Metab 1991; 17: 534 – 537.

[16] Pollard RH, Bridgman JF, North M et al. A Proficiency Score for Assessing the Reliability of Self Blood Glucose Monitoring. Diabetic Med 1988; 5: 489 – 493.

[17] Ross D, Heinemann L, Chantelau EA. Short-term evaluation of an electro-chemical system (Exac-Tech) for blood glucose monitoring. Diabetes Res Clin Pract 1990; 10: 281–285.
[18] Schöffling K, Bachmann W, Drost H et al. Wie zuverlässig sind ambulante Blutzucker-Kontrollmethoden in der Hand des Patienten? Dtsch med Woschr 1982; 107: 605–609.
[19] Skyler JS, Skyler DL, Seigler DE et al. Algorithms for adjustment of insulin dosage by patients who monitor blood glucose. Diabetes Care 1981; 4: 311–318.
[20] Unger H, Willms B. Blutzuckerselbstkontrolle mit einem neuen Blutzuckerteststreifen. Dtsch med Woschr 1980; 105: 566–570.
[21] Willms B, Schumann E, Koberstein R. Prüfung eines neuen Glukosereflektometers (Reflolux® II) im Labor und in der Diabetikerselbstkontrolle. Akt Endokr Stoffw 1987; 8: 169–172.

Measurements of glycated haemoglobin and other circulating glycated proteins

R. R. Little, D. E. Goldstein

Abstract

Glycated haemoglobin is a reliable index of average blood glucose during the previous 2–3 months and is now used routinely to monitor glycaemic control in diabetic individuals. The most commonly used assay methods include ion-exchange chromatography, electrophoresis, and affinity chromatography. Not all methods measure the same glycated haemoglobin component; assay results vary depending on the component measured, and the particular assay used. The need for standardization of values between laboratories has been recognized but has not yet been implemented.

Glycated serum protein and glycoalbumin measurements provide an index of glycaemia over a 2–4 week period and have been investigated as alternatives for monitoring glycaemic control. The most widely used methods include Nitroblue Tetrazolium Reduction or "fructosamine", and affinity chromatography. The clinical value of these shorter term measurements of glycaemic control is still under investigation.

Glycated protein measurements have been studied for use in diabetes screening. Further studies are needed to determine whether these measures are sensitive enough to identify most individuals at risk for diabetic complications.

Introduction

Diabetes is associated with serious complications of the eyes, kidneys, heart and blood vessels, and other organ systems. The relationship between the development and progression of microvascular complications of diabetes and glycaemic control has been debated for many years. Studies have been hampered by the inadequacy of methods to assess long-term glycaemic control objectively.

Traditional methods of assessing glycaemic control in diabetes, such as taking a medical history, performing a physical examination, and measuring

Offprint from
Research Methodologies in Human Diabetes – Part 1

blood and urine glucose, while extremely important for routine care, have only limited value as indices of long-term glycaemic status. It is only with the development of glycated haemoglobin (GHb) testing that an accurate, objective measure of long-term glycaemic status is possible.

Glycated haemoglobins were discovered over 35 years ago when Kunkel and Wallenius [1] demonstrated that human adult haemoglobin could be separated into fast and slow migrating components based on differences in electrical charge. Further studies by several investigators using cation-exchange chromatography confirmed that adult human haemoglobin was heterogeneous. These studies also demonstrated that the fast moving components identified by Kunkel and Wallenius could be further separated into at least three fractions which were named HbA1a, HbA1b, and HbA1c based on their order of elution. It was not until the late 1960s that studies demonstrated increased levels of these "fast haemoglobins" in persons with diabetes [2].

The human erythrocyte is freely permeable to glucose, and GHb is formed continuously from HbA at a rate proportional to the ambient glucose concentration. Therefore, the amount of GHb is a function of the erythrocyte lifespan and the blood glucose levels to which the erythrocytes have been exposed. Studies indicate that, under most circumstances, GHb measurement provides a reliable index of average blood glucose during the preceding two to three months[3–7]. For routine patient care, GHb is generally tested 3–4 times per year to document the diabetic patient's overall success in adhering to the prescribed treatment regimen. The test often confirms other clinical data but sometimes may be the only information that alerts the physician to the need for a change in therapy or further assessment. The GHb test can also be useful as an educational tool for the patient and family [8]. The American Diabetes Association (ADA) has recommended routine use of the test in all patients with diabetes; first to document the degree of glycaemic control at initial assessment, then as part of continuing care [9].

It has also become clear that many other circulatory and tissue proteins undergo glycation proportional to their surrounding glucose concentrations. Since glycation of proteins is ubiquitous, some investigators questioned whether excessive glycation might alter function, perhaps providing a link between longstanding hyperglycaemia and the development of diabetic complications. Glycated products have been demonstrated in collagen [10], albumin [11], nerve myelin [12], and proteins of the red cell membrane [13]. Recent chemical studies of glycation have focused on new glycation adducts called advanced glycation endproducts, which form very slowly through a series of further reactions and rearrangements. These adducts, once formed, accumulate indefinitely on long-lived proteins. Physiologic processes shown to be altered by non-enzymatic glycation include enzyme activity [14], binding of critical regulatory molecules [15], crosslinking of proteins [16], susceptibility to proteolysis [17], nucleic acid function [18], macromolecular recognition and endocytosis [19], and immunogenicity [20].

Chemical structure and nomenclature of glycohaemoglobin

The term "glycated haemoglobin" – also called glycohaemoglobin or glycosylated haemoglobin – refers to a series of stable minor haemoglobin components that are formed slowly and nonenzymatically from haemoglobin and glucose. The process is a multistep condensation reaction of glucose with an amine moiety of haemoglobin. The sequence is initiated by the condensation of a free primary amine on haemoglobin with the carbonyl of the glucose resulting in the formation of a Schiff base. This Schiff base is not stable and may either dissociate or undergo an Amadori rearrangement to form a stable ketoamine (Fig. 1) [5].

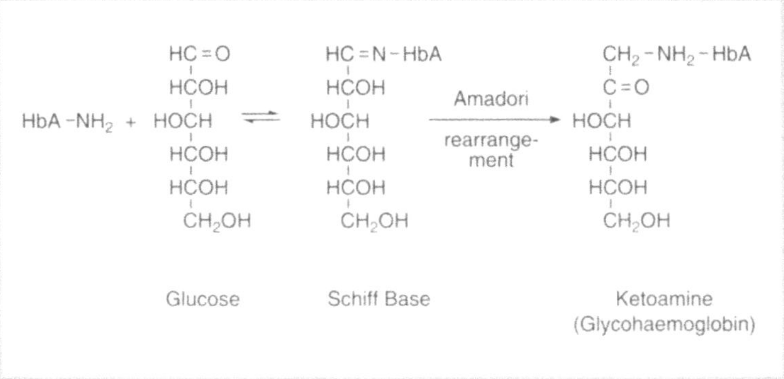

Fig. 1 The formation of glycohaemoglobin

Of the fast moving haemoglobins identified in the 1950s, HbA1c is present in greatest quantity in both normal and diabetic individuals. HbA1c is a specific GHb formed by the interaction of glucose and the amino-terminal valine of one or both beta chains of HbA [21] Glycation of haemoglobin also takes place at sites other than the ends of the beta chains, such as the epsilon amino groups of lysine residues and the amino-terminal valines of the alpha chains. Glycation at these sites (glycated HbA0) may represent as much as 50% of the total GHb in both normal and diabetic subjects [22]. These glycated haemoglobins, unlike HbA1 or HbA1c, cannot be separated from nonglycated haemoglobins by methods that separate molecules based on charge differences.

History of clinical laboratory methods

The early GHb methods, based on the work of Trivelli, et al measured HbA1c by cation exchange column chromatography [23]. The method was somewhat cumbersome for routine use in the clinical laboratory, however, and was subsequently modified for routine use in the late 1970s. These simplified, commercially available assays initially took the form of disposable mini columns which separated HbA1 (the "fast haemoglobins") from HbA0. Although these methods were prone to poor reproducibility, they became widely used for routine laboratory analysis [24]. Soon afterwards, a commercial kit incorporating the agar gel electrophoretic method of Allen et al [25] became commercially available for the measurement of HbA1. Methods for measuring HbA1c by isoelectric focusing were also described at about this time. It became clear in the early 1980s that interference by labile aldimine (Schiff base) was important and several methods for its removal were reported [26]. Soon other ion exchange mini column methods were described which allowed the separation of HbA1a + b from HbA1c [27, 28]. In 1981, Mallia, et al [29] described a boronic acid affinity support for the separation of glycated haemoglobins. A commercial affinity chromatography mini column method was soon available for the quantification of "total GHb" by affinity chromatography [30]. Modifications of the original procedure now include affinity HPLC [31] and affinity binding by two-dimensional centrifugation [32]. In the late 1980s, dedicated, automated HPLC systems measuring HbA1c became available [33, 34] and in the late 1980s to 1990, methods for measurement of HbA1c by immunoassay were described which are now commercially available [35, 36].

Glycated haemoglobin methodology

The major assay methods can be divided into three major categories based on the manner in which glycated and non-glycated haemoglobin components are separated. Within these categories, methods can measure different glycated haemoglobin components (HbA1c, HbA1, or total GHb).

Methods based on charge differences

*Cation-exchange chromatography:*Ion-exchange chromatography is based on the exchange of charged ions between a mobile phase and charged functional groups (ligand) which are covalently attached to a stationary phase. Many GHb species, including HbA1c, are less positively charged at neutral pH than HbA0, and bind less tightly to a negatively charged resin. Typically, haemolysate is applied to a column filled with resin, at least two buffers differing in ionic strength are applied to the resin, and the eluate is collected. The minor haemoglobin components, primarily HbA1a, A1b, and A1c, elute before the more positively charged main haemoglobin fraction, HbA0, and their percentages of total haemoglobin can be easily determined using a spectrophotometer. Some procedures separate only HbA1 (HbA1a + b + c) from HbA0, while others separate the various minor haemoglobin components from one another allowing quantification of HbA1c specifically. Procedures range from disposable mini or micro columns to expensive automated HPLC systems. At least one HPLC system also separates HbF which otherwise co-elutes with HbA1c [33].

Ion-exchange chromatographic methods are affected greatly by temperature and pH; these factors must be tightly controlled to achieve optimum accuracy and precision. The labile Schiff base intermediate co-chromatographs with the stable ketoamine and must be removed prior to assay. Although some ion-exchange methods can detect the presence of certain haemoglobinopathies, most commonly used methods do not give an accurate measure of glycated haemoglobin if a haemoglobinopathy is present. Ion-exchange methods are also generally quite sensitive to sample storage conditions.

Electrophoresis: HbA1 or HbA1c can be separated from HbA0 by electrophoresis. A haemolysate is applied to a suitable support medium and a potential is applied across the support. The most commonly used electrophoresis methods separate HbA1 as a single peak utilizing an agar gel. The gel contains negatively charged groups that interact with the various haemoglobin components. The HbA1 fraction migrates on the cathodic side of haemoglobin A0. Quantification is accomplished most easily by scanning the gel using a densitometer.

Electrophoresis methods are relatively insensitive to variations in buffer pH, ionic strength, and temperature. As with ion-exchange chromatography, the labile Schiff base intermediate co-migrates with the stable ketoamine and must be removed prior to assay. Some electrophoresis methods can give accurate measures of glycohaemoglobin in the presence of some haemoglobinopathies such as HbS or HbC trait. Some abnormal haemoglobins (e.g.

HbF), however, interfere with glycohaemoglobin measurement. As with ion-exchange methods, electrophoresis is quite sensitive to sample storage conditions.

Methods based on structural characteristics

Boronate affinity chromatography: Affinity chromatography is a technique capable of separating large molecules based on their chemical structure. The stationary phase, usually packed in a column, consists of an insoluble inert matrix with an appropriate ligand attached. When the mobile phase containing the substances to be separated is passed through the column, substances are separated by their differing interactions with the ligand. For GHb, m-aminophenyl boronic acid (ligand) coupled to agarose, cellulose or other polymer resin (matrix) binds to the cis-diol groups in glucose modified haemoglobin to form a reversible 5-membered ring complex [29]. For affinity chromatography, haemolysate can be prepared directly from whole blood, applied to an equilibrated column and washed with two buffers. The first buffer elutes the non-glycated haemoglobin fraction that does not have cis-diol groups and, therefore, does not bind to the boronic acid; glycated components are retained on the column. The bound fraction is then eluted with the second buffer which contains a counter-ligand that displaces the glycated material from the boronic acid binding sites. Relative ratios of bound (glycated) to non-bound (non-glycated) haemoglobin fractions can be quantified spectrophotometrically at 414 nm. Affinity chromatography separates not only HbA1c, but also other glycohaemoglobins that cannot be separated by differences in their charge. Kits containing prepacked columns and the appropriate buffers are available from several manufacturers. An automated affinity chromatographic HPLC system [31] and an affinity binding by two-dimensional centrifugation methods [32] are also available.

Affinity binding and affinity chromatographic methods are less sensitive to small variations in temperature and pH than ion-exchange methods. Unlike methods that separate glycohaemoglobin components based on differences in charge, affinity methods are not affected by labile GHb intermediates or the presence of haemoglobinopathies and is relatively insensitive to sample storage factors.

Immunoassay: A few immunoassay methods for measurement of GHb have been described [35, 36]; at least two of these are commercially available and measure HbA1c. However, the exact specificities of the antibodies, and therefore, each assays interferences may be different [37]. The Miles DCA2000 immunoassay is based on inhibition of HbA1c-specific antibody agglutination [35]. HbA1c specific antibody was developed using monoclonal antibody technique. An agglutinator, which is a synthetic polymer containing a plurality of a HbA1c-like glycopeptide, causes agglutination of the antibody-latex, which is inhibited by HbA1c in unknown blood samples. This inhibition is quantified by a descrease in absorption using an automated photometer. This particular immunoassay appears to be very specific for HbA1c and is not affected by most abnormal haemoglobins or labile Schiff base intermediates. The method is also relatively insensitive to sample storage conditions.

Methods based on chemical reactivity

Hydroxymethylfurfural-thiobarbituric acid colorimetry: The major chemical method that has been used, mainly in research laboratories, is the hydroxymethylfurfural-thiobarbituric acid (HMF-TBA) method. Glycoamino groups on protein (e. g. Hb) are converted to 5-HMF by heating in a weak acid. The 5-HMF can be measured by HPLC or, more commonly, by photometry, after reacting with a color development reagent such as TBA. This method determines glyco groups on both valine and lysine residues. One important advantage of this method is that pure fructose can be included as an assay standard. Unlike most other GHb methods, assay results are expressed as a quantity of HMF, absorbance, or fructose equivalents.

The HMF-TBA method is not affected by the presence of labile Schiff base intermediates or haemoglobinopathies. This method is minimally affected by sample handling and storage conditions. However, the assay does require removal of free glucose from samples and careful standardization of assay conditions.

Selection of a glycohaemoglobin assay method

Each general method category and its many variations has specific advantages and disadvantages for the clinical laboratory; none should be considered the "best" method. Despite the fact that different methods often produce different absolute test results, results of methods currently available usually correlate well and provide useful clinical information if performed properly. For each laboratory the choice of a method will depend on a number of factors including set-up costs, number of samples to be analyzed, desired turn-around time, sample handling constraints, and patient population characteristics (prevalence of haemoglobinopathies).

Inter-laboratory standardization of glycated haemoglobin

Each type of assay method measures GHb in a slightly different way and assay conditions will differ from laboratory to laboratory. In addition, there is no consensus on either a reference method or a single GHb standard or calibrator that can be used with all available methods. Thus, absolute numbers generated in one laboratory cannot be compared easily to numbers generated in another laboratory, even if both use the same basic assay method. This is shown in Table 1, using data taken from a recent College of American Pathologists Survey. The interlaboratory CV for one HbA1 ion-exchange method was over 14.5%. Furthermore, excluding outliers, a single quality control sample gave mean values ranging from 9.26% (Bio Rad HbA1c columns) to 16.76% (Helena Glyco-Tek measuring total GHb) depending on the glycohaemoglobin component measured and the specific assay method used. Under these circumstances, each laboratory that performs determinations of GHb must work closely with clinicians to ensure proper interpretation of results.

Because the GHb test is used primarily to monitor individual patients over time, a high degree of long-term assay precision is essential. In addition to long-term precision within each laboratory, the need for interlaboratory comparisons and standardization of values between laboratories is increasing, both for patient care and research studies.

Table 1 Inter-laboratory comparison of assay methods: College of American Pathologists 1992: survey results

Method	Mean	%CV
HbA1 Electrophoresis		
*Corning Glytrac	12.15	11.1
*Helena Rep	14.08	8.9
HbA1 Ion-exchange		
*Helena Glyco Hb Quik	10.42	14.5
HbA1c Ion-exchange		
Bio-Rad Diamat HPLC	11.23	5.0
Bio-Rad HbA1c columns	9.26	9.1
HbA1c Electrophoresis		
*Beckman Diatrac	10.93	9.6
Total gHb Affinity		
*Isolab Glyc-Affin	16.32	5.9
*Helena Glyco-Tek	16.76	5.0

* calibrators are not provided

Table 2 Standardization of glycohaemoglobin measurement: summary of methods

Method	Method Type	Component Measured	Auto/ Manual Assay	Standard* Material type, storage	Standardization Format*
Reference	Ion-Ex. HPLC	HbA1c	semi-A	EH (RL), −70 °C	
Diamat (Bio-Rad)	Ion-Ex. HPLC	HbA1c	A	LEH (Bio-Rad), 4 °C R, −20 °C	1 pt, each run
Glyc-Affin (Isolab)	Aff. Chr. mini-col	Total GHb	M	EH (RL), −70 °C	4 pt, each run
GlycoTest (Pierce)	Aff. Chr. mini-col	Total GHb	M	EH (RL), −70 °C	3−4 pt, each run
Vision GHb (Abbott)	Affinity Binding	Total GHb	A	EH (RL), −70 °C	4 pt, each lot of 2° std.
CLC330 HPLC (Primus)	Affinity HPLC	Total GHb	A	LEH (Primus), 4 °C R, −70 °C	2 pt, each 500 injections
REP Glyco-30 (Helena)	Electr.	HbA1	semi-A	LEH (Sherwood), 4 °C R, −70 °C	3 pt, each run
Diatrac HbA1c (Beckman)	Electr.	HbA1c	semi-A	EH (Beckman), −20 °C	3 pt, each run
DCA2000 (Miles) (bar code calibration)	Immunoassay	HbA1c	A	EH (Miles), 4 °C	12 pt, each lot of reagents

* All values for standards were assigned by the Reference HPLC method.

A = automated
M = manual
EH = erythrocyte haemolysate
LEH = lyophilized erythrocyte haemolysate
R = reconstituted
RL = Reference Laboratory
WBH = whole blood haemolysate

This table was adapted from Little et al., Clin Chem 1992; 38: 2472−2478.

Recent studies indicate that standardization among laboratories using a variety of assay methods is feasible. In a recent study [38] two clinical laboratories performed GHb analyses by several different methods (Table 2). A third, reference laboratory, performed GHb analyses by an ion-exchange HPLC method. This reference HPLC method is a two-buffer, step-gradient HPLC assay for HbA1c which has been previously described [39]. The column consisted of a BioRex 70, 400-mesh resin (Bio-Rad, Richmond, CA) packed in a glass column that was temperature-controlled. A liquid-chromatographic system was used to separate, measure (at 410 nm), and quantify the differentially eluted haemoglobin fractions. A single calibrator was included in each run and the system's variables were adjusted, if necessary, so that the

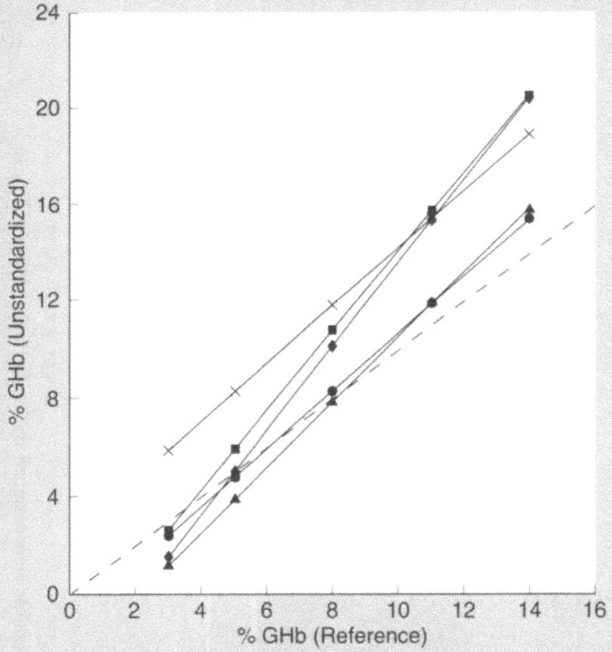

Fig. 2 Relation between Diamat HPLC and uncalibrated GHb values from five different GHb assay methods. --- unity line; —— regression lines: (–■–) Glyc-Affin (n = 125, r = 0.99), (–▲–) GlycoTest (n = 100; r = 0.98), (–◆–) CLC330 HPLC (n = 144, r = 0.99), (–×–) REP Glyco-30 (n = 121, r = 0.96), (–●–) Diatrac HbA1c (n = 123, r = 0.99). (From Clin Chem 1992; 38: 2472, ref # 38.)

value was within acceptable limits of a previously established value (+/ – 1 SD). This assay system, which has been on-line since 1978, is rigorously controlled and can deliver reproducible results over the long-term; the inter-assay CV for this method has been consistently < 3%.

A variety of calibration materials were used in the clinical laboratories (Table 2); all were erythrocyte haemolysates with the labile Schiff base fraction removed. For some methods, the calibrator was supplied by the manufacturer of the particular GHb assay method and for other methodos, the calibrator was either prepared at the reference laboratory [39] or purchased from Sherwood Medical (St. Louis, MO) (see Table 2). All calibration materials were assigned GHb (HbA1c) values by the reference method. Assigned values were based on the mean of > 10 runs by the reference method. Calibrators were then analyzed along with patient specimens by the methods to be evaluated, and calibrated GHb values for samples were obtained either by a standard curve or by a single point calibration procedure. The comparison methods studied are shown in Table 2.

The Diamat HPLC (Bio-Rad, Hercules, CA) was used as a secondary reference method because of its suitability for large-scale sample comparisons. As with the other clinical laboratory methods, the Diamat calibrator value was assigned by the Reference HPLC. All comparison samples analyzed by the other methods were also analyzed by Diamat HPLC in order to monitor the effectiveness of GHb standardization.

Fig. 2 shows the regression analyses between GHb values obtained by uncalibrated assays and values from the Diamat HPLC. The Abbott Vision Glycated Hb method and the Miles DCA 2000 immunoassay method are both calibrated internally and report only calibrated values. Although there is good agreement in absolute values for the two affinity chromatography methods, there are large differences in values among other methods. For example, a patient with an HbA1c value of 10% by the Diamat method could be reported as having 10.3 total GHb by the Pierce GlycoTest II method or 14.2% HbA1 by REP electrophoresis. Fig. 3 shows regression analyses between GHb values from the Diamat HPLC and seven different methods after calibration. An HbA1c value of 10% by the Diamat HPLC would measure between 9.5% and 10.2% by the other standardized methods, a substantially narrower range (0.7% GHb) than the range obtained by using uncalibrated values (4.2% GHb) from the five methods shown in Fig. 2.

A comparison of interassay imprecision, with and without calibration (for those GHb methods for which uncalibrated values were available) showed substantial improvement in between-assay precision after calibration of assay results. Estimates of imprecision for one affinity chromatography method

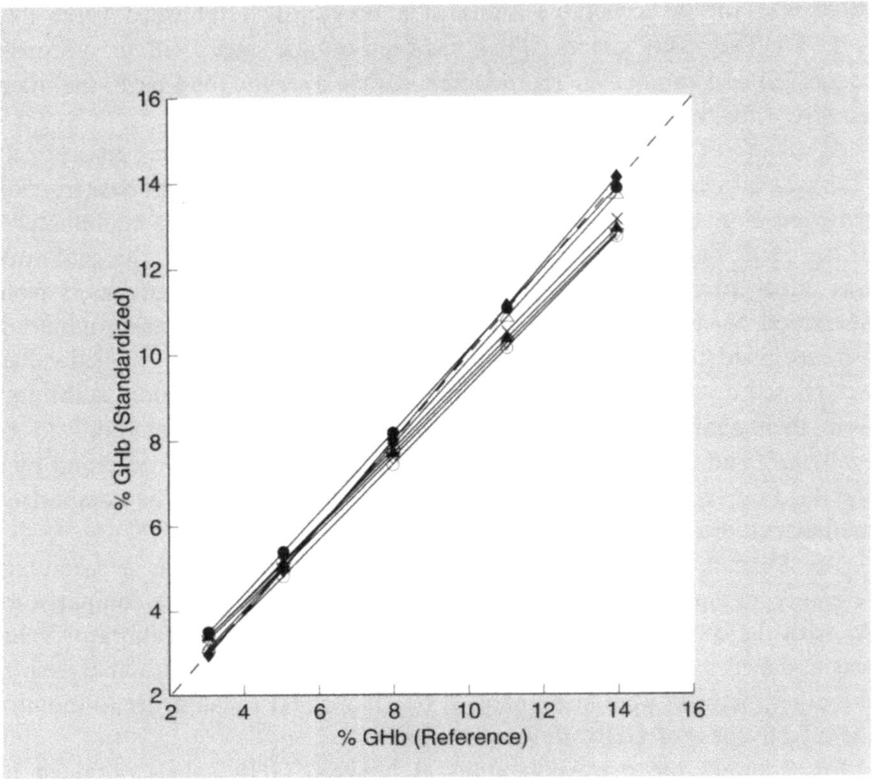

Fig. 3 Relation between Diamat HPLC and calibrated GHb values from seven different GHb assay methods. --- unity line; —— regression lines (–■–) Glyc-Affin (n = 125, r = 0.99), (–▲–) GlycoTest (n = 100, r = 0.99), (–◆–) CLC330 HPLC (n = 144, r = 0.99), (–×–) REP Glyco-30 (n = 87, r = 0.98), (–●–) Diatrac HbA1c (n = 123, r = 0.99), (–⧖–) Vision GHb (n = 135, r = 0.98), (–☆–) DCA2000 (n = 197, r = 0.99). (From Clin Chem 1992; 38: 2472, ref # 38.)

over a 5 year period using several reagent lots and two different affinity resin formulations showed a considerable improvement with the CV for uncalibrated results (using a normal range quality control specimen) being 10.3% compared to a CV of 4.3% for calibrated GHb results.

Most clinicians (and patients with diabetes) do not know how to relate their own laboratory's GHb results to average blood glucose concentration. Because there is currently no standardization, results in the literature relating blood glucose and GHb concentrations [40] cannot be used to help the medical practitioner and diabetic patient interpret the GHb test results, except in a very general way. There are still many widely used methods that do not include calibrators and do not have an internal mechanism for calibration of the assay method (see Table 1). A broadly based system of standardization would allow development of uniform goals for blood glucose control in persons with diabetes as well as improved surveillance of assay quality. Large-scale standardization efforts are anticipated.

Intermediate-term glucose monitoring

The degree of glycation of serum proteins (GSP) provides an index of glycaemia over a shorter period of time (2–4 weeks) than glycation of haemoglobin. GSP and glycated serum albumin correlate well with GHb and have been suggested as alternative methods of monitoring diabetic control.

Several methods have been described which measure either GSP or glycoalbumin. Methods based on separation due to charge differences have not found wide application in the measurement of GSP because of the lack of significant charge differences between the glycated and nonglycated components.

Methods based on chemical reactivity

Hydroxymethylfurfural-thiobarbituric acid (HMF-TBA) colorimetry: This method can be used for GSP and Glycoalbumin in the same way that it is used for measurement of GHb. For measurement of GSP, the only sample preparation required prior to assay is removal of glucose by either dialysis or by protein precipitation. For specific measurement of glycoalbumin, albumin must first be separated from other serum proteins by e. g. DEAE-cellulose and affigel blue chromatography. This method has not been routinely used in the clinical laboratory.

Nitroblue tetrazolium ("fructosamine") method: In 1982, Johnson, et al [41] described a method based on the ability of ketoamines or "fructosamines" to act as reducing agents in alkaline solution. The term "fructosamine" was introduced into the clinical chemistry literature as a general term for glycated protein. However, it has come to be associated specifically with the analyte measured in the nitroblue tretrazolium (NBT) assay, and this assay method has come to be known as the fructosamine assay. Basically, serum was added to carbonate buffer and NBT at 37 °C. NBT is reduced to a formazan dye which absorbs in the range of 550 nm. Absorbance was measured at 10 and 15 min and compared to standards containing a synthetic ketoamine product. The assay became commercially available for use on several chemistry analyzers a few years after the initial report.

Since the initial description of this method there have been a large number of reports of interferences (e. g. uraemia, lipaemia, bilirubin, ascorbate, haemolysis). Other problems include standardization and matrix problems, dependence on buffer pH and assay timing, as well as influence of protein concentration. There are now many reports describing modifications in the assay, and an improved version is also now commercially available from at least one manufacturer [42].

Methods based on structural characteristics

Boronate affinity chromatography: Affinity chromatography has been used for separation and measurement of both GSP and glycoalbumin. Protein determination after separation on affinity columns is accomplished by UV absorbance at 280 nm or Coomassie Blue reagent at 595 nm. Albumin in glycated and nonglycated fractions can be determined with bromcresol green or ELISA [43]. Alternatively, albumin can first be separated by Affi-Gel Blue affinity chromatography or anion exchange HPLC [44] and boronate affinity chromatography can then be used to determine the glycated albumin fraction. Boronate affinity chromatography methods for measurement of GSP or glycoalbumin are commercially available in the form of minicolumns and automated HPLC.

Immunoassay: Glycoalbumin or GSP can also be measured by immunoassay in which glycoalbumin or GSP binds with an antibody specific for the glycated moieties on albumin or all serum proteins [45]. An ELISA method which uses a peroxidase-bound second antibody to quantitate the amount of glycoalbumin bound to a monoclonal antibody is commercially available.

Use of glycated haemoglobin/proteins for diabetes screening

The oral glucose tolerance test (OGTT) is still considered the "gold standard" for diagnosing diabetes. Performance of a complete OGTT is not only time-consuming and expensive but is physically demanding on the individual being tested. It also requires fasting before the test and cooperation in the collection of blood samples for 2 h during the test [46]. Furthermore, results of the test vary with age, activity level, metabolic stress, time of day, and other factors [47]. Measurement of GHb or GSP has been suggested as an alternative to OGTT for diabetes screening, offering some practical advantages over measurement of serum or plasma glucose; it is not influenced by recent activity levels, metabolic stress, or food intake [48]. Because these factors do not affect glycoprotein measurement, patient cooperation is minimal; the test can be performed in nonfasting subjects from one small blood sample.

Many reports have explored the possibility of using GHb and GSP for diagnosis and/or screening for diabetes [49 – 54]. Results have been conflicting and difficult to compare because of differences in characteristics of the patient populations studied, testing procedures and criteria for diagnosis. Overall, most studies suggest that neither GHb nor GSP would be a reliable substitute for the OGTT for diabetes diagnosis. Some studies, however, show that precise measures of both GHb and glycoalbumin may be useful in screening for those at greatest risk for diabetic complications [54, 55]. A recent study also showed that in 54 Pima Indians (a population with a very high prevalence of diabetes) with impaired glucose tolerance (IGT), GHb was a better predictor of progression to diabetes than 2 hour plasma glucose [56]. Further studies are necessary to determine whether subjects with a diagnosis of diabetes who have normal GHb are truly at a lower risk of developing chronic diabetic complications than diabetic subjects with abnormal GHb. Further studies are also needed to determine whether subjects with IGT who have persistently high GHb/GSP are at a significantly greater risk for developing complications than subjects with normal GHb/GSP.

Conclusions

Glycohaemoglobin is a valuable tool for assessing glycaemic control and is used routinely in the care of persons with diabetes. Measurement of GHb has also shown useful research applications, facilitating studies requiring objective assessment of long-term glucose control. A recent report by Larsen et al [57] showed that regular monitoring of GHb in persons with diabetes can lead to changes in diabetes treatment and improvement of metabolic control. The Diabetes Control and Complications Trial (DCCT), a large scale, long-term study involving 1400 subjects in 27 clinical centers, demonstrated that intensive therapy resulted in a substantial decrease in GHb as well as a reduction in proliferative and non-proliferative retinopathy, laser therapy, microalbuminuria, and clinical neuropathy [58].

The diversity of GHb methods currently in use, combined with the lack of available standards for use with many types of assays, makes it exceedingly difficult to compare results between laboratories. Thus, we must recognize that the usefulness of GHb measurement in diabetes care and the potential for its use in establishing uniform care goals will depend on our ability to standardize its measurement.

With respect to use of GHb for screening and diagnosis, long-term studies are necessary to determine if individuals with persistent normal GHb values but abnormal glucose tolerance test results are at increased risk for diabetic complications.

The value of GSP or glycoalbumin as a shorter-term measure of glycaemic control for use in routine patient care is still unclear, especially in light of at least one report that GHb can change much more rapidly than is generally appreciated [59]. A few studies examining different measures of short-term control by analysis of either glycated plasma or serum proteins or glycated albumin show that these measures may not be more sensitive than GHb for diabetes screening [55–60]. The recent availability of improved assays for GSP may clarify the usefulness of this measure both for patient care and diabetes screening.

Acknowledgments: Portions of this report were adapted from Little, RR and Goldstein, DE. Long term glucose monitoring with glycated proteins. Lab Med 1992; 23: 533–538.

References

[1] Kunkel HG, Wallenuis G. New hemoglobins in normal adult blood. Science 1955; 122: 288.
[2] Rahbar S. An abnormal hemoglobin in red cells of diabetics. Clin Chim Acta 1968; 22: 296–298.
[3] Jovanovic L, Peterson CM. The clinical utility of glycosylated hemoglobin. Am J Med 1981; 70: 331–338.
[4] Goldstein DE, Little RR, Wiedmeyer HM et al. Glycated hemoglobin: methodologies and clinical applications. Clin Chem 1986; 32: B64–70.
[5] Bunn HF. Nonenzymatic glycosylation of protein: relevance to diabetes. Am J Med 1981; 70: 325–330.
[6] Baynes JW, Bunn HF, Goldstein DE et al. National Diabetes Data Group: report of the expert committee on glucosylated hemoglobin. Diabetes 1984; 7: 602–606.
[7] Nathan DM, Singer DE, Hurxthal K et al. The clinical information value of the glycosylated hemoglobin assay. N Engl J Med 1984; 310: 341–346.
[8] Goldstein DE, Little RR, Wiedmeyer HM et al. Educational Uses of Glycated Hemoglobin Determinations. In: Ryall RG, ed. Glycated Proteins in Diabetes Mellitus. Proceedings of an International Symposium. Adelaide, South Australia: CSR Ltd Sugar Division, 1990; 165–177.
[9] American Diabetes Association Clinical Practice Recommendations: Standards of medical care for patients with diabetes mellitus. Diab Care 1991; 14: 10–13.
[10] Monnier VM, Kohn RR, Cerami A. Accelerated age-related browning of human collagen in diabetes mellitus. Proc Natl Acad Sci USA 1984; 81: 583–587.
[11] Baynes JW, Thorpe SR, Murtiashaw MH. Nonenzymatic glucosylation of lysine residues in albumin. Methods in Enzymol 1984; 106: 88–98.
[12] Vlassara H, Brownlee M, Cerami A. Excessive nonenzymatic glycosylation of peripheral and central nervous system myelin components in diabetic rats. Diabetes 1983; 32: 670–674.
[13] Miller JA, Gravallese E, Bunn HF. Nonenzymatic glycosylation of erythrocyte membrane proteins: relevance to diabetes. J Clin Invest 1980; 65: 896–901.
[14] Eble AS, Thorpe SR, Baynes JW. Nonenzymatic glucosylation and glucose-dependent cross-linking of protein. J Biol Chem 1983; 258: 9506–9512.

[15] Brownlee M, Vlassara H, Cerami A. Inhibition of heparin-catalyzed human antithrombin III activity by nonenzymatic glycosylation: possible role in fibrin deposition in diabetes. Diabetes 1984; 33: 532–535.
[16] Stevens VJ, Rouzer CA, Monnier VM et al. Diabetic cataract formation: potential role of glycosylation of lens crystallins. Proc Natl Acad Sci USA. 1978; 75: 2918–2922.
[17] Lubec G, Pollak A. Reduced susceptibility of nonenzymatically glucosylated glomerular basement membrane to proteases: is thickening of diabetic glomerular basement membranes due to reduced proteolytic degradation? Renal Physiol 1980; 3: 4–8.
[18] Bucala R, Model P, Cerami A. Modification of DNA by reducing sugars: a possible mechanism for nucleic acid aging and age-related dysfunction in gene expression. Proc Natl Acad Sci USA 1984; 81: 105–109.
[19] Williams SK, Devenny JJ, Bitensky MW. Micropinocytic ingestion of glycosylated albumin by isolated microvessels: possible role in pathogenesis of diabetic microangiopathy. Proc Natl Acad Sci USA 1981; 78: 2393–2397.
[20] Witzum JL, Steinbrecher UP, Fisher M et al. Nonenzymatic glycosylation of homologous low density lipoprotein and albumin renders them immunogenic in the guinea pig. Proc Natl Acad Sci USA 1983; 80: 2757–2761.
[21] Bookchin RM, Gallop PM. Structure of hemoglobin Alc: nature of the N-terminal beta chain blocking group. Biochem Biophys Res Comm 1968; 32: 86–93.
[22] Shapiro R, McManus MJ, Zalot C et al. Sites of non-enzymatic glycosylation of human hemoglobin A. J Biol Chem 1980; 255: 3120–3127.
[23] Trivelli LA, Ranney HM, Lai HT. Hemoglobin components in patients with diabetes mellitus. N Engl J Med 1971; 284: 353–357.
[24] Schellekens APM, Sanders GTB et al. Sources of variation in the column-chromatographic determination of glycohemoglobin (HbA1). Clin Chem 1981; 27: 94–99.
[25] Allen DW, Schroeder WA, Balog J: Observations of the chromatographic heterogeneity of normal adult and fetal hemoglobin. J Am Chem Soc 1958; 80: 6065–6069.
[26] Bannon P, Joly JG, Lessard F et al. Comparison of three methods for the elimination of the labile fraction of HbA1. Clin Biochem 1985; 18: 114–117.
[27] Jaynes PK, Willis MC, Chow PP. Evaluation of a mini-column chromatographic procedure for the measurement of hemoglobin A1c. Clin Bioch 1985; 18: 32–36.
[28] Jones MB, Koler RD, Jones RT. Micro-column method for the determination of hemoglobin minor fractions A1a + b and A1c. Hemoglobin 1978; 2: 53–58.
[29] Mallia AK, Hermanson GT, Krohn DK et al. Preparation and use of a boronic acid affinity support for separation and quantitation of glycosylated hemoglobins. Anal Lett 1981; 14: 649–661.
[30] Klenk DC, Hermanson GT, Krohn RI et al. Determination of glycosylated hemoglobin by affinity chromatography: comparison with colorimetric and ion-exchange methods, and effects of common interferences. Clin Chem 1982; 28: 2088–2094.
[31] Scott BK, Peterson CM. Evaluating glycated protein by high-performance boronate affinity chromatography. Diabetes Professional 1990; summer: 20–24.
[32] Fiechtner M, Ramp J, England B et al. Affinity binding assay of glycohemoglobin by two-dimensional centrifugation referenced to hemoglobin A1c. Clin Chem 1992, 38: 2372–2379.
[33] Lim GI, Koay ESC, Aw TC. The Bio-Rad Diamat analyser: an automated liquid chromatography system for haemoglobin A1c (HbA1c) determination. Ann Acad Med 1989; 18: 357–362.
[34] Diamandis EP, Ellis G. Liquid chromatography of glycated hemoglobins with the Daiichi HA-8110 automated analyzer. Clin Chem 1984; 30: 503–504.
[35] Knowles BJ, Haigh WB, Michand GC et al. A monoclonal antibody based immunoassay for glycosylated A1c. Diabetes 1986; 35, suppl. 9: 4–5.
[36] John WG, Gray MR, Young DM et al. An enzyme immunoassay for HbA1c: a new generation in diabetic monitoring. Diabetic Med 1990; 7, suppl 2: 8A.

[37] Weykamp CW, Penders TJ, Muskiet FAJ et al. Glycohemoglobin: influence of hemoglobin-variants and derivatives, as investigated by 102 laboratories using 16 different methods. Clin Chem 1993; 39: 1717–1722.
[38] Little RR, Wiedmeyer HM, England JD et al. Interlaboratory standardization of measurements of glycohemoglobins. Clin Chem 1992; 38: 2472–2478.
[39] Goldstein DE, Little RR, England JD et al. Methods for quantitating glycosylated hemoglobins: high performance liquid chromatography and thiobarbituric acid colorimetry. In: Clarke WL, Larner J, Pohl SL, eds. Methods in diabetes research. Vol. 2: Clinical methods. New York: John Wiley, 1986, 475–504.
[40] The DCCT Research Group. Diabetes control and complications trial (DCCT): results of feasibility study. Diabetes Care 1987; 10: 1–9.
[41] Johnson RN, Metcalf PA, Baker JR. Fructosamine: a new approach to the estimation of serum glycosylprotein. An index of diabetic control. Clinica Chimica Acta 1982; 127: 87–95.
[42] Cefalu WT, Bell-Farrow AD, Petty M et al. Clinical validation of a second-generation fructosamine assay. Clin Chem 1991; 37: 1252–1256.
[43] Rendell M, Brannan C, Nurenberg J et al. Fingerstick glycosylated hemoglobin, plasma protein, and albumin. Diab Care 1987; 10: 629–632.
[44] Shima K, Ito N, Abe F et al. High performance liquid chromatographic assay of serum glycated albumin. Diabetologia 1988; 31: 627–631.
[45] Cohen MP, Hud E. Measurement of plasma glycoalbumin levels with a monoclonal antibody based ELISA. J Immunol Methods 1989; 122: 279–283.
[46] WHO Expert Committee on Diabetes Mellitus: Second Report. Geneva: World Health Org., 1980 (Tech Rep Ser 646).
[47] Sherwin RS: Limitations of oral glucose tolerance test in diagnosis of early diabetes. Primary Care 1977; 4: 255–266.
[48] Gabbay KH, Sosenko JM, Banuchi GA et al. Glycosylated hemoglobins: increased glycosylation of hemoglobin A in diabetic patients. Diabetes 1979; 28: 337–340.
[49] Ferrell RE, Hanis CL, Aguilar L et al. Glycosylated hemoglobin determination from capillary blood samples; utility in an epidemiologic survey of diabetes. Am J Epidemiol 1984; 119: 159–166.
[50] Bolli G, Compagnucci P, Cartechini MG et al. HbA1 in subjects with abnormal glucose tolerance but normal fasting plasma glucose. Diabetes 1980; 29: 272–277.
[51] Kesson CM, Young RE, Talwar D. Glycosylated hemoglobin in the diagnosis of non-insulin-dependent diabetes mellitus. Diabetes Care 1982; 5: 395–398.
[52] Lester E, Frazer AD, Shepherd CA et al. Glycosylated haemoglobin as an alternative to the glucose tolerance test for the diagnosis of diabetes mellitus. Ann Clin Biochem 1985; 22: 74–78.
[53] Hall PM, Cook JGH, Sheldon J et al. Glycosylated hemoglobins and glycosylated plasma proteins in the diagnosis of diabetes mellitus and impaired glucose tolerance. Diab Care 1984; 7: 147–150.
[54] Little RR, England JD, Wiedmeyer HM et al. Relationship of glycosylated hemoglobin to oral glucose tolerance: implications for diabetes screening. Diabetes 1988; 37: 60–64.
[55] Shima K, Abe F, Chikakiyo H et al. The relative value of glycated albumin, hemoglobin A1c and fructosamine when screening for diabetes mellitus. Diab Res Clin Pract 1989; 7: 243–250.
[56] Little RR, England JD, Wiedmeyer HM et al. Glycated hemoglobin (GHb) predicts development of diabetes in persons with impaired glucose tolerance (IGT) (abstr). Diabetes 1990; 39 Suppl 1: 204A.
[57] Larsen ML, Horder M, Mogensen ER. Effect of long-term monitoring of glycosylated hemoglobin levels in insulin-dependent diabetes mellitus. New Engl J Med 1990; 323: 1021–1025.

[58] The DCCT Research Group: The effect of intensive treatment of diabetes on the development and progression of long-term complications in insulin-dependent diabetes mellitus. New Engl J Med 1993; 329: 977–986.
[59] Goldstein DE, Oermann CM, Madsen RW et al. Glycated hemoglobin kinetics: predicted and actual rates of change (abstr.). Diabetes 1989; 38 (suppl 2): 459.
[60] Little RR, Wiedmeyer HM, Wilke AA et al. Evaluation of glycohemoglobin (GHB) and glycated plasma proteins (GPP) for diabetes screening: ROC Curve analysis (abstr.). Diabetes 1993; 42 (suppl 1): 199 A.

Research methodologies in evaluating patient education in diabetes – to reflect on the goals of patient education

I. Mühlhauser, U. Bott

The changing scene in evaluating diabetes education

Concepts of evaluating diabetes education have progressed in recent years. Traditionally, evaluation studies have focused on the assessment of patients' knowledge about and adherence to dietary treatment prescriptions and the degree of metabolic control was used as the principal outcome measure [4]. However, many evaluation studies have failed to demonstrate the impact of diabetes education on metabolic control [5, 16, 29]. The inability to document improvements of glycaemic control following various educational efforts has led to far-reaching considerations and suggestions, such as to question the justification for third-party reimbursement for out-patient education [28] or the use of glycaemic control as a principal outcome measure and eventually substitute it by other parameters, such as quality of life measures, serum-cholesterol levels, or smoking habits [20, 22].

Recently, comprehensive concepts of evaluation have been proposed, which take into account all possible aspects of the diabetic life, including environmental and social variables (social support, living situation, clinic organisation, etc.), process and mediating variables (knowledge, attitudes, self-efficacy or sense of control, health beliefs, personal models, problem-solving or coping skills, intentions, etc.), short-term health outcomes (GHb, blood glucose variability, hypoglycaemic episodes, serum-cholesterol levels, blood pressure, smoking habits, body weight, quality of life, functional limitations, psychological factors), patient characteristics (target population, demographics, medical history, cognitive functioning, co-morbidity, participation rate, attrition rate, etc.), diabetes management (lifestyle change including dietary intake, eating behaviour, exercise, medical self-care including glucose testing, medical adherence, insulin-self-regulation, foot care and safety, patient-provider interaction including patient activity level, degree of patient-provider congruence), long-term health outcomes (complications including retinal, neuro-

Offprint from
Research Methodologies in Human Diabetes – Part 1

pathic, renal, sexual, stroke, mortality including diabetes-related and all causes), and, finally, analyses of the cost-effectiveness of the programme [22]. Although such complex models of evaluation represent more realistic reflections of the many facets which might be of relevance for the outcome of diabetes education, it remains to be shown whether such a holistic approach is widely practicable and to what degree it will help to improve diabetes care. It is worth noting that a recent study on the evaluation of an outpatient education programme for insulin-treated patients, which considered a substantial number of these factors, including quality of life measures, was not able to show a decrease of GHb values or a reduction of hospitalisation days, although some aspects of self-perceived quality of life appeared to have improved [16]. Thus, even a comprehensive evaluation concept, based on a sophisticated model of health behaviour [1], leads to disappointing results in main outcome parameters if ineffective insulin treatment regimens are used [40]. It has been argued, however, that for any rational education and nutritional counselling, an improvement of health status *has to be* documented, and that the (cost-)effectiveness of these services has to be proven [28]. In addition, it has been urged that other dimensions of patient education such as psychological and psychosocial interventions are also studied according to adequate scientific rules [47]. Although the psychosocial research in diabetes expanded substantially during the 1980s [14, 21, 33, 42, 44, 45, 47], there is still a lack of meaningful psychometric scales which are able to demonstrate possible and convincing associations between attitudes, health beliefs or coping strategies and glycaemic control.

If education does not work...

The short history of evaluation of diabetes education is characterised by a number of misconceptions about what diabetes education is and what it can achieve [40]. One fundamental misconception about the role of diabetes education is to understand education primarily as a tool to motivate the patient to change attitudes and behaviour in order to adhere to treatment prescriptions. Such a concept is based on the assumption that the patient agrees to the treatment prescription. However, in many instances he/she does not, and quite often rightly so. The history of diabetes treatment has experienced a series of erroneous concepts, the most persistent ones being the impositions of dietary restrictions such as the total prohibition of any sugar. Another problem in diabetes education is related to the frequent lack of defining treatment goals for individual patients or patient groups such as the indiscriminate call for normalisation of blood glucose levels in every diabetic patient, e. g. irrespective of the age of the patient. Frequently, educational interventions do not, for example, differentiate between the type 1 diabetic patient without complications, whose only medical problem is the lack of insulin, and the obese type 2 diabetic patient with a complex metabolic syndrome. For these patients, completely different treatment goals and therapeutic options need to be applied. A further problem concerning the evaluation of diabetes education arises if the education is separated from, rather than integrated into, the treatment programme, i. e. the treatment is prescribed by the physician, and at some later stage, the patient is referred to an educational programme. Often, the goals of the education programme cannot be achieved with the treatment prescribed [16, 29]. For example, if an insulin-dependent patient wants to achieve near-normal blood glucose values, but still is on a once- or twice-daily insulin regimen, he or she will not be able to reach this goal, even with the most sophisticated teaching programme. Likewise, if the patient is not trained to use daily metabolic self-monitoring and adaptation of insulin dosages accordingly on a day-to-day basis he/she will not be able to achieve and maintain optimal blood glucose control [49]. A further problem is an unstructured educational approach, which is frequently mistaken for individualised care. Many health care providers set up and use their own educational approaches instead of using established and structured teaching programmes, which have already been evaluated and shown to be effective. Structured intervention programmes which effectively combine the treatment and teaching parts of patient care and which have been shown to be effective, have been available for quite some time [2, 23, 24, 27, 30, 37]. In other fields of medicine it is customary to use structured and systematically evaluated treatment programmes, e. g. when applying chemotherapy in oncology. But, in the field of diabetes care, evaluated education programmes are only reluctantly accepted. A considerable amount of unnecessary work could be avoided if physicians would use established programmes, adapt them to their local needs and concentrate research on the further improvement of programmes which already exist. The importance of various aspects of diabetes education, e. g. the patient-physician relationship, knowledge, attitudes, skills such as insulin dose adaptation, sense of control, health beliefs, coping strategies, group interaction, social support etc. have already been well accepted by specialists in education, psychologists, etc. This holds true although studies of educational and psychosocial interventions have demonstrated divergent results [41], due to the use of different theoretical concepts and different assessment methods.

Education programmes affect numerous aspects of psychosocial functioning which have the potential to influence metabolic parameters, but we need a theoretical framework and educational models in order to understand the complex relationships between knowledge, psychosocial aspects, behaviour and metabolic control (Fig. 1). The Health Belief Model [3, 43] is a model which seems to be applicable in the field of diabetes and especially useful for explaining regimen adherence in type 2 diabetic patients [25]. Specific health beliefs were also identified as significant predictors of GHb in type 1 diabetic patients [6, 11]. However, there are many methodological problems in evaluating psychological instruments of clinical relevance [47].

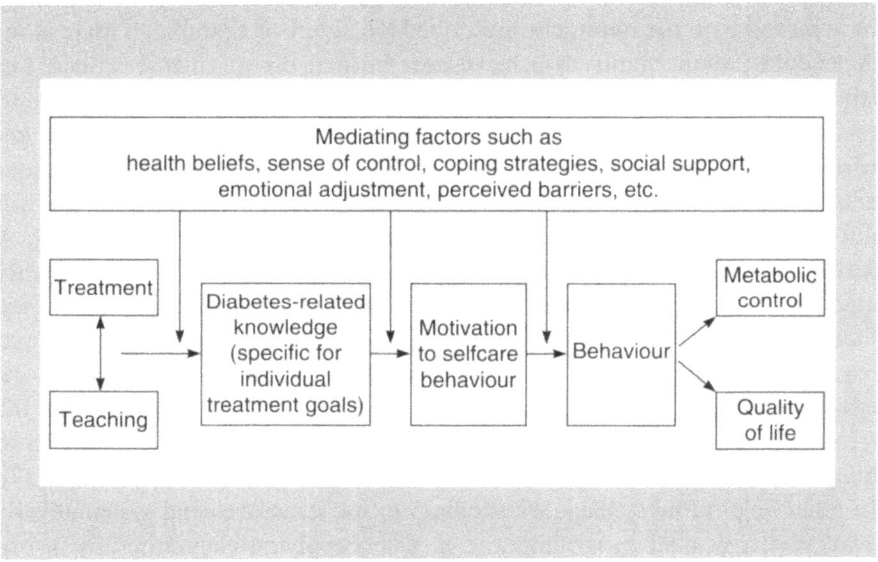

Fig. 1 Model of the relationship between knowledge, psychosocial aspects, behaviour and metabolic control

Defining the objectives of treatment-education-evaluation

Diabetes education is an integral part of diabetes treatment. Hence, the evaluation of diabetes education cannot be separated from the evaluation of diabetes treatment as such. Evaluation of diabetes education is always an evaluation of the diabetes treatment programme as a whole. The goals of diabetes education are part of the goals of diabetes treatment, and these goals have to be defined by each patient with the support of the medical team. Likewise, the possibilities of achieving these goals have to be made known to the patient, so the patient can make an informed decision on which treatment is most appropriate for him/her under the present circumstances, in order to best accomplish his/her treatment goals. Goals and modes of therapy may change during different life situations. Thus, the objectives of diabetes education should be defined as the empowerment of the patient to make an informed decision about his/her treatment goals, to formulate reasonable and achievable short and long-term objectives, to choose a treatment strategy and to carry out the therapy effectively and safely without undue dependence on medical institutions. Accepting such a definition of diabetes education, the teaching process has to become an integral part of any therapy for any patient.

Although individual treatment objectives differ, general characteristics are applicable for different groups of patients. Education programmes have to be tailored to the needs of the different patient groups. Likewise, each teaching programme has to be evaluated separately against the goals of diabetes therapy.

Evaluating treatment and teaching programmes for patients with type 1 diabetes

The insulin-dependent patient wants the insulin to be substituted in a way that does not interfere with life style, that allows them to continue family, social, professional life, leisure time activities as usual, with the confidence of remaining healthy despite diabetes. In practical terms, this means achievement and maintenance of a degree of glycaemic control that prevents hypo- and hyperglycaemic symptoms and, in the long-term, the avoidance of visual impairment, renal failure, foot amputation etc.; at the same time this calls for the least possible restriction with regard to eating habits [12], leisure time activities, professional life etc. Since continuous optimal glycaemic control can be achieved only at the expense of daily metabolic self-monitoring and day-to-day adaptations of insulin dosages according to eating habits, physical exercise etc., a certain risk of hypoglycaemia, and some restrictions in daily life, the patient has to have the opportunity to decide what degree of glycaemic control at what expense would be most appropriate under the present life situation. The role of the medical team is to help the patient to define realistic goals and to provide the knowledge, skills and empathic support to accomplish these goals.

The patient who manifests type 1 diabetes is usually a lay person with limited medical knowledge. Students who want to become physicians have to pass innumerable examinations and physicians, who want to treat diabetic patients are expected to have an additional training in diabetology. It appears self-evident that a lay person who manifests diabetes will have to receive extensive training in order to be able to carry out insulin therapy effectively and safely. It is also clear that the education programme has to include a substantial amount of knowledge and skills and to provide the competence and self-confidence to perform the treatment without undue dependence on medical institutions.

The main objective of evaluation is to assess to what extent the treatment goals have been achieved by the patient. The most successful treatment and teaching program will be the one that achieves the best possible degree of metabolic control at the least frequency of severe hypoglycaemia with the least restrictions of the patients' lifestyle and with the patients feeling competent and confident in the management of their diabetes. Under the assumption of a successful programme, it would be sufficient to measure HbA1(c) levels, frequency of severe hypoglycaemia and some parameters on quality of life, e. g. hospitalisation days, sick leave days [2] perceived restrictions with regard to eating habits [13], leisure time activities, etc.

However, if the treatment and teaching goals are not achieved, a more comprehensive approach of evaluation is necessary, in order to identify the possible reasons for the lack of success, and to evaluate whether these factors could be modified either on the part of the health care providers or on part of the patient.

Such a comprehensive evaluation has to include, first of all, a critical analysis of the medical treatment strategies [40]. Unphysiological insulin prescriptions, e. g. only one or two insulin injections per day, predominant use of long-acting insulin preparations, etc. are major obstacles for the achievement of optimal glycaemic control and interfere with usual eating habits and other lifestyle activities. Unnecessary treatment prescriptions will interfere with patient compliance to efficient performance. On the other hand, patients have to be trained in day-to-day adaptations of insulin dosages based upon daily metabolic (blood-glucose) self-monitoring. Just providing the patient with a leaflet on algorithms is not sufficient. In addition, frequently, inadequate algorithms are used, e. g. reduction of insulin dosages by only 2–4 units before strenuous and prolonged exercise or increase of insulin dosages by only 2–4 units in case of illness. Some basic knowledge in insulin treatment apparently has not yet been included in clinical practice at all places, such as the necessity to reduce insulin dosages also after strenuous and prolonged exercise [36]. Competence in insulin-dose adaptation can only be acquired (be it the medical team or the patient) by practical training related to real-life situations. How insulin can be substituted effectively and safely has been shown repeatedly and adherence of the medical team to established standards of insulin therapy is indispensable [2, 12, 13, 23, 24, 27, 30, 37].

Blood glucose self-monitoring is a further prerequisite for type 1 diabetic patients who strive for near-normoglycaemia. It is of note, however, that daily metabolic self-monitoring is useful only if patients are competent to immediately react to each single measurement by adapting insulin dosages or by making other treatment decisions. Thus, it is not surprising that studies, in which patients had not been taught to make immediate treatment decisions, failed to show an effect of blood glucose self-monitoring on metabolic control [49]. Likewise, it appears useless to ask patients to perform blood glucose profiles once or twice per week in order to present them to the treating physician during the next consultation.

A further objective of evaluation is the process of teaching, the interaction between the physician, the teachers and the patient. Important research has investigated this aspect of diabetes care, and various approaches are available for assessment [2, 31].

A further aspect of comprehensive evaluation of diabetes education is the assessment of knowledge transfer and training in skills. In contrast to the present tendency to disregard the importance of knowledge, in our view, diabetes-related knowledge is an essential basis for effective treatment of type 1 diabetes. Although several studies have failed to demonstrate a relationship between diabetes-related knowledge and glycosylated haemoglobin values, such an association does exist, if various prerequisites are fulfilled [7, 9]. Thus, the test has to measure aspects which are relevant to the achievement of good metabolic control, e. g. daily life decisions for adaptation of insulin dosages rather than general knowledge, e. g. about (patho-) physiology. The test has to represent the main objectives of the education programme and be tailored to patient groups homogeneous with respect to treatment goals and treatment strategies. Thus, existing knowledge tests [17, 18] are not generally applicable, in contrast to what has recently been suggested [48]. Initial reliability analyses of the diabetes knowledge scales by Dunn [17] indicated that test results depend on local conditions of education programmes. Therefore, test results will not be comparable if educational programmes lack standardisation with respect to methods and objectives.

It is worthy of note that the association of diabetes-related knowledge and metabolic control is not always linear, indicating that the application of simple correlation analysis is not always the appropriate statistical method. Lockington et al. [34, 35] performed quintile grouping of knowledge scores and found patients in the lowest scoring group to have the highest HbA1(c) values, whereas the other four groups had comparable glycaemic control. In a recent analysis we found diabetes-related knowledge to be significantly associated with lower GHb values in a large number of type 1 diabetic patients after participation in an intensive treatment and teaching programme [9] Nevertheless, we agree with Lockington et al. [34, 35] that there seems to be a 'threshold' of knowledge above which further increases in knowledge do not lead to further improvement of glycaemic control. Beyond this threshold, other factors (i. e. attitudes, motivation) are likely to be of greater importance.

Therefore, it appears worthwhile to examine psychosocial aspects (emotional adjustment, coping strategies, self-efficacy, perceived control, health beliefs, social support, treatment satisfaction) as mediating factors and predictors of knowledge transfer to increased diabetes self-care behaviour and improved metabolic control [9]. If such variables can be identified and reliably measured, it should be possible to improve teaching and treatment programmes by developing and applying new educational and behavioural techniques in order to affect emotional adjustment and health beliefs in a more structured way. The validity of such psychometric scales appears to be specific for certain patient groups under certain life conditions. We cannot assume that attitudes, burdens and coping strategies of diabetic patients will be identical in different countries with their different lifestyles, health care systems and different patient education programmes. Thus, it is not surprising that the ATT39 test [18, 19] demonstrated different results and factor structures in different studies [8, 46].

Due to the failure of some education programmes to demonstrate an association between the intervention programme and metabolic control, it has been suggested to shift emphasis to measures of quality of life. However, generally applicable tools are missing. The DCCT quality of life measure [15] appears particularly related to the specific health care structures and modes of therapy used in the DCCT, although parts of the questionnaire could be transferable to other treatment conditions. Bradley and Lewis [10, 32] have developed psychological outcome measures of well-being and treatment satisfaction, and have evaluated them in tablet-treated type 2 diabetic patients [10]. The test was reported to be reliable and of validity, according to psychometric-statistical criteria. However, in contrast to what was expected, for patients with substantial retinopathy or acute foot ulcers, depression and anxiety scores were lower whereas positive well-being and general well-being scores were greater than for respondents without these complications, casting doubt on the methodology used. Since the assessment of general quality of life (e. g. anxiety, depression, positive well-being) is complex and difficult, scales should focus on diabetes-related aspects such as treatment satisfaction, dietary and other lifestyle restrictions, etc. Scores on general quality of life scales appear to be affected by many other factors beyond diabetes therapy which makes interpretation of test results more speculative.

Finally, it has to be stressed, that the prerequisite for any meaningful evaluation of diabetes treatment and diabetes education is a written curriculum, which comprises all treatment and teaching objectives, as well as respective contents and methods, the staff responsibility, and clinic organisation. In addition, it has to be guaranteed that the curriculum is followed by all members of the medical team, and that changes are made only if the decision has been made by all the members of the team. Thus, a written curriculum is basic for the quality control in diabetes education. A certain structure, which has been proven to be effective, can be maintained independently from changes in staff or environmental aspects. On the other hand, only if the objectives are precisely defined can they be evaluated. Furthermore, a written curriculum makes education programmes comparable and transferable. The feasibility of effective and safe transfers of structured diabetes treatment and teaching programmes to non-specialised general hospitals and to the offices of general practitioners, respectively, has been recently shown [24, 27]. Thus, the quality of diabetes care can be improved and decentralised, if established programmes are well documented. If treatment and teaching goals are not achieved the curriculum should be reviewed systematically. This review should involve all members of the medical team who are involved in the performance of the programme.

Evaluating treatment and teaching programmes for patients with type 2 diabetes

The young type 2 diabetic patient can develop hyperglycaemic-related microvascular and neuropathic complications and, therefore, has to be informed about these sequelae in order to make informed decisions about short- and long-term treatment goals and intensity of treatment interventions.

The elderly patient who manifests type 2 diabetes – in developed countries the majority of diabetic patients are older than 60 years when diabetes is diagnosed – will not be threatened by debilitating microvascular complications. Thus, for these patients normoglycaemia is no longer the primary therapeutic goal. Rather, the patient wants to be free of symptoms, be it hyperglycaemic- or treatment-related, nor is normalisation of body weight a therapeutic goal. Frequently, the loss of only a few kilos of body weight will help in achieving and maintaining a clinical state free of hyperglycaemic symptoms. On the other hand, in the elderly patient prevention of foot complications and in the majority of cases treatment of hypertension are major objectives of treatment and education.

A major problem arises when defining other, more controversial treatment and teaching goals for patients with type 2 diabetes, e. g. normalisation of cholesterol levels. More research is urgently needed on how to present to type 2 diabetic patients real risks and possible benefits of treating alleged risk factors, such as high cholesterol levels in an unbiased way. The patient should be able to make an informed decision on whether treatment of "risk factors" appears worthwhile and practicable under his/her life conditions.

Blood glucose testing is rarely necessary in type 2 diabetic patients, however, glucosuria testing is essential for the patient to be able to observe his or her efforts to improve glucose control [24, 30]. Simple dietary recommendations emphasising restriction of caloric intake are usually sufficient for patients treated without oral sulphonylureas. Thus, the necessary knowledge about diabetes is limited when compared to the patient with type 1 diabetes. Outcome measures have to be oriented against individual treatment goals, rendering HbA1 levels of secondary importance.

Evaluating teaching and treatment programmes for patients with late complications

Treatment and teaching goals may change, if patients develop diabetic late complications. Treatment of hypertension may become the primary medical problem. Substantial research has been carried out on problems of physicians' and patients' compliance to the diagnosis, initiation of treatment and adherence to treatment in non-diabetic persons with hypertension. For the diabetic patient, hypertension presents a second medical problem which requires continuous attention. Diagnosis of hypertension frequently means diagnosis of nephropathy and may induce substantial depression in these patients, which, in turn, will interfere with effective treatment. In contrast to the abundant research on new antihypertensive drugs, only limited efforts have been made to evaluate the overall quality of hypertension care in diabetic patients. Frequently, blood pressure is not measured at all, and if measured, treatment is often not initiated and if initiated, patients frequently fail to reach optimal blood pressure values.

Structured hypertension treatment and teaching programmes for patients with and without diabetes have been developed and evaluated [38, 39]. These programmes are based upon increased involvement of the patients in control and treatment of their hypertension, including blood pressure self-monitoring and participation in treatment decision making. However, not all patients succeed in coping with hypertension and their medical condition rapidly deteriorates to endstage renal failure [38]. Thus, further research could be helpful to improve hypertension care in diabetes.

References

[1] Ajzen, I, Fishbein M. Understanding attitudes and predicting social behavior. Englewood Cliffs, NJ: Prentice Hall, 1980.

[2] Assal JP, Mühlhauser I, Pernet A et al. Patient education as the basis for diabetes care in clinical practice and research. Diabetologia 1985; 28: 602–613.

[3] Becker MH, Maiman LA. Strategies for enhancing patient compliance. Journal of Community Health 1980: 6: 113–135.

[4] Beeney LJ, Dunn SM. Knowledge improvement and metabolic control in diabetes education: approaching the limits? Patient Educ Couns 1990; 16: 217–229.

[5] Bloomgarden ZT, Karmally W, Metzger MJ et al. Randomized, controlled trial of diabetic patient education: improved knowledge without improved metabolic status. Diabetes Care 1987; 10: 263–272.

[6] Bond GG, Aiken LS, Somerville SC. The health belief model and adolescents with insulin-dependent diabetes mellitus. Health Psychology 1992; 11: 190–198.

[7] Bott U, Scholz V, Grüßer M et al. Evaluation of a knowledge test with 546 Type 1 (insulin-dependent) diabetic patients in 10 centres. Diabetologia 1988; 31: 473A.

[8] Bott U, Scholz V, Mühlhauser I. Emotional adjustment in 687 Type 1 diabetic patients measured using the ATT39 scale. Diabetes 1990; 39: 643A.

[9] Bott U, Jörgens V, Grüßer M et al. Predictors of glycemic control in Type 1 diabetic patients after participation in an intensified treatment and teaching program. Diabetic Med 1994; 11: in press.

[10] Bradley C, Lewis KS. Measures of psychological well-being and treatment satisfaction developed from the responses of people with tablet-treated diabetes. Diab Med 1990; 7: 445–451.

[11] Brownlee-Duffeck M, Peterson L, Simonds JF et al. The role of health beliefs in the regimen adherence and metabolic control of adolescents and adults with diabetes mellitus. Journal of Consulting and Clinical Psychology 1987; 55: 139–144.

[12] Chantelau EA, Frenzen A, Gösseringer G et al. Intensive insulin therapy justifies simplification of the diabetes diet: a prospective study in insulin-dependent diabetics. Am J Clin Nutr 1987; 45: 958–962.

[13] Chantelau E. Relation of dietary barriers in patients with insulin-dependent diabetes mellitus to different modes of treatment. J Am Dietetic Assoc 1992; 92: 1129–1131.

[14] Davis WK, Hess GE, Hiss RG. Psychological correlates of survival in diabetes. Diabetes Care 1988; 11: 538–545.

[15] DCCT Research Group. Reliability and validity of a diabetes quality-of-life measure for the diabetes control and complications trial (DCCT). Diabetes Care 1988; 11: 725–732.

[16] DeWeerdt I, Visser AP, Kok GJ et al. Randomized controlled multicentre evaluation of an education programme for insulin-dependent diabetic patients: effects on metabolic control, quality of life, and costs of therapy. Diab Med 1991; 8: 338–345.

[17] Dunn SM, Bryson JM, Hoskins PL et al. Development of the diabetes knowledge (DKN) scales: forms DKNA, DKNB, and DKNC. Diabetes Care 1984; 7: 36–41.

[18] Dunn SM. Reactions to educational techniques: coping strategies for diabetes and learning. Diab Med 1986; 3: 419–429.

[19] Dunn SM, Smartt HH, Beeney LJ et al. Measurement of emotional adjustment in diabetic patients: validity and reliability of ATT39. Diabetes Care 1986; 9: 480–489.

[20] Dunn SM. Rethinking the models and modes of diabetes education. Patient Educ Couns 1990; 16: 281–286.

[21] Glasgow RE, McCaul KD, Schafer LC. Barriers to regimen adherence among persons with insulin-dependent diabetes. J Behavioral Med 1986; 9: 65–77.

[22] Glasgow RE, Osteen VL. Evaluating diabetes education. Are we measuring the most important outcomes? Diabetes Care 1992; 15: 1423–1432.

[23] Glasgow RE, Toobert DJ, Hampson SE et al. Improving self-care among older patients with Type 2 diabetes: the "sixty something..." study. Patient Educ Couns 1992; 19: 61–74.
[24] Grüßer M, Bott U, Ellermann P et al. Evaluation of a structured treatment and teaching program for non-insulin treated Type 2 diabetic outpatients in Germany after the nationwide introduction of reimbursement policy for physicians. Diabetes Care 1993; 16: 1268–1275.
[25] Harris R, Linn MW. Health beliefs, compliance and control of diabetes mellitus. Southern Medical Journal 1985; 78: 162–166.
[26] Johnson SB. Methodological issues in diabetes research. Measuring adherence. Diabetes Care 1992; 15: 1658–1667.
[27] Jörgens V, Grüßer M, Bott U et al. Effective and safe translation of intensified insulin therapy to general internal medicine departments. Diabetologia 1993; 36: 99–105.
[28] Kaplan RM, Davis WK. Evaluating the costs and benefits of outpatient diabetes education and nutrition counseling. Diabetes Care 1986; 9: 81–86.
[29] Korhonen T, Huttunen JK, Aro A et al. A controlled trial on the effects of patient education in the treatment of insulin-dependent diabetes. Diabetes Care 1983; 6: 256–261.
[30] Kronsbein P, Jörgens V, Mühlhauser I et al. Evaluation of a structured treatment and teaching programme on non-insulin-dependent diabetes. Lancet 1988; 2: 1407–1411.
[31] Lacroix A, Assal JP. Peut-on améliorer les prestations pédagogiques des médecins qui enseignent aux malades? Analyse comparative des mêmes cours donnés avant et après une formation pédagogique. Diabete & Metabolisme 1992; 18: 387–394.
[32] Lewis KS, Bradley C, Knight G et al. A measure of treatment satisfaction designed specifically for people with insulin-dependent diabetes. Diab Med 1988; 5: 235–242.
[33] Lloyd CE, Matthews KA, Wing RR et al. Psychological factors and complications of IDDM. The Pittsburgh epidemiology of diabetes complications study. VIII. Diabetes Care 1992; 15: 166–172.
[34] Lockington TJ, Farrant S, Meadows KA et al. Knowledge profile and control in diabetic patients. Diabetic Medicine 1988; 5: 381–386, 1988.
[35] Lockington TJ, Powels S, Meadows KA et al. Attitudes, knowledge and blood glucose control. Diab Med 1989; 6: 309–313.
[36] MacDonald M. Postexercise late-onset hypoglycemia in insulin-dependent diabetic patients. Diabetes Care 1987; 10: 584–588.
[37] Mühlhauser I, Bruckner I, Berger M et al. Evaluation of an intensified insulin treatment and teaching programme as routine management of Type 1 (insulin-dependent) diabetes. The Bucharest-Düsseldorf Study. Diabetologia 1987; 30: 681–690.
[38] Mühlhauser I, Sawicki P, Didjurgeit U et al. Uncontrolled hypertension in Type 1 diabetes: assessment of patients' desires about treatment and improvement of blood pressure control by a structured treatment and teaching programme. Diab Med 1988; 5: 693–698.
[39] Mühlhauser I, Sawicki PT, Didjurgeit U et al. Evaluation of a structured treatment and teaching programme on hypertension in general practice. Clin and Exper Hypertension 1993; 15: 125–142.
[40] Mühlhauser I, Berger M. Diabetes education and insulin therapy: when will they ever learn? J Intern Med 1993; 233: 321–326.
[41] Padgett D, Mumford E, Hynes M et al. Meta-analysis of the effects of educational and psychosocial interventions on management of diabetes mellitus. J Clin Epidemiol 1988; 41: 1007–1030.
[42] Peyrot MF, McMurry JF. Stress buffering and glycemic control Diabetes Care 1992; 15: 842–846.
[43] Rosenstock IM. Understanding and enhancing patient compliance with diabetic regimens. Diabetes Care 1985; 8: 610–616.
[44] Rubin RR, Peyrot M. Psychological problems and interventions in diabetes. A review of the literature. Diabetes Care 1992; 15: 1640–1657.
[45] Songer TJ, DeBerry K, LaPorte RE et al. International comparisons of IDDM mortality. Diabetes Care 1992; 15 (Suppl 1): 15–21.

[46] Welch G, Smith RBW, Walkey FH. Styles of psychological adjustment in diabetes: a focus on key psychometric issues and the ATT39. J Clin Psychol 1992; 48: 648–658.
[47] Williams G, Pickup J, Keen H. Psychological factors and metabolic control: time for reappraisal? Diab Med 1988; 5: 211–215.
[48] World Health Organization. Guidelines for education programmes. In: Diabetes care and research in Europe: the St. Vincent declaration action programme. Krans HMJ, Porta M, Keen H, eds. WHO, Regional Office for Europe, Copenhagen; EUR/ICP/CLR 055/3; 1992: 15–18.
[49] Worth R, Home PD, Jonston DG et al. Intensive attention improves glycaemic control in insulin-dependent diabetes without further advantage from home blood glucose monitoring: results of a controlled trial. Br Med J 1982; 285: 1233–1240.

Research methodologies in diabetic retinopathy

E. M. Kohner, V. Patel, R. Chibber

The retina is the only part of the body where the vessels and a deep tissue can be observed in life directly, repeatedly and non invasively. It is for this reason that there are many detailed descriptions of appearances in health and diesease of the retina. In contrast to obtain tissue for examination in life is difficult, and even today is usually done during operations. Biopsies of the vitreous and of the anterior chamber fluid have become more common in recent years, and are used as diagnostic procedures, especially when infection or tumour is suspected.

Because of the ability to observe the changes in life, the lesions of diabetic retinopathy have been well described. Serial observations allowed for description of the natural history of the lesions. Unfortunately the pathogenic mechanisms which lead up to the earliest lesions and which determine whether retinal lesions change little over the years (Fig. 1 a, b) or advance rapidly (Fig. 2 a, b) remain a mystery. It is for this reason that continued research is

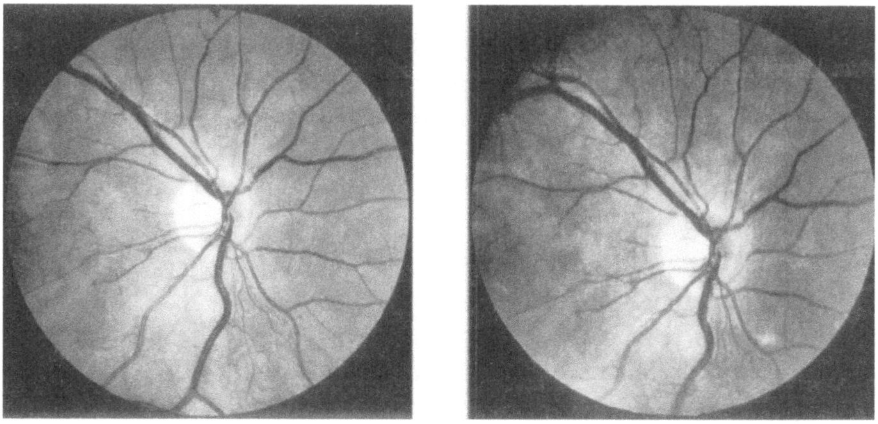

Fig. 1 a Right disc area of patient with mild retinopathy. Only few microaneurysms seen
b. Same as 1 a but 2 years later. There are now more haemorrhages and microaneurysms, a few hard exudates and a cotton wool spot

Offprint from
Research Methodologies in Human Diabetes – Part 1

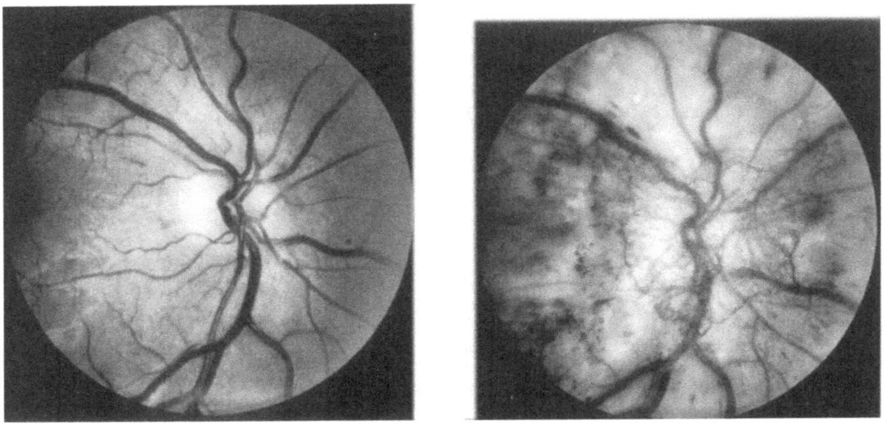

Fig. 2a Patient with non-proliferative retinopathy, dilated veins, microaneurysms and haemorrhages
b Same as 2a but 9 months later. There are extensive new vessels arising from the disc, there are gross venous changes and an ischaemic retina

important. The research procedures are clinical or experimental. Much of the experimental work is based on animal studies, although animals do not usually develop all the features of diabetic retinopathy.

In this chapter we review the most important research methods, as used in studying retinal disease and will relate them to some of the findings in diabetic retinopathy.

Assessment of retinal photographs

Retinal photographs can be colour photographs, red free or monochromatic photographs and fluorescein angiograms. All have their special place in research.

Colour photographs

Colour photographs are used in assessment of treatment effects. They are an essential part of any prospective study using new methods of treatment and are particularly useful in the study of early diabetic retinopathy. Photography is essential, as it is difficult to remember individual eyes and lesions.
Photographic grading: The majority of assessments are based on grading retinal photographs, a semiquantitative method, which compares lesions seen in a patient with those seen on 'standard' photographs. Careful selection of

the standards is therefore important. Too many standards make the process complicated and too few standards make it difficult to differentiate between lesions which are clinically important from those which are not important.

The first widely used grading system was described by Oakley et al [1] and was developed specially for the evaluation of the then only treatment for sight threatening diabetic retinopathy, pituitary ablation. It is based on 4 main lesions seen on retinal photographs, and for each of the lesions (microaneurysms and haemorrhages, hard exudates, new vessels and fibrous retinitis proliferans) there are 4 standard photographs allowing for 6 grades of severity including absence of lesions. The grading is still used for the clinical evaluation of patients attending the Hammersmith Hospital.

The Airlie House grading system was developed by a panel of experts at the first meeting on diabetic retinopathy, held in 1968 [2]. The system was never really used, but became important because it forms the basis of the

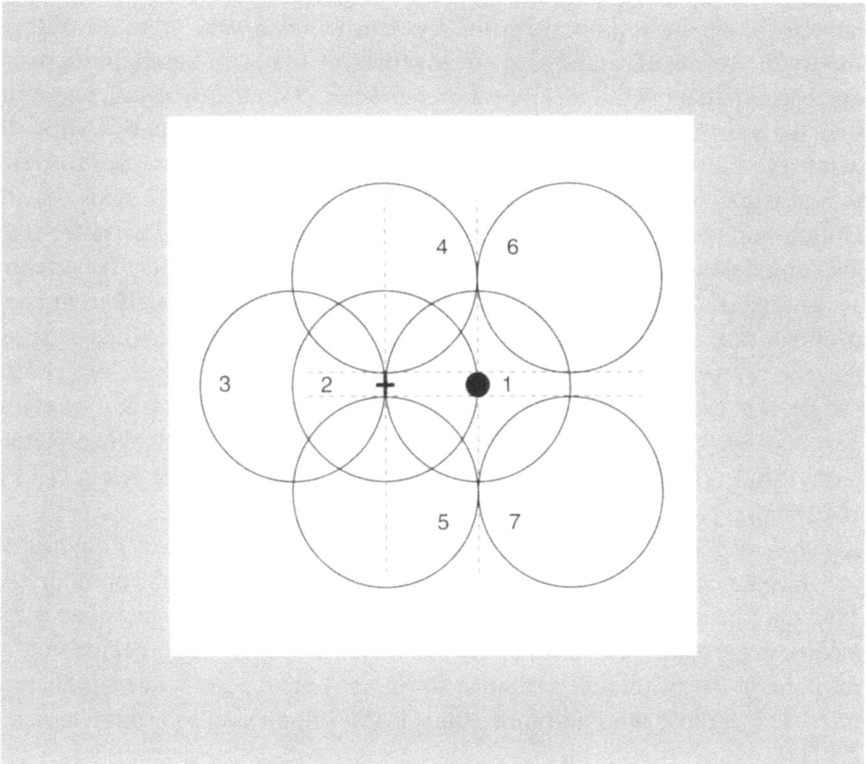

Fig. 3 Seven standard fields photographed in stereo pairs. 1 = disc, + = fovea, 2 = field centred on fovea

most widely used grading system, the Wisconsin system [3]. The Wisconsin system was based initially on 191 patients with diabetic retinopathy, who were followed for a 6 year period. The retinal lesions were grouped according to their prognostic significance primarily for the evaluation of development of neovascularisation. The fields photographed are 7 standard fields (Fig. 3), taken as stereo pairs, which allows estimation of macular oedema as retinal thickening and position of new vessels and fibrous tissue in relation to the plain of the retina. For each lesion there are 3 standard photographs, and the lesions include arterial and venous abnormalities and cotton wool spots. The lesions are then grouped according to severity giving retinopathy levels between 10 and 41 for increasingly severe non proliferative or background retinopathy, between 41 and 60 preproliferative retinopathy, and over 60 varying severity of proliferation. Levels are also given for non assessable eyes secondary to vitreous haemorrhage.

This grading system is very time consuming and since it has 64 standard photographs in stereo pairs, it is really complicated. Special grading centres have to be set up to cope with this system. It has 3 very great advantages. Firstly the two eyes can be assessed together, by a system based on the worse eye, e. g. a patient could have a grading of 40/< 40 in the two eyes, suggesting that the worse eye has quite severe non proliferative retinopathy, while the better eye is milder. The second advantage is that it can be adapted for fewer retinal fields. Thus the Eurodiab study used only 2 standard fields and the United Kingdom Prospective Diabetes Study uses 4 fields. The latter study also emphasizes macular lesions, as it studies NIDD patients. The greatest advantage is that researchers from different centres and even different countries can talk to each other, and know exactly what is meant when a patient has e. g. a retinopathy level of 30. The first major study in which this grading system was used was the Diabetic Retinopathy Study (DRS) study on retinal photocoagulation [4] followed by the Early Treatment of Diabetic Retinopathy Study (ETDRS) [5–8]. The epidemiological studies of Klein et al [9, 10] are also based on this grading system.

Accurate quantitation of lesions: The lesions which are commonly quantitated are microaneurysms (MA). MAs can be counted from retinal photographs. This may be useful in early retinopathy, where increase in microaneurysms means progression of retinopathy. Klein et al found that progression of retinopathy to proliferative lesions during a 4 year period was significantly increased in those who had more than 11 MA in an eye, to a relative risk of 2.8 [11].

There have been studies trying to quantitate hard exudates, but this is more difficult, because even if they apparently have well defined edges their colour merges gradually into the background of the retina. Also small hard exudates are numerous, larger plaques are far fewer.

Red free photographs

Red free photographs show up the vessels and some of the lesions far better than colour photographs, as the background of the red retina is eliminated. Red free photographs are commonly used when densitometric methods are used to measure retinal vessel diameter. This is important in all methods of blood flow studies.

The densitometric profile allows for the measurement of the half height vessel width [12]. This is used by most observers because it is more reproducible than that taken lower down, where the vessel width is largest. This is because of the variable density of the background makes vessel diameter measurement difficult. More recently the densitometric half height method was improved to allow computer driven assessment of vessel diameter [13]. It must be remembered that this method only measures the red blood column width. Vessel wall diameter measurements have been reported recently [14].

Fluorescein angiograms

Fluorescein angiograms are used in research procedures to count MAs, look at the size of non perfused areas and to measure leakage. The very detailed method of counting MAs in the field centred on the fovea as described by Baudoin et al [15] was improved to allow computer assisted method [16]. Completely automated methods have been described, but are not universally available, as they have been worked out for specific computers. Progression of microaneurysm numbers in early retinopathy is an indication of further occlusion of vessels, and is particularly useful in studies where antiplatelet drugs are used.

Fully automated method for measuring non perfused areas is in progress. Small areas are now measured quite accurately. Other uses of image analysis technology is developing rapidly at present and include filling pattern of retinal vessels [17] aswell and measurement of leakage from fluorescein angiograms [18]. The latter should be a good measure of blood retinal dysfunction in early retinopathy, and if a medical treatment would be possible for maculopathy, it would be a method of choice.

Analysis of fluorescein angiograms from cine films or scanning laser ophthalmoscope are used for measurement of retinal blood flow, and are discussed later.

Retinal photography demonstrates the anatomical lesions. Functional lesions are important in the development of retinopathy. The next two sections deal with the most important ones, leakage and haemodynamic changes, as studied in clinical diabetes.

Vitreous fluorophotometry

Vitreous fluorophotometry was introduced by Cunha-Vaz in 1975 [19]. It is a sensitive method to measure leakage from the retinal vessels into the vitreous cavity. It was thought to show leakage even before the development of clinically obvious retinopathy. The initial methods were unsatisfactory, but eventually the Fluorotron Master was developed, with which it was possible to get reproducible and valid measurements.

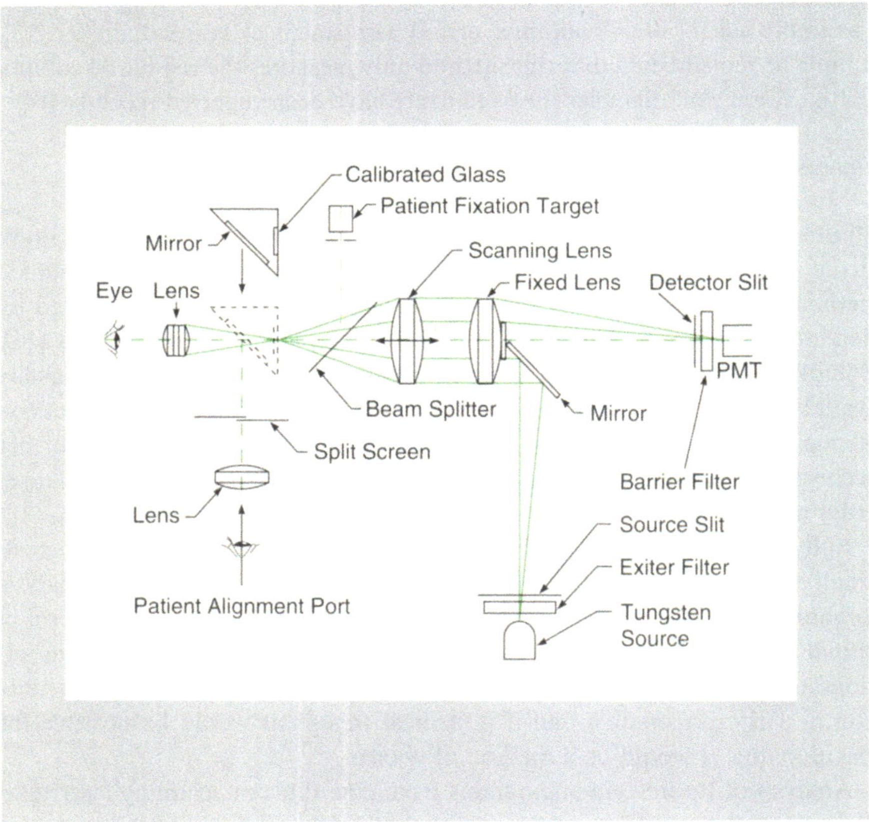

Fig. 4 Line diagram of Fluorotron-master

The Fluorotron Master is a commercially available instrument (Coherent Radiation, Palo Alto, California, USA). A schematic representation of the unit is shown in Fig. 4. A halogen light source with double barrier and excitor filters produces a beam of blue light with a wavelength of 480 nm which is transmitted by one part of the lens system into the eye. The light excites the fluorescence and the emitted green light of 520 nm is directed through the lens system into a photomultiplier. Each photon of light is converted into an electrical impulse and these are counted over a given time interval. Low intensity impulses generated by noise are cut out by the equipment. The optical electronic unit is linked to a computer visual display unit, printer and data storage unit.

Using this equipment it became obvious that there was no leakage from retinal vessels before the development of retinopathy [20, 21]. It also became evident that in its original form the equipment really only measures fluorescein leakage in the visual axis, and therefore in early retinopathy leakage is only seen if it originates in the macular region [21]. Through cooperative work in the EEC funded by this organisation the methodology and analysis throughout Europe is now standardised. Since leakage through the tight junctions or through the endothelial cells is one of the early and important functional abnormalities in diabetic retinopathy this method will be of value in studying drugs which may reduce leakage, such as ACE inhibitors, and other hypotensive agents.

Haemodynamic changes in diabetic retinopathy

While leakage probably does not occur until some anatomical lesions of retinopathy are seen, haemodynamic flow changes occur early.

The retinal circulation affords the only direct access to visualization of the microangiopathic manifestations of diabetes mellitus. Many techniques have been utilised to measure retinal blood flow in diabetes, most are still in use today.

Quantification of retinal blood flow

Mean transit time of fluorescein

Hickam and Frayser [22] measured the mean transit time taken by fluorescein to appear in the retinal vein from its visualisation in the retinal artery. In an adaptation of this method, high speed fluorescein cine-angiography was used to measure the retinal artery fluorescein front advance rate Dollery [23], Hill and Young [24]. There are several problems with this method. Even though the arterio-venous transit time can be accurately measured, in order to calculate the volume flow rate, the total volume of the retinal vasculature needs to be determined. Bulpitt and Dollery [25] described a method for estimating this from the arterial and venous diameters at different orders of retinal vessel branching. An acceptable degree of accuracy was difficult to attain however. In diabetic retinopathy there is a breakdown of the blood retinal barrier and any leakage of fluorescein from the retinal vessels would lead to an erroneous determination of the mean transit time of fluorescein. Nonetheless it was with this technique that Kohner et al [26] and Cunha-Vaz and Lima [27] conducted the earliest studies on the quantification of retinal blood flow in diabetic retinopathy.

Radio-labelled microspheres
In the animal setting Alm and Bill [28] used radioactive microspheres to quantitate the retinal blood flow. The basic principle is that following injection of the microspheres into the left the number embolising in a given tissue, after the first transit, will be proportional to its blood flow. The radioactivity in the dissected tissue is then compared to the radioactivity in a known volume of blood which acts as the reference. This technique, although widely regarded as the gold standard for measuring retinal blood flow, was limited in scope because of its application requires the sacrifice of the animal under study.

Blue light entoptic phenomenon
The original idea that retinal capillary blood flow could be measured by estimating the speed of the white cell perceived by the entoptic phenomenon was by Vierordt in 1862 and quantitated by Riehm et al in 1972 [29]. This phenomenon, known as the blue light entoptic phenomenon, relies on assessment of the speed of the white cells that are normally seen one looks into a deep blue light or a cloudless blue sky. The explanation for this effect is that red blood cells, but not the white cells, will absorb most of the blue light approximating to 430 nm. The white cells alone are then able to stimulate adjacent photoreceptors and be perceived as moving white corpuscles. As this is a colour vision phenomenon it is the macular white cells that are seen and therefore the inner macula or the perifoveal flow that can be estimated. Earlier quantification of the blue light entoptic phenomenon relied on subjects tracking a single white cell as it traversed a length of capillary. This unsatisfactory assessment was superseded by Riva's technique which allowed the subject to estimate the speed of their entoptically perceived white cells and match them to computer simulation of white cells moving at various speeds [30].

Scanning laser ophthalmoscopy

Scanning laser ophthalmoscopy allows direct quantification of red blood cell velocity in the perifoveal capillaries [31]. Since measurement of blood flow require both the velocity and cross sectional area of the vessels, this technique is at present limited in scope. Nevertheless the scanning laser ophthalmoscope has increased the accuracy with which the fluorescein dye advance front and the arterio-venous passage time can be assessed [32]. The increased sensitivity of the technique leads to a paradoxical loss of specificity in determining the retinal arterio-venous passage time. In the original mean circulation time of fluorescein determination, a bolus of fluorescein was injected and the dye concentration versus time plotted through the artery and then the vein. The time between the maximas of dye concentrations in the artery and vein is then the mean transit time. With the scanning laser ophthalmoscope, the first appearance of fluorescein in the retinal artery near the optic disc margin to the first appearance of dye in the adjacent retinal vein is timed. In a healthy retina the dye will be able to cross to the retinal vein via the first retinal capillary network distal to the retinal artery under study. Where there is capillary closure, such as in diabetic retinopathy, the arteriovenous passage time will be prolonged because the fluorescein has to take a longer course to enter the retinal venous circulation. The arterio-venous passage time therefore becomes dependent on the degree of capillary closure as well as the velocity of retinal blood flow. Bertram et al [32] demonstrated a significant increase in the arteriovenous passage time using this technique in diabetic retinopathy.

Targeted dye delivery

This is a recent exciting technique that allows quantification of retinal blood flow, so far it has only been evaluated in lower primates [33]. Basically fluorescein is encapsulated into 0.2 μm diameter temperature sensitive liposomes and injected intravenously. Using a retinal camera setup, an argon laser is used to increase the temperature of a segment of retinal vessel. The increase in temperature releases fluorescein from the liposomes which then produce a sharply defined fluorescein dye front that can be measured to provide the retinal vessel transit time. This technique may be refined in the future for use in humans.

Laser Doppler velocimeter

The retinal laser Doppler velocimeter (LDV) was invented by Riva's group and presented to the scientific community in 1972 [34]. Tanaka et al [35] of the same group reported the first measurements in the human retinal circulation. In the last 20 years laser Doppler velocimetry, allowing reproducible and non-invasive measurements, has become the method of choice for investigating retinal blood flow in disease and health. Laser Doppler velocimetry relies on the Doppler effect. The fundamental principle is that the shift in frequency, that a wavelength undergoes after reflecting off a moving object, is directly proportional to its velocity. For the purpose of the retinal circulation the instrumentation uses a laser beam to provide the waveforms which are then focused and processed after reflecting from the red blood cells.

Components of the bidirectional laser Doppler velocimeter: The bidirectional laser Doppler velocimeter is based upon a Topcon retinal fundus camera (Topcon TRC-FE, Tokyo, Japan) with special adaptions to allow the retinal camera to be used to measure retinal vessel velocity. The LDV instrumentation as a complete unit is manufactured by Oculix Inc. (Philadelphia, USA).

A Helium-Neon laser is used to as the waveform that undergoes the Doppler shift. It is 632.8 nm wavelength, linearly polarized with a power of 0.8 mW, equivalent to a maximum retinal irradiance of 80 mW/cm^2 (Melles Griot, Irvine, USA). This level of retinal irradiance is completely safe and has no known sequelae affecting retinal function, it is also within the limits of safety defined by Sliney and Freasier for extended retinal irradiation [36]. The range through which the laser beam can be focused onto the retinal vessel is -4 to $+4$ dioptres for ametropic eyes.

Principles of LDV operation: The basic principle of the LDV is shown in Fig. 5a and b. The early models of the LDV were only able to give comparisons of velocities rather than absolute determinations. This was because the instrumentation was such that reflected light was collected by one light sensitive probe only. This problem was overcome by the introduction of the bidirectional laser Doppler velocimeter by Riva's group in 1979 [37]. In this technique the Doppler shifted scatter is collected along two distinct directions with a known angle of separation to their respective photodetectors. The two photodetectors have a different frequency shift, since each detects a different velocity vector. However, knowing the fixed predetermined angle of separation of the two beams allows the calculation of the theoretical maximum frequency shift. This will therefore be independent of the exact orientation of the retinal blood vessel and the angle of the incident beam with respect to the flow direction. The determination of the Vmax has been automated over the last few years due to the availability of customised software from Petrig and Riva [38]. The photomultiplier signal is processed by the computer (Masscomp MCS-561 microsupercomputer, Masscomp Inc., Massachusetts, USA) and the spectra of frequency shifts is displayed. To calculate the Vmax of the red

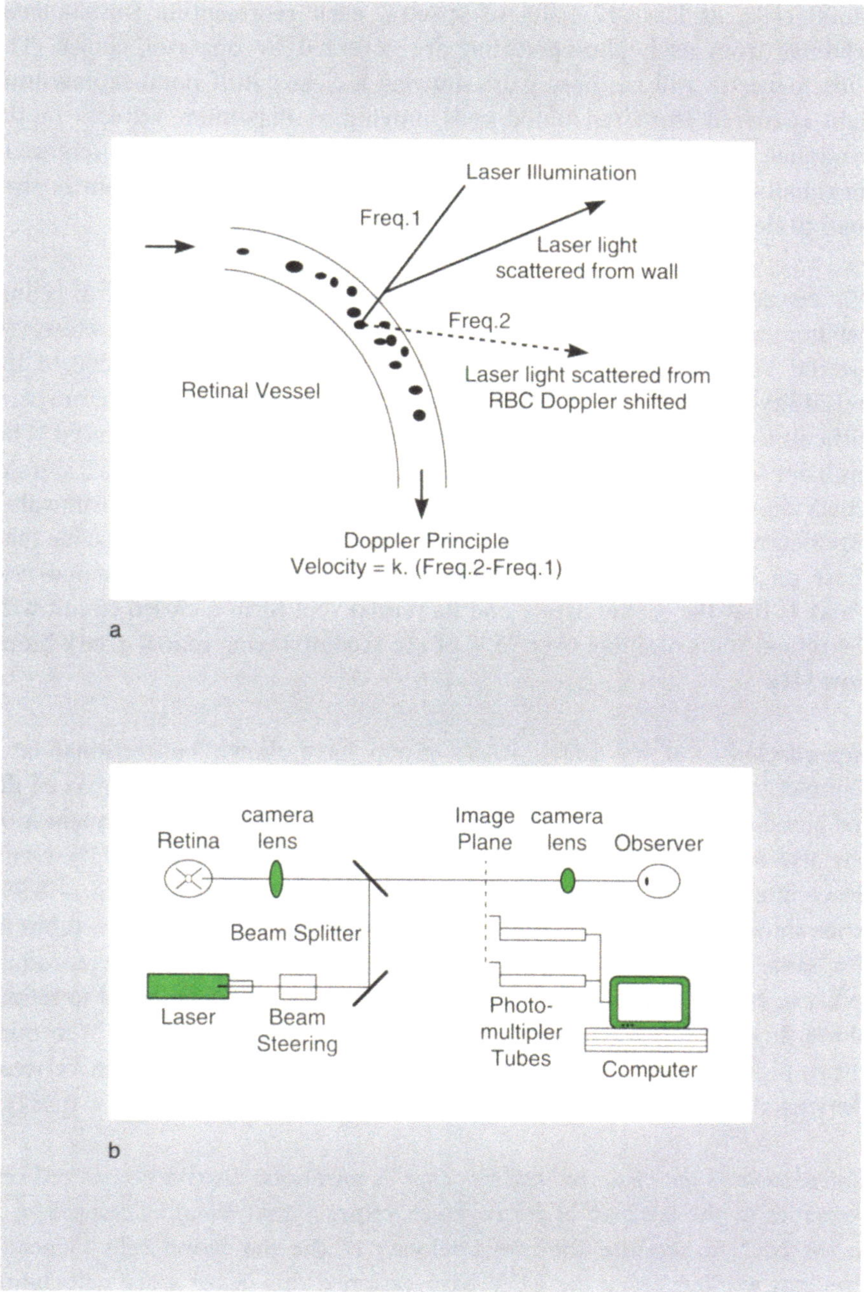

Fig. 5 a The Doppler principle on which laser Doppler velocimetry is based
b Line diagram of principle of bidirectional laser Doppler velocimetry

blood cells, at least 12 pairs of spectra, each representing simultaneous readings from each photodetector, are collected by operator choice. The chosen spectra will be those pairs showing a clear cutoff point representing light scattered from red blood cells moving at maximum velocity in the centreline axial flow. The computer then determines the average difference in maximally shifted spectra from each photodetector. An algorithm is then used to determine the Vmax using the above equation.

The choice of retinal vein Vmax measurement: Ideally in the study of retinal haemodynamics, retinal artery blood flow should be determined. However, arterial Vmax varies considerably throughout the cardiac cycle due to the pulsatility of the retinal arterial flow. An average Vmax is therefore very difficult to select from the heterogeneity of the power spectra produced. This problem led Feke to use retinal artery pulsatility, defined as Vmax systole/Vmax diastole as a haemodynamic parameter [39]. It was also Grunwald's experience that retinal vein LDV measurements were more reproducible than those on retinal arteries [40]. A further justification for using retinal vein Vmax is that the retinal artery and its retinal vein form a closed circuit with the retinal veins draining over 95% of the accompanying retinal artery blood flow [41].

Reproducibility of the LDV: Rivs's group have shown bidirectional laser Doppler velocimetry to be reproducible for the determination of Vmax of the red blood cells [42]. The reproducibility and validation of this instrumentation has also been determined by Sullivan et al [43]. They found the 95% confidence intervals for the reproducibility of the LDV to be +8.9% to − 8.9% when initial measurements were repeated two weeks later in human subjects. The same study in miniature pigs showed the 95% interval for the reproducibility to be + 9.8% to − 9.8%. The LDV technique was compared to retinal blood flow measurement using radio-labelled microspheres (Sn 113) in miniature pigs [43]. There was a very high and significant correlation between the retinal blood flows measured the two techniques ($r = 0.99$, $p < 0.001$).

Calculation of the mean red cell velocity: A parabolic distribution of red cell velocities in the laminae of microvessels requires that Vmax is divided by a factor of 2 to produce the mean velocity of the red blood cells (Vmean). Previous workers using the LDV have assumed this factor when calculating the Vmean [41, 43]. Riva et al [42] use a factor of 1.6 do divide the Vmax and translate it to the Vmean. Their argument was based on work showing that blood flowing in glass capillaries, with internal diameters encompassing the range of diameters of retinal vessels, has a Vmax to Vmean ratio of 1.6 : 1 [44, 45]. These experiments show that the parabolic distribution of the velocities is blunted in the centreline region of flow resulting in a net increase in the Vmean.

Limitations of the LDV: The presence of lens opacities, a particular problem with diabetic patients with their increased incidence of cataract formation, leads to scattering of the laser beam before it can be point-focused onto a retinal vessel. Accurate measurement of the Vmax is then not possible. Another problem associated with older subjects is that they are more likely to have impaired vision and are therefore unable to fixate on the target and the LDV technique is limited with the internal fixation device to subjects with a visual acuity of 6/12 or better. The technique remains labour intensive as one operator is required to operate the retinal camera and another to work the computer.

Retinal haemodynamic changes in diabetes mellitus

Abnormal reactivity of the diabetic retinal circulation to stresses such as hyperoxia and hypercapnia have been known for a long time [46]. Retinal blood flow was found to be elevated by Kohner et al [26] using the mean circulating time of fluorescein. Using vitreous fluorophotometry, Cunha-Vaz et al [19] demonstrated a breakdown in the blood-retinal barrier in diabetes. A later longitudinal study showed that the development of the retinal lesions of diabetic retinopathy paralleled an increase in retinal vessel permeability [27]. Increased viscosity was found in diabetic subjects in comparison to non-diabetic controls by McMillan [47]. This in conjunction with the phenomenon of reduced red cell deformability [48] could potentially reduce retinal capillary blood. Bar intuitative speculation the role of these haemodynamic alterations has not been defined. A recent study using laser Doppler velocimetry showed that retinal blood flow is significantly increased in all forms of untreated diabetic retinopathy [49]. Retinal blood flow was found to be similar in non-diabetic control subjects and diabetic subjects without diabetic retinopathy. In comparison to these groups retinal blood flow was significantly increased in background retinopathy by 33.2%, pre-proliferative retinopathy by 69.4% and 50.1% in proliferative retinopathy. Following successful panretinal photocoagulation for proliferative retinopathy, flow was significantly reduced.

Vascular reactivity

The ability of the retinal vessels to react to various stimuli will depend on the basal blood flow, on the strength of the stimulus and most importantly on the ability of the retinal vessel to respond. Blood flow in tissues is regulated by central and local mechanisms, the latter being known as autoregulation. Autoregulation has been defined as the ability of the vessel to alter its diameter in such a way that blood flow remains constant under varying perfusion pressure [50]. The concept of autoregulation has been expanded by Guyton [51] to mean that blood flow to tissues will be regulated according to their metabolic needs. In different tissues the most powerful stimuli are different. Thus in the cerebral circulation CO_2 is the most powerful stimulus, while in the retinal circulation hypo and hyperoxia have been found to be most effective in altering blood flow. Autoregulation is particularly important in the retinal circulation, because the retinal vessels do not have functioning autonomic innervation. In diabetes autoregulation is thought to be impaired because of the abnormal glucose levels. This can be tested by raising the blood pressure by isometric exercise, or infusion of tyramine, a naturally occurring vasoactive peptide. Blood flow can be measured when the perfusion pressure is raised to various levels above baseline. This study has been done in normal controls and diabetics with early retinopathy. It showed, that autoregulation breaks down in the normal controls at around 40% rise in mean blood pressure, while in diabetics with normal blood glucose level it already breaks down at 30% rise of blood pressure. In the presence of hyperglycaemia there is no autoregulation even at only 15% rise in mean blood pressure. These results suggest, that vessel reactivity is impaired even when the glucose is normal, but is much more damaged in the presence of high glucose [52]. Similarly breathing 100% oxygen significantly reduced blood flow in the normal controls by 63%, but much less in diabetics, the reactivity decreasing with increasing severity of retinopathy [53]. Grunwald et al also found that in badly controlled diabetics blood flow was increased and oxygen reactivity reduced, but when their blood glucose was normalised flow reduced and oxygen reactivity increased [54].

While abnormalities of autoregulation are important in the development and progression of diabetic retinopathy, there is further evidence implicating haemodynamic factors in the pathogenesis of diabetic retinopathy. Thus raised intraocular pressure and unilateral carotid stenosis, both of which reduce retinal blood flow tend to protect against the development of diabetic retinopathy. In contrast, four factors that increase the risk of progression of diabetic retinopathy, hyperglycaemia, hypertension, pregnancy and autonomic neuropathy, have all been shown to increase retinal blood flow [49].

Further research in retinal haemodynamics should be directed towards determining the effects of commonly used antihypertensive and cholesterol lowering agents, and any other vasoactive drugs. Agents such as methylguanidine have already been shown to reduce retinal blood flow in diabetic rats [55]. The potential therefore exists for pharmacological manipulation of the retinal circulation to mitigate against an adverse haemodynamic milieu in the diabetic patient.

Cell culture in the study of pathogenic mechanisms in diabetic retinopathy

While the studies described so far are important in clinical research the basic underlying abnormalities require laboratory studies. In recent years cell biology has been extended to the field of retinal vessels.

The major problem in understanding the pathogenic mechanisms in diabetic retinopathy is the lack of a suitable in vivo model which develop the morphological changes characteristic of retinopathy. To overcome this problem, various laboratories have now established an in vitro cell culture model for examining putative mechanisms involved in diabetic retinopathy.

Cell culture is defined as the growth of a specific cell type under in vitro conditions [55]. The technique allows the isolation of a pure cell population, its serial propagation, and identification. The major disadvantages in using cell culture for any investigation is that cells are not in their normal environment, and the close interactions with other cells which exist in vivo are absent. Great care has to be exercised when attempting to extrapolate results from in vitro studies to the in vivo situation. Despite the limitations, cell culture continues to make a major contribution to the study of diabetic retinopathy.

For most studies bovine or human retinal microvascular cells have been used. The technique for isolating retinal capillary pericytes and endothelial cells have now been well established [55–59]. For the most part, these procedures involve digestion of the microvessels from postmortem retinas with collagenase-dispase and adding these to tissue culture flasks. To culture endothelial cells the plastic surface has to be pre-coated with either gelatin or fibronectin to facilitate cell attachment. Cellular outgrowth from attached microvessels occurs in a few days to give small colonies of cells which then grow to fill the flask (Fig. 6). Cells can then be passaged by trypsinization and used for experimentation. The identity of endothelial cells and pericytes is assessed by morphological criteria (Fig. 6) and by assaying for the presence

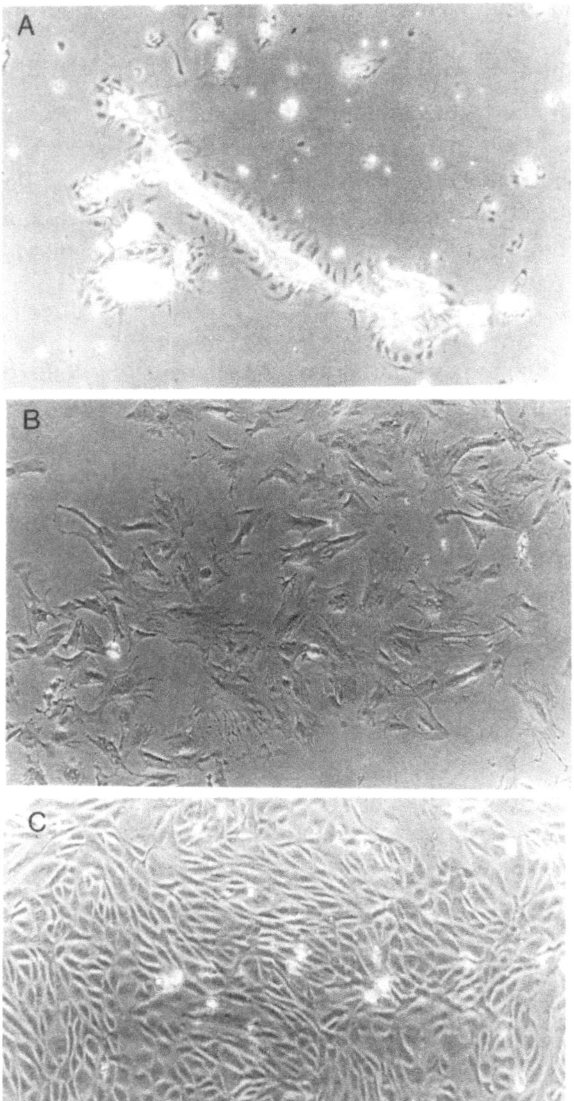

Fig. 6 Phase contrast micrograph of retinal vascular cells in tissue culture; A collagenase-digested capillary fragment attached to fibronectin-coated tissue culture flask showing migrating cells; B preconfluent cultures of retinal pericytes. The cells are large and multipolar; C confluent culture of endothelial cells
Magnification × 100

of cell specific markers [58, 59]. The technique for isolating and maintaining other retinal cells has also been described [60, 62]. The rest of this section will describe briefly how these isolated retinal cells are being used in the field of diabetic retinopathy to examine the nature of glucose toxicity, regulation of capillary permeability, role of haemodynamics, and the mechanisms of retinal neovascularization.

Glucose toxicity: The ability to culture retinal vascular cells has greatly helped in understanding the metabolic activity of these cells. The pericytes have been shown to synthesise collagen [63], and glycosaminoglycans [64]. As in situ, the enzyme aldose reductase has also been localised in cultured pericytes and endothelial cells [65, 66]. The presence of this enzyme has been associated with early loss of pericytes and the development of diabetic retinopathy [67]. Some evidence for the suggestion that pericyte can autoregulate microvascular flow has been provided by in vitro studies. Pericytes have been shown to contain muscle and non-muscle actin [68], and contract in vitro both spontaneously and in response to endothelin and vasoactive agents [69–71].

Using in vitro cell culture model, metabolic conditions that exist in diabetic patients have been tested for their effects on the growth of retinal capillary pericytes and endothelial cells. Cells grown in tissue culture dishes can be exposed to high glucose concentrations and the effect on their replication determined by cell counting using haematocytometer and/or thymidine incorporation into newly formed DNA. High glucose has been shown to reduce the replication of pericytes and endothelial cells [72, 73], and induce the synthesis of basement membrane components [72, 74]. Other effects of high glucose concentrations on cultured pericytes and endothelial cells have been reviewed by Lorenzi et al [75].

Although, the question whether retinal pericytes and endothelial cells replicate in vivo remains to be resolved [75] cell culture offers the opportunity of examining the therapeutic potential of drugs designed to prevent diabetic complications. Decreased thymidine incorporation caused by high glucose in pericytes has been shown to be prevented by adding an aldose reductase inhibitor to the growth medium [76].

Retinal angiogenesis: A variety of bioassays have been used to test the vasoproliferative activity of retinal tissue samples, including, endothelial cell migration [77] and proliferation [78] in vitro, and capillary growth in vivo in the developing chick chorioallantoic membrane (CAM) [79] and the corneal pocket [80]. Although, various angiogenic factors have been identified, further work is still required to establish their role in vivo angiogenesis. The possibility that endothelial cells themselves might regulate angiogenesis has been examined in vitro. Endothelial cells have been shown to synthesise substantial amounts of bFGF [81] which in vitro has been found to be mitogenic [82] and chemotactic [83] for endothelial cells. It has also been found to induce capillary endothelial cells to form capillary-like tubes [84]. However, how bFGF causes angiogenesis in vivo is unclear since this growth factor lacks a signal peptide and is not secreted [85]. Some mechanisms by which bFGF may be released by cells have been reviewed by D'Amore [86].

The hypothesis of Michaelson that hypoxia is an important stimulus for neovascularization can be tested using cultured cells [87]. Rosen et al [88] have studied the effect of various oxygen tension on the proliferative capacity of retinal vascular cells. The results showed that oxygen tension can directly alter the proliferation of endothelial cells. However, the minimum oxygen tension used in these experiments were 80 mm Hg which is more or less in the physiological range of the retina. The results of Shreeniwas et al [89] and Shotliff et al (in preparation) demonstrate a decrease in endothelial cell proliferation under hypoxic conditions ($<$ 18 mm Hg). Although, hypoxia decreased the proliferation of endothelial cells the receptors for bFGF appeared to be upregulated [89] suggesting perhaps a paracrine role for bFGF in retinal angiogenesis. This can be examined by studying the effect of hypoxia on endothelial cell proliferation in co-culture with other retinal vascular cells.

Cell culture has also been used to study the formation of microvessels by isolated endothelial cells in response to extracellular matricies [84] and angiogenic factors [90]. The suggestion that angiogenesis is regulated by cell-cell interaction in vivo, namely, the interaction between endothelial cells and other cells, such as, pericytes, smooth muscle cells and glia, can also be investigated in vitro. Using a co-culture model, Orlidge and D'Amore [91] were able to demonstrate that pericytes can exert a control over the proliferation of endothelial cells but only when the two cells are in direct contact. Interesting findings on cell-cell interaction has recently been reported by Sakada et al [92] showing that conditioned medium removed from smooth muscle cells grown under hypoxic conditions stimulates cultured endothelial cells to form capillary-like structures.

In addition to in vivo models of proliferative vitreo retinopathy [93], Forrester et al [94] have recently reported on an in vitro model system for the study of proliferative retinopathy. Bovine retinal explants were cultured in collagen gels to mimic the vitreoretinal interface. Endothelial cell out growth from the retinal explant was shown to occur and the results further suggested a close involvement of glia cells in the formation of vessel like tubular structures. A quantitative measure of angiogenesis in vitro using

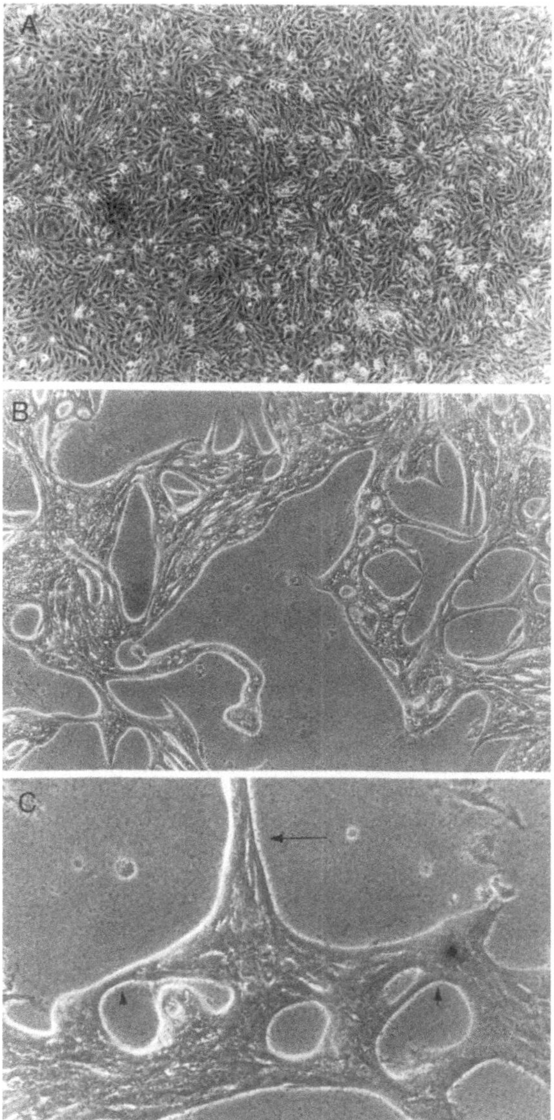

Fig. 7 Phase contrast micrograph of retinal capillary endothelial cells cultured within human plasma clot; A confluent culture of endothelial cells on gelatin-coated dish (magnification × 40); B endothelial cells showing capillary-like structures when cells are overlayed with clotted human plasma (magnification × 100); C capillary-like structures showing the formation of "lumen" (arrowhead) and capillary chord (arrow)

microvessels has been described [95] and is useful in examining the effect of angiogenic agonist and antagonists. Recent studies (Chibber et al, in preparation) have also shown that retinal capillary endothelial cells cultured within plasma clot tends to from capillary-like structures very rapidly (Fig. 7) offering a cost-effective in vitro model to study mechanisms involved in retinal angiogenesis.

Minakawa et al [90] have established an in vitro angiogenic model which allows the examination of the interactions that take place between astrocytes and pericytes with capillar-like structures of brain microvessels. This in vitro system could also be useful in examining the association of pericytes and glia with capillary-like structures in retinal angiogenesis.

Role of haemodynamics in retinopathy: To complement in vitro haemodynamic studies, recent work has shown that endothelial cells can be grown on glass capillary tubes or glass slides pretreated with gelatin and then exposed to varying degrees of shear stress using flow chamber perfused via a control head recirculating flow pump. This in vitro model has proved useful in examining the effect of shear stress on, membrane phospholipid metabolism [97], the production of endothelin, ATP [98], prostacyclin [99], and migration and proliferation of endothelial cells [100].

Permeability studies: Factors responsible for causing increased capillary permeability during the evolution of retinopathy are not known. In order to study this King et al [101] have used an in vitro cell culture model that possess permeability characteristics that are very similar to the endothelium in vivo. Endothelial cells are grown as a confluent culture on a fibronectin-coated spectroscopic porous membrane which has an exclusion size of M 50,000. Growth media with or without added macromolecules can be placed on the upper chamber and their movement through the monolayer determined. The model resembles the in vivo endothelium and shows intercellular junctions, restricts the movement of certain macromolecules and the passage of electrical current [102]. Using this model King et al [103] showed that endothelial cells are responsible for most of the vascular permeability and that hyperglycemia or diabetic conditions does not affect the barrier properties. This work has been suggested already by work using vitreous fluorophotometry. Audus et al [104] have recently discussed the use of the in vitro biological barrier for drug transport and metabolism studies.

It is hoped that using these methods and applying others we will soon be able to fully understand the pathogenesis of diabetic retinopathy. We will then be able to find effective treatment for its prevention.

References

[1] Oakley N, Hill DW, Joplin G et al. Diabetic Retinopathy: I. Assessment of severity and progression by comparison with a standard set of photographs. Diabetologia 1967; 3: 402–405.
[2] David MD, Norton EWD, Myers FL. The Airlie Classification of diabetic retinopathy. In: Goldberg MF, Fine SL, eds. Treatment of diabetic retinopathy. Arlington: US Dept of Health Education & Welfare, Public Health Services, 1969; 7–22.
[3] Klein BE, David MD, Segal P et al. Diabetic retinopathy: Assessment of severity and progression. Ophthalmology 1984; 91: 10–17.
[4] Diabetic Retinopathy Study Research Group. Preliminary report on effect of photocoagulation therapy. Amer J. Ophthalmol 1976; 81: 383–397.
[5] Early Treatment Diabetic Retinopathy Study Research Group. Photocoagulation for diabetic macular oedema: ETDRS report No 1. Arch Ophthalmol 1985; 103: 1796–1806.
[6] Early Treatment Diabetic Retinopathy Study Research Group. Design and baseline characteristics: ETDRS report No 7. Ophthalmology 1991; 98: 741–756.
[7] Early Treatment Diabetic Retinopathy Study Research Group. Grading diabetic retinopathy from stereoscopic colour fundus photographs and extension of the modified Airlie House Classification: ETDRS report No 10. Ophthalmology 1991; 98: 786–806.
[8] Early Treatment Diabetic Retinopathy Study Research Group. Fundus photographic risk factors for progression of diabetic retinopathy: ETDRS report No 12. Ophthalmology 1991; 98: 823–833.
[9] Klein R, Klein BEK, Moss SE et al. The Wisconsin Epidemiological Study of Diabetic Retinopathy: II. Prevalence & risk of diabetic retinopathy when age at diagnosis is less than 30 years. Arch Ophthalmol 1984; 102: 520–526.
[10] Klein R, Klein BEK, Moss SE et al. The Wisconsin Epidemiological Study: III. Prevalence of risk of diabetic retinopathy when age at diagnosis is 30 or more years. Arch Ophthalmol 1984; 102: 527–532.
[11] Klein R, Meuer SM, Moss SE et al. The relationship of retinal microaneurysm counts to the 4 year progression of diabetic retinopathy. Arch Ophthalmol 1989; 107: 1780–1785.
[12] Brinchmann-Hansen O. Heier H, Myhre, K. Fundus photography of width and intensity profiles of the blood column and light reflex in retinal vessels. Acta Ophthalmol (Copenh) suppl 1986; 179: 20–8.
[13] Newsom RSB, Sullivan PM, Rassam SMB et al. Retinal vessel measurement: comparison between observer and computer driven methods. Graefe's Arch Clin Exp Ophthalmol 1992; 230: 221–225.
[14] Patel V, Rassam SMB, Brinchmann-Hansel O et al. A new concept in accurately measuring vessel diameter from transmittance and densitometry profiles of fundus photographs. Invest Ophthalmol Vis Sci 1992; 33–804.
[15] Baudoin CE, Passa P, Sharp P et al. for the DAMAD Study Group. Affect of Aspirin alone and Aspirin plus Dipyridamole in early diabetic retinopathy. Diabetes 1989; 38: 491–498.
[16] Baudoin CE, Lay BJ, Klein JC. Automatic detection of microaneurysms in diabetic fluorescein angiography. Rev Epidem et Sante Publ. 1984; 32: 245–261.
[17] Jagoe R, Arnold J, Blauth C et al. Measurement of capillary dropout in retinal angiograms by computerised image analysis. Pattern Recognition Letters 1992; 13: 143–157.
[18] Phillips RP, Ross PG, Sharp PF et al. Use of temporal information to quantify vascular leakage in fluorescein angiography of the retina. Clin Phys Physiol Meas 1990 Supp A; 11: 81–85.
[19] Cunha-Vaz J, de Abreu F, Campos AJ et al. Early breakdown of the blood retinal barrier in diabetes. Brit J Ophthalmol 1975; 59: 649–656.
[20] Chahal PS, Fallon TJ, Jennings SJ et al. Vitreous fluorophotometry in patients with no or minimal diabetic retinopathy. Diabetes Care 1986; 9: 134–139.

[21] Bek T, Lund Andersen H. Localised blood retinal barrier leakage and retinal light sensitivity in diabetic retinopathy. Brit J Ophthalmol 1990; 74: 388–391.
[22] Hickam JB, Frayser R. A photographic method for measuring the mean retinal circulation time using fluorescein. Invest Ophthalmol Vis Sci 1965; 4: 876–84.
[23] Bulpitt CJ, Dollery CT. Estimation of retinal blood flow by measurement of the mean circulation time. Cardiovas Res 1971; 5: 406–12.
[24] Dollery CT. Dynamic aspects of the retinal microcirculation. Archiv Ophthalmol 1968; 79: 536–9.
[25] Hill DW, Young S. Arterial inflow studies of the cat retina using high speed cine-angiography. Exp Eye Res 1976; 23: 35–45.
[26] Kohner EM, Hamilton AM, Saunders SJ et al. The retinal blood flow in diabetes. Diabetologia 1975; 11: 27–33.
[27] Cunha Vaz JG, Fonseca JR, de Abreu JRF et al. Studies on retinal blood flow: II. Diabetic retinopathy. Arch Ophthalmol 1978; 96: 809–811.
[28] Alm A, Bill A. The oxygen supply to the retina. (II) Effects of high intraocular pressure and of increased arterial carbon dioxide tension on uveal and retinal blood flow in cats. Acta Physiologica Scandanavica 1972; 84: 306–19.
[29] Reihm E, Podesta HH, Bartsch C. Untersuchungen über die Durchblutung in Netzhautkapillaren bei interocularen Drucksteigerungen. Ophthalmologica 1972; 164: 249–255.
[30] Riva CE, Petrig BL. Blue field entoptic phenomenon and blood velocity in the retinal capillaries. J Opt Soc Am 1980; 70: 1234–38.
[31] Wolf S, Arend O, Toonen H et al. Retinal capillary blood flow measurement with a scanning laser ophthalmoscope. Preliminary results. Ophthalmology 1991; 98: 996–1000.
[32] Bertram B, Wolf S, Fiehofer S et al. Retinal circulation times in diabetes mellitus type 1. Brit J Ophthalmol 1991; 75: 462–65.
[33] Guran T, Zeimer RC, Shadidi M et al. Quantitative analysis of retinal haemodynamics using targeted dye delivery. Invest Ophthalmol Vis Sci 1990; 31: 2300–6.
[34] Riva CE, Roberts PW, McMeel JW et al. Laser Doppler measurements of blood flow in capillary tubes and retinal arteries. Invest Ophthalmol Vis Sci 1972; 11: 936–44.
[35] Tanaka T, Riva CE, Ben-Sira I. Blood velocity measurements in human retinal vessels. Science 1974; 18: 830–831.
[36] Sliney DH, Freaseier BC. Evaluation of optical radiation hazards. Applied Optics 1973; 12: 1–24.
[37] Riva CE, Feke GT, Eberli B et al. Bidirectional LDV system for absolute measurement of blood speed in retinal vessels. Applied Optics 1979; 18: 2301–6.
[38] Petrig BL, Riva CE. Retinal laser Doppler velocimeter: towards its computer-assisted clinical use. Applied Optics 1988; 27: 1126–1134.
[39] Feke GT, Tagawa H, Yoshida A et al. Retinal circulatory changes related to retinopathy progression in insulin-dependent diabetes mellitus. Ophthalmology 1985; 92: 1517–22.
[40] Grunwald JE, Riva CE, Brucker AJ et al. Laser Doppler velocimetry study of the retinal circulation in diabetes mellitus. Arch Ophthalmol 1986; 104: 991–996.
[41] Feke GT, Tagawa H, Deupree DM et al. Blood flow in the normal human retina. Invest Ophthalmol Vis Sci 1989; 30: 58–65.
[42] Riva CE, Grunwald JE, Sinclair SH et al. Blood velocity and volumetric flow rate in human retinal vessels. Invest Ophthalmol Vis Sci 1985; 26: 1124–32.
[43] Davies EG, Sullivan PM, Fitzpatrick M et al. Validation & reproducibility of bidirectional laser Doppler velocimetry for the measurement of retinal blood flow. Curr Eye Res 1992; 11: 633–640.
[44] Baker M, Wayland H. On-line volume flow rate and velocity profile measurement for blood in microvessels. Microvas. Res. 1974; 7: 131–143.
[45] Damon DN, Duling BR. A comparison between mean blood velocities and central line red cell velocities as measured with a mechanical image streating velocimeter. Microvas Res 1979; 17: 330–332.

[46] Hickam JB, Frayser R. Studies of the retinal circulation in man. Circulation 1966; 33: 302–15.
[47] McMillan DE. The effect of diabetes on blood flow properties. Diabetes 1983; 32: Suppl 2; 56–63.
[48] Juhan I, Vague P, Buonocore M et al. Abnormalities of erythrocyte deformability and platelet aggregation in insulin-dependent diabetics corrected by insulin in vivo and in vitro. Lancet 1982; (i): 535–537.
[49] Patel V, S. Rassam, R. Newsom et al. Retinal blood flow in diabetic retinopathy. BMJ 1992; 305: 678–683.
[50] Johnson PC, Wayland H. Regulation of blood flow in single capillaries. Am J Physiol 1967; 212: 1405–1415.
[51] Guyton AC, Carrier O, Walker JR. Evidence for tissue oxygen demand as the major factor causing autoregulation. Circ Res 1964; 14: 60–69.
[52] Rassam SMB, Patel V, Kohner EM. The effect of hypertension on retinal vascular autoregulation in diabetes mellitus. Submitted for publication.
[53] Grunwald JE, Riva CE, Bruckner AJ et al. Altered retinal vascular response to 100% oxygen breathing in diabetes mellitus. Ophthalmology 1984; 91: 1447–1452.
[54] Grunwald JE, Riva CE, Martin DR et al. Effect of an insulin induced decrease in blood glucose on the human retinal circulation. Ophthalmology 1987; 94: 1614–1620.
[55] Paul J. Cell and Tissue cultures. Edinburg, London, New York: Churchill Livingstone Press, 1975.
[56] Wong HC, Boulton M, Marshall J et al. Growth of retinal capillary endothelia using pericyte conditioned medium. Invest Ophthalmol Vis Sci 1987; 28: 1767–1775.
[57] Su T, Gillies MC. A simple method for the in vitro culture of human retinal endothelial cells. Invest Ophthalmol Vis Sci 1992; 33: 2809–2813.
[58] Buzney SM, Massicotte SJ, Hetu N et al. Retinal vascular endothelial cells and pericytes. Invest Ophthalmol Vis Sci 1983; 24: 470–480.
[59] Gitlin JD, D'Amore PA. Culture of retinal capillary cells using selective growth media. Microvas Res 1983; 26: 74–80.
[60] Savage FJ, Day JE, Hogg P et al. Tissue culture of retinal glial cells. Eye 1988; 2: S164–S179.
[61] Boulton MC, Marshall J, Melleno J. Retinitis pigmentosa: A preliminary report on tissue culture studies of retinal pigment epithelial cells from eight affected human eyes. Exp Eye Res 1983; 37: 307–318.
[62] Burke JM, Foster SJ. Cultures of rabbit retinal glial cells: Methods and cellular orgin of explant outgrowth. Curr Eye Res 1982; 337: 138–141.
[63] Cohen MP, Frank RN, Khalifa AA. Collagen production by cultured retinal pericytes. Invest Ophthalmol Vis Sci 1980; 19: 90–94.
[64] Stramm LE, Li W, Aguire GD et al. Glycosaminoglycans synthesis and secretion by bovine retinal capillary pericytes in cultures. Exp Eye Res 1987; 44: 17–28.
[65] Hohman TC, Nishimura C, Robison WG. Aldose reductase and polyol in cultured pericytes of human retinal capillaries. Exp Eye Res 1989; 48: 55–60.
[66] Lee TS, MaCregor LC, Fluharthy SJ et al. Differential regulation of protein kinase C and (Na, K)-adenosine triphosphatase activities by elevated glucose levels in retinal endothelial cells. J Clin Invest 1989; 83: 90–94.
[67] Frank RN. On the pathogenesis of diabetic retinopathy. Ophthalmol 1991; 48: 586–593.
[68] Herman IM, D'Amore PA. Microvascular pericytes contain muscle and nonmuscle actin. J Cell Biol 1985; 101: 43–52.
[69] Kelley C, D'Amore P, Hechtman HB et al. Microvascullar pericyte contractibility in vitro: Comparison with other cells of the vessel wall. J Cell Biol 1987; 104: 483–490.
[70] Kelley C, D'Amore P, Hechtman HB et al. Vasoactive hormones and cAMP affect pericyte contraction and stress fibres in vitro. J Muscle Res Motil 1988; 9: 184–194.
[71] Das A, Frank RN, Weber ML et al. ATP causes retinal pericytes to contract in vitro. Exp Eye Res 1988; 46: 349–362.

[72] Li W, Shen S, Khatami M et al. Stimulation of retinal capillary pericyte protein synthesis and collagen synthesis in culture by high glucose concentrations. Diabetes 1984; 33: 785–789.
[73] Lorenzi M, Cagliero E, Toledo S. Glucose toxicity for human endothelial cells in culture: Delayed replication, disturbed cell cycle, and accelerated cell death. Diabetes 1985; 34: 621–627.
[74] Cagliero E, Roth T, Roy S et al. Characteristics and mechanisms of high glucose-induced overexpression of basement membrane components in cultured human endothelial cells. Diabetes 1991; 40: 102–110.
[75] Lorenzi M. Glucose toxicity in the vascular complications of diabetes: The cellular perspectives. Diabetes Metabol Rev 1992; 8: 85–103.
[76] Li W, Tang L, Zhou Q et al. DNA-synthesis regulation and correlation with inositol triphosphate levels in cultured retinal capillary pericytes. Exp Eye Res 1989; 49: 677–683.
[77] Glaser BM, D'Amore PA, Seppa H et al. Adult tissues contain chemoattractments for vascular endothelial cells. Nature 1980; 288: 483–484.
[78] Chen CH, Chen SC. Angiogenic activity of vitreous and retinal extract. Invest Ophthalmol Vis Sci 1980; 19: 596–602.
[79] Glaser BM, D'Amore PA, Micheli RG et al. Demonstration of vasoproliferative activity from mammalian retina. J Cell Biol 1980; 84: 298–304.
[80] Federman JL, Brown GC, Feldberg NT et al. Experimental ocular angiogenesis. Am J Ophthalmol 1989; 89: 231–237.
[81] Schweigerer L, Neufeld G, Friedman J et al. Capillary endothelial cells express basic fibroblast growth factor, a mitogen that promotes their own growth. Nature 1987; 325: 257–259.
[82] Thomas KA. Fibroblast growth factors. FASEB J 1987; 1: 434–440.
[83] Terranova VP, Diflorio R, Lyall RM et al. Human endothelial cells are chemotactic to endothelial cell growth factor and heparin. J Cell Biol 1985; 101: 2330–2334.
[84] Madri JA, Williams SK. Capillary endothelial cell cultures: Phenotypic modulation by matrix components. J Cell Biol 1983; 97: 153.
[85] Jaye M. Howk R, Burgess W et al. Human endothelial cell growth factor: Cloning, nucleotide sequence, and chromosome localization. Science 1986; 233: 541–545.
[86] D'Amore PA. Modes of FGF release in vivo and in vitro. Cancer and Metastasis Res 1990; 9: 227–238.
[87] Michaelson IC. The mode of development of the vascular system of the retina, with some observation on its significance for certain retinal diseases. Trans Ophthalmol Soc UK 1948; 137–180.
[88] Rosen P, Boulton ME, Moriaty P et al. Effect of varying oxygen concentrations on the proliferation of retinal vascular cells in vitro. Exp Eye Res 1991; 53: 597–602.
[89] Shreeniwas R, Ogawa S, Cozzolino F et al. Macrovascular and microvascular endothelium during long-term hypoxia: alteration in cell growth, monolayer permeability, and cell surface coagulant properties. J Cell Physiol 1991; 146: 8–17.
[90] Montesano R, Vassall JD, Baird A et al. Basic growth factor induces angiogenesis in vitro. Proc Natl Acad Sci 1986; 83: 7297–7301.
[91] Orlidge A, D'Amore PA. Inhibition of capillary endothelial cell growth by pericyte and smooth muscle cells. J Cell Biol 1987; 105: 1455–1462.
[92] Sakada H, Nakashima Y, Kumyama S et al. Media conditioned by smooth muscle cells cultured in a variety of hypoxic environments stimulates in vitro angiogenesis. Am J Pathol 1992; 141: 1507–1516.
[93] Yeo JH, Sadegl J, Campochiaro PA et al. Intravitreous fibronectin and platelet-derived growth factor: A new model for traction retinal detachment. Arch Ophthalmol 1986; 104: 417–422.

[94] Forrester JV, Chapman A, Kerr C et al. Bovine retinal explant cultured in collagen gels: A model system for the study of proliferative retinopathy. Arch Ophthalmol 1990; 108: 415–420.
[95] Nicosia RF, Ottineth A. Growth of microvessels in serum-free matrix cultures of rat aorta: A quantitative assay of angiogenesis in vitro Lab Invest 1990; 63: 115–122.
[96] Minakawa T, Bready J, Berliner J et al. In vitro interaction of astrocytes and pericytes with capillary-like structures of brain microvessel endothelia Lab Invest 1991; 65: 32–39.
[97] Bhagyalakshmi A, Berthiaum F, Reich KM et al. Fluid shear stress stimulates membrane phospholoipid metabolism in cultured human endothelial cells. J Vasc Res 1992; 29: 443–449.
[98] Milner P, Bodin P, Loesch A et al. Increased shear stress leads to differential release of endothelin and ATP from isolated endothelial cells from 4- and 12-month old rabbit aortas. J Vasc Res 1992; 29: 420–425.
[99] Grabowski EF, Jaffe EA, Webster BB. Prostacyclin production by cultured endothelial cell monolayer exposed to step increases in shear stress. J Lab Clin Med 1985; 103: 36–43.
[100] Ando J, Nomum H, Kamiya A. The effect of fluid shear stress on the migration and proliferation of cultured endothelial cells. Microvas Res 1987; 33: 62–70.
[101] King GL, Berman AB, Bonner-Weir BL et al. Regulation of vascular permeability in cell culture. Diabetes 1987; 36: 1460–1467.
[102] Furie MB, Cramer EB, Naprstek BL et al. Cultured endothelial cell monolayer that restricts the transendothelial passage of macromolecules and electrical current. J Cell Biol 1984; 98: 1033–1041.
[103] Andus KL, Bartel RC, Hadalgo IJ et al. The use of cultured epithelial and endothelial cells for drug transport and metabolism studies. Pharm Res 1990; 7: 435–450.

Methodologies to assess renal function in diabetes mellitus

S. L. Jones, G. C. Viberti

Introduction

The main functions of the kidney are the excretion of soluble waste products from the body and the regulation of water and salt homeostasis, processes that require both glomerular filtration and tubular reabsorption and secretion. The kidney is also an important site of production and secretion for several hormones such as renin, erythropoeitin, the active form of vitamin D, 1,25-dihydroxycholecalciferol, and autocoids such as prostaglandins. These substances act at distal sites as well as locally in the regulation of renal function. The glomerular membrane acts as a size, charge and shape selective barrier, permitting the free passage of water, electrolytes, small solutes and plasma proteins of less than 2.0 nm in molecular radius, which, along the nephron, undergo different degrees of tubular reabsorption. The filtration of larger proteins and macromolecules is greatly restricted unless there has been damage to the glomerular membrane. Tubular damage results in disturbances of water and acid-base metabolism and in excretion of predominantly smaller molecular weight proteins. The principal methods for the physiological assessment of renal function therefore comprise measurements of glomerular filtration rate, of urinary proteins and ionic solutes.

Kidney disease is a major complication of both insulin-dependent (IDDM) and non-insulin-dependent diabetes mellitus (NIDDM) and represents approximately one third of all new cases of end stage renal failure (ESRF). The development of renal disease in diabetes is a slow process which requires several years but abnormalities of renal function are detectable early in the evolution of this process.

Increased GFR in diabetes was first described in 1952 by Fiaschi, Grassi and Andres [1] and subsequently by Stadler in 1959, in insulin treated children of short diabetes duration [2]. These observations were confirmed in adult diabetic patients of both short and long duration [3, 4]. GFR is generally

Offprint from
Research Methodologies in Human Diabetes – Part 1

increased by 10–15% in IDDM patients without proteinuria and the frequency distribution curve is overall shifted to the right with a right sided skewness compared to the non-diabetic population [5]. In NIDDM the presence or absence of glomerular hyperfiltration has been more controversial [6–8]. The level of GFR may be related to the duration of diabetes, with higher GFR being found in those NIDDM patients of shorter duration. The need to adjust GFR for age and the difficulties of estimating duration of diabetes in these patients has added to the problem. Ethnic differences may also exist [8, 9]. Altered systemic and renal haemodynamics and local structural changes have been postulated to play a role in the initiation and progression of diabetic renal disease [10]. Glycaemic control, familial predisposition, renal and glomerular enlargement, as well as dietary protein intake, systemic and intraglomerular hypertension may all be contributory [5]. Glomerular hyperfiltration itself is largely driven by increases in plasma flow and capillary pressure. This abnormality of renal vasoregulation is probably derived from alterations in several metabolic and hormonal vasoactive control systems which include glucose, ketone bodies, glucagon, prostaglandins, atrial natriuretic factor, kinins and the renin-angiotensin system. Glomerular hyperfiltration has been proposed as a risk factor for the later development of nephropathy [11] but this suggestion has been variably confirmed or refuted in subsequent studies [12–14], and whether high GFR *independently* determines subsequent renal injury remains uncertain.

Renal haemodynamics

GFR does not usually fall until persistent proteinuria develops. In IDDM patients with proteinuria, GFR, in the absence of intervention, is thought to decline linearly, but the actual rate varies between patients. Levels of blood pressure and of protein intake affect the rate of decline of GFR, blood glucose control appears to have a limited impact on this process at this stage [15, 16].

Conventionally GFR is corrected for body surface area and normalised to 1.73 m^2 to take into account the relationship between renal size and body size and permit comparisons between and within groups. GFR in the general population increases until the age of 2 years and starts to fall steadily from the age of 35 years, at a rate of approximately 2 ml per decade which increases to around 4 ml per decade after the age of 60 years.

Renal plasma flow is often measured in conjunction with GFR and tends to follow the same course [17, 18] with initial hyperfunction and decline after the onset of proteinuria. Renal vascular resistance (RVR) tends to increase with progressive loss of renal function.

Kidney size is increased in IDDM patients with approximately 40% of patients having kidneys larger than normal. Increased kidney volume is a prerequisite for glomerular hyperfiltration [19].

Information as to glomerular barrier function can be further obtained from the study of the clearance rates of molecules of different sizes and charge. These include the fractional clearances of albumin, IgG subclasses of similar size but differing charge, and of neutral dextrans of graded size [20, 21]. Using these techniques in diabetic patients with AER > 30 mg/24 hours loss of glomerular charge selectivity has been suggested with pore size selectivity defects appearing at a more advanced stage of heavier albuminuria (AER > 300 mg/24 hrs) [21].

Protein excretion

Persistent clinical albuminuria (AER > 300 mg/24 hrs, corresponding approximately to a total protein excretion of > 500 mg/24 hrs) heralds progressive renal disease. The detection of proteinuria has important therapeutic implications aimed at reducing the rate of decline of GFR.

The development of a sensitive assay for urinary albumin in the early 1960's [22], allowed the detection of elevations of urinary albumin excretion above the range for healthy non-diabetic individuals but below those levels associated with clinical proteinuria. These intermediary levels of AER from 30 to 300 mg/24 hrs were defined as microalbuminuria and were shown in several longitudinal studies to be predictive of the later development of clinical diabetic nephropathy in IDDM patients [23–25]. In NIDDM patients microalbuminuria has been shown to be predictive not only of heavier proteinuria, but also of increased cardiovascular mortality [26, 27]. In the non-diabetic elderly population microalbuminuria is associated with cardiovascular disease and in patients with essential hypertension with a number of risk factors for coronary heart disease [28, 29].

In both IDDM and NIDDM microalbuminuria has been found to be associated with a higher blood pressure [30], lipid and coagulation factor abnormalities [31, 32], markers of endothelial dysfunction [33], reduced insulin sensitivity and left ventricular hypertrophy. All these factors may in part account for the increased cardiovascular risk of these individuals. Moreover patients with microalbuminuria also have an increased frequency of other diabetic complications including retinopathy and neuropathy [34, 35]. Microalbuminuria is associated with significant structural renal lesions and should be regarded as an indicator of early (but established) renal disease. Its detection has become of great importance for therapeutic programmes of secondary prevention of overt nephropathy. Recent studies have revealed the level of blood pressure, the actual level of AER (though still within the normal range), the quality of blood glucose control and smoking as determinant factors for the progression from normoalbuminuria to microalbuminuria. These observations, combined with a growing knowledge of the familial factors predisposing to diabetic kidney disease open up the prospect for primary prevention therapies in the future [36–38].

In diabetic kidney disease tubular function as well as glomerular function can be affected. Small molecular weight proteins, which are freely filtered at the glomerulus, are reabsorbed in the tubules and tubular secretion of protein into the lumen also occurs.

In normoalbuminuric diabetic patients tubular proteinuria is unusual, unless there is severe metabolic dysregulation [5]. Increased urinary excretion of a number of proteins such as β_2-microglobulin, retinal binding protein and N-acetyl-beta-glucosaminidase (NAG) has been described in diabetic patients with microalbuminuria. This tubular dysfunction appears to be transitory as it is promptly controlled by improvement of metabolic control [39–41]. Tubular function appears to be consistently disrupted after GFR declines below 40 ml/min. Whether this tubular proteinuria is the result of protein overload or of direct disease induced tubular injury remains however uncertain.

Renal excretion of electrolytes and small solutes in the early stages of diabetes is largely under the influence of glycaemic control. Maximum rates of glucose reabsorption are elevated in poorly controlled diabetic patients as are the absolute rates of sodium reabsorption. The latter is probably due, at least in part, to the proximal tubular cotransport of sodium with glucose. Enhanced proximal tubular reabsorption could decrease distal sodium delivery and thereby trigger a tubuloglomerular feedback mechanism which would lead to augmentation of glomerular filtration rate. Insulin also has a direct effect on distal sodium reabsorption. Phosphate reabsorption is diminished in insulin-dependent patients [5, 42].

Renal biopsy studies have demonstrated a relationship between degrees of albuminuria and structural morphological lesions in the diabetic kidney. GFR is closely related to the available glomerular filtration surface area, and to the extent of glomerular occlusion [43, 44]. Measurement of urinary albumin and other urinary proteins are therefore of the utmost importance for the detection, monitoring and treatment of renal disease in diabetes.

Renal haemodynamics and kidney volume

Glomerular filtration rate

One fifth of the cardiac output flows through the kidneys. The glomerular filter retains within the circulation all the cells and restricts passage of plasma proteins exceeding 2 nm in molecular radius but allows free passage of water and solutes. Approximately 180 – 200 l of filtrate is formed each 24 hrs. Four factors determine GFR: (1) the glomerular plasma flow; (2) the hydrostatic capillary pressure; (3) the ultrafiltration coefficient which is the product of the permeability of the capillary wall to water and the capillary filtration surface area; (4) the oncotic pressure. In humans of all these factors only GFR, renal plasma flow (RPF) and oncotic pressure are measureable. Filtration fraction (FF) is calculated as the GFR/RPF ratio and represents the determinants of GFR not accounted for by glomerular plasma flow, i. e. the ultrafiltration coefficient and the transglomerular pressure gradient.

The ideal substance to measure GFR must meet the following criteria: it must be freely filtered at the glomerulus, not reabsorbed or secreted by the renal tubules, not metabolised, have no extrarenal route of excretion and be non-toxic. Unfortunately no naturally occuring substance exactly satisfies these conditions. Inulin a disperse polymer of fructose represents the best approximation to such a substance and in humans the renal clearance of inulin is accepted as the gold standard and reference method for the measurement of GFR.

Renal clearance techniques – inulin clearance: The amount of a substance such as inulin excreted in the urine (UV, where U is the concentration in urine and V the urine flow) equals that filtered at the glomerulus over the same period of time. If the plasma level is constant and there is no other route of excretion the clearance of the substance (UV/P where P is the concentration in plasma) then equals the filtration of water, thus the GFR.

A stable plasma concentration of inulin is achieved, in normal individuals, following a primed (3.5 g in 35 ml water), constant infusion (40 mg/min in NaCl 0.9%) after approximately 45 – 60 minutes equilibriation. To calculate the GFR urine is collected at accurately timed intervals for determination of the excretion rate of inulin and a plasma sample taken at the mid point of each interval for measurement of inulin concentration. Studies are usually carried out under a steady state of water diuresis to ensure accurate urine collection volumes. At least three 30 minute collection periods are used.

Urine collections are not always required for the measurement of inulin GFR. Once equilibriation has been achieved and a stable plasma inulin concentration ($\approx$ 30 mg/100 ml) obtained the urinary excretion rate of inulin (UV) equals its infusion rate and can be calculated from it. This inulin constant infusion technique, without urine collection, allows measurements of GFR under steady state conditions but is unsuitable for physiological studies where GFR changes are induced.

Methodological problems: The technique requires that constant plasma inulin levels are maintained. This needs the use of an accurate infusion pump. This technique is relatively labour intensive and is time consuming. Some patients do not easily tolerate the water loading and accurate urine collection may present a problem in the diabetic patient with a degree of autonomic neuropathy affecting bladder control. In these patients the period-to-period coefficient of variation of inulin clearance can be as high as 30%. Calculations made by integrating values from multiple successive urine collections are meant to minimise this variation.

Laboratory problems: Inulin, a disperse polymer of fructose derived from the dahlia root, is relatively insoluble and heating is required to get it into solution. Commercial preparations contain some free fructose. A polyfructosan (Inutest, Boehringer Mannheim, Mannheim, Germany) is now available which is easily water soluble at room temperature. All methods of measuring inulin depend upon hydrolysis and measurement of the resulting free fructose making plasma and urine blank measurements of particular importance. Chemical methods for inulin determination may produce high plasma and urine blank measurements. These inconveniences have been reduced by the use of more specific enzymatic methods which measure sorbitol [45, 46] or hydrolyse inulin to fructose [47, 48]. These methods have been automated and nowadays the coefficient of variation for inulin determination is less than 5%.

Plasma clearance techniques: Several radiolabelled chelates which are believed to be cleared entirely or almost entirely by glomerular filtration have been used to assess GFR in man. ^{51}CrEDTA, ^{125}I-iothalamate and ^{99}Tcm-DTPA can be used as substitutes for inulin in constant infusion renal clearance techniques. More interest has, however, centered with these compounds on the use of alternative techniques which avoid the need for constant infusion and for urine collection. These methods rely on the disappearance rate of the substance in question from the circulation. The rate of appearance of a substance in urine following an intravenous bolus injection can provide an alternative method to the rate of plasma disappearance for determination of GFR, but this technique has found little use. The method of GFR measurement should be named on the basis of the technique used (e. g. renal clearance vs. plasma clearance) rather than the substance used (e. g. inulin vs. ^{51}CrEDTA).

Calculation of GFR by the single injection method relies on mathematical interpretation of the plasma disappearance curve of the substance employed. For ^{51}CrEDTA, for instance, after an intravenous injection of 70 µCi (2.6 MBq), conventionally blood is sampled from the contralateral arm at 2, 3 and 4 hours or at longer intervals for patients with impaired renal function and simple monoexponential analysis of the plasma disappearance curve applied. This gives a good approximation to inulin GFR for GFRs in the normal and low ranges [49]. The injection of radioisotope must be accurately quantitated and given into a vein with good flow. This technique tends to be preferred by patients and medical/paramedical personel alike. There are however a number of problems: (1) an overestimate of approximately 22% of the volume of distribution arises from oversimplification of the monoexponential approach; (2) a discrepancy of approximately 5% between inulin and ^{51}CrEDTA clearances is caused by tubular reabsorption of the chelate; (3) a higher concentration of chelate in venous blood compared to arterial blood. For these reasons a correction factor of 0.87 needs to be applied to make the ^{51}CrEDTA plasma clearance GFR more comparable with the inulin renal clearance GFR. To avoid the need for correction in the simple monoexponential analysis some authors take additional samples during the initial equilibration period and use a two-compartment model for analysis or base their calculations on the whole area under the disappearance curve [50, 51].

Although a good comparability between methods of plasma and renal clearance is obtained for GFR in the normal and low range of GFR, poorer results are obtained for supranormal GFR. In 100 IDDM patients without proteinuria GFR was measured by a single injection technique of ^{51}CrEDTA and multiple blood sampling; the plasma disappearance curve was analysed by both simple monoexponential analysis and a more complex curve fitting procedure [50]. In a subset of patients GFR was also measured by renal clearance of inulin to provide the reference standard data. GFR ranged between 83 and 196 ml/min/1.73 m^2. The estimate of GFR by complex curve fitting analysis compared closely to inulin renal clearance GFR. A comparison of ^{51}CrEDTA GFR's analysed by the simple monoexponential analysis and the complex curve fitting procedure showed overestimation of GFR by the simple technique, progressively above 100 ml/min/1.73 m^2 (Fig. 1).

Recent developments in the measurement of inulin at low concentration have enabled the use of this substance in single injection techniques avoiding exposure of the subjects to radioactivity which is of obvious importance,

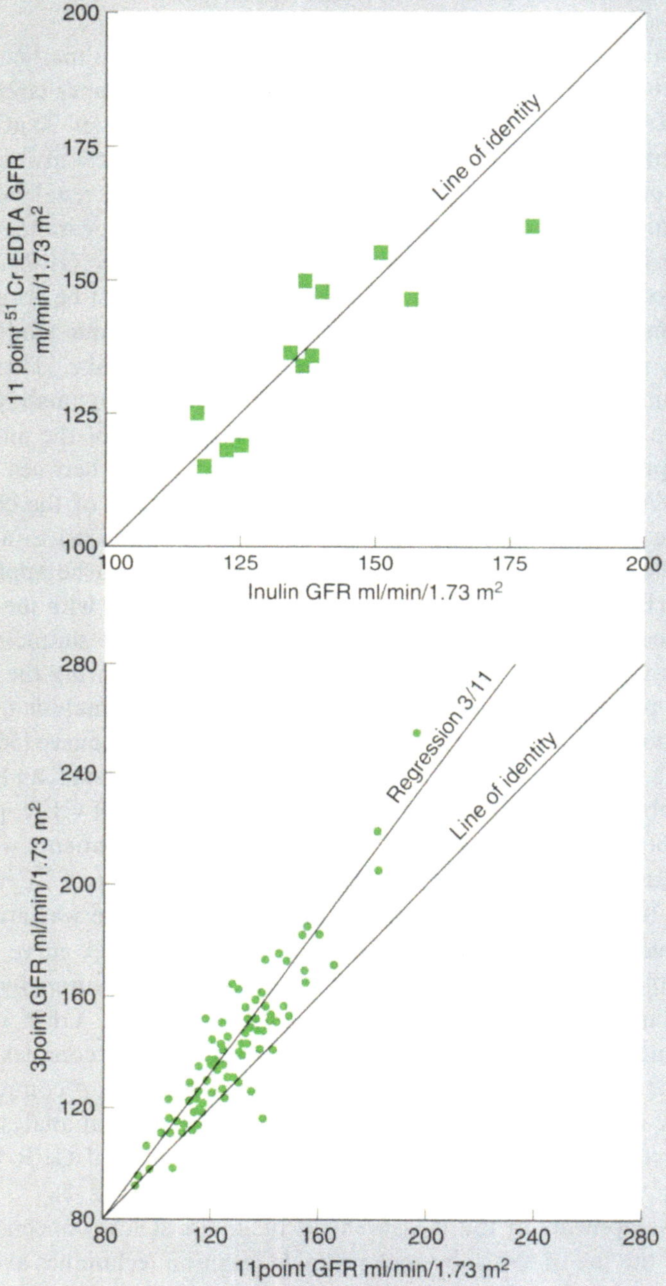
200
175
150
125
100
11 point 51 Cr EDTA GFR ml/min/1.73 m2
Line of identity
100
125
150
175
200
Inulin GFR ml/min/1.73 m2
280
240
200
160
120
80
3point GFR ml/min/1.73 m2
Regression 3/11
Line of identity
80
120
160
200
240
280
11point GFR ml/min/1.73 m2

particularly when applied to repeated measurements in children and in pregnant women [52]. The radiocontrast medium iohexol has also recently been proposed as a substance for estimation of GFR without the need for urine collection [53].

In conclusion accurate determination of GFR in diabetic patients requires the use of renal clearance methods or the employment of the multiple early and late sampling (for ^{51}CrEDTA at 5, 15, 30, 50, 90, 120, 180, 240, 300, 360 and 405 minutes) and complex plasma disappearance curve analysis when plasma clearance methods are used.

Creatinine clearance and serum creatinine as a measure of GFR: The estimation of GFR by creatinine clearance is a simple, widely used and cheap method. It requires the collection of a blood sample and one, but preferably more, accurately timed 24 hour urine collection. It can be performed on an outpatient basis. A number of problems however are associated with the measurement:

1. The generation rate of creatinine varies: serum creatinine may double after a meat meal and is muscle mass and gender dependent.
2. The accurate measurement of serum creatinine to eliminate interference of other chromogens requires the use of reaction rate methods, or HPLC methods, which are not available everywhere and are more expensive [54, 55].
3. Creatinine is secreted by the renal tubules. The use of creatinine clearance thus leads to an overestimation of GFR by a factor of 1.2 or greater.
4. The coefficient of variation for urinary creatinine excretion in a single individual is never less than 6% and may be greater than 20%.
5. In advanced renal failure extrarenal clearance of creatinine occurs.
6. Complete accurately timed 24 hour urine collections are difficult to obtain.

To overcome some of these shortcomings Cockroft and Gault [56] have devised a formula for estimation of GFR based on measurement of serum creatinine alone. This method when adjusted for gender obtains a reasonably good approximation of the GFR for levels in the depressed range. The relationship between serum creatinine and GFR however has the general

---

←

Fig. 1 Upper panel: Comparison between GFR measured by renal clearance of inulin and plasma clearance of ^{51}CrEDTA by multiple sampling (11 point) and complex curve fitting analysis. Lower panel: Comparison of GFR measured by plasma clearance of ^{51}CrEDTA computed by standard simple monoexponential analysis (3 point GFR) or complex curve fitting analysis (11 point GFR). Simple monoexponential analysis progressively overestimates GFR for values exceeding 100 ml/min characteristics of an asymptotic function. Serum creatinine is therefore a poor reflection of GFR for changes in the range of normal to modestly reducted values (i. e. for GFR > 50 ml/min) [57].

The reciprocal or the log of serum creatinine is used to assess glomerular function once serum creatinine has exceeded 200 μmol/l. In progressive renal failure serial plots closely mimic the rate of decline of the GFR. It is a convenient method for long term monitoring of progressive renal impairment in the clinic and especially useful for predicting the onset of end stage renal failure [58]. Some of the limitations mentioned for creatinine clarance apply to serum creatinine measurements. Because of its dependency on animal protein intake levels of serum creatinine become an unreliable measure of GFR when therapy with low protein diet is instituted. Under these conditions the creatinine pool may require up to 4 months to regain homeostasis.

β_2-Microglobulin: β_2-microglobulin, a circulating plasma protein of 1.6 nm radius, is nearly freely filtered and almost totally reabsorbed (approximately 99.9%) by the proximal tubule. It is degraded in the tubular cells and is not recycled. Under normal circumstances its production rate is constant, not dependent on muscle mass and not affected by protein intake. It is considered a reliable plasma measure of GFR [59]. Serum β_2-microglobulin level rises progressively as GFR falls below 80 ml/min and its logarithm is linearly related to GFR changes. Serum β_2-microglobumin concentrations are however time consuming and relatively expensive to measure. Moreover its concentration can rise because of increased production due to a number of disease states such as tumours especially of the lymphoid cell line and inflammatory diseases such as SLE, rheumatoid arthritis and Sjogren's syndrome.

Which method for determination of GFR?: The renal clearance of inulin remains the standard by which other methods are compared. Renal clearance techniques are the only method sensitive to changing haemodynamic parameters during the course of a few hours. Inulin is cheap to measure and, apart from the water loading and the need to produce urine frequently on demand, the method is not unpleasant for the patient.

The single injection techniques are useful for long term follow-up of patients and simpler to perform. The traditional radioisotopic methods do however involve radiation exposure, albeit very small, and are not favoured in children or pregnant women. Newer methods using single dose inulin (or iohexol) would be preferable in these groups. The effective radiation dose from ^{51}CrEDTA in an adult with normal renal function after an injection of 70 uCi

(2.6 MBq) of ^{51}CrEDTA has been estimated to be 7 μCi which is approximately equivalent to the daily dose from background radiation sources.

The inverse of serum creatinine is a simple and cheap way to follow renal function in patients with renal impairment but is not useful until serum creatinine has risen above 200 μmol/l and unreliable when the patient is on low protein diet.

Renal plasma flow

Para-aminohippurate renal clearance: The clearance of p-aminohippurate (PAH) by a primed (600 mg in 3 ml water), constant infusion (14 mg/min in NaCl 0.9%), is the classical method of measuring renal plasma flow. As for inulin clearance an equilibration period of approximately 60 minutes is required and a stable plasma concentration of $\approx$2 mg/100 ml is needed. At low concentrations PAH is removed by filtration and secretion in a single circulation through the kidney. Renal blood flow is calculated from renal plasma flow and haematocrit (Hct); RBF = RPF/(1-Hct). The laboratory method to determine PAH employs N-(1-napthyl) ethylenediamine hydrochloride coupling following diazotization as described by Bratton and Marshall [60].

Methodological problems: PAH is incompletely extracted in a single passage through the kidney. Studies using renal artero-venous PAH gradient suggest that only approximately 85% on average is removed. The measured clearance is not therefore a true reflection of renal plasma flow. Some investigators apply corrective factors of 0.7 for normal individuals, 0.8 for patients with kidney disease, while other workers prefere to use the crude data and to apply the term 'effective renal plasma flow' (ERPF) [61].

Laboratory problems: In the presence of glycosuria Schiff-base formation between the N-terminal of PAH and glucose takes place. This glucose adduct of PAH is not detected by chemical determination and results in an apparent reduction in urinary PAH concentration. This problem can be overcome by collecting the urine into alkali or by acid hydrolysis of the urine before measurement of the PAH [62].

^{131}I hippuran: Isotopic methods of measurement of renal plasma flow are also available. The isotope most commonly used is ^{131}I hippuran, a compound which approximates the criteria required for measurement of renal plasma flow. Both renal and plasma clearance techniques have been described with this compound and have been used for the estimation of renal plasma flow [63].

Other haemodynamic parameters: Filtration fraction (FF) and renal vascular resistance (RVR) are variables derived from the values of GFR, RPF and arterial pressure. FF = GFR/RPF and reflects the determinants of GFR not represented by the glomerular plasma flow, i. e. the transglomerular pressure gradient and the ultrafiltration coefficient. RVR = MBP × (1-Hct)/RPF, where MBP indicates mean blood pressure, that is diastolic blood pressure plus one third of pulse pressure (systolic minus diastolic pressure).

Other measurements of kidney function and assessment of kidney size

Radioisotopic imaging of the kidney provides a means of studying both structure and function. With ^{99}Tcm-DTPA a gamma camera image of the kidneys themselves can be obtained and GFR is calculated from these sequences [64]. These methods are also applied to detect renal artery stenosis which is prevalent in older diabetic patients. The scintigraphic images can be analysed visually for a vascular renal perfusion phase (upslope, phase 1), a parenchymal phase (maximal activity, phase 2), and an excretory phase (downslope, phase 3). Other parameters can be calculated such as time to maximal activity, paraenchymal transit time, split function index between right and left kidneys and residual cortical count. Unilateral renal artery stenosis is considered present if the total uptake is less than 42% and the time to peak 60 seconds longer than in the contralateral side or over 270 seconds [65, 66]. The method has sensitivity and specificity of approximately 86% and 89%. The combination of ^{99}TcmDTPA scanning with captopril administration is used to improve the sensitivity of detection and to assess the likely response to surgery.

For this test diuretics should be stopped at least 3 days prior to the study and angiotensin converting enzyme (ACE) inhibitors at least one week previously. Blood pressure is monitored and 25 mg captopril given with blood pressure monitoring continuing at ten minute intervals until ^{99}TcmDTPA is injected and the scanning performed one hour later. Deterioration of the renogram following captopril challenge is the hallmark of haemodynamically significant renal artery stenosis. A renal artery stenosis that is not significant will be associated with a normal mean parenchymal transit time (MPTT). Whilst it is easiest to detect unilateral stenosis, bilateral stenosis can also be detected from analysis of the MPTT. A captopril-stimulated renogram has a sensitivity of between 80 and 90% and a specificity 85 to 100% depending on the criteria used [65]. The captopril renogram can be completed first without a baseline study, if normal the interpretation may be reported as low-probability for renal artery stenosis and a baseline study need not be obtained.

Renal arteriography remains the gold standard for diagnosing renal artery stenosis and permits localisation of the lesion; it is however invasive and not without risk. Digital subtraction angiography represents an improvement in the imaging technique. The contrast medium can be given peripherally, the procedure is less expensive and can be done on an outpatient basis; the risk of contrast induced renal failure and atheroemboli however persists.

Renal volume is measured by a number of techniques. Plain radiography is not sufficiently accurate in view of the 3 dimensional nature of the kidney. Alternative methods include ultrasonography [19, 67], computerised tomography and nuclear magnetic resonance imaging. Computer reconstruction and subsequent estimation of kidney volume are possible with these latter techniques. Enlargement of the kidney is found in diabetes and measurements of kidney size are sometimes performed. Nephromegaly may be related to the development of kidney disease [68] and diabetic patients with renal failure have comparatively larger kidneys.

Albumin excretion

Definitions

Overt proteinuria, the hallmark of clinical diabetic nephropathy is usually diagnosed when albumin excretion rate (AER) exceeds 200 μg/min or 300 mg/24 hours. In a healthy non-diabetic population the normal range for albumin excretion is between 1.5 and 20 μg/min with a geometric mean of 6.5 μg/min. By convention microalbuminuria is defined as an AER between 20 and 200 μg/min.

Urinary total protein excretion in excess of 0.5 g/24 hrs has classically been used for the diagnosis of renal disease in diabetes mellitus. However, the variability of this measurement is high, proteins of both glomerular and tubular origin are detected and there is no specificity. In the last 10 years it has become recognised that the best, most reliable marker of impaired renal function in diabetes is urinary albumin excretion.

Variations of urinary albumin excretion

Albumin concentration in the urine is affected by a number of factors including strenuous physical exertion [69], poor metabolic control [70], protein intake [71], water loading [72], posture, pregnancy and urinary tract infection. AER in both normal and diabetic patients tends to be 25% higher during the day than at night [73], and has an average day to day variation of about 40% [74]. Conditions for the collection of urine for the measurement of albumin must therefore be standardised.

Urine collection for AER

Twenty-four hour urine collection has been used to measure albumin excretion. Accurate compliance with this procedure is not simple, standardisation of collection conditions is difficult and acceptability to the patients low. A timed overnight urine collection is easier to perform and standardize and is more readily accepted by patients, it has come to be adopted by many investigators. In an effort to further reduce the influence of extrarenal factors and improve compliance some authors have used short-term supervised timed collections. This procedure does not seem to improve on overnight urine collection and is more demanding on both patient and nursing time and may be limited by clinic space.

In view of the day to day variability of AER, accurate determination requires at least 3 urine collections over a period of 2–3 months, before microalbuminuria is diagnosed. On any collection urinary tract infection should be excluded by nitrite testing or microscopy and culture.

Screening for albuminuria

Albustix has traditionally been used for the rapid bedside detection of proteinuria. It is highly sensitive for the diagnosis of albumin concentration > 200 mg/l [75], but has low sensitivity and specificity for lower albumin concentrations.

When screening large populations of diabetics for microalbuminuria it is generally considered impractical to request timed urine collections from all subjects even using the relatively straight forward overnight collection. A number of alternatives have been suggested. The measurement of albumin concentration or preferably of albumin/creatinine ratio (to reduce the influence of urine flow rate) in a first morning urine sample has been found to relate closely with an overnight AER. Similar measurements have also been used on random spot urine samples, but the correlation with AER appears less satisfactory. It has become practice to screen using first morning urine A/C ratio and to proceed to a timed collection only in those patients with an increased probability of having microalbuminuria. Gatling et al found an albumin/creatinine ratio of > 2 to predict an AER > 30 µg/min with a sensitivity of 96% and a specificity of 99.7% [76], and Hutchinson reported an albumin concentration of > 17 mg/l to have a sensitivity of 96.8% and a

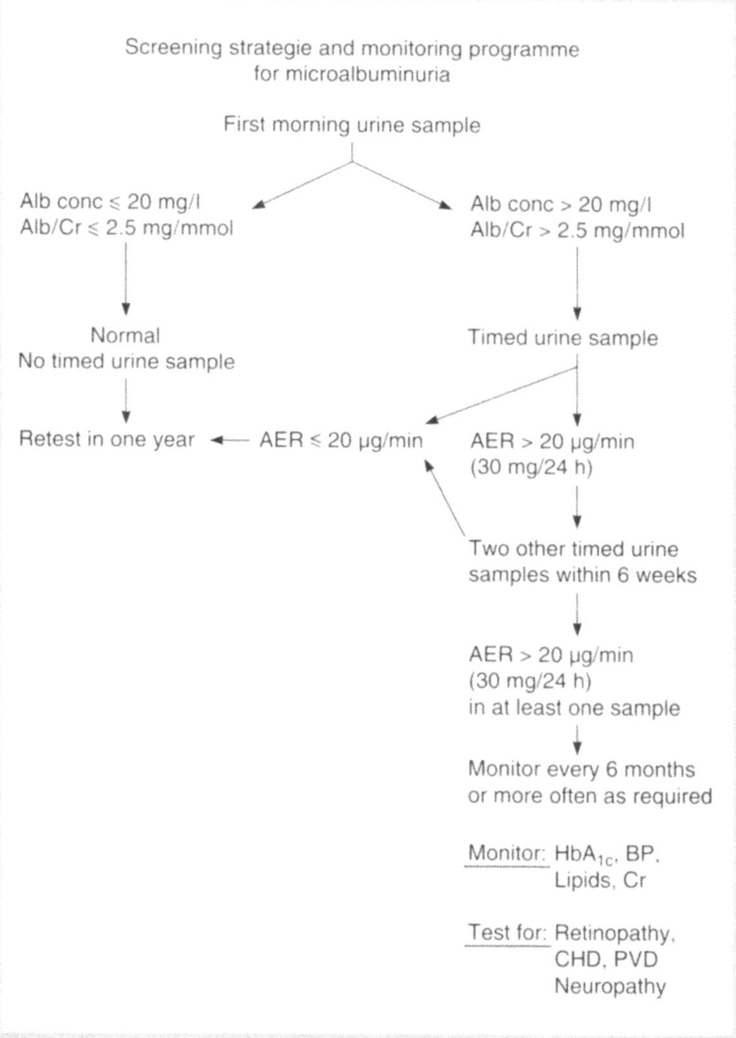

***Fig. 2** Flow diagram illustrating the St. Vincent Declaration action programme recommendations for screening and follow-up of early diabetic nephropathy*

specificity of 90% [77]. The type of measurement and the cut off levels used are to some extent determined by the aims of screening (e.g. population prevalence, recruitment for clinical studies or preventative treatment programmes). A number of recommendations have recently been made by the St. Vincent Declaration implementation programme for the screening of diabetic patients with albuminuria and their subsequent monitoring and treatment [78]. It is recommended that all patients with IDDM above the age of 12 years and of 5 or more years duration and all NIDDM patients should be screened annually, by albumin concentration or A/C ratio on a morning sample. Those with albumin concentration > 20 mg/l or A/C ratio > 2.5 mg/mmol should have a subsequent measurement of AER on a timed overnight sample and, if found elevated, microalbuminuria should be confirmed on at least one of two subsequent urine collections. If the patient has normal AER on initial screening this should be repeated at yearly intervals, those with microalbuminuria should be followed at 6 monthly intervals or more often and screened for other risk factors for diabetic complications and for cardiovascular disease (Fig. 2).

Methods for determination of albumin in urine at low concentrations

Laboratory methods: Radial immunodiffusion was one of the first antigen-antibody reaction based methods described for the specific measurement of albumin in the urine [79]. However, while useful, it is too insensitive for the measurement of albumin concentrations in the range of 'microalbuminuria'. Sensitive radioimmunoassays were developed for the detection of albumin at low concentrations. The first of these methods was published in 1963 by Keen and Chlouverakis [22] and was based on a double antibody system. In brief, in this assay one hundred microlitres of appropriately dilute radioactive ^{125}I labelled human albumin were added to polystyrene tubes, 100 µl of standard solutions of known albumin concentrations were added to a set of tubes (for the standard curve) and the same quantity of urine of unknown albumin concentration to the remaining tubes. All tubes were incubated for 18 hours at room temperature with 100 µl of appropriately diluted guineapig anti-human-albumin serum sufficient to complex with 30–50% only of the added ^{125}I albumin. 100 µl of appropriately diluted rabbit anti-guineapig-globulin serum was then added as precipitant, the reagents mixed and incubated for a further hour at the same temperature. The precipitated complex was then separated from the free albumin in solution by filtering the contents of the tubes through cellulose-acetate-membrane filters. Precipitates were counted in a well-type scintillation counter, a standard curve spanning the range of albumin concentration from 3 to 60 mg/100 ml drawn and the concentration of the samples derived by interpolation. (An example of this original standard curve is reported in Fig. 3.) The sensitivity of this assay was approximately 1.5 mg-100 ml. The double antibody method has undergone subsequent modifications. A single antibody assay has been described [80] and other authors have replaced the second antibody precipitation with PEG precipitation [81]. The standard curve of these assays has been expanded to cover the range 0.25 to 160 mg/l. In the following years a number of other antigen antibody based reaction methods were developed including immunofluorescence, immunoturbidimetry and immunonephelometry. With the current methods the within assay coefficients of variation (CV) vary between 2% and 5%, and

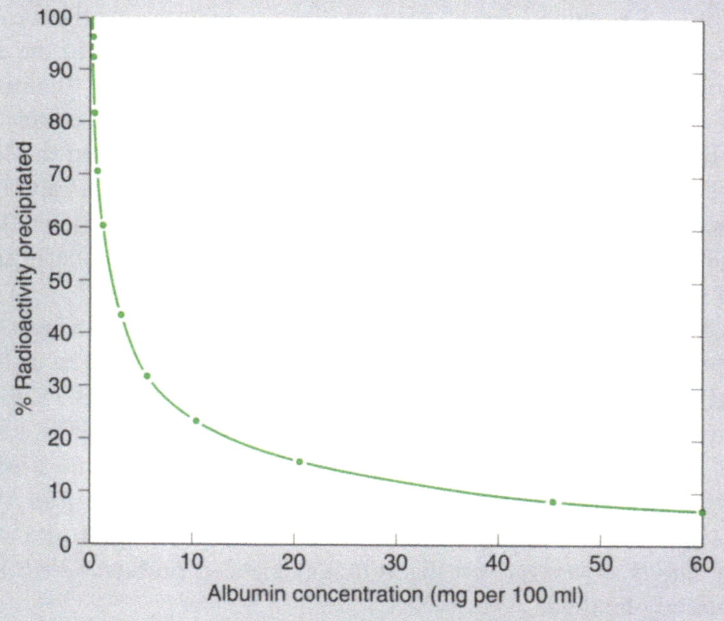

Fig. 3 Precipitation curve relating the proportion of radioactivity precipitate to the concentration of albumin (Keen and Clouverakis, 1963)

between assay CVs between 4% and 9.6% in the range 0.25 – 160 mg/l. The assay sensitivities vary between 0.5 to 1.5 mg/l. Some of these methods have been automated and are now routinely used in laboratories.

Immunoturbidometric (IT) and nephelometric (IN) assays: The immunoturbidometric method is based on the reduction of light transmission caused by an antibody-antigen reaction in solution. Adjustment of PEG concentration and particle linking to latex beads can increase speed and sensitivity of the assay [81, 82]. Most immunoglobulins are precipitated by 20% PEG while smaller antigens like albumin are quite soluble at this concentration, such antigens will be precipitated once complexed to antibodies. Binding of albumin to latex beads can increase the refraction index of the antigen-antibody complex. The nephelometric methods is similar in principle but based on the light scattering properties of the antibody-antigen complex rather than reduction in light transmission. In both methods non-specific light absorption or scattering is corrected automatically by blank or initial reaction readings. The assays read over an albumin concentration range up to 100 mg/l and are sensitive down to less than 1.5 mg/l. They are precise, accurate, economical and rapid with a running time of approximately 8 minutes. Antigen excess (i. e. albumin concentration > 100 mg/l) may prevent formation of the antigen-antibody complex and give a so called 'hook effect' with diminished signal and erronoeusly low results. Although with automated methods this should be detected and flagged by the analyser, it is recommended to screen the urine with dipsticks before the assay and to dilute the urine appropriately. PEG accelerated immunoturbidometric and immunonephelometric methods are suitable for the assay of large numbers of samples, particularly if an automated spectrophotometric system is available [82].

ELISA (enzyme linked immonosorbent assay) methods have also been used for the detection of albumin in urine at low concentrations [83]. The walls of polystyrene microtitre plates are coated with albumin. Diluted urine is mixed with rabbit antiserum against albumin and then with alkaline phosphatase conjugated anti-rabbit immunoglobulins. Following incubation and washing substrate is added and the enzyme activity measured photometrically [84]. Though very sensitive, reading concentrations as low as 15 µg/l, the assay has, in the hands of several investigators, experienced problems with non-specific antibody binding.

Problems with laboratory measurement of urinary albumin: The lack of a standard albumin reference preparation makes comparison of results between laboratories difficult. Preparations available include lyophilised purified human albumin powder, commercial liquid preparations of human albumin or calibrated human serum. Extent of polymerisation, water content and fatty acid content differ between these preparations. Dilution of calibrants with buffer alone may also lead to losses due to adsorption onto container surfaces, unless prevented by the addition of Triton X-100 or BSA. A quality assurance scheme for urinary albumin has been established in the UK and participation of laboratories in such a scheme will undoubtedly lead to improved comparative procedures. The type of container used to store the urine sample, the temperature and length of storage and subsequent treatment of the sample may potentially affect albumin concentration. Though loss of albumin during storage has been reported by a number of authors, recent studies indicate that urine collected in polypropyline tubes can be stored at 4 °C or at room temperature for up to on week and at − 20 °C or − 40 °C for up to 6 months without any reduction in albumin concentration. Samples can be thawed up to 6 times without any loss in albumin concentration. Once thawed centrifugation is not needed but thorough mixing is important [85].

Office/bedside methods for the assessment of albumin at low concentration: A number of rapid assays for the detection of microalbuminuria have been developed. Micral-Test (Boehringer) is a dipstix test based on an immunocapture technique, NycoCard U-Albumin (Nycomed pharma) a 3-drop test based on a solid phase ELISA, Rapitex (Behring) is based on an agglutination test and Albumin Screen (Sclavo) relies on an agglutination inhibition principle (Table 1). These new tests have the advantage of making the results available immediately, and could be used for population screening purposes. The cost however is still relatively high at approximately £1 per test. Two of these new methods are described briefly.

Micral-Test: Micral-Test is a specific test strip method in which the colour reaction is mediated by an antibody bound enzyme. The white fleece of the test strip serving as a reservoir is dipped into the urine for 5 seconds upto just beneath the blue test zone, then laid down horizontally. The absorbed urine entres a zone on the strip containing a soluble antibody-enzyme which specifically binds to urinary albumin. Excess conjugate is retained in a separation zone containing immobilised human albumin so that only the conjugated immunocomplex is mobile and can pass through the matrix with the fluid flow and reach the reaction zone. Here the enzyme B-galactosidase reacts with a substrate, producing a red dye, the intensity of which after exactly 5 minutes is directly related to the albumin content of the urine. Micral-Test yields semiquantitative results reflected by five colour blocks on the vial label. Depth of dipping the strip and timing of reading of the colour development are critical and sticks should be protected from extremes of temperature. Micral test has been compared with both RIA and immunotur-

Table 1 *Test principal, performance, detection limit for and problems of not and four office/bedside methods for the measurement of albumin levels in urine, at low concentration*

Test name	Manufacturer	Test principal	Test performance	Detection limit mg/l	Problems
Micral Test	Boehringer	Immunocapture	semiquant	10	Dipping procedure fiddly – reading time critical
Nycocard-U Albumin	Nyomed-Pharma	ELISA	semiquant	20	Pipetting volume critical
Rapitex	Behring	Latex agglutination	qualitative	20	Qualitative. Negative results for alb conc > 200 mg/l. Requires positive and negative standards
Albumin Screen	Sclavo	Latex agglutination inhibition	semiquant	25	Small semiquantitative range 25–50 mg/l. Requires positive and negative standards

Table 2 Sensitivity, specificity, positive and negative predictive value and efficiency of Nycocard U-Albumin measurements for the detection of urinary albumin concentrations of 20, 40 and 80 mg/l and over (RIA) in 134 diabetic patients

	Nycocard U-Albumin		
	20 mg/l	40 mg/l	80 mg/l
Sensitivity %	100	100	100
Specificity %	70	82	94
Positive predictive value %	79	70	82
Negative predictive value %	98	100	100
Efficiency	85	87	96

Sensitivity is number of positive Nycocard results divided by number of positive results by RIA, specificity number of negative Nycocard results divided by number of positive RIA results, positive predictive value number of true positive results divided by the total number of positive results, negative predictive value the number of true negative results divided by the total of negative results, the efficiency the number of true positive plus true negative results divided by the total number of tests

bidometric assays. Setting the level of microalbuminuria at 20 mg/l the test has been reported to have a sensitivity varying between 90 and 100% and a specificity varying between 91 and 100% by different authors [86, 87].

NycoCard U-Albumin: Nycocard U-Albumin is a 3 drop test based on a solid phase ELISA. The test kit includes a test card containing immobilised anti-human albumin antibodies on a porous membrane and conjugate albumin specific antibodies with microsized colloidal gold. The albumin molecules in the sample are trapped by the membrane bound antibodies and subsequently bind to the coloured conjugate antibodies. Excess of coloured conjugate is removed by washing solution and the colour intensity (proportional to the albumin concentration) on the sample evaluated using a reference colour chart. The test takes 2 minutes and the colour development in the Nycocard U-Albumin is stable and can be read at any time after the procedure is completed. A close correlation between albumin concentration measured by NycoCard U-Albumin and by RIA in the range 20 to 80 mg/l is found (Table 2). The results were not affected by storage of the urine at 22 °C for up to 5 days.

Tubular function

Sodium excretion

Sodium homeostasis is often altered in diabetes and patients with proteinuria and microalbuminuria have been reported to have increased tubular sodium reabsorption and to have an expanded exchangeable sodium pool [42]. The excretion and reabsorption of sodium along the tubules in animals can be measured directly by micropuncture technique but in man is only assessable indirectly. Tests of tubular function can be divided into those measuring proximal function and those measuring distal function. In practice however there is often substantial overlap, especially with the more commonly used tests of sodium reabsorption, urinary concentrating ability and urinary acidification. Sodium is absorbed in the proximal tubule but some is believed also to be absorbed in the thick ascending limb and a small amount in the collecting duct. In the proximal tubule lithium is absorbed at the same rate as sodium and under normal circumstances, is not handled by the distal nephron. This however seems to change during hyperglycaemia and glycosuria [88]. The lithium clearance, measured by administering 600 mg lithium carbonate orally, approximately 12 hours before the clearance study, gives some estimate of proximate tubular reabsorption of sodium and water. The difference between sodium and lithium clearance represents distal sodium absorption [89]. These methods are mainly used for research purposes and it should be remembered that glycosuria and changes in urinary glucose excretion will affect proximal tubular sodium handling and alter distal sodium absorption [89]. Standardisation of experimental conditions are therefore required and allowance for confounding factors made when studying tubular sodium handling in diabetes.

Tubular proteins

Measures of tubular function include the measurement of the urinary excretion of small molecular weight proteins such as β^2-microglobulin (β^2-m), retinal binding protein (RBP) and N-acetyl-β-D-glucosaminidase (NAG). All are measured by RIA [41, 90]. β^2-microglobulin is lost in acid urine (pH < 5.5) and for a true reflection of its excretion the urine must be alkalinised. Most workers alkalinise the urine in the container, however the ideal method would require alkalinisation of the patient as breakdown of β_2-microglobulin is believed to occur in the bladder at low pH [41].

Methods of assessing glomerular barrier integrity

Fractionated neutral dextran clearance represents the best available method for determination of glomerular size selectivity in the clinical setting. Dextran is a polysaccharide tracer which it is not reabsorbed by the tubules. Narrow size fractionation enables studies of barrier size selectivity over a wide range of molecular radii, from 2.0 to around 7.2 nm. Several studies of dextran clearance have been conducted in diabetes [20, 21] and the results interpreted using a theoretical mathematical model of glomerular pore size distribution. With the development of proteinuria, the glomerular barrier loses its size selectivity properties and a small proportion of large pores develops (the so called "shunt-pathway") which allows the preferential filtration of macromolecules the size of 5.6 nm or greater. Studies of charge selectivity barrier properties in man have been hampered by the availability of safe anionic tracers. Sulphated dextran which has been used in animal studies is not suitable for human use. To obviate this problem several investigators have used the clearance of endogenous proteins such as albumin, IgG and IgG subclasses to address the issue of the glomerular membrane charge selectivity changes induced by diabetic nephropathy. Authors who have used the albumin/IgG clearance ratio or the clearances ratio of the similarly sized but differently charged IgG subclasses (IgG/IgG_4) have come to the conclusion that the early proteinuria and microalbuminuria of diabetes are the results of a loss of charge selectivity of the glomerular barrier [21, 91]. Although with heavier proteinuria a close correlation is found between clearance of neutral dextrans and clearance of IgG and albumin, for lesser degrees of proteinuria several problems of interpretation exist. Both albumin and IgG are almost entirely (95–97%) reabsorbed in the tubules and unless tubular reabsorption capacity is saturated, urinary excretion is not a reliable representation of glomerular filtration but reflects the composite actions of glomerular and tubular function. Moreover IgG is produced post-glomerularly and secreted by the kidney. Dextrans are also not devoid of problems. The random coiling nature of the molecule makes them able to pass through pores that would restrict the passage of spherical proteins. These methods have important applications in the studies of the pathophysiology of proteinuria but have limited clinical use.

References

[1] Fiaschi E, Grassi B, Andres G. La funzione renale nel diabete mellito. Rassegna Fisiopatologica. Clinica e Terapeutica 1952; 4: 373–410.
[2] Stadler G, Schmid R. Severe function disorders of glomerular capillaries and renal haemodynamics in treated diabetes mellitus during childhood. Ann Paediat 1959; 193: 129.
[3] Ditzel J, Schwarz M. Abnormally increased glomerular filtration rate in short-term insulin treated diabetic subjects. Diabetes 1967; 16: 264–267.
[4] Mogensen CE. Glomerular filtration rate and renal plasma flow in short-term and long-term juvenile diabetes mellitus. Scand J Lab Clin Invest 1971; 28: 91–100.
[5] Pinto JR, Viberti GC. The patient with diabetes in Textbook of Clinical Nephrology. Ed Cameron S, Davison AM, Grunfeld JP, Kerr D, Ritz E. Oxford Medical Publications 1992; 505–545.

[6] Vora JP, Dolben J, Dean JD et al. Renal haemodynamics in newly presenting non-insulin dependent diabetes mellitus. Kidney Int 1992; 41: 829–836.
[7] Schmitz A, Christensen T, Taagehoej Jensen F. Glomerular filtration rate and kidney volume in normoalbuminuric non-insulin-dependent diabetics – lack of glomerular hyperfiltration and renal hypertrophy in uncomplicated NIDDM. Scand J Clin Lab Invest 1989; 49: 103–108.
[8] Fabre J, Balant LP, Dayer PG et al. The kidney in maturity onset diabetes mellitus: A clinical study of 510 patients. Kidney Int 1982; 21: 730–738.
[9] Palmisano JJ, Lebowitz HE. Renal function in black americans with type 2 diabetes. Journal of diabetic complications 1989; 3: 40–44.
[10] Hostetter RH, Renke HG, Brenner BM. The case for intrarenal hypertension in the initiation and progression of diabetic and other glomerulopathies. Am J Med 1982; 72: 375–380.
[11] Mogensen CE. Microalbuminuria as a predictor of clinical diabetic nephropathy. Kidney Int 1987; 31: 673–689.
[12] Lervang H-H, Jensen S, Brochner-Mortensen J et al. Early glomerular hyperfiltration and the development of late nephropathy in type 1 (insulin-dependent) diabetes mellitus. Diabetologia 1988; 31: 723–729.
[13] Jones SL, Wiseman M, Viberti GC. Glomerular hyperfiltration as a risk factor for diabetic nephropathy: Five year report of a prospective study. Diabetologia 1991; 34: 59–60.
[14] Rudberg S, Persson B, Dahlquist G. Increased glomerular filtration rate as a predictor of diabetic nephropathy – A 8-year prospective study. Kidney Int 1992; 41: 822–829.
[15] Viberti GC, Bilous RW, Mackintosh D et al. Long term correction of hyperglycaemia and progression of renal failure in insulin-dependent diabetes. Br Med J 1983; 286: 598–602.
[16] Bending JJ, Viberti GC, Watkins PJ et al. Intermittent clinical proteinuria and renal function in diabetes: evolution and the effect of glycaemic control. Br Med J 1986; 292: 83–86.
[17] Christiansen JS, Gammelgaard J, Frandsen M et al. Increased kidney size, glomerular filtration rate and renal plasma flow in short term insulin-dependent diabetes. Diabetologia 1981; 20: 451–456.
[18] Christiansen JS. On the pathogenesis of the increased glomerular filtration rate in short-term insulin-dependent diabetes. Thesis. University of Copenhagen 1984.
[19] Wiseman MJ, Viberti GC. Kidney size and GFR in type 1 (insulin-dependent) diabetes mellitus revisited. Diabetologia 1983; 25: 530.
[20] Scadling JD, Myers BD. Glomerular size-selectivity and microalbuminuria in early diabetic glomerular disease. Kidney Int 1992; 41: 840–847.
[21] Deckert T, Kofoed-Enevoldsen A, Vidal P et al. Size- and charge selectivity of glomerular filtration in type 1 (insulin-dependent) diabetic patients with and without albuminuria. Diabetologia 1993; 36: 244–251.
[22] Keen H, Chlouverakis C. An immunoassay method for urinary albumin at low concentrations. Lancet 1963 ii; 913–4.
[23] Viberti GC, Hill RD, Jarrett RJ et al. Microalbuminuria as a predictor of clinical neuropathy in insulin-dependent diabetes mellitus. Lancet 1982 i; 1430–1432.
[24] Mogensen CE, Christensen CK. Predicting diabetic nephropathy in insulin-dependent patients. N Engl J Med 1984; 311: 89–93.
[25] Mathiesen ER, Oxenboll B, Johansen K et al. Incipient nephropathy in type 1 (insulin-dependent) diabetes. Diabetologia 1984; 26: 406–410.
[26] Mattock MB, Morrish NJ, Viberti GC et al. Prospective study of microalbuminuria as predictor of mortality in NIDDM. Diabetes 1992; 41: 736–741.
[27] Schmitz A, Veath M. Microalbuminuria: a major risk factor in non-insulin-dependent diabetes. A 10-year follow-up study of 503 patients. Diabetic Medicine 1988; 5: 126–34.
[28] Damsgaard EM, Froland A, Jorgensen OD et al. Microalbuminuria as a predictor of increased mortality in elderly people. Brit Med J 1990; 300: 297–300.
[29] Yudkin JS, Forrest RD, Jackson CA. Microalbuminuria as predictor of vascular disease in non-diabetic subjects. Islington Diabetes Survey. Lancet 1988; 2: 530–3.

[30] Wiseman M, Viberti GC, Mackintosh D et al. Glycaemia, arterial pressure and microalbuminuria in type 1 (insulin-dependent) diabetes mellitus. Diabetologia 1984; 26: 401–405.
[31] Jones SL, Close CF, Mattock MB et al. Plasma lipid and coagulation factor concentrations in insulin-dependent diabetics with microalbuminuria. Br Med J 1098; 298: 487–490.
[32] Jensen T, Stender S, Deckert T. Abnormalities in plasma concentrations of lipoproteins and fibrinogen in type 1 (insulin-dependent) diabetic patients with increased urianry albumin excretion rates. Diabetologia 1988; 31: 142–145.
[33] Jensen T. Albuminuria – a marker of renal and generalised vascular disease in insulin-dependent diabetes mellitus. Danish Medical Bulletin 1991; 38 (2): 134–144.
[34] The Microalbuminuria Collaborative Study Group. Microalbuminuria in type 1 (insulin-dependent) diabetes: Prevalence and clinical characteristics. Diabetes Care 1992; 15: 495–501.
[35] Parving H-H, Hommel E, Mathiesen E et al. Prevalence of microalbuminuria, arterial hypertension, retinopathy and neuropathy in patients with insulin-dependent diabetes. Br Med J 1988; 296: 156–160.
[36] Earle K, Walker J, Hill C et al. Familial clustering of cardiovascular disease in patients with insulin dependent diabetes and nephropathy. New Engl J Med 1992; 326: 673–677.
[37] Dahl-Jorgensen K, Bjoro T, Kierulf P et al. Long-term glycaemic control and kidney function in insulin-dependent diabetes mellitus. Kidney Int 1992; 41: 920–923.
[38] Messent JWC, Elliott TG, Hill RD et al. Prognostic significance of microalbuminuria in insulin-dependent diabetes mellitus: A twenty-three year follow-up study. Kidney Int 1992; 41: 836–840.
[39] Watts GF, Vlitos MA, Morris RW et al. Urinary N-acetyl-beta-D-glucosaminidase excretion in insulin-dependent diabetes mellitus: relation to microalbuminuria, retinopathy and glycaemic control. Diabete et Metabolism 1988; 14: 653–8.
[40] Watanabe Y, Nunoi K, Maki Y, Nakamura Y, Fujishima M. Contribution of glycaemic control to the level of N-acetyl-B-D-glucosaminidase and serum NAG in type 1 (insulin-dependent) diabetes mellitus without proteinuria. Clin Nephrol 1987; 28: 227–31.
[41] Watts GF, Powell M, Rowe DJ et al. Low-molecular weight proteinuria in insulin-dependent diabetes mellitus: a study of the urinary excretion of beta 2-microglobulin and retinol binding protein in alkalinized patients with and without microalbuminuria. Diabetes research 1989; 12: 31–6.
[42] Fioretto P, Muollo B, Faranota PP et al. Relationship among natriuresis, atrial natriuretic peptide and insulin in insulin-dependent diabetes. Kidney Int 1992; 41: 813–822.
[43] Osterby R, Parving HH, Nyberg G et al. A strong correlation between glomerular filtration rate and filtration surface in diabetic nephropathy. Diabetologia 1988; 31: 265–270.
[44] Walker JD, Close CF, Jones SL et al. Glomerular structure in type-1 (insulin-dependent) diabetic patients with normo- and microalbuminuria. Kidney Int 1992; 41: 741–749.
[45] Gutmann I, Bergermeyer HU. Inulin. In: Bergermeyer HU, ed. Methods of enzymatic analysis. 2nd ed. Vol. 111. Weinheim: Verlag Chemie; New York: Academic press, 1974; 1149–1150.
[46] Dalton RN, Turner C. A sensitive and specific method for the measurement of inulin. Ann Clin Biochem 1987; 24 Suppl. 1: 231.
[47] Day DF, Workman WE. A simple assay for renal clearance determination using immobilised B-furanidase. Annals of the New York Academy of Science 1984; 434: 504–507.
[48] Degenaar CP, Frenken LAM, van Hooff JP. Enzymatic method for determination of inulin. Clin Chem 1987; 33: 1070–1071.
[49] Chantler C, Garnett ES, Parsons et al. Glomerular filtration rate measurement in man by the single injection method using 51CrEDTA. Clin Sci 1969; 37: 169–180.
[50] Veall N, Gibbs GP. The accurate determination of tracer clearance rates and equilibrium distribution volumes from single injection plasma measurements using numerical analysis. In: Joakes AM, Constable AR, Brown NJG, Tauxe WN, eds. Radionuclides in Nephrology. London: Academic Press, Grune and Stratton, 1982; 125–130.
[51] Hagstom KE, Nordenfelt I, Svesson L et al. Comparison of different methods for determination of glomerular filtration rates in disease. Scand J Clin Lab Invest 1974; 34: 31–36.

[52] Mantini G, Dalton RN, Tomlinson PA et al. The estimation of glomerular filtration rate from single injection plasma inulin measurements using numerical analysis. Abst Paediatr nephrol 1989; 3: c128 (Abstract).
[53] Stake G, Monn E, Rootwell IT et al. The clearance of isohexol as a measure of glomerular filtration rate in children with chronic renal failure. Scand J Clin Lab Invest 1991; 51: 729–734.
[54] Spencer K. Analytical reviews in clinical chemistry: the estimation of creatinine. Annal of Clin Biochem 1986; 23: 1–25.
[55] Ambrose RT, Ketchum DF, Smith JW. Creatinine determined by high performance liquid chromatography. Clin Chem 1983; 29: 256–259.
[56] Cockcroft DW, Gault MH. Prediction of Creatinine Clearance from serum creatinine. Nephron 1976; 16: 31–41.
[57] Shemesh O, Golbetz H, Kriss JP et al. Limitations of serum creatinine as a filtration marker in glomerulopathic patients. Kidney Int 1985; 28: 830–838.
[58] Mitch WE. Measuring the rate of progression of renal insufficiency. In: Mitch WE, ed. The progressive nature of kidney disease. New York: Churchill-Livingstone, 1986; 167–187.
[59] Trollfors B, Norrby R. Estimation of glomerular filtration rate by serum creatinine and serum B2-microglobulin. Nephron 1981; 28: 196–99.
[60] Bratton AC, Marshall EK. A new coupling component for sulphanilamide determination. J Bio Chem 1938; 128: 537–550.
[61] Nyberg G, Granerus G, Aurell M. Renal extraction ratios for 51Cr-EDTA, PAH, and glucose in early insulin-dependent diabetic patients. Kidney Int 1982; 21: 706–708.
[62] Dalton RN, Turner C, Green SA et al. Schiff base formation between glucose and para-aminohippurate in frozen samples. Ann Clin Biochem 1987; 24 (Suppl. 1): 238–9.
[63] Schlegel JU, Halikiopoulos HL, Prima R. Determination of filtration fraction using the gamma camera. J Urology 1979; 122: 447–450.
[64] Rehling M, Moller ML, Lund LO et al. ^{99}mTc-DTPA gamma-camera renography: normal values and rapid determination of single kidney glomerular filtration rate. European Journal of Nuclear Medicine 1985; 11: 1–6.
[65] Vidt DG. The diagnosis of renovascular hypertension. Am J Hypertens 1991; 4: 663S–668S.
[66] Al-Nahhas A, Marcus AJ, Bomanji J et al. Validaty of the mean paranchymal transit time as a screening test for the detection of functional renal artery stenosis in hypertensive patients. Nuclear Medicine Communications 1989; 10: 807–815.
[67] Rasmussen SN, Haase L, Kjeldsen H et al. Determination of renal volume by ultrasound scanning. JCU 1978; 6: 160–164.
[68] Inomata S. Renal hypertrophy as a prognostic index for the progression of diabetic renal disease in non-insulin-dependent diabetes mellitus. J Diabetic Complications 1993; 7: 28–33.
[69] Viberti GC, Jarrett RJ, McCartney M et al. Increased glomerular permeability induced by exercise in diabetic subjects. Diabetologia 1978; 14: 293–300.
[70] Bangstaad H-J, Hanssen KF, Keirulf P et al. Elevated albumin excretion rate is common among poorly controlled adolescent insulin dependent diabetics. Diabetes Res 1987; 6: 43–46.
[71] Viberti GC, Bognetti E, Wiseman MJ et al. Effect of protein-restricted diet on renal response to a meat meal in humans. Am J Physiol 1987; 253: F388–F393.
[72] Viberti GC, Mogensen CE, Keen H et al. Urinary excretion of albumin in normal men: The effect of water loading. Scand J Clin Lab Invest 1982; 42: 147–151.
[73] Eshoj O, Feldt-Rasmussen B, Larsen ML et al. Comparison of overnight, morning and 24 hour urine collections in the assessment of diabetic microalbuminuria. Diabetic Med 1987; 4: 531–533.
[74] Cohen DL, Close CF, Viberti GC. The variability of overnight albumin excretion in insulin-dependent diabetics and normal subjects. Diabetic Med 1987; 4: 437–440.
[75] Gatling W, Knight C, Hill RD. Testing for urinary protein: Comparison of Albustix and laboratory albumin determination. Practical Diabetes 1985; 2: 38–41.

[76] Gatling W, Knight C, Mullee MA et al. Microalbuminuria in diabetes: a population study of the prevalence and an assessment of three screening tests. Diabetic Med 1988; 45: 343–347.
[77] Hutchison AS, O'Reilly DSJ, MacCuish AC. Albumin excretion rates, albumin concentration and albumin/creatinine ratio compared for screening diabetics for slight albuminuria. Clin Chem 1988; 34: 2019–21.
[78] Diabetes Care and research in Europe. Krans HHJ, Porta M, Keen H. Copenhagen: WHO, 1992; 29–32.
[79] Mancini G, Carbonara AO, Heremans JF. Immunochemical quantitation of antigen by single radial immunodiffusion. Immunochemistry 1965; 2: 235–239.
[80] Miles DW, Mogensen CE, Gundersen HJG. Radioimmunoassay for urinary albumin using a single antibody. Scand J Clin Lab Invest 1970; 26: 5–11.
[81] Creighton WD, Lambert PH, Miescher PA. Detection of antibodies and soluble antigen-antibody complexes by precipitation with polyethylene glycol. J Immunol 1973; 111: 1219–1227.
[82] Kearney EM, Mount JN, Watts GF et al. Simple method for determining urinary albumin at low concentrations using Cobas-Bio centrifugal analyser. J Clin Pathol 1987; 40: 465–468.
[83] Medcalf EA, Newman DJ, Gorman EG et al. Rapid, robust method for measuring low concentrations of albumin in urine. Clin Chem 1990; 36: 446–449.
[84] Torffvit O, Weislander J. A simplified enzyme-linked immunosorbent assay for urinary albumin. Scand J. Clin Lab Med 1986; 46: 545–548.
[85] Collins ACG, Sethi M, MacDonald FA et al. Temperature of storage and differing methods of sample preparation in the measurement of albumin in urine. Submitted March 1993.
[86] Marshall SM, Shearing PA, Alberti KG. Micral-test strips evaluated for screening for albuminuria. Clinical Chemistry 1992; 38 (4): 588–91.
[87] Jury DR, Mikkelsen DJ, Glen D et al. Assessment of Micral-Test microalbuminuria test strip in the laboratory and in diabetic outpatients. Annals of Clinical Biochemistry. 1992; 29: 96–100.
[88] Skott O, Btuun NE, Giese J et al. What does lithium clearance measure during osmotic diuresis. Clin Sci 1987; 73: 126–127.
[89] Koomans HA, Boer WH, Mees EJD. Evaluation of lithium clearance as a marker of proximal tubular handling. Kidney Int 1989; 36: 2–12.
[90] Feldt-Rasmussen B, Deckert M, Dineson B. Beta-2-microglobulin in urine and serum determined by a micro-ELISA technique. Scand J Clin Lab Invest 1986; 46: 791–793.
[91] Tomlanovich S, Deen WM, Jones HW et al. Functional nature of glomerular injury in progressive diabetic glomerulopathy. Diabetes 1987; 36: 556–565.

Conducting clinical trials in diabetic eye disease

R. Klein, B. E. K. Klein, S. E. Moss

Introduction

Diabetic eye disease is a leading cause of blindness in the United States [1]. The primary cause of loss of vision in people with insulin-dependent diabetes is diabetic retinopathy while in diabetic people who are not insulin-dependent, cataract, glaucoma, and macular degeneration also contribute in a significant way to loss of vision [2].

A number of clinical trials have examined medical and surgical interventions designed to prevent development or progression of retinopathy and loss of vision. These have led to new observations regarding the relationships of glycaemia, aldose reductase inhibitors, aspirin, and other drugs to diabetic retinopathy [3–6].

Prior to the Diabetes Control and Complications Trial (DCCT), clinical trials had not consistently demonstrated that control of hyperglycaemia prevented the development or progression of retinopathy [3, 4]. Data from the DCCT demonstrated a beneficial effect of tight glycaemic control on the incidence and progression of retinopathy in people with insulin dependent diabetes [7]. The Veterans Administration Trial on the Control and Complications in Noninsulin Dependent Diabetes is currently examining the relationship of metabolic control to the primary or secondary prevention of retinopathy in diabetic people with non-insulin-dependence [8]. Additional trials studying aldose reductase inhibitors, antiplatelet drugs, growth factor antagonists, and antihypertensive drugs in primary and secondary prevention of diabetic retinopathy have either just been completed or are in progress. At present, there are no proven medical interventions which prevent or decrease the progression of diabetic retinopathy and loss of vision. Three multicentered, randomized, controlled clinical trials, the Diabetic Retinopathy Study (DRS, to evaluate panretinal photocoagulation for the treatment of proliferative diabetic retinopathy) [9]; the Early Treatment Diabetic Retinopathy Study (ETDRS, to evaluate focal photocoagulation for macular oedema, panretinal photocoagulation for nonproliferative and early proliferative ret-

Offprint from
Research Methodologies in Human Diabetes – Part 1

inopathy, and aspirin for progression of retinopathy) [6]; and the Diabetic Retinopathy Vitrectomy Study (to evaluate vitrectomy for vitreous hemorrhage) have demonstrated the efficacy of photocoagulation and vitrectomy for diabetic patients with late stages of retinopathy [10].

This chapter examines methodologic approaches currently used in designing clinical trials of diabetic retinopathy. Insights are drawn from a population-based cohort study of diabetic retinopathy as well as from previous clinical trials. Data from one population-based cohort study of diabetic retinopathy, the Wisconsin Epidemiologic Study of Diabetic Retinopathy (WESDR), will be used to provide estimates of sample size for future trials involving diabetic retinopathy as an endpoint [11–14].

Background

Brief overview of natural history of diabetic retinopathy

Usually the first ophthalmoscopically detectable lesions of diabetic retinopathy are retinal microaneurysms. Prior to their appearance, abnormalities in the blood-retinal barrier and retinal blood flow may occur. After the appearance of retinal microaneurysms, retinopathy may progress with the appearance of other nonproliferative abnormalities such as retinal hard exudates (lipid exudate deposits), cotton wool spots (small localized infarctions of the nerve fiber layer of the retinal, intra-retinal microvascular abnormalities (collateral dilated capillary channels in areas of retinal ischaemia), and venous beading (irregular dilation of retinal veins associated with significant retinal ischaemia). Diabetic patients may progress to the proliferative stage with the development of new blood vessels and fibrous tissue at the optic disc or near venules elsewhere in the retina. These new blood vessels may bleed and the fibrovascular tissue can cause traction on the macula with loss of vision. Spontaneous regression may occur at any stage. Macular oedema (thickening of the retina in the macular area) may also develop. Visual loss may result from macular oedema or proliferative retinopathy.

Pathogenesis

The pathogenesis of diabetic retinopathy is poorly understood. A number of possible mechanisms have been suggested [15–17]. Hyperglycaemia is thought to be an important initiator of these disease processes, which include biochemical changes (increased aldose reductase, changes in myo-inositol phosphatidyl-inositol metabolism, increases in 1,2-diacyl-sn-glycerol, nonenzymatic glycosylation, increased protein kinase C, decreased heparin sulphate proteoglycan, increased auto-oxidation, and changes in vasoactive substances such as endothelin, prostanoids, nitrous oxide, and histamine), physiological changes (increased retinal small blood vessel resistance, decreased retinal blood flow velocity, compensatory vasodilation, increased permeability, and loss of autoregulation), rheological changes (increased blood viscosity, increased platelet adhesiveness and clotting, decreased red blood cell deformability, increased red blood cell aggregation, and increased binding of macrophages), and growth factor changes (increased fibroblast, transforming-β, and insulin-like growth factors, and increased growth hormone). These abnormalities are associated with the development of a number of anatomic changes in the diabetic retina which include pericyte loss, endothelial cell abnormalities, acellular capillaries, increased basement membrane thickness, and retinal pigment epithelial abnormalities.

It is likely that the initiation and progression of retinopathy is due to a complex relationship among a number of these factors which vary at different stages in the natural history of retinopathy and from individual to individual.

Epidemiology

Epidemiologic population-based studies have provided important information on the incidence and progression of diabetic retinopathy, as well as potentially intervenable risk factors such as glycosylated haemoglobin and blood pressure. The WESDR has provided data on the prevalence and severity of retinopathy by duration of diabetes (Fig. 1, 2) and the four-year incidence and progression of diabetic retinopathy by age, sex, and duration of diabetes (Table 1) in younger-onset persons (diagnosis of diabetes less than 30 years of age and taking insulin) [11–14]. The prevalence of diabetic retinopathy varied from 17% in those with diabetes for less than five years to 98% in those with diabetes for 15 or more years; proliferative retinopathy was absent in those with shorter duration of diabetes, but present in 48% in those with 15 or more years of diabetes. For older-onset persons (diagnosis of diabetes at 30 years of age or older and either taking or not taking insulin) the prevalence of any retinopathy varied from 28% to 78% and proliferative retinopathy from 2% to 16% with diabetes for less than five years and 15 or more years, respectively.

In the younger-onset group, the highest four-year incidences of retinopathy occurred between 3 and 10 years of diabetes, the highest rates of progression of retinopathy occurred between 3 and 19 years of diabetes, and the highest rates of progression to proliferative retinopathy were between 11 and 19 years of diabetes.

Table 1 Four-year incidence of any retinopathy, improvement or progression of retinopathy, or progression to PDR by age and by duration of diabetes at baseline WESDR examination*

Group	Age or duration of diabetes at baseline examination, y	No. at risk	Incidence of any retinopathy, %	No. at risk	Improvement, %	No. at risk	No change, %	Progression, %	Progression to PDR*, %
Younger-onset	By age								
	0–9	26	15.4	0	–	27	96.3	3.7	0
	10–12	42	54.8	2	–	48	70.8	27.1	0
	13–14	25	48.0	2	–	32	62.5	37.5	3.1
	15–19	66	72.7	56	7.1	140	47.9	49.3	10.0
	20–24	42	64.3	81	3.7	130	48.5	49.2	11.5
	25–29	25	72.0	67	6.0	101	49.5	46.5	15.8
	30–34	34	61.8	57	8.8	102	52.0	43.1	11.8
	35+	11	63.6	111	8.1	133	60.2	33.1	12.8
	35–39	7	–	40	5.0	51	56.9	39.2	9.8
	40–44	3	–	21	4.8	25	56.0	40.0	16.0
	45+	1	–	50	12.0	57	64.9	24.6	14.0
	By duration of diabetes								
	0–2	69	37.7	4	–	75	80.0	18.7	0
	3–4	68	61.8	5	–	84	64.3	34.5	1.2
	5–6	60	65.0	30	3.3	103	54.4	44.7	3.9
	7–8	32	68.8	37	5.4	85	40.0	57.6	8.2
	9–10	23	73.9	53	5.7	84	54.8	41.7	11.9
	11+	19	73.7	–	–	–	–	–	–
	11–12	–	–	43	0	54	44.4	55.6	22.2
	13–14	–	–	38	7.9	43	30.2	62.8	27.9
	15–19	–	–	68	2.9	79	55.7	41.8	16.5
	20–24	–	–	39	15.4	42	57.1	28.6	14.3
	25–29	–	–	32	9.4	34	61.8	29.4	14.7
	30+	–	–	27	14.8	30	56.7	30.0	16.7

Table 1 (continued)

Group	Age or duration of diabetes at baseline examination, y	No. at risk	Incidence of any retinopathy, %	No. at risk	Improvement, %	No. at risk	No change, %	Progression, %	Progression to PDR*, %
Older-onset	By age								
Using insulin	30–44	18	50.0	6	16.7	26	57.7	38.5	3.8
	45–59	47	59.6	70	5.7	135	54.1	43.0	8.9
	60–74	61	45.9	119	17.6	202	58.4	31.2	8.9
	75+	28	28.6	20	35.0	55	67.3	20.0	10
Not using	30–44	14	50.0	4	25.0	19	63.2	31.6	5.3
	45–59	83	30.1	21	4.8	114	68.4	30.7	4.4
	60–74	168	32.7	48	20.8	257	73.2	23.0	1.9
	75+	55	41.8	28	28.6	96	69.8	21.9	0
	By duration of diabetes								
Using insulin	0–4	48	27.1	19	15.8	77	77.9	18.2	0
	5–9	48	70.8	19	10.5	78	47.4	50.0	5.1
	10–14	24	54.2	38	21.1	73	50.7	38.4	5.5
	15+	34	38.2	139	14.4	190	57.4	32.1	12.1
Not using	0–4	155	31.0	24	16.7	201	79.1	18.9	2.0
	5–0	99	32.3	29	27.6	152	69.1	25.7	2.0
	10–14	29	37.9	15	6.7	52	63.5	34.6	0
	15+	37	51.4	33	21.2	81	59.3	32.1	4.9

* PDR indicates proliferative diabetic retinopathy.

† From Klein R, Klein BEK, Moss SE et al. Wisconsin Epidemiologic Study of Diabetic Retinopathy. IX. and X. Arch Ophthalmol 1989; 107: 237–243, 244–249.

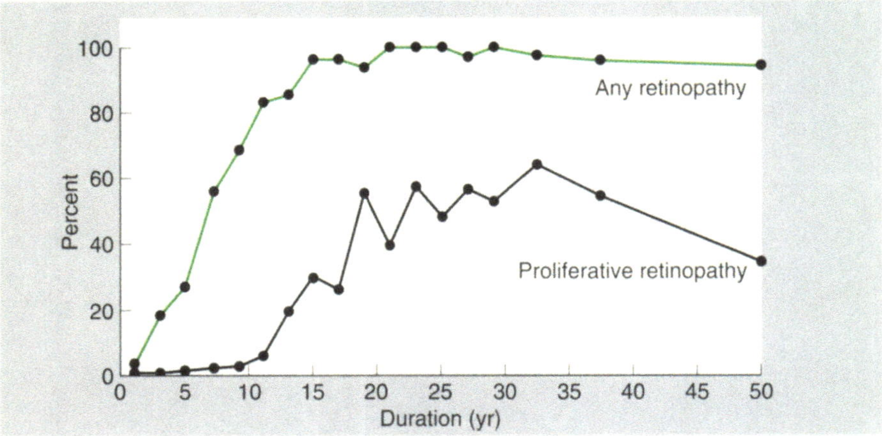

Fig. 1 The frequency of retinopathy or proliferative retinopathy by duration of diabetes (years) in 996 insulin-taking persons diagnosed to have diabetes before 30 years of age who participated in the Wisconsin Epidemiologic Study of Diabetic Retinopathy (WESDR) 1980–1982. Source: Klein R, Klein BEK, Moss SE et al. The Wisconsin Epidemiologic Study of Diabetic Retinopathy. II. Prevalence and risk of diabetic retinopathy when age at diagnosis is less than 30 years. Arch Ophthalmol 1984; 102: 520–526. Copyright American Medical Association. Reproduced with permission

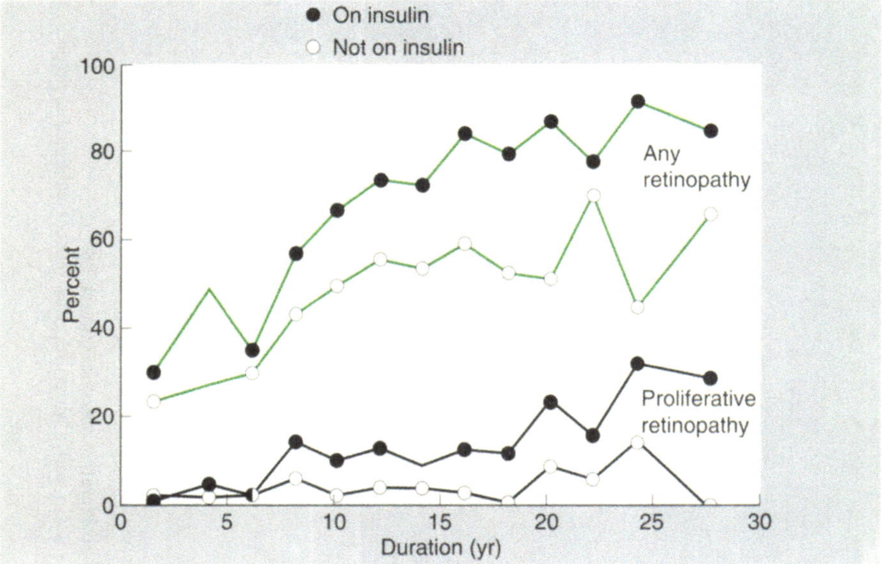

Fig. 2 The frequency of retinopathy or proliferative retinopathy by duration of diabetes (years) in 674 people taking insulin and 696 people not taking insulin diagnosed after 29 years of age who participated in the WESDR, 1980–1982. Klein R, Klein BEK, Moss SE et al. The Wisconsin Epidemiologic Study of Diabetic Retinopathy. III. Prevalence and risk of diabetic retinopathy when age at diagnosis is 30 or more years. Arch Ophthalmol 1984; 102: 527–532. Copyright American Medical Association. Reproduced with permission

Data from the WESDR suggested a strong dose-response relationship between glycosylated haemoglobin measured at baseline and the four-year incidence and progression of retinopathy in both younger- and older-onset groups [18]. Blood pressure was associated with increased risk of incidence and progression of retinopathy in only the younger-onset group [19].

Study design considerations in clinical trials of diabetic retinopathy

The specific study design adopted for a clinical trial of diabetic retinopathy will depend, in part, on the specific drug or intervention to be evaluated. The discussion which follows provides general rather than specific study design approaches.

What is the optimal time in the course of diabetes to intervene with a specific drug?

The optimal time in the course of diabetes to apply the intervention can be estimated from four-year incidence and rates of 2 or greater step progression in the WESDR [13, 14]. For example, peak 4-year incidence of retinopathy in people with younger-onset insulin-dependent diabetes is expected in those with 3 to 10 years of diabetes. Those with 11 to 19 years of diabetes and with moderate to severe nonproliferative retinopathy are at highest risk to progress to proliferative retinopathy. However, variations in covariates, such as glycaemia, which have a significant effect on these relationships may affect these estimates of incidence or rates of progression of retinopathy. If the DCCT reports a positive finding and if these results are applied in practice with a resultant decrease in glycaemia, there may be a delay in incidence or progression of diabetic retinopathy.

Inclusion and exclusion criteria for trials with diabetic retinopathy as an endpoint

Trials of primary prevention of retinopathy, by definition, usually exclude people with retinal microaneurysms in either eye. In secondary prevention trials, the choice of the range of severity of retinopathy included in the study will depend, in part, on whether the intervention is specific for a given severity of retinopathy, the toxicity of the drug to be tested, the length of time it takes to reach a meaningful endpoint (such as two or greater step progression), sample size considerations, and the availability of subjects. A pragmatic approach, when relatively little is known about the relationship of a medical intervention to the pathogenesis of retinopathy, is to include a broad range of nonproliferative retinopathy (Level 20 to Level 47 on the ETDRS scale, see below).

Other ocular exclusion criteria in trials of diabetic retinopathy may include conditions which affect the quality of the fundus photographs and the ability to detect retinopathy, such as cataracts or other opacities in the media (such as corneal scarring or vitreous haemorrhage). Eyes with high intraocular pressure or glaucoma, age-related macular degeneration, high myopia, or those which have had intraocular surgery or photocoagulation are also often excluded.

How long should the trial last?

A larger sample size may shorten the time necessary to demonstrate the effect of an intervention. However, regardless of the sample size, an adequate period of time is usually necessary before the intervention may exert a beneficial effect on the incidence or progression of retinopathy. For example, it may take a certain period of time before reduction of blood sugar results in slowing the rate of progression of retinopathy. In both the Steno and Kroc clinical trials, the experimental group, treated with insulin pumps to achieve rapid glycaemic control, initially experienced a transient worsening of retinopathy over the first four to six months of the trials [3, 4]. Thereafter, the rates of progression appeared similar for the treated and control arms of the trials [20]. Similar changes were seen in the DCCT [7].

Because of the high costs of clinical trials, investigators are usually interested in determining the affect of the intervention in the shortest period of time possible, such as 6 months to 2 years. However, there is general consensus, especially in trials of primary prevention or secondary intervention of early diabetic retinopathy, of the need for such trials to last at least 3 or more years.

Endpoints

Endpoints should have clinical relevance in terms of functional impairment. The most meaningful endpoint in trials of diabetic eye disease is significant loss of vision. In the DRS, a clinical trial designed to evaluate the effect of an intervention, panretinal photocoagulation, in eyes with proliferative retinopathy in which there is a high likelihood of loss of vision, a significant decrease in the visual acuity, defined as a decrease to 5/200 or worse at two consecutive study visits, was used as the endpoint. In the ETDRS, which was designed to evaluate the benefit of focal photocoagulation treatment of macular oedema, doubling of the visual angle (i. e., 20/20 at baseline to 20/40 at follow-up) was used to define an event. However, in trials of primary prevention or secondary intervention of diabetic retinopathy, such as the DCCT, loss of vision, such as doubling of the visual angle, is not an appropriate primary endpoint because of the relative rarity of such events over the 7 to 10 year duration of the trial. Instead, surrogate endpoints, such as the development of a two or greater step progression in the severity of diabetic retinopathy have been accepted as clinically meaningful. Development of proliferative retinopathy or clinically significant macular oedema are also clinically meaningful endpoints.

Data from the WESDR suggest that changes in the number of retinal microaneurysms (e. g., tripling of the count from baseline) may be a clinically meaningful endpoint [21]. In this study, after controlling for other risk factors, eyes with tripling of the microaneurysm count were more likely to develop more severe retinopathy associated with loss of vision than eyes in which the microaneurysm count did not change. Change in the microaneurysm counts have been included as an endpoint in a number of trials [22, 23]. However, microaneurysm counts have not gained widespread acceptance as a meaningful endpoint in clinical trials of diabetic retinopathy.

Methods of detection of diabetic retinopathy

Direct and indirect ophthalmoscopy, and biomicroscopy with contact lens examination have been employed to detect diabetic retinopathy and macular oedema in clinical trials. While these techniques are less expensive and permit visualization of the periphery of the retina, they require a trained observer, do not provide a permanent record, and make it difficult to monitor quality control and minimize observer bias.

The development of fundus photography provided an objective, sensitive, and reproducible approach for detecting and documenting retinopathy. Color stereoscopic 30 degree fundus photographs of seven standard fields, as described in the DRS has become the standard approach to document the severity and progression of diabetic retinopathy in clinical trials [24].

Fluorescein angiography has been used to detect blood flow, capillary closure and leakage of fluorescein. Data from the ETDRS suggest that fluorescein angiography and color fundus photographs are similar in terms of prediction of progression of retinopathy [25]. Because fluorescein angiography is an invasive procedure and has been associated with allergic side effects, including anaphylaxis, and because there is also difficulty in maintaining consistent quality of the angiograms over time, it is not as often used to measure the progression of retinopathy in epidemiologic studies and clinical trials.

Vitreous fluorophotometry is used to quantitate fluorescein leakage into the vitreous cavity [26]. It involves a slit lamp photometric determination of fluorescein concentration in the vitreous. It is a sensitive and objective measure of fluorescein leakage. However, few studies have examined the relationship of increased vitreous fluorescence and the progression of retinopathy. One such study suggests that increased vitreous fluorescence, as determined by vitreous fluorophotometry, is not predictive of progression of retinopathy in those with no or minimal diabetic retinopathy at baseline [27]. Furthermore, because vitreous fluorophotometry is not routinely used by ophthalmologists in the clinical care of diabetic patients, vitreous fluorophotometers may not be available in some study sites.

Tests of retinal blood flow and electrophysiologic tests, such as electroretinography and visual evoked responses have been suggested as useful adjuncts to fundus photography for determining the risk of progression of retinopathy [28, 29]. However, to date, they have not been routinely used in clinical trials of diabetic retinopathy. Detailed descriptions of these approaches and their limitations appear elsewhere [28, 29].

How many color fundus photographs and how often to photograph

Most clinical trials use seven standard photographic fields (see Fig. 3) to document progression of diabetic retinopathy. While fewer fields may improve compliance and reduce the costs of photography and grading, they may result in reduced sensitivity in detection of retinopathy. Moss et al [30] have demonstrated that for eight retinopathy levels, the rate of agreement with seven fields ranged from 80% for two fields to 91% for four fields. In that study, the rate of agreement was also dependent on the specific retinopathy severity levels of interest, with markedly less sensitivity of fewer fields when proliferative retinopathy was the endpoint of interest. While the sensitivity of fewer fields for detection of retinopathy may be considered good, over the course of a trial, the overall sensitivity of fewer fields may be low, resulting in the need for an increased number of study subjects. This may outweigh the savings resulting from the use of fewer photographic fields.

The frequency of fundus photography is optimally determined by the rate of progression of retinopathy. In many clinical trials of diabetic retinopathy, fundus photography is suggested at 6 month or yearly intervals. However, in

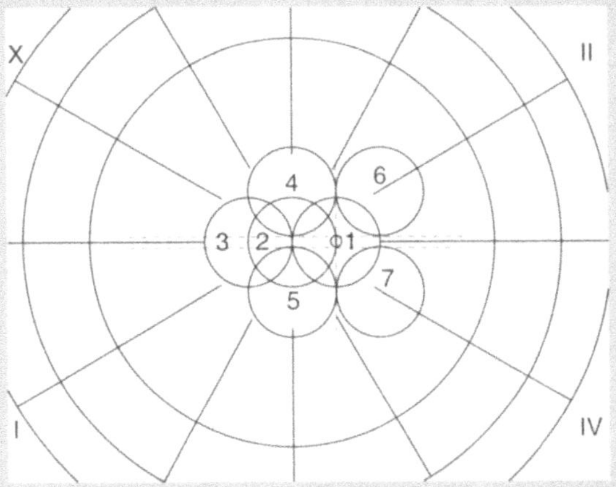

Fig. 3 Schematic diagram of the seven standard fields of the retinal fundus

primary prevention studies of diabetic people who are not insulin-dependent, photography every two years may be more practical because of the slower rates of progression of retinopathy.

Classification systems

Classification systems for diabetic retinopathy, based on the natural history of diabetes, have been used in clinical studies since 1890. The modified Airlie House Scheme of grading and the Early Treatment Diabetic Retinopathy Study Classification scheme for severity of retinopathy have been used in recent clinical trials [24, 31]. The severity scales are presented in Table 2. The ETDRS demonstrated that the more severe the level of retinopathy at baseline, the higher the likelihood of progression to proliferative retinopathy four year later [32]. The "internal" validity of one such scale used in the WESDR has been demonstrated [33]. In that study, there was a significant trend for increasing four-year incidence of doubling of the visual angle with increasing severity of retinopathy at baseline.

*Table 2 ETDRS final retinopathy severity scale (for individual eyes)**

Level	Severity	Definition
10	DR absent	Microaneurysms and other characteristics absent
14†	DR questionable	HE, SE, or IRMA definite; microaneurysms absent
15†	DR questionable	Haemorrhage(s) definite; microaneurysms absent
20	Microaneurysms only	Microaneurysms definite, other characteristics absent
35‡	Mild NPDR	One or more of the following: Venous loops $\geq$ D/1; SE, IRMA, or VB = Q; Retinal haemorrhages present; HE $\geq$ D/1; SE $\geq$ D/1
43	Moderate NPDR	H/Ma = M/4–5 – S/1 or IRMA = D/1–3 (not both)
47	Moderately severe NPDR	Both L43 characteristics and/or one (only) of the following: IRMA = D/4–5; H/Ma = S/2–3; VB = D/1
53	Severe NPDR‡	One or more of the following: $\geq$ 2 of the 3 L47 characteristics; H/Ma $\geq$ S/4–5; IRMA $\geq$ M/1; VB $\geq$ D/2–3
61	Mild PDR	FPD or FPE present with NVD and NVE absent; or NVE = D
65	Moderate PDR	Either of the following: (1) NVE $\geq$ M/1 or NVD = D; and VH and PRH = A or Q; (2) VH or PRH = D and NVE < M/1 and NVD absent
71	High-risk PDR	Any of the following: (1) VH or PRH $\geq$ M/1; (2) NVE $\geq$ M/1 and VH or PRH $\geq$ D/1; (3) NVD = 2 and VH or PRH $\geq$ D/1; (4) NVD $\geq$ M
75	High-risk PDR	NVD $\geq$ M and VH or PRH $\geq$ D/1
81	Advanced PDR: fundus partially obscured, center of macular attached	NVD = cannot grade or NVD < D and NVE = cannot grade in $\geq$ 1 field and absent in all others; and retinal detachment at center of macula < D
85	Advanced PDR: posterior fundus obscured, or center of macula detached	VH = VS in fields 1 and 2; or retinal detachment at center of macula = D
90	Cannot grade, even sufficiently for level 81 or 85	

DR = diabetic retinopathy, HE = hard exudates, SE = soft exudates, IRMA = intraretinal microvascular abnormalities, NPDR = nonproliferative DR, VB = venous beading, H/Ma = haemorrhages/microaneurysms, PDR = proliferative DR, NVE = new vessels elsewhere (> 1 DD

Grading methods

Trained graders are masked concerning the treatment group to which the trial subjects belong. This may be difficult in trials in which photocoagulation treatment is being evaluated and the treatment scars are apparent in the involved eye. This is less of a problem in trials involving medical interventions.

Graders usually use standard light boxes and viewers to examine the stereoscopic color slide transparencies [31]. The viewers provide stereopsis and magnification of the image. Right and left eyes are often graded separately. Photographs are usually graded independently, from study visit to visit. Direct comparison of fundus photographs may improve accuracy by detecting grader errors or errors resulting from poor photographic technique (poorly defined photographic fields from visit to visit, poor stereopsis, and poor focus) [34]. However, the independent grading method is usually favored in most trials of diabetic retinopathy as it is more convenient and less subject to observer bias.

At present, most grading is done on line into a computer with built in checks for internal consistency and errors. In some trials, photographs are graded separately by two graders working independently of each other using standard grading forms. These gradings may then be compared by computer, and differences in the evaluation of any lesion or overall level are resolved by a third, more senior grader.

In addition to providing data regarding progression of retinopathy, grading of fundus photographs is often used to determine eligibility according to the criteria of the trial, monitor the quality of the photographs for providing feedback to photographers during the trial, and for providing feedback information to the investigators if proliferative retinopathy or macular oedema occurs.

Most grading systems have a quality control program in place to monitor inter- and intraobserver variation of the graders. Feedback is provided to the

---

from disc), NVD = new vessels disc (within 1 DD of disc margin), FPD = fibrous proliferations disc, FPE = fibrous proliferations elsewhere, VH = vitreous haemorrhage, PRH = preretinal haemorrhage. Definitions of severity grades: A = absent, Q = questionable, D = definite, M = moderate, s = severe

* *From Early Treatment Diabetic Retinopathy Study Research Group. Fundus photographic risk factors for progression of diabetic retinopathy. ETDRS Report number 12. Ophthalmology 1991; 98 (Suppl): 823–833 with permission from Ophthalmology.*

† *Levels 14 and 15 are not considered separate steps in the scale, but are pooled with level 10 or 20*

‡ *NPDR levels 35 and above all require presence of microaneurysms*

graders through regular meetings and comparisons of their scores with those of other graders and a more senior grader. This is especially important in long trials where drift in the gradings of retinopathy may have an adverse affect in terms of the trial.

Sample size

One of the most important considerations in planning the trial is that it have enough statistical power to detect differences of clinical importance among groups being compared [35]. Estimation of sample size must take into account the statistic to be used, the degree of difference in the event rate (e. g. incidence of retinopathy, two or more step progression of retinopathy, progression to proliferative retinopathy, doubling of the visual angle, etc) considered clinically meaningful, the significance level (α) of a false positive occurrence in the trial (Type I error), and the power ($1\text{-}\beta$) of finding statistically significant differences between the event rates given that a difference actually exists. The sample size estimate must also take into account estimates of noncompliance and drop-out from the study, and other variations of the estimates in the group to be studied from the groups from which the estimates of the event rate were used (such as systematic differences of glycosylated haemoglobin at baseline, ethnic differences, etc).

Estimates of sample sizes for four-year incidence, two or more step progression, progression to proliferative diabetic retinopathy, and incidence of clinically significant macular oedema, are provided from the WESDR population in Tables 3 and 4, with various assumptions in α ($p = .05$ and $p = .01$), power ($1-\beta$, of 0.80 and 0.90) for differences in the response (δ) of the event rate which is to be detected for given durations and baseline

Table 3 Four-year incidence of any retinopathy, progression of retinopathy, progression to proliferative retinopathy and incidence of clinically significant macular oedema in the WESDR

Event	Younger-onset (%)	Older-onset	
		Taking insulin (%)	Not taking insulin (%)
Incidence of retinopathy	59	43	34
Two-step progression of retinopathy	41	34	25
Progression to proliferative diabetic retinopathy	11	7	2
Incidence of clinically significant macular oedema	4	5	1

Table 4 Sample size estimates per group

Rate in control group, %	Change in rate, %	α = .05		α = .01	
		Power = 80%	Power = 90%	Power = 80%	Power = 90%
5	50	1627	2125	2346	2945
	75	817	1059	1166	1457
	100	511	659	725	902
10	50	764	996	1099	1378
	75	381	493	543	677
	100	237	305	335	416
40	20	652	856	947	1193
	30	302	393	434	544
	40	176	227	251	312
	50	116	149	164	203
60	20	276	358	395	494
	30	124	158	174	216
	40	69	87	96	118
	50	44	54	60	72

retinopathy levels [13, 14, 36]. The sample size calculations assume the endpoints as dichotomous response variables. More specific sample size estimates can be developed specifying inclusion and exclusion criteria. Trials in which retinopathy is more severe at baseline will more likely have a large drop-out rate due to increased mortality.

Other considerations

New findings from current clinical trials and epidemiologic studies may have an impact on the outcome of trials which are underway because of the possibility of altering the natural history of retinopathy. The advent of multiple daily injections of insulin and tailored regimens of insulin and self blood glucose monitoring, have resulted in a significant decrease in hypergly-caemia. In addition, because the DCCT has demonstrated a significant effect of glycaemic control on the progression of retinopathy, there may be a further reduction of hyperglycaemia in the diabetic population. From the WESDR, we have estimated that for every 1% absolute decrease in glycosylated haemoglobin there is a 35% decrease in the four-year incidence of proliferative retinopathy in the population [18]. Moreover, more aggressive treatment of blood pressure using new drugs such as angiotensin converting enzyme inhibitors may also result in reduced rates of progression of retinopathy or incidence of macular oedema. Investigators planning clinical trials should take these changes into account when planning their trials.

Summary

Grading of color stereoscopic fundus photographs using standardized protocols provides an objective approach for determining retinopathy in clinical trials. Two or more step progression, development of proliferative retinopathy or macular oedema, or loss of vision are acceptable endpoints in such trials. Data from recent epidemiologic studies can be used to determine sample size estimates and also suggest optimal times for interventions.

References

[1] Klein R, Klein BEK. Vision disorders in diabetes. In: Hamman RF, Harris MI, eds. Diabetes in America, Diabetes data compiled 1984. Bethesda, MD: U.S. Public Health Service, 1985 (DHHS NIH publ. no. 85–1468).

[2] Klein R, Klein BEK, Moss SE. Visual impairment in diabes. Ophthalmology 1984; 91: 1–9, 1984.

[3] The Kroc Collaborative Study Group. Blood glucose control and the evolution of diabetic retinopathy and albuminuria: A preliminary multicenter trial. N Engl J Med 1984; 311: 365–372.

[4] Lauritzen T, Frost-Larsen K, Larsen HW et al. Steno Study Group. Two-year experience with continuous subcutaneous insulin infusion in relation to retinopathy and neuropathy. Diabetes 1985; 34 (Suppl 3): 74–79.

[5] Sorbinil Retinopathy Trial Research Group. A randomized trial of sorbinil, an aldose reductase inhibitor in diabetic retinopathy. Arch Ophthalmol 1990; 108: 1234–1244.

[6] Early Treatment Diabetic Retinopathy Study Research Group: Photocoagulation for diabetic macular edema. Early Treatment of Diabetic Retinopathy Study Report No. 1. Arch Ophthalmol 1985; 103: 1796–1806.

[7] The DCCT Research Group. The effect of intense treatment of diabetes on the development and progression of long-term complications in insulin-dependent diabetes mellitus. New Eng J Med 1993; 329: 977–86.

[8] Abraira C, Emanuele N, Colwell et al. Glycemic control and complications in type 2 diabetes. Design of a feasibility trial. Diabetes Care 1992; 15: 1560–1571.

[9] Diabetic Retinopathy Study Group. Photocoagulation treatment of proliferative diabetic retinopathy: Clinical application of Diabetic Retinopathy Study (DRS) findings. DRS Report No. 8. Ophthalmology 1981; 88: 583–600.

[10] Diabetic Retinopathy Vitrectomy Study Group. Two-year course of visual acuity in severe proliferative diabetic retinopathy with conventional management. Ophthalmology 1985; 92: 492–502.

[11] Klein R, Klein BEK, Moss SE et al. The Wisconsin Epidemiologic Study of Diabetic Retinopathy: II. Prevalence and risk of diabetic retinopathy when age at diagnosis is less than 30 years. Arch Ophthalmol 1984; 102: 520–526.

[12] Klein R, Klein BEK, Moss SE et al. The Wisconsin Epidemiologic Study of Diabetic Retinopathy: III. Prevalence and risk of diabetic retinopathy when age at diagnosis is 30 or more years. Arch Ophthalmol 1984; 102: 527–532.

[13] Klein R, Klein BEK, Moss SE et al. The Wisconsin Epidemiologic Study of Diabetic Retinopathy: IX. Four-year incidence and progression of diabetic retinopathy when age at diagnosis is less than 30 years. Arch Ophthalmol 1989; 107: 237–243.
[14] Klein R, Klein BEK, Moss SE et al. The Wisconsin Epidemiologic Study of Diabetic Retinopathy: X. Four-year incidence and progression of diabetic retinopathy when age at diagnosis is 30 years or more. Arch Ophthalmol 1989; 107: 244–249.
[15] Frank RN. On the pathogenesis of diabetic retinopathy. A 1990 update. Ophthalmology 1991; 98: 586–593.
[16] Kohner EM, Porta M, Hyer SL. The pathogenesis of diabetic retinopathy and cataract. In: Pickup J, Williams G, eds. Textbook of diabetes. Vol. 2. Oxford, England: Blackwell Scientific Pub, 1991; 564–574.
[17] Tilton RG, Chang K. Hasan KS et al. Prevention of diabetic vascular dysfunction by guanidines. Inhibition of nitric oxide synthase versus advanced glycation end-product formation. Diabetes 1993; 42: 221–232.
[18] Klein R, Klein BEK, Moss SE et al. Glycosylated hemoglobin predicts the incidence and progression of diabetic retinopathy. JAMA 1988; 260: 2864–2871.
[19] Klein R, Klein BEK, Moss SE et al. Is blood pressure a predictor of the incidence or progression of diabetic retinopathy? Arch Intern Med 1989; 149: 2427–2432.
[20] The Kroc Collaborative Study Group. Diabetic retinopathy after two years of intensified insulin treatment: Follow-up of the Kroc Collaborative Study. JAMA 1988; 260: 37–41.
[21] Klein R, Meuer SM, Moss SE et al. The relationship of retinal microaneurysm counts to the 4-year progression of diabetic retinopathy. Arch Ophthalmol 1989; 107: 1780–1785.
[22] The DAMAD Study Group. Effect of aspirin alone and aspirin plus dipyridamole in early diabetic retinopathy: A multicenter randomized controlled clinical trial. Diabetes 1989; 38: 491–498.
[23] TIMAD Study Group. Ticlopidine treatment reduces the progression of nonproliferative retinopathy. Arch Ophthalmol 1990; 108: 1577–1583.
[24] Diabetic Retinopathy Study Research Group. Report 7. A modification of the Airlie House classification of diabetic retinopathy. Invest Ophthalmol Vis Sci 1981; 21: 210–226.
[25] Early Treatment Diabetic Retinopathy Study Research Group. Fluorescein angiographic risk factors for progression of diabetic retinopathy. ETDRS report number 13. Ophthalmology 1991; 98 (Suppl): 834–840.
[26] Waltman SR. Vitreous fluorophotometry. In: Little HL, Jack RL, Patz A et al, eds. Diabetic retinopathy. New York: Thieme-Stratton Inc., 1983; 72–81.
[27] Engler C, Krogsaa B, Lund-Andersen H. Blood-retina barrier permeability and its relation to the progression of diabetic retinopathy in type 1 diabetics. An 8-year follow-up study. Graefe Arch Clinic Exp 1991; 229: 442–446.
[28] Grunwald JE, Riva CE, Sinclair SH et al. Laser doppler velocimetry study of retinal circulation in diabetes mellitus. Arch Ophthalmol 1986; 104: 991–996.
[29] Bresnick GH, Palta M. Predicting progression to severe proliferative diabetic retinopathy. Arch Ophthalmol 1987; 105: 810–814.
[30] Moss SE, Meuer SM, Klein R et al. Are seven standard photographic fields necessary for classification of diabetic retinopathy? Invest Ophthalmol Vis Sci 1989; 30: 823–828.
[31] Early Treatment Diabetic Retinopathy Study Research Group. Grading diabetic retinopathy from stereoscopic color fundus photographs – an extension of the modified Airlie House classification. ETDRS report number 10. Ophthalmology 1991; 98 (Suppl): 786–806.
[32] Early Treatment Diabetic Retinopathy Study Research Group. Fundus photographic risk factors for progression of diabetic retinopathy. ETDRS Report number 12. Ophthalmology 1991; 98 (Suppl): 823–833.
[33] Moss SE, Klein R, Klein BEK. The incidence of vision loss in a diabetic population. Ophthalmology 1988; 95: 1340–1348.

[34] Davis MD, Hubbard LD, Trautman J et al. Studies of retinopathy. Methodology for assessment and classification with fundus photographs. Diabetes 1985; 34 (Suppl 3): 42–49.
[35] Friedman LM, Furber CD, DeMets DL. Fundamentals of clinical trials. 2nd Ed. Littleton, Mass: PSG Publishing Co., 1985.
[36] Fleiss JL. Statistical methods for rates and proportions. 2nd Ed. New York: Wiley, 1981, 33–49.

Economic analysis in diabetes

A. Haddix, E. Dasbach, S. Teutsch

Introduction

Economic analysis is one of a series of tools available to policy makers that combines information about the benefits of a therapeutic intervention with the costs incurred. When resources are unlimited, it is natural to do everything for a patient when the health benefits exceed the health risks. However, when resources are limited, it becomes imperative that these resources be used as judiciously as possible to provide the greatest benefit possible commensurate with the resources available. Economic analyses are useful to help allocate resources wisely and allow for a comparison of the benefits achieved with the costs incurred among a series of alternate treatment or preventive strategies for a single problem; among different strategies for different problems; or among different strategies for entirely different outcomes, e. g., should resources be devoted to health or education. This information can serve as an additional piece of information when recommending appropriate care and in developing guidelines for public health and clinical practice.

Because economic analyses are used as part of policy decision making, e. g., should a medical procedure be covered by insurance or should an education program be supported, they should be part of answers to a series of questions, such as

- What is the magnitude of the problem (incidence or prevalence)?
- How well does the intervention work (effectiveness)?
- How much does the intervention cost (cost analysis)?
- What alternative strategies are there and how do they compare (decision analysis)?
- How much do I gain for additional expenditures (cost-effectiveness, cost-benefit, or cost-utility analysis)?

Economic analyses of technologies (preventive and therapeutic interventions) include *cost-analysis (CA), cost-effectiveness (CEA), cost-benefit (CBA), and cost-utility (CUA) analysis.* All but cost analysis require a measure of the effectiveness of the technology. The natural history of the development of technologies leads to progressively more refined measures of effectiveness [1].

Offprint from
Research Methodologies in Human Diabetes – Part 1

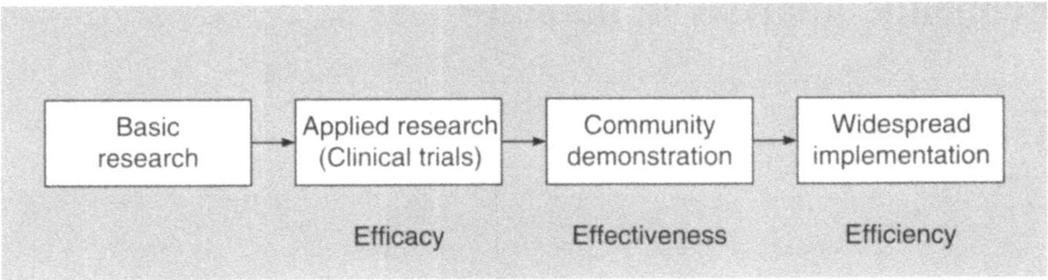

Fig. 1 Relationship between the stage of development of a technology and the assessment of its impact

As technologies are developed and implemented, they progress through a series of stages (Fig. 1). Clinical research generally provides information regarding the *efficacy* of a treatment modality, or how well the therapy works under ideal circumstances, where patients are carefully selected, providers have particular interest and skills in the treatment under investigation, and care of the patient is greatly facilitated.

One rarely is able to achieve the same level of benefit in community-based settings, where all patients must be considered, access to care may be less than ideal, adherence to clinical regimens may be compromised, and motivation of providers and patients may be more modest. In this situation, the magnitude of the benefits achieved is called the *effectiveness* of the treatment or prevention modality. Information on effectiveness should be generated from community-based settings. Developing such information may require population-based studies or databases that contain information on clinical services rendered and health outcomes achieved. Computerized medical records and data bases linking information on individuals may be of particular value in assessing medical effectiveness.

Because economic analysis compares the benefits of treatment with the costs incurred, it is important to properly identify the technology to be evaluated and to what it is to be compared. In most cases, the comparison is between one treatment and another or no treatment at all. In general, one wants to assess the costs and benefits in practical community-based settings, and, consequently, the economic impact should be based on the effectiveness, rather than the efficacy of therapy.

Methods of economic analysis

Before an economic evaluation is conducted, the method and scope of the study must be clearly defined.

Evaluation method

Four types of economic evaluations are commonly conducted to assist in the selection of appropriate health care programs; *cost-analysis (CA), cost-effectiveness analysis (CEA), cost-utility analysis (CUA), and cost-benefit analysis (CBA).*

Cost analysis: A CA is conducted to calculate the net cost of an intervention, treatment course, or to determine the cost of an illness.

Cost-effectiveness analysis: CEA compares the costs of alternative interventions or treatment courses per health outcome achieved. CEA is the most frequently used technique to compare alternative treatment courses or interventions [2]. Four scenarios for which CEA is most suited are [3]:

- comparing alternative treatments for an identical goal;
- determining the most effective utilization of funds earmarked for a specific population;
- providing empirical support for the adoption of previously underfunded medical programs with low cost-effectiveness ratios; and
- identifying care practices which are not worth their cost.

A health outcome often used in cost-effectiveness analyses is the life year saved. Other outcome measures include lives saved, cases prevented, and cases identified.

Cost-utility analysis: CUA is a special case of CEA, whereby the benefits are measured in standardized units allowing comparison across a wide range of diseases. This standard metric should have the ability to measure effectiveness of health programs that improve length of life as well as quality of life. To meet these requirements, the health economics field adopted the quality adjusted life year (QALY) as a standard metric from which to conduct CUAs. The QALY integrates quality of life with length of life by discounting length of life by the quality of life expected using a multiplicative formula. Several methods have been developed for adjusting life expectancy by quality of life [4–7]. Both CEA and CUA have cost as a numerator and health effects as the denominator. They are the most suitable methods for the health sector.

Cost-benefit analysis: CBA is an economic evaluation in which all costs and benefits are measured in monetary terms and expressed as dollars of benefit per dollar expended. CBAs are conducted when the net resource cost of a program is the desired outcome measure. CBAs, however, are often difficult to conduct when evaluating health programs. The economic and ethical difficulties associated with measuring health outcomes in monetary terms limit the usefulness of this evaluation method.

Scope

Once the appropriate method of analysis has been selected, the scope of the evaluation must be defined. The scope dictates what costs and consequences should be included in the analysis. Defining the scope of the analysis involves defining both the economic perspective and the time frame of the analysis.

Perspective: To define the perspective, the question, "who is responsible for the costs and consequences of the services being evaluated?", needs to be answered. For example, will society, the Federal Government, a State Government, an employer, a private health insurer, or an individual be responsible for the costs and consequences of the service? These are just a handful of the many economic viewpoints that can be adopted in an economic evaluation. Each viewpoint may require measuring different costs and consequences. Measuring the cost of blindness from the viewpoint of the U.S. Federal Government, for instance, should include at least the cost of assistance provided through Social Security Disability Income (SSDI) and Supplemental Security Income (SSI). A private health insurer, on the other hand, is not responsible for paying SSDI or SSI to their beneficiaries. As a consequence of adopting this narrower perspective, the resulting policies may not be optimal for the health of the general public. Instead, a more useful perspective to adopt is one that considers all the costs to the entire health care system because the resulting policies will maximize the efficiency of the health care system for the general public [8]. Economic analyses typically use the societal perspective. This approach includes all social and program costs regardless of who pays for or receives the benefits.

Time frame: The second step in defining the scope is to define the time frame in which program costs and consequences will occur. Studies may cover one or more years in which the intervention or treatment course is delivered. The time frame of the analysis should include and be limited to the time period when the intervention or the treatment costs are incurred and benefits realized.

A one-year time frame is often practical. Data from health-care facilities are often available for a calendar or a fiscal year, e. g., the number of tests or persons participating in a program may be available for a one year period.

Use of data for a full year smoothes out any seasonal variation on participation. A multi-year time frame may be more appropriate when there is an extended start-up time, high initial cost, or the treatment course is long. A multi-year time frame is also appropriate for interventions with high initial costs.

In multi-year evaluations and in evaluations in which the disease or complications averted occur in future years, the *present value* of costs and benefits *discounted* to the base year of the analysis is used. Discounting is a method for adjusting the value of future costs and benefits. Discounting – expressed as the present value of a dollar – is based on the time-value of money, i. e., a dollar today is worth more than it will be a year from now (even if inflation is not considered). Further discussion of discounting, the calculation, and selection of a discount rate is presented elsewhere [9, 10].

Similarly in a CBA, the net present value (NPV) of costs [(costs-benefits)/ $(1 + r)^t$] where r is the discount rate and t is the time period is preferred to the cost-benefit ratio since many factors may be included as either a cost or a negative benefit. Hence, researchers using the same data might find different cost-benefit ratios.

Measuring costs

The cost of a program should reflect the *opportunity cost* of the resources expended. The opportunity cost of a program represents the foregone benefits of not using the resources on the next best alternative program. When comparing the costs of alternative health programs, the appropriate method is to use marginal or net costs rather than average costs. Net costs provide the ability to set priorities when allocating resources to health programs.

$$\text{Net Cost} = \text{Cost}_{\text{Intervention}} + \text{Cost}_{\text{Sideeffects}} - \text{Cost}_{\text{Disease}} - \text{Cost}_{\text{Indirect}}$$

Costs are broken down into the cost of the intervention ($Cost_{Intervention}$), the costs of the side effects of the intervention ($Cost_{Sideeffects}$), less the costs of diagnosis and treatment associated with the disease ($Cost_{Disease}$) which was avoided as a result of the intervention, and the indirect costs ($Cost_{Indirect}$) saved or incurred as a result of changes in productivity resulting from morbidity or premature mortality.

Intervention costs: Every intervention or treatment course requires resources for implementation and maintenance. These include direct labor for services rendered, facilities and utilities, equipment and supplies, and administrative support. Intervention costs may be categorized as either *fixed* or *variable costs.* Fixed costs are those that do not vary in the short run. They are independent of the quantity of the intervention delivered. Examples of fixed costs include rent, equipment lease payments, salaries, and administrative overhead. Variable costs are the costs associated with the delivery of a unit of the intervention. Examples of variable costs include laboratory tests, physician visits, and drug costs. Categorization of fixed and variable costs becomes important in the computation of incremental costs for CEA and CUA.

One category of fixed cost that deserves mention is *capital costs* [11, 12]. Capital costs represent an investment in an asset which is used over time. Capital costs either may be recorded in the year expended or may be amortized over the life of the asset.

Cost of side effects: Costs of side effects of the intervention include the expenses associated with incidental findings and hazards and psychological effects associated with the intervention itself. Costs may include medical expenses and the value of lost productivity as a result of the side effect.

Cost of disease averted: Cost of disease averted includes the direct costs of medical care that would have been associated with management had the disease or complications not been prevented.

Indirect costs: Indirect costs measure the effect of changes in health status that result from the intervention or treatment course on an individual's productivity. These are costs to society of premature morbidity and mortality associated with illness. Thus, if one can avert disease, one averts the morbidity and mortality that occur with that disease. Two methods of determining the monetary value of morbidity and mortality are the *human capital* and the *willingness-to-pay* approaches. The human capital approach values this loss as the income not earned by these individuals. The willingness-to-pay approach values this loss as what someone might be willing to spend to avert this particular event. The inclusion of indirect costs in economic evaluation is not universally accepted. To address this issue, studies may report results of analysis with and without the indirect costs. Details of the calculation of indirect costs can be found elsewhere [13–15].

Sensitivity analysis: Sensitivity analyses are conducted to examine the magnitude and direction of effects when one or more variables are changed to reflect the range of uncertainty about their estimates.

Examples of economic analysis

This section reviews examples of economic evaluations of diabetes health programs published in the literature. We have selected three examples of economic evaluations of diabetes health programs to review for this section. Each article exemplifies a different type of economic evaluation: a *CEA*, a *CBA*, and a *CUA*.

Cost-effectiveness analyses

CEAs represent the majority of the economic evaluations of diabetes health programs published in the literature. Of these evaluations, many have focused on assessing the cost-effectiveness of alternative strategies for detecting and treating diabetic retinopathy [15–23]. The following reviews one of these studies.

Alternatives: This economic evaluation compared six alternative strategies for detecting and treating diabetic retinopathy. A baseline case represented the natural progression of diabetic retinopathy [18]. Each of the six alternatives represented a combination of administering one of three imaging examinations either annually or biannually. The three imaging examinations included opthalmoscopy through a dilated eye, non-mydriatic fundus photography, and mydriatic photography. Studies [24, 25] have established the operating characteristics of these three diagnostic techniques. The Diabetic Retinopathy Study established that timely laser therapy was an efficacious intervention for reducing the risk of vision loss in persons with diabetic retinopathy [26].

Perspective: The economic evaluation adopted an economic viewpoint of that of a state or national initiative that was responsible for the cost and consequences of detecting and treating diabetic retinopathy.

Costs, Consequences, and time frame: The cost of each alternative was based on the resources required to provide the diagnostic and treatment service. For example, the study derived the cost of the ophthalmoscopy screening visit by determining the cost of the labor, supplies, materials, and overhead required to provide the service. The cost of not providing ophthalmologic care included the rehabilitative and maintenance costs associated with blindness. The benefits of detection and treatment were measured in sight-years. The analysis computed the total costs and benefits for each alternative by simulating the progression of diabetic retinopathy in three hypothetical cohorts of persons with diabetes (i. e., persons with insulin-dependent diabetes mellitus (IDDM), those with non-insulin-dependent diabetes mellitus (NIDDM) taking insulin, and those with NIDDM not taking insulin) and accruing the costs and benefits over a 60-year period. To accrue costs and sight years, the analysis discounted costs and sight years to 1989 values at an annual rate of 5%. Incremental costs were computed by subtracting the costs of the baseline case from the costs of an alternative.

Benefits were measured in sight years. In particular, sight years gained were computed by subtracting the number of sight years realized with an alternative from the number of sight years realized by the baseline case. The analysis measured economic efficiency in units of incremental cost per sight year gained.

Results: The results of the economic evaluation indicated that biannual and annual detection programs can be cost saving in the two insulin-taking cohorts. In other words, biannual and annual detection and treatment programs were more effective and less expensive than the baseline alternative. For instance, annual screening in the IDDM cohort with a mydriatic camera saved $ 3,200 for every sight year gained. These cost savings were realized because detection and treatment prevented blindness and the rehabilitative and maintenance costs associated with blindness. For the NIDDM cohort not taking insulin, only biannual ophthalmoscopy was cost saving. The other alternatives were all more effective, but more costly than the baseline case. For example, annual screening with a mydriatic camera cost $ 6,540 for every sight year gained. This finding, however, does not mean that the biannual and annual programs are not worth the cost in the NIDDM cohort. How much one is willing to pay for the added benefit is a policy decision.

Sensitivity analyses: Sensitivity analyses indicated that the results of the evaluation were fairly robust even when the prevalence of those individuals with retinopathy at a high risk for visual loss decreased to 1% in the population. In addition, biannual mydriatic photography was found to be more effective than annual screening by the other two modalities if the sensitivity of the other two modalities decreased below 65%.

This study is just one of many that have examined the cost effectiveness of strategies for detecting and treating diabetic retinopathy. Others [16, 17, 20] have reported similar findings. We encourage the reader to review these other studies as well other cost-effectiveness analyses such as one of the cost-effectiveness of screening and early treatment of nephropathy in persons with IDDM [27].

Cost-benefit analyses

Only a small number of CBAs of diabetes health programs have been reported in the literature. The following reviews a cost-benefit analysis of a preconception care program.

Alternatives: One study [28] assessed the costs and benefits of a preconception care program aimed at recruiting pre-pregnant women with diabetes and providing comprehensive prenatal care. The costs of this program were compared with the cost of not providing this type of care to pregnant women with diabetes. Previous research had established that preconception care can reduce the complications associated with diabetes in pregnancy [29].

Perspective: The analysis did not explicitly state the economic viewpoint. However given the nature of the data collected in the study, a reasonable viewpoint from which to interpret the results might be from a third party payer such as a state Medicaid program or a private health insurer.

Costs, consequences, and time frame: The scope of the economic evaluation included the time from initiation of preconception care to post-delivery hospitalization discharge. Thus, only short-term costs were included and long-term medical costs due to adverse birth outcomes were excluded. The costs of the preconception care program were computed by determining the labor and overhead required to provide the service. The benefits of the preconception care program were derived by calculating the hospitalization savings realized by reducing the length of hospitalization for labor and delivery of women who had received preconception care relative to the length of hospitalization of women who had not received preconception care. The study collected total charges from the billing histories for all mothers in the two intervention groups. Charges incurred over the duration of pregnancy, for delivery, and for neonatal care from birth to discharge were included in the analysis. Given the preconception care program savings were realized some time after the preconception care was initiated, the study discounted the savings to present value at an annual rate of 8%. Costs and benefits were combined as the ratio of benefits to costs in dollar units.

Results: The preconception are program had a benefit-cost ratio of 5.19 to 1. In other words, for every dollar spent on the preconception care program, there is an estimated savings of $ 5.19. These short-term economic savings are primarily realized by the shorter length of stay experienced by mothers and their babies who participated in the preconception care program relative to the length of hospital stay of the mothers and babies who had not participated in the preconception care program.

Sensitivity analyses: The benefit-cost ratio reported was a conservative estimate. The savings depended greatly on when women enroll in the preconception care program as well as on the severity of the diabetes of the women who enrolled. Specifically, greater savings can be realized in women with severe diabetes who enroll before conception. The annual savings attributable to the preconception care program in California ranges from $ 14 million to $ 19 million, depending on how many women enroll in the program before conception.

Cost-Utility analyses

We were able to locate only one CUA of a program for preventing diabetic complications in the literature. It reported the results of a cost-utility analysis of a diet and exercise intervention aimed at improving quality of life in persons with NIDDM [30]. This cost-utility analysis was a secondary study within a larger clinical trial aimed at demonstrating the benefits of dietary changes and exercise in persons with NIDDM.

Alternatives: The clinical trial demonstrated that an intervention consisting of diet and exercise improved quality of life when compared with the control intervention of basic education.

Perspective: The economic viewpoint of the evaluation was not stated.
Costs, consequences, and time frame: The cost of the diet and exercise intervention was based on 1986 clinical charges in the San Diego, California community. Benefits were measured in quality-adjusted life-year (QALY) units. The Quality of Well-Being health utility index [31] was used to derive the QALY benefits associated with each alternative. Costs and QALYs were measured only for the year 1986. Thus, discounting was not necessary. Marginal costs and QALYs gained were computed as net increases over the control program.

Results: This study reported that the marginal cost per QALY gained for the intervention program was $ 10,870. This was comparable to the economic efficiency of other widely advocated health care programs.

Sensitivity analyses: Sensitivity analyses were not reported.

Conclusion

Economic analyses of prevention, treatment, and control of diabetes and its complications are important adjuncts to studies of efficacy and effectiveness. By carefully examining the costs and health outcomes, clinicians, public health practitioners, and health policy markers can make more prudent judgments concerning the appropriateness and relative advantages of alternative therapeutic and preventive care strategies.

References

[1] Teutsch, SM. A framework for assessing the effectiveness of disease and Injury prevention. Morb Mort Weekly Rep 1992; 41: RR–S.
[2] Weinstein MC, Stason WB. Foundations of cost-effectiveness for health and medical practices. N Engl J Med 1977; 296: 716–21.
[3] Emery DD, Schneiderman LJ. Cost-effectiveness analysis in health care. Hastings Center Report, 8–13, July/August 1989.
[4] Froberg DG, Kane RL. Methodology for measuring health state preferences. J Clin Epidemiology 1989; 42 (4, 5, 6, 7).
[5] Torrance GW, Boyle MH, Horwood SP. Application of multi-attribute utility theory to measure of social preferences for health states. Oper Res 1982: 30 (6).
[6] Kaplan RM, Bush JW, Berry CC. Health status: types of validity and the index of well-being. Health Services Res 1976.
[7] Nord E. Methods for quality adjustment of life years. Soc Sci Med 1992; 34 (5): 559–569.
[8] Eddy EM. Assessing Health Practices and Designing Practice Policies. American College of Physicians, 1992.
[9] Drummond MF, Stoddart GL, Torrance GW. Methods for the economic evaluation of health care programmes. Oxford, UK: Oxford University Press, 1987.
[10] Sassone PG, Schaffer WA. Cost-benefit analysis – A handbook. San Diego, California: Academic Press, 1978.
[11] Richardson AW, Gafni A. Treatment of capital costs in evaluating health-care programs. Cost and Management 1983; Nov.–Dec: 26–30.
[12] Levin HM. Cost-effectiveness analysis in evaluation research. In: Guttentag M and Struening EL, eds. Handbook of evaluation research. Vol 2. 1975: 89–122.
[13] Luce BR, Elixhauser A. Standards for socioeconomic evaluation of health care products and services. New York: Springer-Verlag, 1990.
[14] Rice DP, Hodgson TA, Kopstein AN. The economic costs of illness: A replication and update. Health Care Finance Review 1985; 7: 61–80.
[15] Koopmanschap MA, van Ineveld BM. Towards a new approach for estimating indirect costs of disease. Soc Sci Med 1992; 34: 1005–1010.
[16] Javitt JC, Canner JK, Sommer A. Cost effectiveness of current approaches to the control of retinopathy in type 1 diabetics. Ophthalmology 1989; 96: 255–264.
[17] Javitt JC, Canner JK, Frank RG et al. Detecting and treating retinopathy in patients with type 1 diabetes mellitus. Ophthalmology 1990; 97: 483–494.
[18] Dasbach EJ, Fryback DG, Newcomb PA et al. Cost effectiveness of strategies for detecting diabetic retinopathy. Medical Care 1991; 29: 20–39.
[19] Schulpher MJ, Buxton MJ, Ferguson JE et al. A relative cost-effectiveness analysis of different methods of screening for diabetic retinopathy. Diabetic Medicine 1991; 8: 644–650.

[20] Javitt JC, Aiello LP, Bassi LJ et al. Detecting and treating retinopathy in patients with type 1 diabetes mellitus. Ophthalmology 1991; 98: 1565–1573.
[21] Schulpher MJ, Buxton MJ, Ferguson JE et al. Screening for diabetic retinopathy: A relative cost-effectiveness analysis of alternative modalities and strategies. Health Economics 1992; 1: 39–50.
[22] Lairson DR, Pugh JA, Kapadia AS. Cost effectiveness of alternative methods for diabetic retinopathy screening. Diabetes Care 1992; 10: 1369–1377.
[23] Fendrick AM, Javitt JC, Chaing YP. Cost effectiveness of the screening and treatment of diabetic retinopathy. Int J of Technology Assessment in Health Care 1992; 8: 694–707.
[24] Moss SE, Klein R, Kessler OD et al. Comparison between ophthalmoscopy and fundus photography in determining severity of diabetic retinopathy. Ophthalmology 1985; 92: 62.
[25] Klein R, Klein BEK, Neider MW et al. Diabetic retinopathy as detected using ophthalmoscopy, a non-mydriatic camera, and a standard fundus camera. Ophthalmology 1985; 92: 485.
[26] Diabetic Retinopathy Study Group. Photocoagulation treatment of proliferative diabetic retinopathy: Clinical application of diabetic retinopathy study (DRS) findings. (DRS report No. 8) Ophthalmology 1982; 88: 583.
[27] Siegel JE, Krowlewski AS, Warram JH et al. Cost effectiveness of screening and early treatment of nephropathy in patients with insulin-dependent diabetes mellitus. J Am Soc Nephr 1992; 3: S111–S119.
[28] Scheffler RM, Feutchbaum LB, Ciaran SP. Prevention: The cost-effectiveness of the California Diabetes and Pregnancy Program. AJPH 1992; 82: 168–175.
[29] Kitzmiller JL, Gavin LA, Gin GD et al. Preconception care of diabetes: glycemic control prevents congenital anomalies. JAMA 1991; 265: 731–736.
[30] Kaplan RM, Hartwell SL, Wilson DK et al. Effects of diet and exercise interventions on control and quality of life in non-insulin-dependent diabetes mellitus. J Gen Int Med 1987; 2: 220–228.
[31] Kaplan RM, Atkins CJ, Timms RM. Validity of a quality of well-being scale as an outcome measure in chronic obstructive pulmonary disease. J Chron Dis 1984; 37: 85–95.

Research methodologies in connective tissue changes and diabetic skin disease

Th. Danne

Introduction

Diabetes is associated with a variety of connective tissue changes and skin disorders [1]. These disorders can be divided into those associated with diabetes-related neurovascular complications, such occurring in a higher incidence in diabetes due to the metabolic disorder, or alterations resulting from cutaneous complications of treatment. This review will focus on non-invasive research methodologies of connective tissue abnormalities, such as quantitative and qualitative changes of collagen and other components of the extracellular matrix, which are associated with the development of microangiopathy and may therefore serve as markers for its early detection [2]. In human diabetes this can be investigated by clinical examination, by testing of skin microvascular and nerve function and by determinations of matrix components in body fluids. As techniques examining skin microvascular function by percutaneous measurements will be discussed elsewhere, this review will concentrate on the clinical entity described as diabetic "cheiroarthropathy" or "limited joint mobility" (LJM) and deal with methods for blood and urine determination of connective tissue metabolism in human diabetes.

Biochemical changes of extracellular matrix components in diabetes

The extracellular matrix consists of the classical interstitium, which occupies intercellular spaces, and basement membranes, which are sheet-like protein matrices providing structural support for epithelial, endothelial and certain mesenchymal cells contributing to the permselectivity of the capillary wall. As thickening of retinal and glomerular basement membranes (GBM) are regarded as one ultrastructural hallmark of diabetic microangiopathy [3], most of our knowledge on matrix changes in diabetes comes from the investigation of the glomerulus.

Offprint from
Research Methodologies in Human Diabetes – Part 1

The major macromolecular components of the matrix are collagen, glycoproteins and proteoglycans. The distinctive basement membrane collagen (type IV) is its predominant constituent and comprises approximately 70% by weight of the GBM [4]. Collagens are proteins composed of three similar or identical polypeptide chains, called α-chains, folded into a triple helix, which gives the molecule a particular stability. Type IV collagen forms a mesh-like network, which gives structural support to the basement membrane.

The second major group of matrix proteins are glycoproteins constituting key elements in its structural organisation. Laminin is the major glycoprotein of all basement membranes. The molecule has been assigned a central role in anchoring cells to various matrix components, including type IV collagen and heparan sulfate proteoglycan. The protease-resistent P1 fragment of laminin can be determined in serum [5]. Fibronectin, which is widely distributed in interstitial connective tissues and mediates cellular adhesion to the extracellular matrix, exists in both a matrix form and a soluble form in plasma. The plasma form is produced by the reticuloendothelial system and is probably independent from the insoluble matrix form [6].

The third group of basement membrane components are proteoglycans. They are believed to be responsible for the charge selectivity of the GBM. Their quantitative changes in the basement membrane play a central role in the Steno hypothesis for the development of diabetic late complications [7].

The function of the basement membrane depends upon its biochemical integrity and the correct interaction of all structural constituents. Quantitative measurements in tissue samples of patients with diabetes have revealed distinct changes, which represent the biochemical basis for basement membrane thickening and mesangial expansion [2]. Initial evidence for compositional changes came from amino acid analyses indicating that constituents associated with collagen (i.e. proteins rich in hydroxylysine, hydroxyproline etc.) are increased in diabetes [8]. Due to the great difficulty to quantitatively solubilise collagen, to this date no major study has quantitatively determined the type IV collagen content in samples of human GBM. Determinations of other components have been made with immunochemical methods. Recently, type VI collagen has been found to be elevated in the GBM of patients with diabetes [9]. In contrast to collagen, laminin and heparan sulfate have been shown to be decreased while no change was observed for fibronectin [10]. Despite clearcut statistical differences, a considerable overlap exists between the tissue values of these constituents in patients and controls. This may be due in part to the difficulty of solubilisation, but may also reflect differences in responses of matrix producing cells from one individual to another when exposed to the diabetic milieu. In accordance with the scarce data in patients with diabetes, results in animal models with experimental diabetes demonstrate that the outstanding feature of the biochemical changes of matrix metabolism is an increase in the amount of type IV collagen [4].

Clinical examination and classification of diabetic cheiroarthropathy

The association of limited joint mobility to microangiopathy [11] is still controversial and requires additional longitudinal studies [12]. After its first

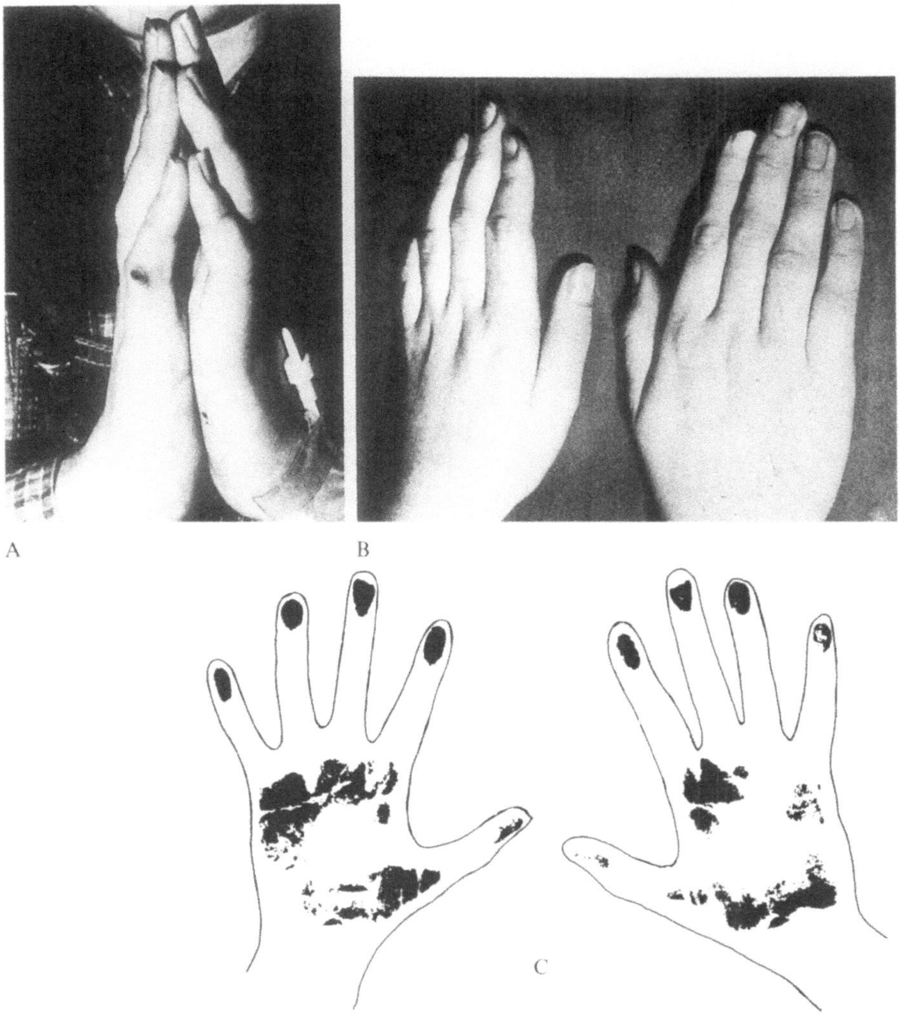

Fig. 1 Examination of active joint movement (A and B) and documentation of total handprints on paper in a patient with LJM grade II (C) (taken from [19] with permission)

Table 1 Classification of diabetes-related cheiroarthropathy

LJM		Functional impairment	Skin	X-Ray
0	hands and fingers normal, no active or passive impairment of mobility	no	negative	negative
I	a active and passive restriction of movement of 1st and 2nd interphalangeal joints on both 5th fingers or	no	minimally thickened cerous skin over the affected joints	negative
	b interphalangeal and metacarpophalangeal joints of the 1st fingers or/and	no	as above	negative
	c the 1st interphalangeal joints of the 4th and the 5th finger or the metacarpophalangeal joints on both hands	no	as above	negative
II	≥ 3 small joints of the fingers with active and passive restriction of movement, plus joints of the wrist and/or cervical vertebrae and/or 1 further big joint, symmetrical bilateral affection	yes	markedly visible skin affection over the affected joints	slightly abnormal positions
III	fixed joint contractures of hands, fingers and further joints	yes	tight, tense, glossy, waxy, thickened, also on trunk and all extremities	joint contractions

description by Rosenbloom et al in 1974 [13], several groups have described LJM in their patient populations. While the initial studies suggested that its occurrence is primarily in young patients with type 1 diabetes, recent studies demonstrate that it may also affect older patients with type 2 diabetes [14]. Further indications that the limited joint mobility reflects a more widespread abnormality of the connective tissue come from findings of thick, tight, waxy skin and abnormal pulmonary function in patients with LJM [15] and from altered levels of blood parameters of connective tissue metabolism [2, 16].

Although subclinical joint abnormalities can already be detected using a goniometer [17], LJM is conventionally studied by clinical examination. However, the classification of the distinct features of cheiroarthropathy in the literature varies and makes comparisons between the published studies difficult. We suggest using a classification similar to that published by Rosenbloom [18], which provides a subdivision into different categories of severity, categorised as stages I, II, and III (Table 1) [19]. For the examination, patients should be asked to approximate the palmar surfaces of their hands with slightly spread fingers or to place their palmar surfaces on a table (Fig. 1). Whenever there is space left between the fingers, the passive extension of the fingers shall be examined by applying gentle pressure on the proximal interphalangeal joints. Severe impairments of function can easily be documented by total handprints on paper (Fig. 1). Rheumatic, traumatic and other reasons for joint contractures have to be excluded by a careful patient history and appropriate laboratory examinations.

Methodologies for the non-invasive monitoring of connective tissue metabolism

Background

Due to the invasive nature of tissue biopsies, it is of great importance for larger clinical studies to find parameters allowing the monitoring of matrix changes with minimal patient discomfort, for example by measurements of matrix components in serum or urine. Novel immunological methods allow the detection of matrix antigens in body fluids and have provided valuable information in patients with matrix-related diseases like rheumatism or fibrotic liver disease [20, 21], growth disorders [22] or kidney diseases [23]. The value of these assays is supported by studies in animals with experimentally induced diabetes revealing increased serum levels of laminin [24] and type IV collagen, which can be corrected by insulin treatment [24], but not by an aldose-reductase-inhibitor [25]. Hypertension [26] and protein rich diets [27] promote further elevation of these antigens. A direct correlation has been described between the incorporation of a radioactive label into the glomerular basement membrane and serum type IV collagen antigens [28]. No evidence has been found for an alteration of the composition or the clearance rate of these antigens in diabetes [29]. Therefore, the serum levels seem to be directly related to the biochemical alterations found in the analysis of the diabetic basement membrane.

General methodological aspects

The theoretical aspects of immunoassays for the connective tissue proteins have been reviewed elsewhere [20], as have practical advice concerning immunisation procedures and setting up an assay [30]. Most methods are

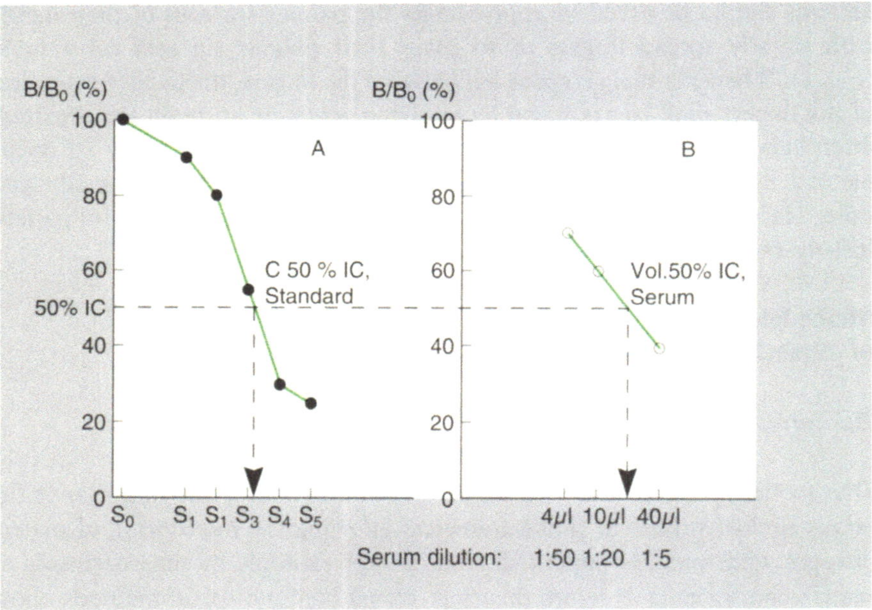

Fig. 2 The 50% intercept method for calculating the result in an immunoassay in which the inhibition curves by the standard antigen (A) and the unknown sample (B) are not parallel. In principle the volume of the unknown sample (empty circles) that gives 50% inhibition of the reaction is assumed to contain the amount of antigen that according to the inhibition curve of the standard (solid circles) causes 50% inhibition. For calculation of the sample concentration, the total volume of the reaction (in the example 200 µl) divided by the volume of the unknown serum at the intercept (Vol. 50% IC) multiplied by the concentration of the standard (C 50% IC) gives the amount of antigen in the unknown sample [31]

established as inhibition assays, either as radioimmunoassay (RIA) or enzyme-linked immunoassay (ELISA). These are usually set up as inhibition assays where the inhibitions achieved by the known standard concentrations are used to construct a standard curve for the estimation of the unknown samples. If the slopes of the inhibition curves for the standard and the unknown sample are parallel, any point of the steep portion of the curve, usually between inhibitions of 20 and 80%, can be used for estimating the antigen concentration of the unknown sample. However, due to the complexity and heterogeneity of many circulating connective tissue protein fragments, a non-parallel inhibition by the samples and the standards is frequently found. It has therefore been suggested that in such situations the apparent concentration of the sample could be calculated from the point where this sample exhibits 50% inhibition, by the so-called 50% intercept method [31] (Fig. 2), although this method is controversial [20]. Another approach to circumvent this problem has been the use of monovalent Fab fragments of the antibodies instead of the polyvalent antiserum [32].

Methods for determination of individual connective tissue proteins and results in human diabetes

Type III collagen: Type III collagen is a collagen found in interstitial connective tissue. The serum levels of the aminoterminal procollagen type III propeptide have been investigated primarily in fibrotic liver diseases [21]. As the aminoterminal propeptide is cleaved in a stoichiometric relationship from the type III collagen molecule prior to the integration into the fibrillar network, it can be used to estimate type III collagen biosynthesis. However, some material may also result from collagen breakdown as the propeptide is incompletely cleaved. The circulating antigen consists of the intact aminoterminal propeptide (molecular weight 45 000 Da), high molecular weight aggregates, as well as lower molecular breakdown products. Recent assay procedures recognise exclusively (PIII – RIA, Farmos, Oulu, Finnland) or predominantly (P – IIIP – RIA "coated tube", Hoechst, Frankfurt, Germany) the intact propeptide [21]. Investigations in diabetes have been carried out with earlier assay systems recognising various species of type III propeptide-related antigens and revealed unaltered levels in type 1 diabetes [33] and elevated levels in patients with type 2 diabetes and vascular complications [34]. In general, type III collagen biosynthesis is closely related to growth, which makes interpretation of values in childhood and adolescence difficult [22].

Table 2 Type IV collagen in serum and urine

Patients	Fragment	Unit	Control*	Diabetes* mellitus	Related to angiopathy	Author (Year) [Reference]
Type 1/2	?	plasma (ng/ml)	76 ± 9 (n = 101)	88 ± 10 (n = 183)	yes	Alland (1984) [42]
Type 1/2	7S	serum (ng/ml)	8 ± 1 (n = 21)	42 ± 5 (n = 70)	yes	Högemann (1986) [37]
Type 1 (children)	NC1	serum (ng/ml)	8 ± 2 (n = 511)	9 ± 2 (n = 110)	no	Danne (1988) [40]
Type 1	NC1	serum (ng/ml)	99 ± 3 (n = 46)	98 ± 5 (n = 36)	no	Torffvit (1989) [36]
		urine (ng/µg creatinine)	1.4 ± 0.2 (n = 54)	2.9 ± 0.3 (n = 59)	yes	
Type 2	7S/NC1	serum (ng/ml)	74 ± 2 (n = 110)	124 ± 4 (n = 137)	yes	Matsumoto (1990) [41]
Type 2	7S?	serum (ng/ml)	9.6 ± 0.3 (n = 53)	20–30 (n = 43)	yes	Watanabe (1991) [43]
		urine (ng/µg creatinine)	500 ± 300 (n = 11)	1000–3200 (n = 36)	yes	
Type 2	7S	serum (ng/ml)	3.4 ± 1.4 (n = 20)	5.3 ± 1.5 (n = 185)	yes	Tomono (1991) [44]
Type 2	7S/NC1	serum (ng/ml)	63 ± 4 (n = 18)	70–144 (n = 72)	yes	Hayashi (1992) [45]
		urine (ng/µg creatinine)	31 ± 3 (n = 36)	45–277 (n = 58)		

* Mean ± 1 SD are given for the patients with diabetes mellitus and controls. When patients with diabetes were divided into groups with different degrees of late complications the range between the mean of the group without to the group with most severe complications is given

Type IV collagen: The type IV collagen molecule contains antigenic determinants in its central triplehelical part and in both of its termini, the aminoterminal 7S domain and the carboxyterminal cross-linking (NC1 = non-collagenous fragment 1) domain. Assays measuring these antigens in human samples have been developed with polyclonal antibodies for NC1 [35, 36] and the 7S domain [37, 38], as well as a sandwich immunoassay system with monoclonal antibodies, which are believed to be directed against the large triple-helical region of type IV collagen [39], but are cross-reacting in part with both 7S and NC1. The NC1 serum levels are independent of growth during childhood after the first two years of life [40] and are therefore suited for studies in children and adolescents with diabetes.

As expected from the results of the animal studies, some cross-sectional studies in adults with diabetes demonstrated elevated levels of type IV collagen associated to the presence of microangiopathy [36, 37, 40–45] (Table 2). The discrepancy in the published concentrations of type IV collagen serum antigens demonstrate that the antibodies used in the various assays appear to differ in their affinity to the various circulating fragments. Clearly, better standardisation has to be achieved. Nevertheless, it appears that assays involving the detection of the 7S fragment show a relationship to microangiopathy and to LJM [16], while human serum NC1 does not. However, recent results of a long-term follow-up study indicate that elevated levels of serum NC1 in patients without complications are indicative of the later development of complications [46].

Assay procedures for NC1 or the central triplehelical part of type IV collagen allow the detection of this fragment in urine. Different urine concentration procedures may have contributed to the variation in urinary levels. In contrast to the serum levels, the urinary NC1 concentrations show an association to microangiopathy and may therefore be a better parameter for the study of glomerular type IV collagen metabolism than serum values [36]. Urinary NC1 levels in patients with glomerulonephritis were independent of kidney function, but related to the degree of proteinuria, thus indicating intrinsic renal disease [23].

Type VI collagen: Recent studies indicate that not only type IV, but also type VI collagen may be involved in diabetic matrix pathology. The quantitation of the type VI collagen content in the glomerular basement membrane revealed a 2.8-fold higher level in diabetic preparations [9]. Similar results were reported for experimental diabetic cardiomyopathy [47]. Furthermore, it was identified to be the molecule responsible for the periodic acid-Schiff (PAS) reactivity of the increased extracellular matrix in both the diabetic kidney and the heart [48].

Type VI collagen can be detected by RIA [49], as well as by an ELISA modification of this assay [50]. The type VI collagen antigen was prepared from extracts of human placenta. These assays recognize fragments of the intact type VI collagen molecule which appear to be liberated into serum through degradation.

Preliminary results in adolescents with diabetes show unaltered serum levels even in patients with early angiopathy, while elevated values are found during diabetic ketoacidosis [51]. However, as type VI collagen is produced in the glomerulus predominantly by mesangial cells [9], and since mesangial expansion is believed to be a central event leading to the loss of kidney function in patients with diabetes, the determination of type VI collagen in urine may reflect better than serum values the mesangial pathology in diabetes. Indeed, the exposure of mesangial cells to high glucose was found to lead to increased type VI collagen production [52].

Laminin: Although studies in experimental diabetes indicate that the laminin synthesis (i. e. steady-state levels of laminin mRNA) is increased in diabetes [53], analyses of diabetic tissue samples found decreased levels of laminin [10]. In view of these observations, elevated levels in serum or urine could reflect either a decreased incorporation into or an accelerated loss of this glycoprotein from the basement membrane.

The non-collagenous basement membrane glycoprotein laminin has major antigenic determinants in its central region (P1 fragment, referring to the liberation of the fragment by pepsin treatment), against which the antibodies in the assay for human samples are directed [38, 54], and in its distal, globular ends of the short arms (P2 fragment) used for the assay in animal studies [20]. Recently, a different assay procedure was published, using antibodies to intact human laminin [55]. Most studies of serum laminin use a commercially available radioimmunoassay for the P1 fragment (Behringwerke, Marburg, Germany) [54] which employs Fab antibody fragments to achieve a linear inhibition of serum antigens. Unfortunately, this assay has been modified several times during the past years, thereby complicating the comparison of the results of different studies performed with this assay. The other laminin P1 assay shows a non-linear inhibition that has to be calculated by the 50% intercept method [38]. Like the other major basement membrane parameter, NC1, laminin P1 is unrelated to growth, and adult levels are reached in children at two years of age [40].

Serum laminin P1 was described to be elevated in both adult patients with type 1 [56] or type 2 diabetes [34], predominantly in patients with nephropathy, but not in those exhibiting retinopathy only. Limited information is available on urinary laminin levels in diabetes [57]. In a cross-sectional study of 218 children and adolescents with diabetes, we found temporarily or permanently elevated serum levels in 28% of the patients [2]. As described in adults, laminin showed a significant relationship to glycaemic control, with elevated levels in 23% of the patients during poor metabolic control. Furthermore, we found a high prevalence of elevated values in patients with LJM, indicating a special susceptibility of these patients to diabetes-related changes in connective tissue metabolism. In contrast to our findings, lower values of laminin were found in children with LJM using the other available RIA for laminin. Furthermore, in that study, the laminin values showed no association to glycaemic control and most values in diabetes were found to be within the reference range [16].

Again, these contradictory results indicate that the antibodies used in the various assays probably recognize different circulating fragments, representing different aspects of the matrix metabolism. These aspects can be elucidated combining molecular sieve chromatography of serum with the radioimmunoassay. Using this approach, the commercial laminin radioimmunoassay was shown to react with two separate laminin antigens with a M_r of 900,000 kD (probably intact laminin) and 300,000 kD (probably degradation products), respectively [54]. Recent preliminary results indicate that these antigens are not elevated proportionally in diabetes, with the fraction of higher molecular weight being increased to a greater extent in patients with diabetic nephropathy [58]. Moreover, structural changes of the laminin molecule in the diabetic milieu have been described *in vitro* [59].

Special problems regarding the interpretation of connective tissue immunoassays

Most connective tissue components are integrated into the matrix in a highly cross-linked fashion and are therefore virtually insoluble. Three possible metabolic mechanisms may contribute to soluble material detectable in serum: firstly, material may be lost from the cell after secretion during matrix synthesis; secondly, propeptide regions may be cleaved off prior to the integration in the matrix, as in case of the aminoterminal propeptide of type III collagen; finally, material from tissue degradation, which is resistant to further breakdown and retains its antigenic determinants, may become measurable in serum. Thus, the amount detected in serum may represent the sum of synthesis and degradation products, although it appears that fragments detected by most assays are predominantly generated *either* by synthesis *or* by degradation [21]. However, a substantial heterogeneity of serum antigens has been described for both type IV collagen [60] and laminin [58]. Additional potential complexity arises from studies of laminin where, under experimental conditions, circulating fragments are removed from the serum by endocytosis of liver endothelial cells at a much slower rate than the intact molecule [61]. Generally, it has to be kept in mind that our limited knowledge on the metabolism about these fragments is derived solely from experimental models. In addition, as outlined above, the protein material for the antibody generation and for the production of standard solutions has been extracted almost exclusively from human placenta. However, recent results indicate that, for example, the immunological properties of the NC1 domain of type IV collagen vary substantially in different basement membranes [62]. Therefore, with respect to diabetic nephropathy, better detection methods could possibly be established with material generated from human glomerular basement membrane.

Outlook

At this time the results of different assay procedures for connective tissue proteins cannot be compared. As outlined in detail above, regarding both antigen concentration in body fluids and the relationship to the clinical situation in diabetes, these procedures show substantial differences. However, as with any other laboratory method introduced in research, increased knowledge will eventually lead to a better standardisation of these procedures. The clinical significance of these methodologies will probably greatly increase, as the establishment of these assays is a logical extension of the experimental biochemical research about the connective tissue changes underlying diabetic microangiopathy to the clinical necessity to identify patients at risk for complications, before they lead to debilitating functional impairment.

References

[1] Feingold KR, Elias PH. Skin problems in the diabetes clinic. In: Mogensen CE, Standl E, eds.: Concepts for the ideal diabetes clinic. Diabetes Forum Series IV. Berlin New York: De Gruyter, 1992; 215–233.

[2] Danne Th, Weber B, Spiro MJ et al. Changes of extracellular matrix metabolism in early diabetic angiopathy. Pediatr Adolesc Endocr 1992; 22: 11–22.

[3] Williamson JR, Tilton RG, Chang K et al. Basement membrane abnormalities in diabetes mellitus: relationship to clinical microangiopathy. Diabetes/Metabolism Rev 1988; 4: 339–370.

[4] Spiro RG. Pathogenesis of diabetic glomerulopathy: a biochemical view. In: Mogensen CE, ed. The kidney and hypertension in diabetes. Boston: Martinus Nijhoff, 1990; 117–130.

[5] Brocks DG, Strecker H, Neubauer HP et al. Radioimmunoassay of laminin in serum and its application to cancer patients. Clin Chem 1986; 32: 787–791.

[6] Danne Th, Borkenstein M, Burger W et al. Plasma Fibronectin and von Willebrand Factor Elevation in IDDM – An Epiphenomenon during poor metabolic control? Pediatr Adolesc Endocrinol 1989; 18: 201–206.
[7] Deckert T, Feldt-Rasmussen B, Borch-Johnsen K et al. Albuminuria reflects widespread vascular damage. The Steno hypothesis. Diabetologia 1989; 32: 219–226.
[8] Beisswenger JP, Spiro RG. Studies on the human glomerular basement membrane: composition, nature of the carbohydrate units and chemical changes in diabetes mellitus. Diabetes 1973; 22: 180–193.
[9] Mohan PS, Carter WG, Spiro RG. Occurrence of type VI collagen in extracellular matrix of renal glomeruli and its increase in diabetes. Diabetes 1990; 39: 31–37.
[10] Shimomura H, Spiro RG. Studies on macromolecular components of human glomerular basement membrane and alterations in diabetes. Decreased levels of heparan sulfate proteoglycan and laminin. Diabetes 1987; 36: 374–381.
[11] Rosenbloom AL, Silverstein JH, Lezotte DC et al. Limited joint mobility indicates risk for microvascular disease. N Engl J Med 1981; 305: 191–194.
[12] Brik R, Berant M, Vardi P. The scleroderma-like syndrome of insulin-dependent diabetes mellitus. Diabetes Metab Rev 1991; 7: 120–128.
[13] Rosenbloom AL, Frias JL. Diabetes mellitus, short stature and joint stiffness. A new syndrome. Clin Res 1974; 22: 92.
[14] Jennings AM, Milner PC, Ward JC. Hand abnormalities are associated with the complications of type II diabetes. Diabetic Med 1989; 6: 43–47.
[15] Buckingham B, Perjda AJ, Sandborg C et al. Skin, joint and pulmonary changes in type 1 diabetes mellitus. Am J Dis Child 1986; 40: 420–423.
[16] Veijola R, Knip M, Risteli L et al. Decreased circulating collagen and laminin metabolites in insulin-dependent diabetic children with joint contractures. Pediatr Res 1993; 33: 501–505.
[17] Tubiana-Rufi N, Prieur AM, Bouden R et al. Early detection of limited joint mobility in diabetic children and adolescents. Diabete Metab 1991; 17: 504–511.
[18] Rosenbloom AL, Silverstein JH, Lezotte DC et al. Limited joint mobility in diabetes mellitus of childhood. Natural history and relationship to growth impairment. J Pediatr 1982; 101: 874–878.
[19] Reimer-Veit M, Burger W, Kroll M et al. Prevalence and development of limited joint mobility in type I diabetic children and adolescents. In: Weber B, ed. Early vascular complications in children with diabetes. Pediatr Adolesc Endocr 1988; 17: 111–121.
[20] Risteli L, Risteli J. Radioimmunoassays for monitoring connective tissue metabolism. Rheumatology 1986; 10: 216–245.
[21] Schuppen D. Connective tissue polypeptides in serum to monitor antifibrotic treatment in hepatic fibrogenesis. J Hepatol; in press.
[22] Danne Th, Grüters A, Schuppan D et al. Procollagen type III propeptide related antigens in serum reflect somatic growth in healthy children and patients with growth disorders. J. Pediatr 1989; 109: 257–260.
[23] Keller F, Lyreal Ser Y, Schuppan D. Raised concentrations of the carboxy terminal propeptide of type IV (basement membrane) procollagen (NC1) in serum and urine of patients with glomerulonephritis. Eur J Clin Invest 1992; 22: 175–181.
[24] Risteli J, Draeger KE, Regitz G et al. Increase in circulating basement membrane antigens in diabetic rats and effects of insulin treatment. Diabetologia 1982; 23: 266–269.
[25] Danne Th, Poulsom R, Schuppan D et al. Streptozotocin-diabetes but not galactose-feeding increases the serum concentration of type IV collagen antigens in rats. Diabetes Research 1990; 14: 1–4.
[26] Hasslacher C, Brocks DG, Mann J et al. Influence of hypertension on serum concentration of type IV collagen antigens in streptozotocin-diabetic and non-diabetic rats. Diabetologia 1987; 30: 344–347.

[27] Kempe HP, Hasslacher C, Engelmann K et al. Einfluß von Diäten mit unterschiedlichem Proteinanteil auf den Typ IV-Kollagenstoffwechsel. Akt Endokr Stoffw 1991; 12: 163 (Abstract).
[28] Hasslacher C, Reichenbacher R, Gechter F et al. Glomerular basement membrane synthesis and serum concentration of type IV collagen in streptozotocin-diabetic rats. Diabetologia 1984; 26: 150–154.
[29] Brocks DG, Neubauer HP, Strecker H. Type IV collagen antigens in serum of diabetic rats: a marker for basement membrane collagen synthesis. Diabetologia 1985; 28: 928–932.
[30] Timpl R: Immunology of the collagens. In: Piez, Reddi, eds. Extracellular matrix biochemistry, New York: Elsevier, 1984; 159–190.
[31] Rohde H, Vargas L, Hahn EG et al. Radioimmunoassay for type III procollagen peptide and its application to human liver disease. Eur J Clin Invest 1979; 9: 451–459.
[32] Rohde H, Langer I, Krieg T et al. Serum and urine analysis of the aminoterminal procollagen peptide III by radioimmunoassay with antibody Fab fragments. Coll Rel Res 1983; 3: 371–379.
[33] Roth J, Ullrich K, Ziegler R et al. Plasma and serum concentrations of fibronectin, laminin and procollagen type III propeptides in juvenile patients with type I diabetes. Pediatr Adolesc Endocrinol 1989; 18: 197–200.
[34] Okazaki R, Matsuoka K, Horiuchi A et al. Assays of serum laminin and type III procollagen peptide for monitoring the clinical course of diabetic microangiopathy. Diab Res Clin Pract 1988; 5: 163–170.
[35] Schuppan D, Besser M, Schwarting R et al. Radioimmunoassay for human type IV (basement membrane) procollagen in body fluids. J Clin Invest 1986; 78: 241–248.
[36] Torffvit O, Agardh CD, Cederholm B et al. A new enzyme-linked immunosorbent assay for urine and serum concentrations of the carboxyterminal domain (NC1) of collagen IV. Application in type I (insulin-dependent) diabetes. Scand J Clin Lab Invest 1989; 49: 431–439.
[37] Högemann B, Voss B, Altenwerth FJ et al. Concentrations of 7S collagen and laminin P1 in sera of patients with diabetes mellitus. Klin Wochenschr 1984; 64: 382–385.
[38] Niemelä O, Risteli L, Sotaniemi EA et al. Type IV collagen and laminin-related antigens in human serum in alcoholic liver disease. Eur J Clin Invest 1985; 15: 132–137.
[39] Obata K, Iwata K, Ichida T et al. One step sandwich immunoassay for human type IV collagen using monoclonal antibodies. Clin Chim Acta 1989; 181: 293–304.
[40] Danne Th, Decker J, Schuppan D et al. Serum Levels of laminin P1 and type IV collagen in healthy children and children with insulin-dependent diabetes mellitus, in: M. Sternberg, MC Gubler, eds. Progress in basement membrane research: Renal and related aspects. London: Libbey, 1988; 315–322.
[41] Matsumoto E, Matsumoto G, Ooshima A et al. Serum type IV collagen concentrations in diabetic patients with microangiopathy as determined by enzyme immunoassay with monoclonal antibodies. Diabetes 1990; 39: 885–890.
[42] Alland A, Hartmann DJ, Loupy G et al. Étude de la fibronectine et du collagène de type IV plasmatiques chez le diabétique. Path Biol 1984; 32: 115–121.
[43] Watanabe T, Negishi K, Katayama S. Serum or urinary concentration of type IV collagen in diabetics. J Diab Compl 1991; 5: 191–192.
[44] Tomono S, Kawazu S, Kato N et al. Clinical implications of serum levels of basement membrane components in diabetic patients with and without albuminuria. J Diab Compl 1991; 5: 193–194.
[45] Hayashi Y, Makino H, Ota Z. Serum and urinary concentrations of type IV collagen and laminin as a marker for microangiopathy in diabetes. Diab Med 1992; 9: 366–370.
[46] Danne Th, Bathke J, Johnston V et al. Predictive value of humoral markers of endothelial and basement membrane metabolism for the development of retinopathy in children with diabetes mellitus. Diabetologia 1992; 35 (Suppl. 1): A142.

[47] Spiro MJ, Crowley TJ. Increased rat myocardial type VI collagen in diabetes mellitus and hypertension. Diabetologia 1993; 36: 93–98.
[48] Spiro MJ, Kumar BRR, Crowley TJ. Myocardial glycoproteins in diabetes: type VI collagen is a major PAS-reactive extracellular matrix protein. J Mol Cell Cardiol 1992; 24: 397–410.
[49] Schuppan D, Rühlmann T, Hahn EG. Radioimmunoassay for human type VI collagen and its application to tissue and body fluids. Anal Biochem 1985; 149: 238–247.
[50] Shahin M, Schuppan D, Waldherr R et al. Serum procollagen peptides and collagen type VI for the assessment of activity and degree of hepatic fibrosis in schistomiasis and alcoholic liver disease. Hepatology 1992; 15: 637–44.
[51] Danne Th, Bathke JM, Gläser I et al. Ist die Serumbestimmung von Kollagen VI zur Früherkennung einer Mikroangiopathie bei Kindern und Jugendlichen mit Diabetes mellitus geeignet? Diabetes und Stoffwechsel 1993; 2: 109 (Abstract).
[52] Pugliese G, Pricci F, Christina G et al. Mechanisms of glucose-enhanced synthesis of extracellular matrix by rat mesangial cells. Diabetologia 1992; 35 (Suppl. 1): All (Abstract).
[53] Poulsom R, Kurkinen M, Prockop DJ et al. Increased steady-state levels of laminin B1 mRNA in kidneys of long-term streptozotocin-diabetic rats. J Biol Chem 1988; 263: 10072–10076.
[54] Brocks DG, Strecker H, Neubauer HP et al. Radioimmunoassay of laminin in serum and its application to cancer patients. Clin Chem 1986; 32: 787–791.
[55] Aoki T, Takasaki T, Miura H et al. Development of a radioimmunoassay of intact laminin and its clinical evaluation as a tumor marker. Chem Pharm Bull Tokyo 1992; 40: 981–985.
[56] Hasslacher Ch, Brocks D. Serum concentration of laminin in type I diabetic patients with and without microangiopathy. Transplant Proc 1986; 18: 1534.
[57] Nakajima C, Shimojo N, Naka K et al. Clinical significance of urinary laminin P1 in diabetic patients. J Diab Compl 1991; 5: 197–198.
[58] Diehl E, Hasslacher Ch. Charakterisierung des Serum-Laminins bei Diabetikern mit und ohne Mikroangiopathie. Akt Endokr Stoffw 1990; 11: 72 (Abstract).
[59] Charonis AS, Reger LA, Dege JE et al. Laminin alterations after in vitro nonenzymatic glycosilation. Diabetes 1990; 39: 807–814.
[60] Yamada S, Kishimoto Y, Suou T et al. Heterogeneity of antigens related to 7S domain of collagen in serum: Application to patients with liver disease. Clin Chim Acta 1992; 212: 73–78.
[61] Smedsrod B, Paulsson M, Johansson S. Uptake and degradation of laminin and nidogen by rat liver cells. Biochem J 1989; 261: 37–42.
[62] Weber M, Pullig O. Different immunologic properties of the globular NC1 domain of collagen type IV isolated from different basement membranes. Eur J Clin Invest 1992; 22: 138–146.

Measurement of extracellular fixed anionically charged molecules

A. Kofoed-Enevoldsen

Introduction

The endothelial glycocalyx, the basal lamina, and many components of the interstitial matrix hold fixed anionically charged molecules. These fixed anionic charges cause a marked restriction of the transcapillary passage of negatively charged macromolecules. Correspondingly, depletion of the fixed anionic charges leads to increased capillary macromolecular permeability. Depletion of fixed anionic charge has been suggested to have an important role in the development of the severe vascular late diabetic complications [1]. Measurement of extracellular fixed anionic charge is therefore of interest in relation to diabetic vascular complications. The clinical usefulness of these measurements as prognostic indicators or as markers of therapeutic outcome still remains to be documented. Thus so far, measurement of fixed anionic charges should be reserved for research purposes. However, since the traditional clinical parameters (e. g. microalbuminuria and blood pressure) may not provide a sufficiently unambiguous characterisation of vascular dysfunction and prognosis, measurement of parameters specifically related to vascular anionic charge density may in future prove to be of use for clinical practise.

This chapter reviews methods for measurement of fixed anionically charged molecules in diabetic patients, and summarises the main results from previous studies. Before breaking into the context of methodology, however, let us briefly discuss the chemical nature and localisation of the fixed anionic charges.

What to measure

The chemical composition of fixed charges

The principal molecular carriers of the fixed anionic charges are carbohydrates and the acid aminoacids (glutamic acid and aspartic acid). Two distinct

Offprint from
Research Methodologies in Human Diabetes – Part 1

categories of the carbohydrates are *sialic acids* and *glycosaminoglycans*. Sialic acids (N-acetylneuramic acids) serve as the terminal residues in the oligosaccharide side chains of glycoproteins and gangliosides. Glycosaminoglycans (acid mucopolysaccharides) are long, unbranched polysaccharide chains composed of repeating disaccharide units (uronic acid linked to N-acetylglucosamine or N-acetylgalactosamine). The negative charge of sialic acids and glycosaminoglycans relates to the ionisation of their carboxyl groups at physiological pH. In addition, sulphation of the glycosaminoglycans (in most cases the amino sugar), results in a further increase in their negative charge. The glycosaminoglycans have the highest density of negative charges of all mammalian macromolecules. All glycosaminoglycans (except hyaluronic acid) are covalently attached to proteins to form *proteoglycans*.

Localisation of fixed charges

Proteoglycans are secreted components of the extracellular matrix or integral components of plasma membranes. Within the basal laminae, a large *heparan sulphate proteoglycan* (Perlecan) constitutes the principal glycosaminoglycan carrier of fixed anionic charge (a review of proteoglycan biochemistry is found in [2]). Within the glycocalyx and the remaining extracellular matrix, other proteoglycans as well as the sialic acids may dominate as carriers of fixed anionic charge.

Functional roles attributed to specific forms of fixed anionically charged molecules

The extracellular matrix forms a complex highly organised basic substance, with profound impact on permeability and multiple cell functions. In a sense, the integrated structural organisation of the extracellular matrix makes it meaningless to speak of an exclusive physiological role for any of its specific carriers of fixed anionic charge. In other words, the absence of any anionic charge component would seem likely to cause the entire compartment to come to a functional break down. Crude neutralisation of the anionic charges by infusion of positively charged substances such as protamine sulphate have been shown to increase capillary permeability [3]. Removal of sialic acids by neuramidase treatment induces proteinuria and morphological derangement of the glomerular filtration barrier [4]. Finally, removal of the fixed anionic charge associated to heparan sulphate induces increased glomerular permeability [5]. Other studies have questioned the role of heparan sulphate sulphation as a major factor for the maintenance of capillary charge selectivity

[6] (for a review of the role of charge in maintaining normal glomerular ultrafiltration see [7]). However controversial this topic may be, measurement of fixed anionic charge related to heparan sulphate has gained considerable interest in diabetes research.

Fixed anionically charged molecules of special relevance to late diabetic vascular complications

Analysis of the biochemical composition of glomerular basement membranes from diabetic patients has shown no reduction in the content of acidic amino acids, whereas a 10% reduction in sialic acids has been found in several studies [8]. Evidence of reduced fixed anionic charge related to heparan sulphate glycosaminoglycan in patients with severe diabetic vascular disease has been found in a number of studies, as discussed below. Although the major contributions to our understanding of the mechanism behind the loss of anionic heparan sulphate glycosaminoglycan comes from animal experiments, a number of methodologies are available for human studies as well.

Methods of measurement

Red blood cell negative charge measured by Alcian blue binding

Measurement of red blood cell (RBC) Alcian blue binding as a marker of capillary wall negative charge was originally proposed by Levin et al. [9]. The proposal was based on the common presence of anionic groups on capillary surfaces and on RBC's. Following their initial demonstration of reduced RBC negative charge in steroid sensitive nephrotic syndrome, a number of studies have suggested a reduction in RBC negative charge in diabetic nephropathy. The biochemical mechanism underlying a reduction in RBC Alcian blue binding may be reduced content or neutralisation of membrane associated sialic acid, which in turn may be caused by impairment of sialyltransferase activity or the presence of a systematically released cationic macromolecule leading to masking of the anionic sites [10]. One study has, however, suggested a reduction in RBC glycosaminoglycan content [11].

Protocol: The principle of the assay is to measure the amount of Alcian blue bound by a known number of erythrocytes. In brief, red blood cells (e. g. $1.2 \cdot 10^9$/ml) washed and suspended in phosphate-buffered saline at pH 7.4 are incubated with 125–250 µg/ml Alcian blue in 25 mmol/l $MgCl_2$ for 30 min at 37° C. After removal of RBC's by centrifugation, the optical density

(650 nm) of the supernatant is measured. Results are expressed as ng Alcian blue bound per 10^6 RBC. A detailed protocol is found in [9], and a modified version in [10].

Results: Typical values for Alcian blue binding are 100–300 ng/10^6 RBC, depending on the initial Alcian blue concentration. The inter-experimental variation is very low (< 5%), and the intraindividual variation (SD/mean) in healthy control subjects is likely to be around 10% (for n = 20–40) [9, 11–13]. Two studies found a 10% reduction in Alcian blue binding in diabetic patients [13, 11] whereas one study found no effect of diabetes [14]. No clear-cut difference has been found between patients with or without diabetic nephropathy. A negative correlation to urinary albumin escape rate (UAE) has been reported in microalbuminuric patients [13], however in the same study, macroalbuminuric patients (UAE > 200 µg/min) showed *increased* Alcian blue binding. Others found a weak negative correlation between UAE and Alcian blue binding within the normal to microalbuminuric range, whereas it disappeared at higher levels of UAE [10, 11].

Comments: The obvious advantage of the RBC Alcian blue binding assay is the accessibility of sample material, and the simple laboratory procedures involved. Drawbacks include the lack of specificity of the assay. Some 80% of the binding relates to sialic acids [9], which again may relate to a number of different groups of macromolecules. The remaining 20% may relate to RBC membrane bound glycosaminoglycans [11]. In consideration of the rather empirically founded type of theory underlying the use of the assay, measurement of these individual components should be included in the protocol. When measured in diabetic patients, RBC sialic acid has been present in normal amounts despite reduced Alcian blue binding, whereas reduced RBC glycosaminoglycan content was suggested in one study [11]. Finally, the calculation of Alcian blue bound per number of erythrocytes does not take into account possible differences in RBC cell surface area.

Glomerular and transcapillary charge selectivity

This indirect measurement of fixed anionic charges is based on the selective capillary filtration of differently charged, identically sized macromolecules. The presumption is that loss of the normal capillary charge selectivity (restricting the passage of the more negatively charged molecules) reflects a loss of fixed anionic charges within the filtration barrier. The method has been used primarily for glomerular charge selectivity, but has recently also been

Table 1 *Endogenous marker-pair molecules used to estimate glomerular charge selectivity in diabetic patients*

Marker-pair	Size (kD)	pI	Ref.
total-IgG:IgG4	156	(6 – 10):5.8	[17, 18, 22, 27]
neutral-IgG:anionic-IgG	156	7.3:4.8	[51]
nonglycated:glycated albumin	69	7.0:6.2	[24, 25]
pancreatic:salivary iso-amylases	54	4.7:(4.0 – 4.7)	[50]

applied to subcutaneous transcapillary filtration. Several different endogenous marker-pairs have been used in human studies (see Table 1). The IgG:albumin index may be considered a hybrid index, subject to influence by both size and charge selectivity. This index was, however, the first to indicate a significant loss of charge selectivity during the development of diabetic nephropathy [15]. The selectivity index (SI) is calculated as the ratio between the clearances of the marker-pair molecules. We prefer to place the most anionic marker in the denominator, so that a *loss* of the ability to discriminate leads to a *reduction* in the nominal value of the selectivity index. The most widely used index for glomerular SI (apart from the hybrid IgG:albumin SI) has been the total-IgG:IgG4 SI ($SI_{total\text{-}IgG:IgG4}$). With regard to the interpretation of the glomerular SI's, the interference with tubular charge selectivity should be observed (see *comments*).

Protocol: Venous blood and a urine specimen are collected. The ratio between the marker-pair plasma concentration must be likely to remain constant during the urine sampling period. With the total-IgG:IgG4 marker-pair, day-to-day and positional (recumbent versus upright position) variation are insignificant (unpublished observation). We used either early morning, spot, or urine specimens collected during forced diuresis. Due to possible systematic differences between these samples, only samples collected under comparable conditions should be used. The stability of the urine sample during storage is a major problem. In common urine specimens stored at $-20°$ C, a progressive decline (10 – 15% per week) in total-IgG content has been observed [16]. Adjustment of pH and addition of exogenous protein may overcome this problem, so that samples can be stored for several months at $-20°$ C. Detailed experimental protocols are found in the following references [16 – 19].

Two recent studies have used the SI principle to study the mechanism behind the generally increased transcapillar escape rate (TER) of albumin in patients with elevated urinary albumin excretion. Two different methods were applied (1) calculation of ratio of TER between non-glycated and glycated albumin [20], and (2) measurement of total-IgG:IgG4 ratio in extracellular fluid [21]. See references for details in the experimental procedures.

Results: Healthy non-diabetic control subjects in our laboratory, have a mean $SI_{total\text{-}IgG:IgG4}$ of 1.5 (cv% 25, n = 10). Normoalbuminuric long-term (>20 years of diabetes duration) diabetic patients seems to follow the same range [17]. Pietravalle et al. reported a disparate and more widespread reference value for $SI_{total\text{-}IgG:IgG4}$ in healthy control subjects (5% and 95% percentile 4 and 14 respectively; recalculated from [18]). This difference is mainly due to differences in the IgG4 measurements resulting in a 3-fold difference in the calculated IgG4 clearances. In patients with elevated urinary albumin excretion rate, the reduction in the $SI_{total\text{-}IgG:IgG4}$ is 20–30%. The shift in SI mimics an "on-of" phenomenon. Only weak correlations with urinary albumin excretion rate have been found, whereas the difference between normoalbuminuric and microalbuminuric (30–100 mg/24 h) patients is significant even within relatively small study populations [17, 22].

No information regarding variation in SI during daily activity is available. However, a considerable day-to-day variation (30–40%) is found in $SI_{total\text{-}IgG:IgG4}$ [23]. A relatively good correlation is found between measurements of $SI_{total\text{-}IgG:IgG4}$ in spot urine specimens and urine collected during forced diuresis (r = 0.72, n = 47) [17]. In IDDM patients with microalbuminuria, $SI_{total\text{-}IgG:IgG4}$ seems influenced by metabolic control [22].

Increased SI has been found in normoalbuminuric diabetic patients using $SI_{IgG:albumin}$ or $SI_{non\text{-}glycated:glycated\ albumin}$ [24–27]. The phenomenon seems related to increased clearance of the most neutral tracer, whereas the anionic is cleared normally. Where indicated in these studies, patients with elevated urinary albumin excretion rate have reduced SI only when compared with normoalbuminuric diabetic patients, not with healthy control subjects. Though a consistent finding in several studies, elevated $SI_{total\text{-}IgG:IgG4}$ or $SI_{IgG:albumin}$ in normoalbuminuric diabetic patients were not found either in our recent study [17], by Pietravalle et al. [18] or by Viberti [15]. In these three studies, SI in patients with elevated UAE was reduced both when compared to healthy control subjects and to normoalbuminuric diabetic patients. In addition, the individual fractional clearances of the two tracers were similar in normoalbuminuric diabetic patients and healthy control subjects.

Studying general transcapillar charge selectivity, Bent-Hansen et al. found a significant, 15% decrease in the ratio of non-glycated:glycated albumin transcapillar escape in patients with elevated UAE [20]. We found, however, no difference in the total-IgG:IgG4 ratio in serum and interstitial fluid between patients with normal an elevated UAE [21]. These findings are not necessarily in conflict, since the possible gel-like performance of the interstitial matrix influencing the later study, may obscure the membrane-like charge selective effect of the capillary filtration barrier (see [21] for a further discussion).

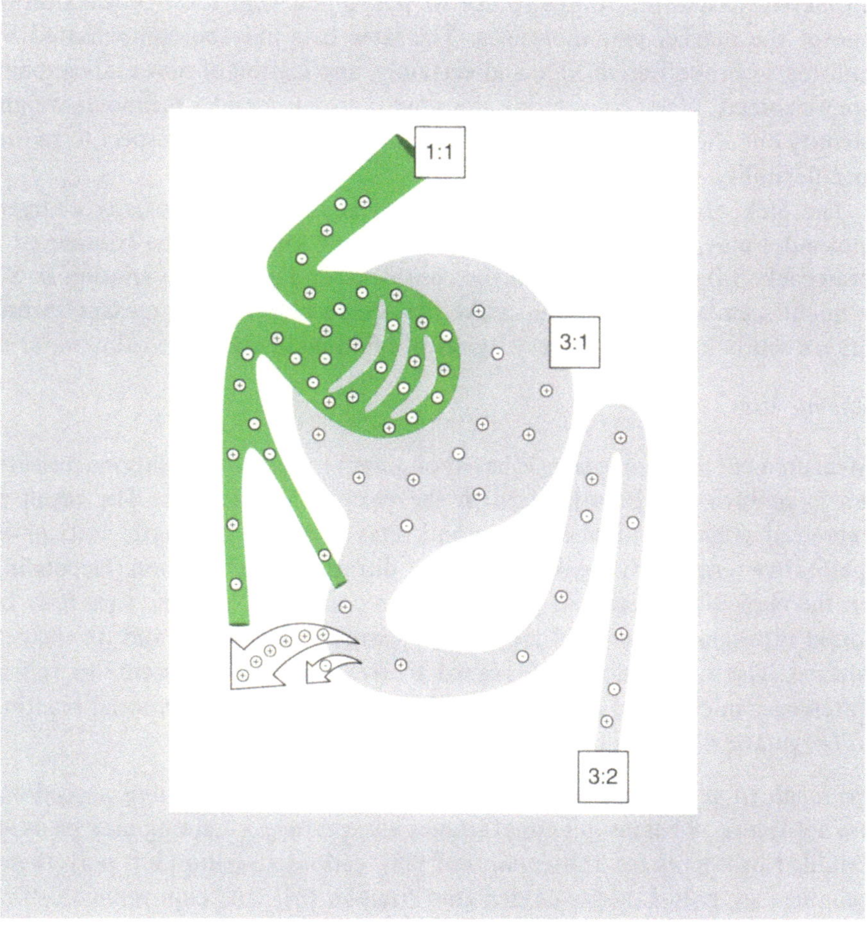

Fig. 1 Schematic drawing illustrating the effect of tubular charge-dependent protein reabsorption on the outcome of the charge selectivity index measurement. The marker-pair molecules are of comparable size, but different charge. The suggestive ratios between cationic and anionic molecules in the three separate compartments (blood; ultrafiltrate; urethral urine) are indicated on the figure. The effect of glomerular charge selectivity causes the cationic:anionic ratio in the ultrafiltrate to increase to 3 : 1. In the tubules, the cationic molecules are preferentially reabsorbed, causing a decrease in the cationic:anionic ratio to 3 : 2. The ratios are arbitrarily chosen and possibly influenced by size and charge characteristics of the marker-pair molecules

Comments: As seen from Fig. 1, tubular charge selective reabsorption significantly influences SI. Indeed, a major drawback related to the measurement of glomerular SI's is that no tubularly inert probe is available. Sulphated dextran has been considered, but may be of only limited use, due partly to the toxicity of their high molecular weight fractions.

Problems may also arise from contamination of the urine specimen with unfiltered plasma or from a source of post-glomerular local production of one of the marker-pair molecules. The later bias may be compensated by utilising several different SI's, and certainly, application of new marker-pairs are welcomed. When considering a new marker-pair, besides the molar-weight identity one should also ensure conformation similarity with respect to radius and flexibility.

The lack of specificity for a distinct type of fixed anionically charged molecules may, as with the Alcian blue binding assay, also be considered a drawback. Taken together with the considerable day-to-day variation in SI, it might seem surprising that, unlike the Alcian blue binding measurements, the reduction in SI still is a very significant finding in relation to albuminuria.

Anionic sites

Measurement of anionic sites is based on their binding to polycationic tracers, which in turn can be visualised in the electron microscope. The result is expressed either as number of anionic sites per area or length unit, or in qualitative terms with regard to size and ultrastructural location. Depending on the choice of tracer and the incubation conditions, anionic sites may be found throughout the basal lamina, the extracellular matrix and on the cell surface. The subdivision with regard to size and location seems to reflect differences in chemical composition, as judged from the differential reaction to enzymatic digestion [28, 29].

Protocol: In general, for human studies only immersion staining procedures are applicable, whereas in animal studies also perfusion staining may be used. Detailed protocols for ruthenium red [30], cationic ferritin [30], polyethyleneimine [28], poly-L-lysine-coated gold complex [31], and cuprolinic blue [29] immersion staining may be found in the references. Cuprolinic blue staining under the "critical electrolyte concentration" conditions enables specific staining of sulphated proteoglycans [32, 34]. It must be borne in mind that the fixation process may significantly influence the structural localisation of the anionic sites, as demonstrated by the differential outcome of cuprolinic blue stained anionic sites after glutaraldehyde or formaldehyde fixation [35]. Recently the so-called "Quick-freezing deep etching" method for tissue processing has been used in combination with polyethyleneimine staining. The method enables three-dimensional ultrastructural visualisation of the anionic sites, and may help to determine their genuine localisation [36].

Results: In spite of the differences between the tracers used, and whether human or animal material is studied, a common pattern of staining of the normal glomerular basement membrane and interstitial capillary basal lamina is found. In the lamina rara externa (LRE) of the glomerular basement membrane and in most capillary basal laminae, staining of a lattice-like array of round oval 15–30 nm sites, spaced 40–60 nm [28–30, 37] is seen. The number of sites at this location is 20–30 per 1000 nm basement membrane (inter-individual cv% around 10% with $n > 20$). In the lamina rara interna (LRI) slightly fewer, less regularly sized and spaced sites are found. Heparitinase treatment removes 80–100% of the LRE anionic sites, whereas slightly fewer (70–80%) are removed from the LRI. Smaller anionic sites (5–10 nm) are distributed randomly over the lamina densa and the mesangial extracellular matrix where also larger sites are found. Using the quick-freezing deep etching method polyethyleneimine particles were found to decorate around fibrils radiating perpendicularly from the lamina densa to podocyte membrane [36].

The first evidence of reduced anionic sites in diabetic nephropathy was provided by Rohrbach [37]. Recently Vernier et al. [29] found a 35% reduction in number of GBM LRE anionic sites in patients with diabetic nephropathy, whereas normoalbuminuric diabetic patients had a normal number of anionic sites. A tendency towards generally smaller sites in diabetic patients was noted in the later study. A reduction of the number of sites in the LRI has also been noted.

Comments: The regular arrangement of the GBM LRE anionic sites seems to enable reproducible quantitation. This does not seem to be the case with anionic sites in other compartments which consequently, until now, has not been thoroughly studied in diabetic patients. Animal experiments indicate, however, that quantitation within most capillary basal laminae is possible [38].

The specificity with regard to the molecular source of the anionic charge is potentially very high. Some scepticism may, however, be raised following the demonstration of the consequences of different fixation processing [35]. It should be considered whether alternative diabetes-related structural alterations of the extracellular matrix (e. g. non-enzymatic glycation) have an effect on the outcome of tissue sample processing. Could it be, that a number of anionic sites in the diabetic basement membrane are lost or rearranged during processing? Indeed, Vernier et al. [29] found a very strong negative correlation between basement membrane width and number of anionic sites. Whereas they preferred to speculate in an in vivo wash-out phenomenon, the possibility of an artificial occurrence still has to be considered.

Measurement of heparan sulphate sulphation

Sulphation of heparan sulphate increases the negative charge. Impairment of heparan sulphate sulphation has been suggested as a key event in the development of diabetic angiopathy. In animal experiments, the most frequently used method has been to measure the incorporation of ^{35}S into heparan sulphate. This approach has only limited use in human studies, although it may be used for in vitro cell culture experiments. An additional way of measuring heparan sulphate sulphation is to analyse the size distribution of oligosaccharide fragments generated by specific digestion of heparan sulphate chains, allowing the cleavage of the chain only at the site of sulphation. These fragments may be quantitated following ^{3}H-glucosamine incorporation, measurement of refractory index measurements (in combination with gel chromatography), or by silver staining (in combination with PAGE electrophoresis).

Protocol: Examples of protocols are found in [39, 40].

Results: Only few, if any, significant abnormalities of proteoglycan metabolism in cell cultures (skin fibroblasts) from diabetic patients have been reported [39, 41–43]. In fibroblast cultures from patients with diabetic nephropathy, we found evidence of reduced heparan sulphate biosynthesis when compared to healthy control subjects, but we found no difference in the degree of sulphation [39].

Comments: Multiple factors may bias in vitro experiments, primarily perhaps the difficulty in establishing a diabetic environment. Other problems relate to the choice of material. Fibroblast cultures have been chosen for their convenience in culturing and their accessibility. Whereas they may not seem very relevant with regard to involvement in the pathogenesis of diabetic vascular complication, recent findings of abnormal growth characteristics and Na^{+}/H^{+} antiport activity indicate that they may still be of relevance for studying genetic abnormalities related to the development of vascular complications [44, 45].

The present lack of a direct demonstration of impairment of heparan sulphate sulphation in diabetic patients, may in future be overcome only if application to human in vivo studies of the methods listed above becomes practicable.

Immunohistochemical quantitation of heparan sulphate glycosaminoglycan

Monoclonal antibodies against human heparan sulphate glycosaminoglycan, workable in immunohistochemical staining and inhibition ELISA, are now available [46]. Such antibodies may be used for in situ quantitation of HS. In combination with antibodies specific for the heparan sulphate proteoglycan core protein, they may be used to explore specific changes in heparan sulphate glycosaminoglycan concentration [47]. In addition, since these antibodies recognise specific epitopes in the glycosaminoglycan chain, they may be used

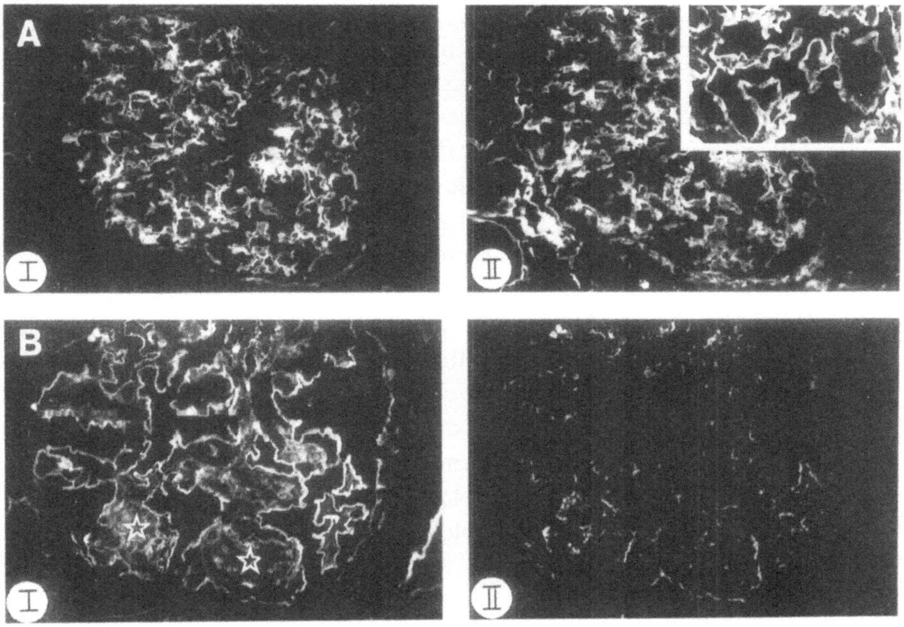

Fig. 2 Indirect immunofluorescence double staining of human glomerular cryostat sections for heparan sulphate proteoglycan core protein (mAb JM-72) (I) and heparan sulphate glycosaminoglycan (mAb JM-403) (II). A (upper panel): Normal control, the insert in II demonstrates the staining of mAb JM-403 at a higher magnification B (lower panel): Patient with diabetic nephropathy, note the strongly decreased staining of mAb JM-403 accompanied with an unaltered mAb JM-72 staining. Asterix in I indicate the staining of the expanded mesangium with mAb JM-72. Reproduced with permission from [47]

for detailed mapping of such epitopes. This could be of relevance when studying the effect of diabetes on heparan sulphate sulphation and other secondary modifications.

Protocol: See references [46] and [47] for detailed protocols.

Results: The monoclonal antibody JM-403 gives rise to subendothelial staining of the human glomerular basement membrane [48] as opposed to the predominantly subepithelial location of anionic sites (see previous paragraph). This may relate to JM-403 recognising an unsulphated epitope [46]. Staining is also seen in other capillary and smooth muscle cell basal laminae.

In patients with diabetic nephropathy, an abnormal segmental or absent staining was found in 8 out of the 10 patients studied [47].

Comments: A major problem is the limited potential for quantitation within the immunohistochemical methodology. Hopefully, the use of computer assisted image analysis will offer scope for more sensitive quantitation. An additional problem in relation to immunohistochemistry is that relevant epitopes may be covered up by other components of the tissue sample, leading to underestimation of target molecule concentration.

Finally, current antibodies are of the IgM type, while antibodies of IgG type seem more feasible for applications like ELISA.

Measurement of heparan sulphate proteoglycan core protein

A review of the methods for measurement of proteoglycan core protein concentration is beyond the scope of this chapter. Further, such measurements only indirectly relate to fixed anionic charges since the core protein itself does not contribute to charge. A number of mono- and polyclonal antibodies has been raised against the many different forms of proteoglycan core proteins. The demand now seems to be to develop sensitive workable assays for nanno-scale measurements in order to enable measurements in biopsy material.

Final remarks

In summary, numerous studies utilising different techniques, have indicated that a reduction in extracellular fixed anionic charge is associated to the development of diabetic vascular complications. Depending on the methodology and specificity of the measurements, the degree of reduction can be estimated to be within the range from 10 to 30%. Recent progress in methods for measurement of anionic charge related to heparan sulphate proteoglycan may hopefully in future enable a more detailed mapping of the possible abnormalities related to this specific component. Animal experiments may also in the near future dominate this area of research, but a considerable number of techniques are now available for much-needed human studies.

References

[1] Deckert T, Feldt-Rasmussen B, Borch-Johnsen K et al. Albuminuria reflects widespread vascular damage. Diabetologia 1989; 32: 219–226.
[2] Kjellén L, Lindahl U. Proteoglycans – Structures and interactions. Ann Rev Biochem 1991.
[3] Kelley VE, Cavallo T. Glomerular permeability – transfer of native ferritin in glomeruli with decreased anionic sites. Lab Invest 1978; 39: 547–553.
[4] Kanwar YS, Rosenzweig LJ. Altered glomerular permeability as a result of focal detachment of the visceral epithelium. Kidney Int 1982; 21: 565–574.
[5] Rosenzweig LJ, Kanwar Y. Removal of sulfated (heparan sulfate) or nonsulfated (hyaluronic acid) glycosaminoglycans results in increased permeability of the glomerular basement membrane to ^{125}I-bovine serum albumin. Lab Invest 1982; 47: 177–184.
[6] Bray J, Robinson GB. Influence of charge on filtration across renal basement membrane films in vitro. Kidney Int 1984; 25: 527–533.
[7] Kanwar YS. Biophysiology of glomerular filtration and proteinuria. Lab Invest 1984; 51; 1: 7–21.
[8] Wahl P, Deppermann D, Hasslacher C. Biochemistry of glomerular basement membrane of the normal and diabetic human. Kidney Int 1982; 21: 744–749.
[9] Levin M, Smith C, Walters MDS et al. Steroid-responsive nephroptic syndrome – A generalised disorder of membrane negative charge. Lancet 1985; ii: 239–242.
[10] Bernard A, Amor AO, Goemare-Vanneste J. et al. Urinary proteins and red blood cell membrane negative charges in diabetes mellitus. Clinica Chimica Acta 1990; 190: 249–262.
[11] Gambaro G, Baggio B, Cicerello E et al. Abnormal erythrocyte charge in diabetes mellitus. Diabetes 1988; 37: 745–748.
[12] Boulton-Jones JM, McWilliams G, Chandrachud L. Variation in charge on red cells of patients with different glomerulopathies. Lancet 1986; ii: 186–188.
[13] Estivi P, Cavallo-Perin P, Pagano G. Electrical anionic charges on red blood cells are reduced in insulin-dependent diabetic patients. J Diab Compl 1989: 3; 45–48.
[14] Mathiesen ER, Smith C, Lauritzen M et al. Surface charge of red blood cells in IDDM patients with incipient and overt nephropathy. Diabetic Medicine 1987; 4: 431–433.
[15] Viberti GC, Mackintosh D, Keen H. Determinants of the penetration of proteins through the glomerular barrier in IDDM. Diabetes 1983; 32 suppl 2: 92–95.
[16] Kofoed-Enevoldsen A, Jensen K, Beck TC. Measuring urinary IgG and IgG_4 excretion (letter). Clin Chem 1991; 37: 1136–1137.
[17] Deckert T, Kofoed-Enevoldsen A, Vidal P Size- and charge selectivity of glomerular filtration in IDDM patients with and without albuminuria. Diabetologia 1993; in press.
[18] Pietravalle P, Morano S, Cristina G et al. Charge selectivity of proteinuria in type 1 diabetes explored by Ig subclass clearance. Diabetes 1991; 40: 1685–1890.
[19] Morano S, Camcelli M, Manusco M et al. Sensitive immunoenzymatic assay for urinary immunoglobulin subclasses of different pH. Diabetes Res 1987; 6: 181–185.
[20] Bent-Hansen L, Feldt-Rasmussen B, Kverneland et al. Plasma disappearance of glycated and non-glycated albumin in type 1 (insulin-dependent) diabetes mellitus -evidence for charge dependent alterations of the plasma to lymph pathway. Diabetologia 1993; in press.

[21] Kofoed-Enevoldsen A, Bent-Hansen L, Deckert. Transcapillary filtration of plasma protein in long-term type 1 (insulin-dependent) diabetic patients. Scand J Clin Lab Invest 1992; 52: 591–597.
[22] Bangstad H-J, Kofoed-Enevoldsen A, Dahl-Jørgensen Ket al. Glomerular charge selectivity and the influence of improved blood glucose control. Diabetologia 1992; 35: 1165–1169.
[23] Kofoed-Enevoldsen A, Jensen K, Deckert T. Glomerular charge selectivity in normoalbuminuric type 1 diabetic patients (Abstract). Diabetologia 1992; 35 suppl 1: A144.
[24] Kverneland A, Feldt-Rasmussen B, Vidal P et al. Evidence of changes in renal charge selectivity in patients with type 1 diabetes mellitus. Diabetologia 1986; 29: 634–639.
[25] Cavallo-Perin P, Chiambretti A, Calefato V et al. The increase in albuminuria induced by exercise is not associated with preferential excretion of glycated albumin in type 1 (insulin-dependent) diabetic patients. Diabetologia 1991; 34: 813–816.
[26] Jerums G, Allen TJ, Cooper ME. Triphasic changes in selectivity with increasing proteinuria in type 1 and type 2 diabetes. Diabetic Medicine 1989; 6: 772–779.
[27] Deckert T, Feldt-Rasmussen B, Djurup R et al. Glomerular size and charge selectivity in insulin-dependent diabetes mellitus. Kidney Int 1988; 33: 100–106.
[28] Vernier RL, Klein DJ, Sisson SP et al. Heparan sulfate-rich anionic sites in the human glomerular basement membrane. N Engl J Med 1983; 309: 1001–1009.
[29] Vernier RL, Steffes MW, Sisson-Ross S et al. Heparan sulfate proteoglycan in the glomerular basement membrane in type 1 diabetes mellitus. Kidney Int 1992; 41: 1070–1080.
[30] Kanwar Y, Farquhar MG. Anionic sites in the glomerular basement membrane. J Cell Biol 1979; 81: 137–153.
[31] Goode NP, Shires M, Davison AM. Preparation and use of the poly-L-lycine gold probe – a differential marker of glomerular anionic sites. Histochemistry 1992; 98: 67–72.
[32] Scott JE. Proteoglycan histochemistry – a valuable tool for connective tissue biochemists. Coll Rel Res 1987; 5: 541–575.
[33] Van Kuppevelt THMSM, Rutten TLM, Kuyper CMA. Ultrastructural localization of proteoglycans in tissue using cuprolinic blue according to the critical electrolyte concentration method. Histochem J 1987; 520–526.
[34] Van Kuppevelt THMSM, Cremers FPM, Domen JGW et al. Staining of proteoglycans in mouse lung alveoli, II Characterization of the cuprolinic-blue positive, anionic sites. Histochem J 1984; 16: 671–686.
[35] Chan FL, Inoue S, Leblond CP. Localization of heparan sulfate proteoglycan in basement membrane by side chain staining with cuprolinic blue as compared with core protein labeling with immunogold. J Histochemistry and Cytochemistry 1992; 40: 1559–1972.
[36] Yoshimura A, Ohno S, Nakano K et al. Threedimensional ultrastructure of anionic sites of the glomerular basement membrane by a quickfreezing and deepetching method using a cationic tracer. Histochemistry 1991; 96: 107–113.
[37] Rorbach R. Reduced content and abnormal distribution of anionic sites (acid proteoglycans) in the diabetic glomerular basement membrane . Virchows Arch Cell Pathol 1986; 51: 127–135.
[38] Chakrabarti S, Ma N, Sima AA. Anionic sites in diabetic basement membranes and their possible role in diffusion barrier abnormalities in the BB-rat. Diabetologia 1991; 34: 301–306.
[39] Deckert T, Horowitz IM, Kofoed-Enevoldsen A et al. Possible genetic defects in regulation of glycosaminoglycans in patients with diabetic nephropathy. Diabetes 1991; 40: 764–770.
[40] Gallagher JT, Turnbull JE, Lyon M. Heparan sulphate proteoglycans – molecular organisation of membrane-associated species and an approach to polysaccheride sequence analysis. Adv Exp Med Biol 1992; 313: 49–57.
[41] Silbert CK, Kleinman HK. Studies of cultured human fibroblasts in diabetes mellitus. Diabetes 1979; 28: 61–64.
[42] Silbert CK, Palmer ME, Humphries DE et al. Production of [^{3}H]hexosamine-labled proteoglycans by cultures of normal and diabetic skin fibroblasts: dilution of exogenous [^{3}H]glucosamine by endogenous hexosamine from glucose and other sources. Arch Biochem Biophys 1989; 268: 393–397.

[43] Silbert CK, Humphries DE, Palmer ME et al. Effects of sulate deprivation on the production of chondroitin/dermatan sulfate by cultures of skin fibroblasts from normal and diabetic individuals. Arch Biochem Biophys 1991; 285: 137–141.
[44] Trevisan R, Li LK, Messent J, Tariq T et al. Na^{+}/H^{+} antiport activity and cell growth in cultured skin fibroblasts of IDDM patients with nephropathy. Diabetes 1992; 41: 1239–1246.
[45] Davies JE, Ng LL, Kofoed-Enevoldsen A et al. Intracellular pH and Na^{+}/H^{+} antiport activity of cultured fibroblasts in diabetic nephropathy. Kidney Int 1992; 42: 1184–1190.
[46] van den Born J, van den Heuvel LPWJ, Bakker MAH et al. A monoclonal antibody against GBM heparan sulfate induces an acute selective proteinuria in rats. Kidney Int 1992; 41: 115–123.
[47] van den Born J, van den Heuvel LPWJ, Bakker MAH et al. Evaluation of the distribution of GBM heparan sulfate proteoglycan core protein and side chains in human glomerular diseases by monoclonal antibodies. Kidney int 1993; in press.
[48] van den Born J, van den Heuvel LPWJ, Bakker MAH et al. Monoclonal antibodies against the core protein and the glycosaminoglycan side chain of glomarular basement membrane heparan sulfate proteoglycan – characterization and immunohistochemical application in human tissues. J Histochem Cytochem 1993; in press.
[49] Vernier RL, Sisson-Ross S, Mauer SM. Cytochemical studies of the anionic charges in the kidney in type 1 diabetes mellitus. Diab Nephrop 1986; 5: 15–18.
[50] Fox JG, Quin JD, Paterson KR et al. Impaired glomerular charge selectivity in microalbuminuria and diabetic nephropathy (Abstract). Diabetologia 1990; 33: A67.
[51] Nakamura Y, Myers B. Charge-selektivity of proteinuria in diabetic glomerulopathy. Diabetes 1988; 37: 1202–1211.

Methods in measuring glucose transporters and insulin receptors in target cells from humans

O. Pedersen, P. H. Andersen, S. Lund, J. F. Bak

Facilitative glucose transporters

Facilitative glucose transporters accelerate the movement of glucose down its concentration gradient (in or out of cells) by energy independent means. cDNAs encoding 5 functional facilitative glucose transporter subtypes have been identified from mammalian tissues. They are named GLUT (the gene symbol for facilitative glucose transporter) and numbered 1 – 5 in the order of their discovery [1 – 4]. The facilitative transporters are broadly alike in structure. Each consists of a polypeptide chain of about 500 amino acids. The amino acid residues at about half of the positions in the five sequences are the same or very similar. The crystallographic (three-dimensional) structure of the facilitative glucose transporters is not known. However, the predicted topology of these transporters suggests an organisation with 25 segments, each coiled into a helix, with 13 largely hydrophilic segments and 12 largely hydrophobic membrane-spanning components [1 – 4]. Both the NH_2^+- and COOH-terminals are on the cytoplasmic side of the plasma membrane. A large exoplasmic loop containing an N-glycosylation site is present between the first and second transmembrane domains. A large cytoplasmic loop is located in the middle of the molecule.

How the glucose transporter polypeptides mediate the entry of glucose into the cell is unknown. It is remarkable, however, that the degree of homology among glucose transporters is not randomly distributed. The most highly conserved regions are the membrane-spanning domains. Thus, the proposed tertiary structure of glucose transporters, and the pattern of amino acids in the transmembrane parts, point to the architecture of a cylinder, which subserves a common function, the formation of a pore for glucose diffusion [1 – 4]. In five transmembrane segments, 3, 5, 7, 8 and 11, the chemically reactive groups of amino acids are hydrophilic on one side of the cylinder and hydrophobic on the other. Bound together with their hydrophobic sides facing away from their common axis, the five segments form a pore whose

Offprint from
Research Methodologies in Human Diabetes – Part 1

inner surface (OH- and $CONH_2$ groups) can participate in hydrogen binding with the many hydroxyl groups on the glucose molecule. Experimental evidence also suggests that the glucose transporter exists in two conformations: one binds glucose on the extracellular side of the membrane, the other on the intracellular side [5]. In other words, it is envisioned that facilitative glucose transporters hold the glucose molecule in weak and transient hydrogen bonds and that they function as conformational oscillators which rapidly shift the binding pocket for glucose between opposite sides of the plasma membrane.

In the following, current techniques for measurements of glucose transport activity and immunoreactive masses of glucose transporters in human adipose and skeletal muscle tissues are discussed.

Glucose transport activity in adipose cells

Human fat cells are fragile, and gentle handling is absolutely necessary to prevent significant cell traumatisation and to ensure insulin responsive cells. The protocol that we use to prepare high-quality cells is described in detail in references 6, 7. Obviously, it may be necessary to make adjustments in procedure to derive optimum conditions given the suppliers and equipment available.

Different hexoses have been used for the study of glucose uptake in fat cells: (a) 3-O-methylglucose, which is only transported and not phosphorylated or further metabolised [7, 8]; (b) 2-deoxy glucose, a non-metabolisable glucose analogue that measures both uptake and phosphorylation [7, 9]; and (c) D-glucose, which measures transport, phosphorylation, and conversion to metabolites [10, 11].

The same basic methodology for measuring initial uptake rate after incubation of cells with trace amounts of hexose for 5–10 sec can be used for each of these hexoses. For studies of insulin dose-response relationships at trace hexose concentration, ^{14}C-D-glucose should be used since it is much cheaper than the other two glucose analogues. Of course, for kinetic studies, the non-phosphorylisable and non-metabolisable 3-O-methylglucose analogue is recommended. The measurement of initial hexose uptake rates after 5–10 sec is a rather difficult technique, however, and recently it was shown that glucose transport can be measured as the uptake of tracer concentrations of D-U-^{14}C-glucose at time intervals up to at least 60 min when diluted cell preparations (volume fractions 0.02–0.05) are used [10, 11]. Although glucose in this time interval is metabolised, glucose transport still is the rate limiting step for glucose processing, and escape of metabolites is insignificant when the glucose concentration is at the trace level. It should be emphasised, however, that at final glucose concentrations exceeding trace level, glucose transport is no longer rate limiting for the glucose processing in human fat cells [11]. No matter which technique is applied for measurement of glucose transport in adipose cells, adenosine deaminase at a final concentration of 5 µg/ml should be included in the incubation buffer to remove endogenously released adenosine.

The mean percentage response of D-glucose uptake to a maximal insulin stimulation is 150–200% above the basal level in normal subjects. The average concentration of insulin giving half-maximal effect on glucose transport is about 80 pM.

Glucose transport activity in skeletal muscle

In vitro techniques are available for measurement of glucose transport in human muscle strips [12, 13]. Samples either of rectus abdominis muscle, obtained during elective abdominal surgery or of vastus lateralis of the quadriceps muscle, obtained from an open biopsy during local anaesthesia are used for preparation of muscle strips. During the surgical procedure, bunches of muscle are mounted at in vivo length by two sets of clamps. About 12 muscle fibre strips, weighing between 20–50 mg can be dissected free from about 1 g of muscle. The excision of the muscle biopsy and the subsequent in vitro handling must be performed with great care to avoid induction of any muscle contractions, which will cause an increase in basal glucose transport activity. The dissection and the following washing and incubation procedures are carried out in an oxygenated Krebs-Henseleit-bicarbonate (KHB) buffer. To measure 3-O-methylglucose uptake, the muscle strips are preincubated with and without insulin for ½ h at 30°C. Subsequently, the muscle strips are blotted briefly on filter paper and incubated with 8 mM 3-O-[^{3}H] methylglucose (437 µCi/mmol) and 32 mM [^{14}C] mannitol (8 µCi/mmol). The accumulation rate for 3-O-methylglucose is linear for 0 min. Following incubation, the muscle strips are blotted on filter paper dampened with incubation medium, trimmed and frozen in liquid nitrogen. The muscle strips are weighed, homogenised in 10% trichloroacetic acid and centrifuged at 1,000 g. Aliquots of the muscle extracts and of the incubation media are counted with channels preset for simultaneous ^{3}H and ^{14}C counting. The amount of each isotope present in the samples is determined and the extracellular space and the intracellular concentration of 3-O-methylglucose are calculated. In muscle strips from young healthy subjects, insulin in maximal concentrations causes a 50–200% increase in 3-O-methylglucose transport activity above basal values. The viability of the muscle strip preparations can be checked by measurements of ATP, phosphocreatine, lactate and glycogen contents before and at the end of the incubation period.

Assessing glucose transporters

Insulin activates glucose transport in skeletal muscle and adipose tissue through a rapid, reversible and concentration-dependent translocation of glucose transporters from an intracellular pool to the plasma membrane [14, 15]. In muscle tissues almost all the increase in glucose transport activity stimulated by insulin can be accounted for by the appearance of active Glut 4 transporters on the cell surface membrane [16]. In adipose cells, Glut 4 is likewise the major insulin regulatable transporter, but Glut 1 also contributes to insulin stimulated glucose transport in these cells [4]. Glucose transporters can be quantitated using different approaches: (a) cytochalasin B binding, a transport inhibitor that binds to glucose transporters without differentiating between glucose transporter subtypes.(b) Western immunoblotting with specific antibodies against different species of glucose transporters, and (c) exofacial photolabelling with sugars that compete for the glucose transporters followed by immunoprecipitation with specific antibodies against glucose transporters. The first and the second approaches can be applied to subcellular fractions of glucose transporters and detailed descriptions of methods for subcellular fractionation are published [17–21]. However, the subcellular fractionation techniques are difficult to apply to studies of glucose transporters in human cells due to the large amount of tissue needed. Moreover, interpretation of results must be balanced by poor recovery of glucose transporter proteins, a high degree of cross-contamination among cellular subfractions, and lack of specific markers for the intracellular pools of glucose transporters.

Cytochalasin B binding

Techniques for measurement of the number of D-glucose-inhibitable cytochalasin B binding sites in subcellular fractions of human adipose cells have been elaborated [18, 19]. In the presence of 5 μM cytochalasin, binding of [^{3}H]-cytochalasin B at 5 ligand concentrations (42–420 nM) is measured at 4° C using 50 μg membrane protein in the absence or presence of 0.5 M D-glucose. Tracer amounts of [^{14}C]urea are included in the assay to correct for unbound cytochalasin trapped in membrane pellets. Even when 5 μM cytochalasin E is included in the binding assay, curvilinear Scatchard plots of cytochalasin B binding are found in plasma membranes from cells prepared in the presence and absence of insulin. However, the inclusion of 0.5 M D-glucose in addition to cytochalasin E further reduces the binding, and subtraction of these data from those obtained in the absence of glucose reveals a single glucose-inhibitable site by Scatchard analysis.

Western immunoblotting of glucose transporters

The immunoreactive glucose transporter contents of muscle or adipose tissues can be estimated using immunoblot analysis on total cellular proteins or subcellular protein fractions [21, 22]. Membrane preparations of protein are subjected to polyacrylamide gel electrophoresis (20 – 50 µg protein/lane) followed by electrophoretical transfer to nitrocellulose filter membranes. The mass of Glut 4 or Glut 1 protein is determined by immunoblotting with specific monoclonal or polyclonal antibodies. Immunolabelled bands are visualised using ECL technique or ^{125}I-protein A. Autoradiograms are quantitated by scanning densitometry.

Exofacial photolabelling of glucose transporters

This technique, which has recently been developed in cultured cells and rat adipose cells, circumvents the problems associated with the subcellular fractionation methods in measuring the amount of glucose transporters on cell surface [22, 23]. An aryl azide derivation of bismannose (ATB-BMPA) which does not penetrate the bilayer of the plasma membrane labels glucose transporters. Subsequent immunoprecipitation of the plasma membrane preparation with specific antibodies allows for a differentiation between the immunoreactive mass of Glut 4 and Glut 1 transporters. We have developed a protocol for exofacial photolabelling of Glut 4 in muscle [16]. Muscle strips are incubated as described above (muscle glucose transport) and transferred to a dark room and further incubated at 18° C for 8 min in KHB buffer containing 1 mCi/ml ATB-[^{3}H]BMPA. Muscles are then irradiated twice for 3 min in a Rayonet RPR 100 photochemical reactor (RPR 3000 lamps), with manual turning over of the muscles after 3 min. Following irradiation, muscles are immediately blotted, trimmed and frozen in liquid N_2. The frozen muscles are weighed and homogenised in 5 ml ice cold 25 mM HEPES, 1 mM NaEDTA, 250 mM sucrose buffer (pH 7.4) containing the following protease inhibitors (1.0 mM pefabloc (AEBSF), 1.0 mM benzamidine and a mixture of leupeptin, pepstatin, aprotinin, antipain each at a final concentration of 10 µg/ml. Then the homogenate is centrifuged for 90 min at 230,000 g_{max}

(4° C), the supernatant is discarded and the pellet resuspended and solubilised in buffer containing 2% $C_{12}E_9$, 0.5% DOC and 0.1% SDS (plus proteinase inhibitors) for 60 min at room temperature. Subsequently the suspension is centrifuged for 30 min at 80.000 g_{max} (4° C). The resulting supernatant is subjected to immunoprecipitation using rabbit antiserum against Glut 4 [22, 23]. The immunoprecipitated glucose transporters are mixed with electrophoresis buffer (10% SDS, 6 M urea and 10% β-mercaptoethanol) and run overnight on a 20 cm long 10% SDS-PAGE gel in Laemmli buffer. Bio-Rad's pre-stained low molecular weight standards are used as molecular weight markers. Gels are briefly stained and destained using Coomassie Blue and then cut into 6 mm slices. The slices are dried at 80° C for 3 h and then dissolved and incubated for 3 h in 1 ml of 30% H_2O_2 containing 2% NH_2OH at 80° C. The levels of radioactivity associated with each peak are obtained by summing the radioactivity in all slices comprising the peak and subtracting background radioactivity which is based on the average radioactivity of the slices on either side of the peak. The values are then normalised per gram of frozen muscle.

Experiments with rat soleus muscle showed that insulin stimulation induced a 6-fold increase in 3-O-methyl-D-glucose uptake and studies using the exofacial labelling revealed a 6- to 7-fold increase in Glut 4 protein content in the total cell surface membrane [16]. Similarly, Glut 4 protein content in the plasma membrane of adipose cells is increased about 20-fold following insulin exposure [22].

The insulin receptor

The insulin receptor is a transmembrane glycoprotein composed of two 130 kDa α-subunits and two 95 kDa β-subunits [24]. The two α-subunits, which are located exterior to the cell membrane, are linked together by disulfide bonds. The α-subunit contains an insulin-binding domain. Each α-subunit is linked to one β-subunit which has an extracellular portion, a hydrophobic membrane-spanning domain and a cytoplasmic extension that contains a tyrosine kinase. The latter is activated after binding of insulin to the receptor. The activated receptor kinase mediates insulin activation of enzyme cascade(s) within the cell. Following the binding of insulin, the receptor-insulin complex is internalised by endocytosis. After degradation of insulin, the insulin receptor may recycle to the plasma membrane.

Insulin receptor binding

Insulin receptor binding may be measured in viable intact cells, in preparations of cellular membranes, and in solubilised insulin receptors.

The binding state of insulin receptors is usually determined with competition assays, i. e. the binding of radiolabelled insulin alone and in competition with various concentrations of unlabelled ligand. Pure preparations of ^{125}I-monoiodo-Tyr^{A14}-insulin are commercially available. This labelled insulin constitutes an almost ideal insulin tracer ligand with respect to homogeneity, stability, and biological activity [25].

The concentration of the radiolabelled insulin 'tracer' should be as low as possible; that is several fold lower than the dissociation constant (K_d) for insulin binding. With about 90% labelling of insulin, the specific activity is approximately 250 µCi/µg. Adequate radioactivity ('counts per minute') in the vials requires a concentration of labelled insulin not less than 0.015 nM. Incubation with labelled insulin may be performed at any temperature between 4 and 37° C. The pH of the incubation buffer should be around 7.6 – 7.8 which is optimal for insulin binding to both cellular and solubilised insulin receptors [6, 26]. A principal step is the separation of free and receptor-bound radioligand following the incubation period (see below). Non-specific binding at trace insulin concentrations, i. e. the percentage of binding of trace concentrations of radiolabelled ligand in the presence of high concentrations of unlabelled ligand divided by the binding of radioligand alone should be as low as possible.

Binding to isolated cells

Insulin binding to receptors of intact cells can be examined if the internalisation of receptor-bound insulin is inhibited. This requires temperatures below 21° C. At 21° C insulin binding has usually come to a steady state after 1 – 2 hr of incubation. Separation of receptor-bound radiolabelled insulin from free (unbound) radioligand in the incubation buffer is achieved either by centrifugation or by using a filter that withholds the cells. By the latter approach, however, non-specific binding may be unacceptably high since insulin may also bind to filters.

Blood cells are readily available to insulin binding studies in man. When the blood sample is loaded upon a Ficoll-Isopaque column, the different cellular constituents of blood are separated by gradient centrifugation. Insulin binding may be measured using erythrocytes [27] or monocytes which account for 80% of the insulin binding by leucocytes [28]. Non-specific insulin binding at tracer insulin concentrations is 20 – 30% in monocytes, and 10–15% in erythrocytes. However, the insulin receptor state in blood cells cannot be extrapolated to insulin target tissues [29, 30]. Accordingly, determination of insulin binding in insulin target cells such as adipocytes and hepatocytes may be more appropriate.

Human adipocytes are prepared from biopsies of human adipose tissue. The adipocytes are isolated during incubation with a mixture of collagenase together with small amounts of unspecified proteolytic enzymes [6]. Gentle centrifugation techniques, in combination with high buffer concentrations of albumin, prevent cell damage during processing of isolated fat cells [6, 30]. Free and adipocyte-bound radiolabelled insulin are separated by centrifugation through silicone oil. Thus, following the incubation period, 10 ml ice-cold saline is added together with 1 ml silicone oil. After low speed centrifugation, the adipocytes (and their receptor-bound insulin) become layered on the top of the oil phase, from which they are transferred to counting vials [6]. Quantitation of insulin binding requires an estimate of adipocyte number and mean adipocyte surface area, which may be calculated from measurements of cell diameters and adipocyte volume fraction ('lipocrit') [6, 30]. Non-specific insulin binding at tracer insulin concentrations is 1–4% in adipocytes [6]. Further details about insulin binding to human adipocytes are given in [6].

There is one published study measuring insulin binding to isolated viable hepatocytes from human liver biopsies obtained during surgery [31].

Binding to isolated membranes

Only a few investigators have measured insulin binding to plasma membranes from human cells. Crude membranes have been isolated from human liver [31, 32] and human muscle [33]. Muscle membranes contain a mixture of cellular membranes. The plasma membrane fraction may be isolated by discontinuous sucrose gradient centrifugation [34]. However, such a purification requires a relatively large tissue sample. Free and membrane-bound radiolabelled insulin are separated by centrifugation. The protein content of the membranes is used for quantitation of insulin binding. Non-specific insulin binding is around 20–40% at tracer insulin concentrations.

Binding to solubilised insulin receptors

Human insulin receptors may be solubilised and purified from placenta [35], erythrocytes [36], monocytes [37], adipocytes [38, 39], hepatocytes [32], and skeletal muscle [40, 41]; references should be consulted for methodological details. Homogenisation of tissue or cells in the presence of a detergent such as Triton X-100 disrupts the membranes and yields solubilised insulin receptors. Ice-chilled homogenators should be used. We have preferred the use of a Potter-Elvehjem homogeniser with a motor-driven Teflon pestle which develops no heat during homogenisation [26]. To preserve the phosphorylation state of the receptor it is recommended to include phosphatase inhibitors such as sodium fluoride, sodium vanadate and sodium pyrophosphate. In addition, the solubilisation buffer should contain protease inhibitors such as bacitracin, benzamidine, aprotinin, phenylmethylsulfonyl fluoride, pepstatin and leupeptin. In addition, the calcium chelator EDTA might be included for inhibition of Ca-dependent enzymes.

Ultracentrifugation (150 000 g) of the detergent-treated homogenate for 60 minutes precipitates non-soluble constituents. Receptor glycoproteins are subsequently partially purified by affinity chromatography using sepharose-coupled wheat germ agglutinin (WGA). The glycoproteins are eluted from the WGA column using a high concentration (0.3 M) of N-acetyl glucosamine. This eluate contains insulin receptors and other glycoproteins (partially purified insulin receptors). Insulin receptors may be further purified using incubation with anti-insulin receptor antibodies and subsequent precipitation with protein A.

Binding of radiolabelled insulin to solubilised insulin receptors can be quantitated after precipitation of the receptor-bound insulin by poly(ethylene glycol) using bovine γ-globulin as a carrier [26]. Applying Scatchard analysis of insulin binding data, the amount of solubilised insulin receptors in the WGA eluate may be estimated. The insulin receptor concentration of the WGA eluate is especially important in relation to quantitation of the receptor kinase activity (see below). However, it is uncertain to draw conclusions about the receptor status of the cell intact system from which it was solubilised.

Kinetics of insulin binding

The analysis of insulin binding data is based upon an assumption of insulin interaction with its receptor being a reversible bimolecular reaction where the association reaction and the dissociation reaction lead to a steady state.

According to these suppositions, the steady state may be considered as:

$$R + L \Leftrightarrow RL \qquad (1)$$

where R is free receptor (i. e. total receptor − occupied receptor), L is free ligand and RL is receptor bound ligand. At steady state the following equation can be derived according to the law of mass action:

$$K_d = [R][L]/[RL] \quad (2)$$

where K_d is the dissociation constant.
The binding of radiolabelled ligand in the presence of various concentrations of unlabelled ligand gives values of bound (B) ligand at different total ligand concentrations. In equation (2) substitution of R with (B_{max} − B), L with F (free ligand), and RL with B gives after transformation:

$$B/F = -1/K_d\,(B - B_{max}) \quad (3)$$

where B_{max} is maximal ligand binding, i. e. an estimate of the total receptor number. According to equation (3) the plot of B/F versus B (Scatchard plot) is supposed to give a straight line where the intercept of the abscissa (B/F = 0) determines B_{max} and the slope of the line is $-1/K_d$. In most insulin binding studies however, the Scatchard plot is curvilinear. Studies of the complicated nature of insulin binding [42, 43] will not be discussed here.

Autophosphorylation and receptor kinase activity

Autophosphorylation

Autophosphorylation of the β-subunit which occurs after insulin binding to the α-subunit – due to a 'release-of-inhibition' mechanism is measureable in solubilised insulin receptors [44]. The holo-receptor is incubated with insulin and [γ-^{32}P]adenosine triphosphate in the presence of $MnCl_2$ and $MgCl_2$ [38, 44]. The latter cations in concentrations of 4–10 mM serve to decrease K_m for ATP. Following the autophosphorylation reaction, the disulfide bonds of the insulin receptors are reduced by 2-mercaptoethanol during boiling and the phosphorylated β-subunits are identified and quantitated by sodium dodecyl sulphate polyacrylamide gel electrophoresis (SDS-PAGE). Autophosphorylation may also be measured in insulin receptors *in situ* in cultured cells by exposing these to [^{32}P]-orthophosphate [45]. Further details are given in references [38, 44–46].

Exogenous substrate phosphorylation

An immediate consequence of insulin-stimulated autophosphorylation of the insulin receptor β-subunit is the activation of its intrinsic protein tyrosine kinase. Recent evidence suggests that a component of a 185 kDa protein may be an endogenous insulin receptor substrate [47]. However, this substrate has not yet been used to determine receptor kinase activity. One synthetic polymer poly(GluNa-Tyr(4:1)) is an excellent exogenous substrate for the insulin receptor tyrosine kinase [48]. Following the addition of insulin to solubilised insulin receptors, poly(GluNa-Tyr(4:1)) (0.2 mg/ml) is added together with $MnCl_2$ and $MgCl_2$ and [γ-^{32}P]ATP (20 µM). After incubation for another 30 minutes at 21° C, an aliquot of the reaction mixture (75 µl) is spotted on Whatmant 31ET filter papers. The filter papers are rinsed for free radioactive ATP by extensive washing in 10% (w/v) trichloroacetic acid. Finally, they are counted for radioactivity, i. e. precipitated [^{32}P]-phosphorylated poly-(GluNa-Tyr(4 : 1)). Histone H2B may also be used as an exogenous substrate of the insulin receptor kinase. The identification of the phosphorylated form of histone H2B however, requires autoradiography using SDS-PAGE [46]. Recently, it has been shown in human insulin receptors solubilised from skeletal muscle biopsies obtained during in vivo insulin stimulation (at pharmacological doses), that the activated state of the insulin receptor was preserved in the detergent-solubilised receptors [49].

References

[1] Mueckler M. Family of glucose transporter genes. Implications for glucose homeostasis and diabetes. Diabetes 1990; 39: 6–11.

[2] Bell GI, Kayano T, Buse JB et al. Molecular biology of mammalian glucose transporters. Diabetes Care 1990; 13: 198–208.

[3] Thorens B, Charron MJ, Lodish HF. Molecular physiology of glucose transporters. Diabetes Care 1990; 13: 209–218.

[4] Kahn BB. Facilitative glucose transporters: regulatory mechanisms and dysregulation in diabetes. J Clin Invest 1992; 89: 1367–1374.

[5] Appleman JR, Lienhard GE. Kinetics of the purified glucose transporter: direct measurement of the rates of interconversion of transporter conformers. Biochemistry 1989; 28: 8221–8227.

[6] Pedersen O, Hjollund E, Beck-Nielsen H et al. Insulin receptor binding and receptor-mediated insulin degradation in human adipocytes. Diabetologia 1981; 20: 636–641.

[7] Pedersen O, Glieman J. Hexose transport in human adipocytes: factors influencing the response to insulin and kinetics of methyl-glucose and glucose transport. Diabetologia 1981; 20: 630–635.

[8] Ciaraldi TP, Kolterman OG, Siegel JA et al. Insulin stimulated glucose transport in human adipocytes. Am J Physiol 1979; 236: 621–625.

[9] Pedersen O, Hjollund E, Lindskov HO. Insulin binding and action on fat cells from young healthy females and males. Am J Physiol: Endocrinol Metab 1982; 243: 158–167.

[10] Kashiwagi A, Verso MA, Andrews J et al. In vitro insulin resistance of human adipocytes isolated from subjects with noninsulin-dependent diabetes mellitus. J Clin Invest 1983; 72: 1246–1254.

[11] Hjollund E, Pedersen O. Transport and metabolism of D-glucose in human adipocytes. Studies of the dependence on medium glucose and insulin concentrations. Biochim Biophys Acta 1988; 937: 93–102.

[12 Dohm GL, Tapscott EB, Pories WJ et al. An in vitro muscle preparation suitable for metabolic studies. J Clin Invest 1988; 82: 486–494.

[13] Andreasson K, Galuska D, Thorne A et al. Decreased insulin-stimulated 3-O-methylglucose transport in in vitro incubated muscle strips from Type II diabetic subjects. Acta Physiol Scand 1991; 142: 255–260.
[14] Wardzala LJ, Cushman SW, Salans LB. Mechanism of insulin action on glucose transport in the isolated rat adipose cell: enhancement of the number of functional transport systems. J Biol Chem 1978; 253: 8002–8005.
[15] Wardzala LJ, Jeanrenaud B. Identification of the D-glucose-inhibitable cytochalasin B binding site as the glucose transporter in rat diaphragm plasma and microsomal membranes. Biochim Biophys Acta 1983; 730: 49–56.
[16] Lund S, Holman GD, Schmitz O et al. Glut 4 content in the plasma membrane of rat skeletal muscle. Comparative studies of the subcellular fractionation method and the exofacial photolabelling technique using ATB-BMPA. FEBS Letter. 1993; 330: 312–318.
[17] Mc Keel DW, Jarett L. Preparation and characterization of a plasma membrane fraction from isolated fat cells. J Cell 1970; Biol 44: 417–438.
[18] Cushman SW, Wardzala LJ. Potential mechanisms of insulin action on glucose transport in the isolated rat adipose cell: apparent translocation of intracellular transport systems to the plasma membrane. J Biol Chem 1980; 255: 4758–4762.
[19] Karniel E, Zarnowski MJ, Hissin PJ et al. Insulin stimulated translocation of glucose transport systems in isolated rat adipose cell. Time course, reversal, and insulin concentration dependence, and relationship to glucose transport activity. J Biol Chem 1981; 256: 4772–4777.
[20] Garvey WT, Maianu L, Huecksteadt TP et al. Pretranslational suppression of a glucose transporter protein causes insulin resistance in adipocytes from patients with non-insulin-dependent diabetes mellitus and obesity. J Clin Invest 1991; 87: 1072–1081.
[21] Lund S, Vestergaard H, Andersen PH, et al. Glut 4 content in the plasma membrane of muscle from patients with noninsulin-dependent diabetes mellitus. Am J Physiol. Endocrinol Metab. 1993; in press.
[22] Holman D, Kozka IJ, Clark AE et al. Cell surface labeling of glucose transporter isoform Glut 4 by bis-mannose photolabel. J Biol Chem 1990; 240: 3493–3500.
[23] Vannucci SJ, Nishimura H, Satoh S et al. Cell surface accessibility of Glut 4 glucose transporters in insulin stimulated rat adipose cells. Biochem J 1992; 288: 325–330.
[24] Kahn CR, White MF. The insulin receptor and the molecular mechanism of insulin action. J Clin Invest 1988; 82: 1151–115.
[25] Gammeltoft S. Insulin receptors: Binding kinetics and structure-function relationship of insulin. Physiol Rev 1984; 64: 1321–1378.
[26] Bak JF, Handberg A, BeckNielsen H et al. Kinetics of insulin binding and kinase activity of the partially purified insulin receptor from human skeletal muscle. Biochim Biophys Acta 1990; 1052: 306–312.
[27] Gambhir KK, Archer JA, Bradley CJ. Characteristics of human erythrocyte insulin receptors. Diabetes 1978; 27: 701–708.
[28] BeckNielsen H, Pedersen O, Kragballe K et al. The monocyte as a model for the study of insulin receptors in man. Diabetologia 1977; 13: 563–569.
[29] Hjollund E, Richelsen B, Pedersen O. Comparative studies of insulin binding to receptor from adipocytes, hepatocytes, monocytes and erythrocytes from the pig. Acta Endocrinol (Cph) 1988; 118: 59–67.
[30] Pedersen O. Studies of insulin receptor binding and insulin action in humans. Dan Med Bull 1984; 31: 132.
[31] Caro JF, Ittoop O, Pories WJ, et al. Studies on the mechanism of insulin resistance in the liver from humans with non-insulin-dependent diabetes. Insulin action and binding in isolated hepatocytes, insulin receptor structure, and kinase activity. J Clin Invest 1986; 78: 249–258.
[32] Arner P, Einarsson K, Ewerth S et al. Studies of the human liver insulin receptor in non-insulin-dependent diabetes mellitus. J Clin Invest 1986; 77: 1716–1718.
[33] Bonen A, Hood DA, Tan MH et al. Insulin binding in human skeletal muscle. Biochim Biophys Acta 1984; 801: 171–176.

[34] Yokono K, Imamura Y, Sakai H et al. Insulin-degrading activity of plasma membranes from rat skeletal muscle. Its isolation, characterization, and biologic significance. Diabetes 1979; 28: 810–817.

[35] Shia M, Rubin JB, Pilch PF. The insulin receptor kinase. Physico chemical requirements for activity. J Biol Chem 1983; 258: 14450–14455.

[36] Suzuki S, Toyota T, Goto Y. Characterization of the insulin receptor kinase from human erythrocytes. Endocrinology 1987;121: 972–979.

[37] Grunberger G, Zick Y, Gorden P. Defect in phosphorylation of insulin receptors in cells from an insulin-resistant patient with normal insulin binding. Science 1984; 223: 932–934.

[38] Handberg A, Gammeltoft S, Juhl H. Protein kinase activity of the partially purified insulin receptor from human adipocytes. Diabetic Med 1987; 4: 446–451.

[39] Freidenberg GR, Henry RR, Klein HH et al. Decreased kinase activity of insulin receptors from adipocytes of non-insulin-dependent diabetic subjects. J Clin Invest 1987; 79: 240–250.

[40] Arner P, Pollare T, Lithell H et al. Defective insulin receptor tyrosine kinase in human skeletal muscle in obesity and Type 2 (non-insulin-dependent) diabetes mellitus. Diabetologia 1987; 30: 437–440.

[41] Bak JF, Schmitz O, Frøkiær J et al. Activity of insulin receptor kinase and glycogen synthase in skeletal muscle from patients with chronic renal failure. Acta Endocrinol (Cph) 1989; 121: 744–750.

[42] De Meyts P, Bianco AR, Roth J. Site-site interactions among insulin receptors. Characterization of the negative cooperativity. J Biol Chem 1976; 251: 1877–1888.

[43] Wang C, Goldfine ID, Fujita-Yamaguchi Y et al. Negative and positive site-site interactions, and their modulation by pH, insulin analogs, and monoclonal antibodies, are preserved in the purified insulin receptor. Proc Natl Acad Sci USA 1988; 85: 8400–8404.

[44] Zick Y, Kasuga M, Kahn CR et al. Characterization of insulin-mediated phosphorylation of the insulin receptor in a cell-free system. J Biol Chem 1983; 258: 75–80.

[45] Kasuga M, Karlsson FA, Kahn CR. Insulin stimulates the phosphorylation of the 95000-Dalton subunit of its own receptor. Science 1982; 215: 185–187.

[46] Burant CF, Treutelaar MK, Landreth GE et al. Phosphorylation of insulin receptors solubilized from rat skeletal muscle. Diabetes 1984; 33: 704–708.

[47] Sun XJ, Rothenberg P, Kahn CR et al. Structure of the insulin receptor substrate IRS-1 defines a unique signal transduction protein. Nature 1991; 352: 73–77.

[48] Braun S, Raymond WE, Racker E. Synthetic tyrosine polymers as substrates and inhibitors of tyrosine-specific protein kinases. J Biol Chem 1984; 259: 2051–2054.

[49] Freidenberg GR, Suter SL, Henry RR et al. In vivo stimulation of the insulin receptor kinase in human skeletal muscle. Correlation with insulin-stimulated glucose disposal during euglycemic clamp studies. J Clin Invest 1991; 87: 2222–2229.

World Medical Association Declaration of Helsinki

Recommendations guiding physicians in biomedical research involving human subjects.

Adopted by the 18th World Medical Assembly, Helsinki, Finland, June 1964, and amended by the 29th World Medical Assembly, Tokyo, Japan, October 1975, and the 35th World Medical Assembly, Venice, Italy, October 1983, and the 41st World Medical Assembly, Hong Kong, September 1989.

Introduction

It is the mission of the physician to safeguard the health of the people. His or her knowledge and conscience are dedicated to the fulfillment of this mission.

The Declaration of Geneva of the World Medical Association binds the physician with the words, "The health of my patient will be my first consideration", and the International Code of Medical Ethics declares that, "A physician shall act only in the patient's interest when providing medical care which might have the effect of weakening the physical and mental condition of the patient."

The purpose of biomedical research involving human subjects must be to improve diagnostic, therapeutic and prophylactic procedures and the understanding of the aetiology and pathogenesis of disease.

In current medical practice most diagnostic, therapeutic or prophylactic procedures involve hazards. This applies especially to biomedical research.

Medical progress is based on research which ultimately must rest in part on experimentation involving human subjects.

In the field of biomedical research a fundamental distinction must be recognized between medical research in which the aim is essentially diagnostic or therapeutic for a patient, and medical research, the essential object of which is purely scientific and without implying direct diagnostic or therapeutic value to the person subjected to the research.

Special caution must be exercised in the conduct of research which may affect the environment, and the welfare of animals used for research must be respected.

Offprint from
Research Methodologies in Human Diabetes – Part 1

Because it is essential that the results of laboratory experiments be applied to human beings to further scientific knowledge and to help suffering humanity, the World Medical Association has prepared the following recommendations as a guide to every physician in biomedical research involving human subjects. They should be kept under review in the future. It must be stressed that the standards as drafted are only a guide to physicians all over the world. Physicians are not relieved from criminal, civil and ethical responsibilities under the laws of their own countries.

Basic principles

1. Biomedical research involving human subjects must conform to generally accepted scientific principles and should be based on adequately performed laboratory and animal experimentation and on a thorough knowledge of the scientific literature.
2. The design and performance of each experimental procedure involving human subjects should be clearly formulated in an experimental protocol which should be transmitted for consideration, comment and guidance to a specially appointed committee independent of the investigator and the sponsor, provided that this independent committee is in conformity with the laws and regulations of the country in which the research experiment is performed.
3. Biomedical research involving human subjects should be conducted only by scientifically qualified persons and under the supervision of a clinically competent medical person. The responsibility for the human subjects must always rest with a medically qualified person and never rest on the subject of the research, even though the subject has given his or her consent.
4. Biomedical research involving human subjects cannot legitimately be carried out unless the importance of the objective is in proportion to the inherent risk to the subject.
5. Every biomedical research project involving human subjects should be preceded by careful assessment of predictable risks in comparison with foreseeable benefits to the subject or to others. Concern for the interests of the subject must always prevail over the interests of science and society.
6. The right of the research subject to safeguard his or her integrity must always be respected. Every precaution should be taken to respect the privacy of the subject and to minimize the impact of the study on the subject's physical and mental integrity and on the personality of the subject.

7. Physicians should abstain from engaging in research projects involving human subjects unless they are satisfied that the hazards involved are believed to be predictable. Physicians should cease any investigation if the hazards are found to outweigh the potential benefits.
8. In publication of the results of his or her research, the physician is obliged to preserve the accuracy of the results. Reports of experimentation not in accordance with the principles laid down in this Declaration should not be accepted for publication.
9. In any research on human beings, each potential subject must be adequately informed of the aims, methods, anticipated benefits, and potential hazards of the study and the discomfort it may entail. He or she should be informed that he or she is at liberty to abstain from participation in the study and that he or she is free to withdraw his or her consent to participation at any time. The physician should then obtain the subject's freely-given informed consent, preferably in writing.
10. When obtaining informed consent for the research project the physician should be particularly cautious if the subject is in a dependent relationship to him or her or may consent under duress. In that case the informed consent should be obtained by a physician who is not engaged in the investigation and who is completely independent of this official relationship.
11. In case of legal incompetence, informed consent should be obtained from the legal guardian in accordance with national legislation. Where physical or mental incapacity makes it impossible to obtain informed consent, or when the subject is a minor, permission from the responsible relative replaces that of the subject in accordance with national legislation.
    Whenever the minor child is in fact able to give a consent, the minor's consent must be obtained in addition to the consent of the minor's legal guardian.
12. The research protocol should always contain a statement of the ethical considerations involved and should indicate that the principles enunciated in the present declaration are complied with.

Medical research combined with professional care (clinical research)

1. In the treatment of the sick person, the physician must be free to use a new diagnostic and therapeutic measure, if in his or her judgement it offers hope of saving life, reestablishing health or alleviating suffering.

2. The potential benefits, hazards and discomfort of a new method should be weighed against the advantages of the best current diagnostic and therapeutic methods.
3. In any medical study, every patient – including those of a control group, if any – should be assured of the best proven diagnostic and therapeutic method.
4. The refusal of the patient to participate in a study must never interfere with the physician-patient relationship.
5. If the physician considers it essential not to obtain informed consent, the specific reasons for this proposal should be stated in the experimental protocol for transmission to the independent committe (1, 2).
6. The physician can combine medical research with professional care, the objective being the acquisition of new medical knowledge, only to the extent that medical research is justified by its potential diagnostic and therapeutic value for the patient.

Non-therapeutic biomedical research involving human subjects (non-clinical biomedical research)

1. In the purely scientific application of medical research carried out on a human being, it is the duty of the physician to remain the protector of the life and health of that person on whom biomedical research is being carried out.
2. The subjects should be volunteers – either healthy persons or patients for whom the experimental design is not related to the patient's illness.
3. The investigator or the investigating team should discontinue the research if in his/her or their judgement it may, if continued, be harmful to the individual.
4. In research on man, the interest of science and society should never take precedence over considerations related to the well-being of the subject.

Subject index

Research Methodologies in Human Diabetes *Part 2*

Scheduled contents

Conducting clinical trials in diabetic neural diseases, including power analysis

Methods in ketone bodies metabolism and intermediary lipid metabolism in diabetes

Methods in protein metabolism in diabetes

Research methodologies in the evaluation of pancreas transplantation and islet cell transplantation

Survival studies related to diabetes: research methodologies

Pitfalls in patient selection and statistical procedures in diabetes research

How to assess efficacy of new oral anti-diabetic drugs?

Research methodologies of eicosanoid biosynthesis and function in diabetes

Measurement of aldose reductase inhibition in humans

Measurement of components of the renin angiotensin system in humans: relationship with diabetic complication and antihypertensive treatment

Research methods of cerebrovascular disease in diabetes

Bei Fragen zur Produktsicherheit wenden Sie sich bitte an:
If you have any questions regarding product safety,
please contact:

Walter de Gruyter GmbH
Genthiner Straße 13
10785 Berlin
productsafety@degruyterbrill.com